2012
YEAR BOOK OF
DERMATOLOGY
AND
DERMATOLOGIC
SURGERY™

The 2012 Year Book Series

Year Book of Anesthesiology and Pain Management™: Drs Chestnut, Abram, Black, Gravlee, Lien, Mathru, and Roizen

Year Book of Cardiology®: Drs Gersh, Cheitlin, Elliott, Gold, Graham, and Thourani

Year Book of Critical Care Medicine®: Drs Dries, Zanotti-Cavazzoni, Latenser, Martinez, Rincon, and Zwank

Year Book of Dermatology and Dermatologic Surgery™: Dr Del Rosso

Year Book of Diagnostic Radiology®: Drs Elster, Abbara, Oestreich, Offiah, Rosado de Christenson, Stephens, and Strickland

Year Book of Emergency Medicine®: Drs Hamilton, Bruno, Handly, Minczak, Mullin, Quintana, and Ramoska

Year Book of Endocrinology®: Drs Schott, Apovian, Clarke, Eugster, Meikle, Oetgen, Ovalle, Schteingart, and Toth

Year Book of Hand and Upper Limb Surgery®: Drs Yao, Adams, Isaacs, Lee, and Rizzo

Year Book of Medicine®: Drs Barker, Garrick, Gersh, Khardori, LeRoith, Panush, Talley, and Thigpen

Year Book of Neonatal and Perinatal Medicine®: Drs Fanaroff, Benitz, Donn, Neu, Papile, Polin, and Van Marter

Year Book of Neurology and Neurosurgery®: Drs Klimo, Minagar, Gandhi, House, Kevill, Liu, Mazia, Panagariya, Ragel, Riesenburger, Robottom, Schwendimann, Shafazand, Uhm, and Yang

Year Book of Obstetrics, Gynecology, and Women's Health®: Drs Dungan and Shulman

Year Book of Oncology®: Drs Arceci, Bauer, Chiorean, Gordon, Lawton, Murphy, Thigpen, and Tsao

Year Book of Ophthalmology®: Drs Rapuano, Cohen, Flanders, Hammersmith, Milman, Myers, Nagra, Nelson, Penne, Pyfer, Sergott, Shields, Talekar, and Vander

Year Book of Orthopedics®: Drs Morrey, Huddleston, Rose, Swiontkowski, and Trigg

Year Book of Otolaryngology-Head and Neck Surgery®: Drs Sindwani, Balough, Franco, Gapany, and Mitchell

Year Book of Pathology and Laboratory Medicine®: Drs Raab and Bissell

Year Book of Pediatrics®: Dr Stockman

Year Book of Plastic and Aesthetic Surgery™: Drs Miller, Gosman, Gurtner, Gutowski, Ruberg, Salisbury, and Smith

Year Book of Psychiatry and Applied Mental Health®: Drs Talbott, Ballenger, Buckley, Frances, Krupnick, and Mack

Year Book of Pulmonary Disease®: Drs Barker, Jones, Maurer, Spradley, Tanoue, and Willsie

Year Book of Sports Medicine®: Drs Shephard, Cantu, Feldman, Galea, Jankowski, Janssen, Lebrun, and Nieman

Year Book of Surgery®: Drs Copeland, Behrns, Daly, Eberlein, Fahey, Huber, Klodell, Mozingo, and Pruett

Year Book of Urology®: Drs Andriole and Coplen

Year Book of Vascular Surgery®: Drs Moneta, Gillespie, Starnes, and Watkins

2012

The Year Book of DERMATOLOGY AND DERMATOLOGIC SURGERY™

Editor-in-Chief

James Q. Del Rosso, DO, FAOCD

Dermatology Residency Director, Valley Hospital Medical Center, Las Vegas, Nevada; Clinical Professor (Dermatology), Touro University College of Osteopathic Medicine, Henderson, Nevada; JDRx Dermatology, Las Vegas Skin & Cancer Clinics, Las Vegas, Nevada, and Henderson, Nevada

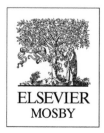

ELSEVIER
MOSBY

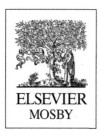

Vice President, Continuity: Kimberly Murphy
Editor: Stephanie Donley
Supervisor, Electronic Year Books: Donna M. Skelton
Electronic Article Manager: Mike Sheets
Illustrations and Permissions Coordinator: Dawn Vohsen

2012 EDITION

Composition by TNQ Books and Journals Pvt Ltd, India

Editorial Office:
Elsevier
Suite 1800
1600 John F. Kennedy Blvd
Philadelphia, PA 19103-2899

International Standard Serial Number: 0093-3619
International Standard Book Number: 978-0-323-08876-3

Printed and bound by CPI Group (UK) Ltd, Croydon, CR0 4YY

Transferred to Digital Print 2012

Editorial Board

Table of Contents

EDITORIAL BOARD vii

JOURNALS REPRESENTED xiii

COLOR PLATE

YEAR BOOK FOCUS: The Clinical Relevance of Maintaining the Functional Integrity of the Stratum Corneum in both Healthy and Disease-affected Skin 1

YEAR BOOK FOCUS: Practical Evaluation and Management of Atrophic Acne Scars: Tips for the General Dermatologist 33

YEAR BOOK FOCUS: Antiperspirant and Deodorant Allergy: Diagnosis and Management 47

STATISTICS OF INTEREST TO THE DERMATOLOGIST 57

CLINICAL DERMATOLOGY 73

1. Urticarial and Eczematous Disorders 75

2. Psoriasis and Other Papulosquamous Disorders 107

3. Bacterial and Fungal Infections 121

4. Viral Infections (Excluding HIV Infection) 133

5. HIV Infection 145

6. Disorders of the Pilosebaceous Apparatus 147

7. Photobiology 193

8. Collagen Vascular and Related Disorders 207

9. Blistering Disorders 229

10. Genodermatoses 237

11. Drug Actions, Reactions, and Interactions 243

12. Drug Development and Promotion 273

13. Miscellaneous Topics in Clinical Dermatology 279

14. Pigmentary Disorders 341

15. Practice Management and Managed Care 355

DERMATOLOGIC SURGERY AND CUTANEOUS ONCOLOGY 361

16. Nonmelanoma Skin Cancer 363

17. Nevi and Melanoma   419
18. Lymphoproliferative Disorders   453
19. Miscellaneous Topics in Cosmetic and Laser Surgery   457
20. Miscellaneous Topics in Dermatologic Surgery and Cutaneous
       Oncology   489

       ARTICLE INDEX   517

       AUTHOR INDEX   533

Journals Represented

Journals represented in this YEAR BOOK are listed below.

Allergy
American Journal of Infection Control
American Journal of Medicine
Annals of Allergy, Asthma & Immunology
Archives of Dermatology
Archives of Disease in Childhood
British Journal of Dermatology
British Journal of Ophthalmology
British Journal of Radiology
British Medical Journal
Burns
Cancer
Cancer Epidemiology, Biomarkers & Prevention
Cardiovascular Pathology
Clinical Infectious Diseases
Contact Dermatitis
Dermatologic Surgery
Dermatologic Therapy
Dermatology
European Journal of Plastic Surgery
Head & Neck
International Journal of Cancer
Journal of Allergy and Clinical Immunology
Journal of Cutaneous Pathology
Journal of Immunology
Journal of Infectious Diseases
Journal of Investigative Dermatology
Journal of Otolaryngology Head & Neck Surgery
Journal of Pathology
Journal of Pediatrics
Journal of Plastic, Reconstructive & Aesthetic Surgery
Journal of Rheumatology
Journal of the American Academy of Dermatology
Journal of the American Medical Association
Journal of the European Academy of Dermatology & Venereology
Laryngoscope
Mayo Clinic Proceedings
Molecular Cancer Therapeutics
Nephrology Dialysis Transplantation Plus
New England Journal of Medicine
Ophthalmology
Oral Oncology
Oral Surgery, Oral Medicine, Oral Pathology, Oral Radiology, and Endodontology
Pediatric Dermatology
Pediatrics

Plastic and Reconstructive Surgery
Seminars In Oncology

STANDARD ABBREVIATIONS

The following terms are abbreviated in this edition: acquired immunodeficiency syndrome (AIDS), cardiopulmonary resuscitation (CPR), central nervous system (CNS), cerebrospinal fluid (CSF), computed tomography (CT), deoxyribonucleic acid (DNA), electrocardiography (ECG), health maintenance organization (HMO), human immunodeficiency virus (HIV), intensive care unit (ICU), intramuscular (IM), intravenous (IV), magnetic resonance (MR) imaging (MRI), ribonucleic acid (RNA), ultrasound (US), and ultraviolet (UV).

NOTE

The YEAR BOOK OF DERMATOLOGY AND DERMATOLOGIC SURGERY™ is a literature survey service providing abstracts of articles published in the professional literature. Every effort is made to ensure the accuracy of the information presented in these pages. Neither the editors nor the publisher of the YEAR BOOK OF DERMATOLOGY AND DERMATOLOGIC SURGERY™ can be responsible for errors in the original materials. The editors' comments are their own opinions. Mention of specific products within this publication does not constitute endorsement.

To facilitate the use of the YEAR BOOK OF DERMATOLOGY AND DERMATOLOGIC SURGERY™ as a reference tool, all illustrations and tables included in this publication are now identified as they appear in the original article. This change is meant to help the reader recognize that any illustration or table appearing in the YEAR BOOK OF DERMATOLOGY AND DERMATOLOGIC SURGERY™ may be only one of many in the original article. For this reason, figure and table numbers will often appear to be out of sequence within the YEAR BOOK OF DERMATOLOGY AND DERMATOLOGIC SURGERY™.

COLOR PLATE I

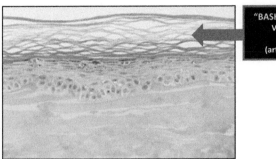

"BASKETWEAVE" HYPERKERATOSIS
Visibly appears as a lattice of
keratin microfibrils
(artifact of histologic processing)

Del Rosso and Levin Fig 1

COLOR PLATE II

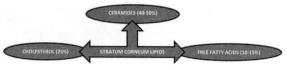

Del Rosso and Levin Fig 3

COLOR PLATE III

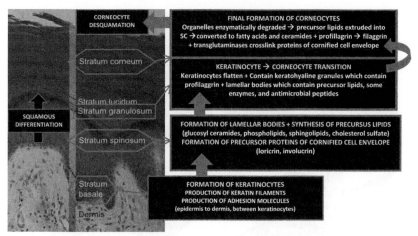

Del Rosso and Levin Fig 4

COLOR PLATE IV

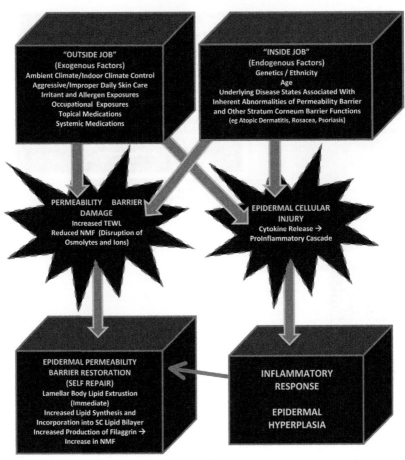

Del Rosso and Levin Fig 5

COLOR PLATE V

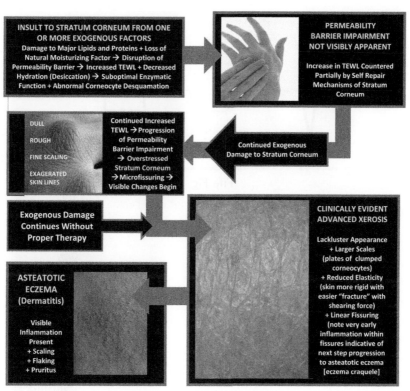

Del Rosso and Levin Fig 6

COLOR PLATE VI

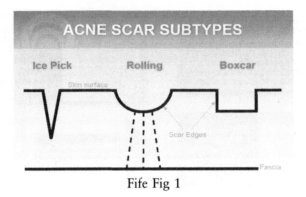

Fife Fig 1

COLOR PLATE VII

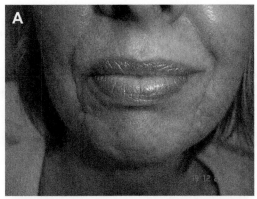

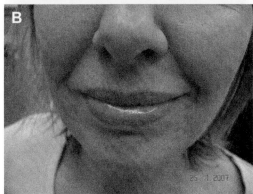

Fife Fig 2 A-B

COLOR PLATE VIII

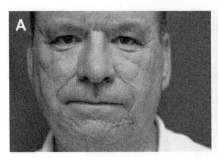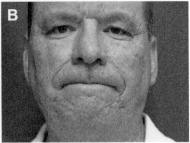

Fife Fig 3 A-B

COLOR PLATE IX

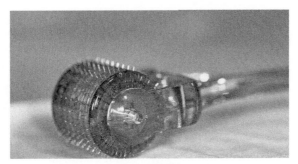

Fife Fig 4

COLOR PLATE X

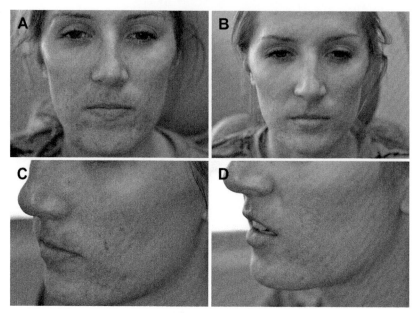

Fife Fig 5 A-D

COLOR PLATE XI

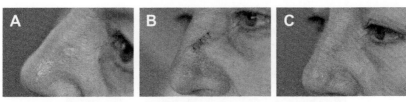

Fife Fig 6 A-C

COLOR PLATE XII

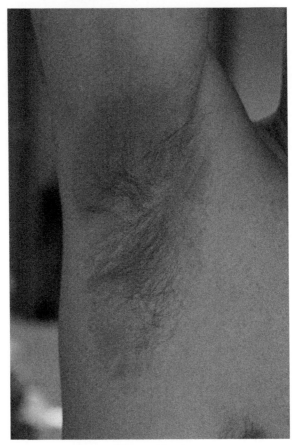

Zirwas Fig 1

COLOR PLATE XIII

Antihypertensives	40 of 117 reported cases: 34·2%
Calcium channel blockers	
Diltiazem[7,10]	6 cases
Verapamil[7,8]	5 cases
Nifedipine[7,10,30]	3 cases
Nitrendipine[31]	1 case
Diuretics	
Hydrochlorothiazide[3,10,22]	10 cases
Hydrochlorothiazide + triamterene[6]	3 cases
Chlorthiazide[5]	2 cases
Beta blockers	
Oxprenolol[32]	4 cases
Acebutolol[33]	1 case
Angiotensin-converting enzyme inhibitors	
Enalapril[16]	2 cases
Lisinopril[19]	1 case
Captopril[34]	1 case
Cilazapril[34]	1 case
Antifungals	30 of 117 reported cases: 25·6%
Terbinafine[12,14–16,35–37]	29 cases
Griseofulvin[13]	1 case
Chemotherapeutics	10 of 117 reported cases: 8·5%
Docetaxel[38]	3 cases
Paclitaxel[24,38]	3 cases
Tamoxifen[39]	2 cases
Capecitabine[40,41]	2 cases
Antihistamines	9 of 117 reported cases: 7·7%
Ranitidine[42]	7 cases
Brompheniramine[42]	1 case
Cinnarizine + thiethylperazine[43]	1 case
Immunomodulators	8 of 117 reported cases: 6·8%
Leflunomide[9,17,25,44]	5 cases
Interferon α and β[10,45]	3 cases
Antiepileptics	3 of 117 reported cases: 2·6%
Carbamazepine[46,47]	2 cases
Phenytoin[48]	1 case
Statins	3 of 117 reported cases: 2·6%
Simvastatin[10,49]	2 cases
Pravastatin[10]	1 case
Biologics	2 of 117 reported cases: 1·7%
Etanercept[50]	1 case
Efalizumab[51]	1 case
Proton pump inhibitors	2 of 117 reported cases: 1·7%
Lansoprazole[52]	2 cases
Nonsteroidal anti-inflammatory drugs	2 of 117 reported cases: 1·7%
Naproxen[53]	1 case
Piroxicam[26]	1 case
Hormone-altering drugs	2 of 117 reported cases: 1·7%
Leuprorelin[19]	1 case
Anastrozole[18]	1 case
Ultraviolet therapy	2 of 117 reported cases: 1·7%
PUVA[54]	1 case
PUVA and UVB[20]	1 case
Others	4 of 117 reported cases: 3·4%
Bupropion[55]	1 case
Tiotropium[56]	1 case
Ticlopidine[57]	1 case
Hay with fertilizer[58]	1 case

The numbers in the table represent citations to references, and the drugs reported to be capable of also producing photosensitivity skin reactions other than SCLE in otherwise healthy individuals are presented in italics. PUVA, psoralen plus ultraviolet (UV) A.

Table 1, Page 210

COLOR PLATE XIV

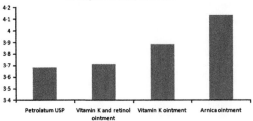

Fig 6, Page 460

COLOR PLATE XV

	Before DS intake		After DS intake	
	Nonexposed skin (n = 16)	UV-DL-exposed skin (n = 16)	Nonexposed skin (n = 16)	UV-DL-exposed skin (n = 16)
Langerhans cells (protein S100)	623 ± 299	416 ± 148[a]	613 ± 270	545 ± 215[bc]
Dermal dendrocytes (factor XIIIa+)	4245 ± 2038	4915 ± 2144	4215 ± 1996	4118 ± 1982[c]
Dermal inflammatory cells (CD45+)	4·4 ± 2·6	8·4 ± 4·0[a]	4·1 ± 2·2	5·9 ± 3·3[ab]
Active melanocytes (tyrosinase)	296 ± 115	331 ± 83[a]	321 ± 109	363 ± 154[a]
Melanin content (Fontana–Masson)	2809 ± 1166	3801 ± 1355[a]	2795 ± 1133	3296 ± 1197[abc]

DS, dietary supplement. Results are shown as mean ± SD. The square of the cell count mm^{-1} length of stratum corneum represents the density of cells mm^{-2} of skin surface. Dermal dendrocyte count was expressed as the number mm^{-2} of factor XIIIa+ cells in the perivascular compartment of the upper dermis. CD45+ cell count was expressed mm^{-2} of skin surface area. Antityrosinase cells were counted in the basal layer of the epidermis. Melanin content was evaluated using digital image analysis after Fontana–Masson staining. [a]Exposed vs. nonexposed area, $P < 0.05$ (Student's t-test), [b]exposed areas before vs. after supplementation, $P < 0.05$ (Student's t-test), [c]comparison of exposed vs. unexposed areas before vs. after supplementation, $P < 0.05$ (Wilcoxon test).

Table 1, Page 198

COLOR PLATE XVI

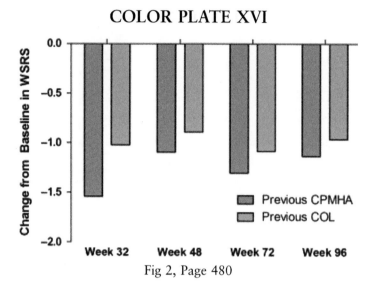

Fig 2, Page 480

COLOR PLATE XVII

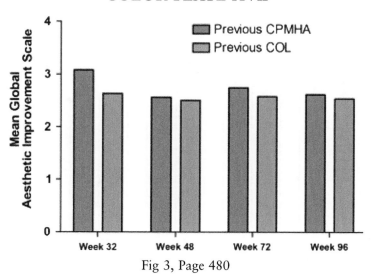

Fig 3, Page 480

COLOR PLATE XVIII

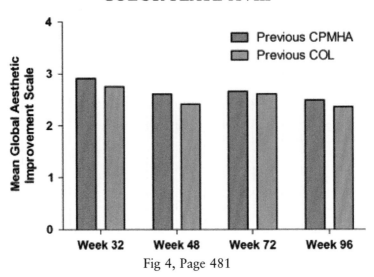

Fig 4, Page 481

COLOR PLATE XIX

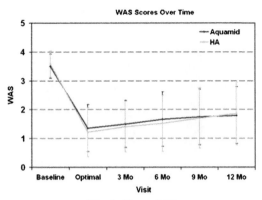

Fig 1, Page 282

COLOR PLATE XX

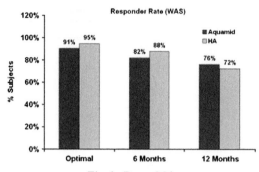

Fig 2, Page 282

COLOR PLATE XXI

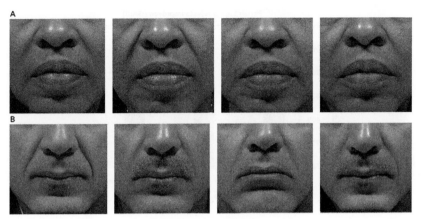

Fig 3, Page 283

COLOR PLATE XXII

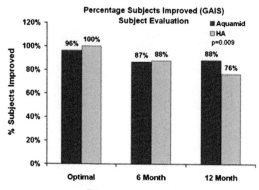

Fig 4, Page 283

COLOR PLATE XXIII

	p-*Value*	
	2 weeks	*3 months*
Body appearance		.05
Satisfaction with weight		.02
Feeling good about one's self	.045	
Physical health	.05	
Household activities	.05	
Overall life satisfaction and contentment		.04

Table 1, Page 286

COLOR PLATE XXIV

	p-Value			
	2 Weeks		3 Months	
	BoNTA	Placebo	BoNTA	Placebo
Body appearance	.01	.025		
Weight			.05	
Less self-consciousness	.03	.03	.01	.01
Perceived self-intellect	.008	.008		
Feeling good about one's self	.002		.002	
Appearance	<.001		<.001	
Confidence in understanding things	.04	.04		.01
Attractiveness			.03	
Total self-esteem	.004		.01	
Social-related self-esteem			.05	
Performance-related self-esteem	.003			
Appearance-related self-esteem	.002		.01	
Mood	.015			
Family relationships	.01			
Overall life satisfaction and contentment	.003		.05	

The results presented represent significant differences from baseline scores for placebo and botulinum toxin type A (BoNTA) groups at 2 weeks or 3 months.

Tabe 2, Page 286

COLOR PLATE XXV

	p-Value	
	2 Weeks	3 Months
Feeling good about one's self	.006	.02
Appearance	.04	.02
Attractiveness	.04	
Sense of doing well	.04	
Total self-esteem	.04	
Mood	.01	
Overall life satisfaction and contentment	.01	.04

The results represent significant differences in change in scores between baseline and 2 weeks and to 3 months. The comparison is made between the resulting change in score, or "change score," for the botulinum toxin type A (BoNTA) and placebo groups.

Table 3, Page 287

COLOR PLATE XXVI

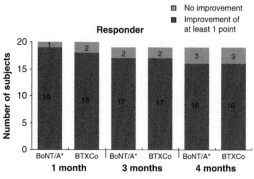

Fig 3, Page 288

COLOR PLATE XXVII

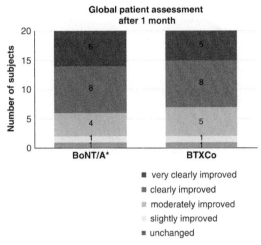

Fig 5, Page 289

COLOR PLATE XXVIII

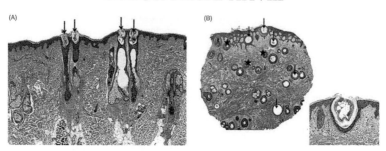

Fig 2 A-B, Page 186

The Clinical Relevance of Maintaining the Functional Integrity of the Stratum Corneum in both Healthy and Disease-affected Skin

James Q. Del Rosso, DO, FAOCD, and Jacquelyn Levin, DO

ABSTRACT

It has been recognized for approximately 50 years that the stratum corneum exhibits biological properties that contribute directly to maintaining and sustaining healthy skin. Continued basic science and clinical research coupled with keen clinical observation has led to more recent recognition and general acceptance that the stratum corneum completes many vital "barrier" tasks, including but not limited to regulating epidermal water content and the magnitude of water loss; mitigating exogenous oxidants that can damage components of skin via an innate antioxidant system; preventing or limiting cutaneous infection via multiple antimicrobial peptides; responding via innate immune mechanisms to "cutaneous invaders" of many origins, including microbes, true allergens, and other antigens; and protecting its neighboring cutaneous cells and structures that lie beneath from damaging effects of ultraviolet radiation. Additionally, specific abnormalities of the stratum corneum are associated with the clinical expression of certain disease states. This article provides a thorough "primer" for the clinician, reviewing the multiple normal homeostatic functions of the stratum corneum and the cutaneous challenges that arise when individual functions of this thin yet very active epidermal layer are compromised by exogenous and/or endogenous factors.

INTRODUCTION

"In my paper of 1964, which established that the horny layer was a tissue made up of corneocytes, I could not have dreamed of the spectacular

---

Dr. Del Rosso is Dermatology Residency Program Director, Valley Hospital Medical Center, Las Vegas, Nevada; Clinical Professor (Dermatology), Touro University College of Osteopathic Medicine, Henderson, Nevada; Las Vegas Skin & Cancer Clinics, Dermatology and Cutaneous Surgery, Las Vegas and Henderson, Nevada. Dr. Levin is PGY-2 (Dermatology), Largo Medical Center, Largo, Florida.

Disclosure: Dr. Del Rosso serves as a consultant, researcher, and/or speaker for Allergan, Coria/Valeant, Galderma, Graceway, Intendis/Bayer, LeoPharma, Medicis, Onset Dermatologics, Ortho Dermatology, Pharmaderm, Promius, Ranbaxy, TriaBeauty, Unilever, and Warner-Chilcott. Dr. Levin reports no relevant conflicts of interest.

Acknowledgment—*Dr. Del Rosso would like to credit Anthony Mancini, MD, a pediatric dermatologist in Chicago, Illinois. A few years ago during a lecture Dr. Mancini was presenting, Dr. Del Rosso heard for the first time the use of the terms "inside job" for endogenous factors, and "outside job" for exogenous factors, applied specifically to atopic dermatitis. Immediately after hearing this, Dr. Del Rosso incorporated Dr. Mancini's description to elucidate these concepts more clearly and informed Dr. Mancini how much he liked these two descriptions from a teaching perspective.

*advances that have been brought to light by an international school of cor-
neobiologists. I did not go any further than asserting that the stratum was
a cellular barrier, the end product of a viable epidermis whose raison d'etre
was to produce the dead stratum corneum...I did not have the vision to
foresee that the stratum corneum would become very much alive."*
                                                      —Albert M. Kligman, MD

The quotation above by Dr. Albert Kligman, which he so brilliantly wrote
in a textbook chapter entitled "A Brief History of How the Stratum Corneum Became Alive," summarizes an important turning point in the history
of dermatological research.[1] A brilliant discovery alone, regardless of how
potentially revolutionary it may become, sits idle in a meaningless void
unless its relevance is recognized and pursued with tenacity. Fortunately,
the science of the stratum corneum (SC) has advanced exponentially due
to the vision and dedication of a collection of leaders in the field of dermatology, referred to by Dr. Kligman as "corneobiologists." Several researchers
and clinicians over the past 5 to 6 decades have contributed to a wide body
of published knowledge that supports our current understanding of how the
SC, once thought to be biologically inert, actively contributes to the physiological homeostasis of skin.[1-3] Additionally, research continues to uncover
specific abnormalities of the SC that contribute to certain dermatological
diseases and/or impaired epidermal functions, and how some topical and
systemic therapies may adversely affect SC integrity and function.[3]

This article reviews the following several subjects: 1) the history of SC
science, 2) the homeostatic mechanisms whereby the SC functions to maintain the structural and functional integrity of skin, 3) impairments of or
changes within the SC that relate to specific dermatological disorders, 4)
endogenous and exogenous factors that create SC dysfunctions, and 5)
our current understanding of clinical approaches to reverse or mitigate SC
abnormalities resulting in improved therapeutic outcomes. It is important
to recognize that "corneobiology," and its many subsets of major clinical
relevance, is in its infancy. Advancements in this field are undoubtedly
part of a major groundswell as more information becomes available from
basic science research. It is readily apparent how this information has
already been incorporated into improved development of skin care products
and better approaches to management of healthy and disease-affected skin.

Early Milestones in the History of Statum Corneum

It was not too long ago that the established belief in dermatology was that
the SC is "a graveyard of insoluble keratin fibrils" that collectively represent
only the lifeless skeleton of what were previously keratinocytes that had
completed their upward journey through the layers of the epidermis prior
to their final destiny of desquamation.[1,2] In the 1950s, the SC, or "horny
layer," was described as the end product of living epidermal cells that disin-
tegrated as they moved up in the process of squamous differentiation, ultimately becoming an "amorphous mass lacking a cellular structure."[2,3]
The concept that the SC is essentially a dead layer devoid of any functional
activity was further entrenched in mainstream thinking by its perfunctory

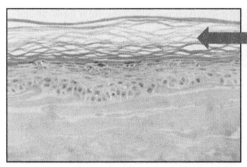

"BASKETWEAVE" HYPERKERATOSIS
Visibly appears as a lattice of keratin microfibrils (artifact of histologic processing)

FIGURE 1.—Note the histologic appearance of the stratum corneum that has classically been described as "basketweave hyperkeratosis." This appearance of the stratum corneum portrays this outermost epidermal layer as a simple lattice of keratin fibrils. In fact, this appearance is an artifact of histologic processing and misrepresents the true *in-vivo* appearance and structural integrity of the stratum corneum. (Reprinted with permission from the Journal of Clinical and Aesthetic Dermatology.)

description as "basketweave hyperkeratosis" when viewed histologically after routine processing (Fig 1).[1,2]

The belief that the stratum corneum was simply the "dead" outermost layer of skin, devoid of biological activity and function, persisted for several years. So how and when were the multiple talents of the SC discovered? The ability to harvest the SC intact and separate it from the remainder of the epidermis led to the belief that the SC was a homogenous Saran™ Wrap-like film that served primarily a protective function.[1,2]

"Perhaps no tissue is so physically maligned by processing for…microscopy…as is the stratum corneum…No tissue of crtitical importance for survival has been so intellectually maligned as well."

—Peter M. Elias, MD

The above quotation by Dr. Peter Elias, which is from a book chapter he authored entitled, "The Epidermal Permeability Barrier: From Saran™ Wrap to Biosensor," succinctly depicts how the significance of the SC was overlooked for decades.[2] Subsequent research and many publications over time led to the progressive recognition of the many physiological functions that occur within the SC, but widespread acceptance of this concept or its clinical relevance did not occur quickly.[3-21] One landmark publication that proved to be a major milestone in the history of relevant SC science was the seminal paper by Dr. Albert Kligman entitled, "Biology of the Stratum Corneum," which was published in 1964.[2] This publication gave the previously ignored SC the respect it had long deserved by refuting prevailing recycled dogma with new information regarding SC structure. Up until this time, the strongly held prevailing belief described the SC as a simple, biologically inactive, outer epidermal layer comprising a fibrillar lattice of dead keratin or the nonviable final product of keratinocyte degradation that immediately precedes normal desquamation.[1,2] In fact, it was noted that the SC is made up of a collection of sturdy cellular-like structures,

Covalently bound lipid   Cornified cell envelope   Intracellular humectants (NMF)

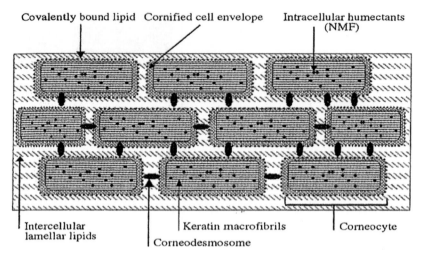

Intercellular lamellar lipids   Keratin macrofibrils   Corneocyte

Corneodesmosome

FIGURE 2.—This figure depicts the "bricks and mortar" structure of the stratum corneum. The corneo-cytes represent the bricks and the intercellular lamellar lipid membrane represents the mortar. Corneocytes comprise primarily keratin macrofibrils, are protected externally by a cornified cell envelope, and are held together by corneodesmosomes. The intercellular lamellar lipid membrane is primarily composed of ceramides, cholesterol, and fatty acids. A mixture of multiple small hygroscopic compounds present within corneocytes, referred to collectively as natural moisturizing factor (NMF), plays a vital role in the physiological maintenance of stratum corneum hydration. (Reprinted with permission from Harding CR. *Dermatol Ther.* 2004;17:6-15.) (Reprinted with permission from the Journal of Clinical and Aesthetic Dermatology.)

with an individual structure being termed a "corneocyte." In time, the concept of the stratum corneum being viewed as "bricks" and "mortar" emerged, with the corneocytes representing the bricks and the intercellular lamellar lipid membrane representing the mortar between the bricks (Fig 2).[6]

The bricks and mortar model of the SC, although it allows for initial conceptualization of the two-compartment macrostructure of the SC, is far too simplistic and does little to relate the constant sequence of varied functional activities that go on within this outermost epidermal layer, which measures just 10 to 20 μm in thickness.[6,22] These diverse yet inte-grated functions of the SC collectively serve to detect, protect, respond, and/or adapt against several exogenous factors. Common exogenous insults to skin include exposure to irritants, allergens, and microbial organisms; climatic changes, especially those which cause low ambient humidity; acute and chronic photodamage; and iatrogenic insults, such as SC abnor-malities associated with certain topical or oral medications. In many cases, the iatrogenic subset of exogenous insults is easily overlooked or not considered by the clinician, except where clinical relevance has been emphasized academically or is well-recognized in practice (i.e., the early irri-tant changes secondary to topical retinoid application). A separate and very relevant category is the endogenous factors, a spectrum of SC abnormalities that are inherently associated with specific disease states, such as atopic dermatitis, rosacea, and psoriasis. Importantly, SC impairments innately associated with specific underlying disease states do not allow for complete

FIGURE 3.—Major stratum corneum lipids and relative content by weight (%). Stratum corneum lipids represent 20% of stratum corneum volume. (Reprinted with permission from the Journal of Clinical and Aesthetic Dermatology.)

TABLE 1.—Synthesis of Stretum Corneum Lipids

Precursor Lipid[a]	Enzymatic Conversion[b]	Final Stratum Corneum Lipid[c]
Glucosylceramide	β-glucosylcerebrosidase	Ceramides
Phospholipid	Phospholipase	Fatty acids
Cholesterol sulfate	Steroid sulfatase	Cholesterol

[a]Precursor lipids that are extruded from lamellar bodies at granular layer into stratum corneum.
[b]enzymatic conversion to final lipid end product.
[c]final lipid deposited into stratum corneum to form the intercellular lamellar lipid membrane (bilayer).

reversal of full SC function as some underlying disorders impart a baseline level of SC impairment even during periods of disease remission.[3,5,7,10,19,26]

MAJOR STRUCTURAL COMPONENTS OF THE STRATUM CORNEUM

The structural components of the SC are depicted in Fig 2. Corneocytes (bricks) comprised primarily of keratin macrofibrils, are protected externally by a cornified cell envelope, and are cohesively held together by corneodesmosomes.[6] The cornified cell envelope is composed predominantly of proteins (e.g., loricin, involucrin) and a covalently bound outer lipid monolayer that is primarily made up of long chain ceramides.[6,22-24] Referred to as the "rivets" of the SC, corneodesmosomes serve to anchor the corneocytes within the SC and are composed of three major specialized proteins (desmoglein-1, desmocollin-1, and corneodesmosin). The primary function of the corneodesmosome is to maintain cohesive force between adjacent corneocytes until which time these rivets are degraded by water-dependent proteolytic enzymes involved in physiological desquamation.[6,22-25]

The intercellular lamellar lipid membrane comprises three major classes of lipid components present in a relative ratio of approximately 3:1:1 based on SC lipid content (% by weight): ceramides (40–50%; multiple subtractions), cholesterol (25%), and fatty acids (10–15%) (Fig 3). These major physiological SC lipids are produced enzymatically within the SC from specific precursor lipids (Table 1).[3,5,6,18,19,22] These precursor lipids are derived from lamellar bodies (LBs) within the granular layer, namely glycosylceramides, sphingomyelin, and phospholipids and are extruded from LBs along with antimicrobial peptides (Fig 3). Upon entry into the SC after extrusion from the LBs, these precursor lipids are enzymatically converted to ceramides 1–7, ceramides 2 and 5, and free fatty acids, respectively.[6,19,22] These two major hydrophobic lipid components of the SC, along with cholesterol, the third major component, and small quantities of other lipids, form a bilayer that comprises the intercellular lamellar lipid membrane.[3,5,22] Collectively, the physiological properties, relative composition, and the specialized intercellular compartmentalization of these physiological lipids within the intercellular lamellar lipid membrane serve to sustain SC water content, regulate water flux, and modify the rate and magnitude of transepidermal water loss (TEWL), all dynamic mechanisms that continuously function to maintain homeostasis.[5,22,26]

As additional information about the SC and its varied functions continue to emerge, it is readily apparent that the SC is not a fixed, nondynamic, nonpliable wall, and its lipid composition is not random and inactive. Rather, the stratum corneum is a factory that is in operation at all times, is always in multi-task mode, and incorporates an array of both adaptive and protective "barrier" properties that are functionally dynamic and continual processes.[1-3,22]

WHAT IS MEANT BY THE TERM "EPIDERMAL BARRIER"?

When people use the term "epidermal barrier," they are almost always referring to the ability of the SC to regulate TEWL, retain moisture for proper enzymatic desquamation, and provide selective permeability of exogenous and endogenous substances.[2,6,22,27] However, these functions are components of just one of the many "barrier" responsibilities that are carried out continuously by the SC, that is, the epidermal permeability barrier. In fact, the SC is multitalented as evidenced by its inherent ability to provide several other barrier properties. Examples include: 1) immunity barrier induced through specific receptor types, cell types, cytokines and chemokines with response via innate and/or cellular immune response patterns; 2) antioxidant barrier which protects against damaging effects of reactive oxygen species (ROS) via superoxide dismutase and other systems; 3) antimicrobial barrier via antimicrobial peptides (AMPs), such as cathelicidins and defensins within the lipid membrane, AMPs in sweat, and AMPs in sebum, and some SC lipids; 4) photoprotection barrier via both light reflectance and ultraviolet (UV) light photoprotectant properties of melanin and other chemicals; and 5) hormone receptor functions, such as peroxisome proliferator-activated receptors (PPARs) and liver X receptors (LXRs).[1-3,6,22,28-30] These different barrier functions of the SC are complexly intertwined with positive and negative feedback loops and biosensors that detect homeostatic abnormalities and stimulate self-repair mechanisms.[1-3,6,22,31-39]

The ability of the SC to quickly adapt and initiate natural physiological recovery of the permeability barrier (self-repair) is demonstrated by the early detection of even modest increases in TEWL, followed by immediate release of lipids stored within existing lamellar bodies, which produces partial reversal of TEWL within minutes, and the marked increase within 2 to 3 hours of precursor lipid production in lamellar bodies that leads to formation of the major SC lipids.[6,22,35,38,39] These replenished SC lipids help to restore the functional integrity of the intercellular lamellar lipid membrane and provide some innate water-binding capacity within the intercellular spaces of the SC.[6,22,35,38,39] Additionally, intracellular SC

TABLE 2.—Relative Concentrations (%) of Components of Natural Moisturizing Factor

40%	Free Amino Acids
12%	Pyrrolidone carboxylic acid
12%	Lactate
9%	Sugars
7%	Urea
6%	Chloride
5%	Sodium
4%	Potassium
2%	Ammonia, uric acid, glucosamine, creatine
2%	Calcium
2%	Magnesium
1%	Phosphate, citrate, formate, other

humectancy and hydration is augmented by an upregulation in filaggrin production and its subsequent conversion into multiple degradation products within the granular layer.[32,34-37] The pivotal step of filaggrin degradation produces free amino acids, pyrrolidone carboxylic acid (PCA), and urocanic acid, which collectively with simple sugars and electrolytes ultimately form a unique hygroscopic "moisturizer" called natural moisturizing factor (NMF), the natural humectant present within corneocytes (Table 2).[1-3,6,37,40]

Although much of our current knowledge and emphasis of the diverse barrier properties of the SC focus on the permeability barrier and its clinical relevance, a thorough understanding of the multiple complex interactions and feedback loops of the SC overall and recognizing specific abnormalities in the SC that contribute to unhealthy skin or diseased skin opens a door of opportunity to optimize SC repair by designing novel therapeutic approaches that target certain abnormalities or deficiencies.[1,3-6,14,15,18,19,22]

The next step in appreciating the multiple roles of the SC in maintaining the functional health and integrity of both normal and disease-affected skin is to develop a thorough overall understanding of SC formation, its major functional components, and its adaptive physiology in healthy skin.

FORMATION OF THE STRATUM CORNEUM

The SC represents the most superficial and final layer of maturation of the epidermis. However, where does the journey of the epidermis begin? The sequence of events occurs as keratinocytes traverse upward after their formation through the different layers (stratum) of the epidermis (Fig 4). Once arriving at a specialized zone of transition, the stratum granulosum, keratinocytes are sequentially modified and then converted to corneocytes, which comprise the SC prior to a final destiny of desquamation. The sequence of epidermal transition and the corresponding layers are 1) cellular proliferation with formation of keratinocytes within the basal layer (stratum basale); 2) keratinocyte squamous differentiation within the spinous layer (stratum spinosum); 3) formation of SC through transition of keratinocytes to corneocytes within the granular layer (statum granulosum) and the compacting layer (stratum compactum); 4) SC maturation

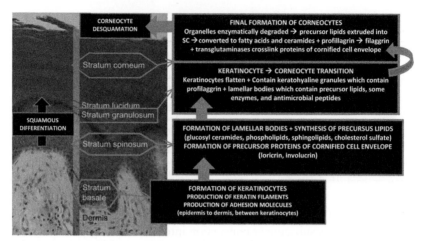

FIGURE 4.—The "Epidermal Factory": Progressive layers and corresponding production steps. (Reprinted with permission from the Journal of Clinical and Aesthetic Dermatology.)

with formation of the permeability barrier as corneocytes interdigitate with proper spatial relationship and cohesion in coordination with the intercellular lamellar lipid membrane (stratum corneum); 5) enzymatic corneocyte separation (stratum disjunctum); and 6) desquamation (into the atmosphere).[6,18,31,41,42]

Importantly, the time course from the start of the journey at the basal cell layer to the endpoint of corneocyte desquamation is generally estimated to take approximately four weeks, with the turnover of the SC being approximately half this duration. This is clinically relevant as therapies directed at modifying visible abnormalities within the SC (e.g., pitted keratolysis) may exhibit a lag time before improvement is apparent. This occurs as new "nondiseased" SC must first be formed before replacing previously "diseased" SC.

During the upward migration of epidermal cells, a stepwise sequence of active biological processes occurs that involves synthesis of specific structural protein, lipids, and enzymes; formation of structures integral to SC function; and activation of key enzymes, such as proteases, lipases, and transglutaminases, all of which impact directly upon SC health and functional integrity.[6,18,31,41-43] Basal keratinocytes of the stratum basale synthesize keratin filaments, adhesion molecules that attach the epidermis to the dermis, interkeratinocyte adhesion molecules, and cytokines and growth factors that regulate the proliferation and differentiation of the epidermis. After upward progression into the stratum spinosum, postmitotic keratinocytes continue the synthesis of keratin filaments, produce LBs composed of precursor lipids (glucosyl ceramides, phospholipids, sphingolipids, cholesterol sulfate), and form precursor proteins of the cornified envelope, which is comprised predominantly of loricrin (70%), and also contains other proteins (involucrin, cornifin, elafin, type II keratins, filaggrin, desmoglein, envoplakin, and small proline-rich proteins [SPRs]).[23,24,31,44] On the exterior surface of the cornified envelope surrounding each corneocyte, ceramides ultimately play an additional role in SC structural integrity as omega-hydroxyceramides form the corneocyte-lipid envelope, which osmotically maintains contents within the corneocyte and contributes to SC adhesion and lamellar organization. Once the synthesis of these multiple structural proteins and lipid precursors is completed, the keratinocytes are then prepared to move upward into the stratum granulosum, the zone of transition into the SC.

In the stratum granulosum, keratinocytes undergo a major "makeover" in preparing to become corneocytes. Within this layer, keratinocytes become flattened and contain specific organelles that serve to prepare the SC in maintaining the stability of the permeability barrier and other homeostatic functions. These organelles include keratohyalin granules, which contain profilaggrin, and LBs, which contain precursor lipids, certain protease enzymes, and AMPs. In the stratum granulosum, the LBs are positioned at the apical surface where they are in a "ready position" for exocytosis of contents into the lipid phase of the SC, which is the next layer of progression in the epidermal cell journey. However, an exception occurs in palmoplantar skin, where there is first cellular progression through an additional layer, the stratum lucidum, before becoming the SC.

Several major biological events occur upon transition from the stratum granulosum to the SC. At this point, keratinocytes become corneocytes after lysosomal degradation of their organelles. Also, there is extrusion by exocytosis of precursor lipids from the LBs into the lipid phase of the SC where they are subsequently enzymatically transformed into fatty acids and ceramides (Fig 4). These fatty acids and ceramides are then incorporated into the intercellular lamellar lipid membrane. Inside the corneocytes, profilaggrin, which originated from within the keratohyalin granules, is converted enzymatically to the protein filaggrin. Filaggrin subsequently migrates toward the periphery of the corneocyte and intermingles with keratin filaments to form the filament-matrix complex. On the surface of the corneocytes, calcium-dependent transglutaminases crosslink the proteins of the cornified cell envelope developing highly insoluble gamma glutamyl-lysine bonds. In the SC, the corneocytes are tightly adhered to each other by the cross-linked extracellular cornified envelope, desmosomal remnants, and the intracellular filament-matrix complex. Ultimately, a healthy SC continually performs several protective and adaptive physiological functions including mechanical shear and impact resistance, regulation of water flux and hydration, resistance to microbial proliferation and invasion, capacity to initiate inflammation via cytokine activation or dendritic cell activity, and selective permeability with exclusion of toxins, irritants, and allergens.[1,22,44]

UNDERSTANDING THE COMPLEXITIES OF THE STRATUM CORNEUM

The first step in understanding the complexities and interactions among the structural components and adaptive physiological functions of the SC is to focus first on the permeability barrier and responses that occur within healthy or "normal" skin. Through maintenance of both proper skin hydration and resistance to shearing forces, the structural integrity of the SC is sustained from day to day, thus allowing other "barrier responsibilities," such as immune surveillance and response, antimicrobial functions, and antioxidant activities to proceed. The ability of the SC to detect subtle changes in its own hydration status, that is, function as its own biosensor, is critical to the maintenance of its functional integrity and the overall appearance of healthy skin.[1-3,6,22] A variety of exogenous ("outside job") and endogenous ("inside job") factors, or both in combination, can contribute to altering the hydration status and integrity of the SC, as reviewed in more detail later.* Nevertheless, when there is either acute insult to the SC or chronic factors that increase TEWL and promote SC desiccation, the SC incorporates several adaptive mechanisms to restore its structural and functional integrity (Fig 5).[1-3,6,18,19,22,31-36,40-45]

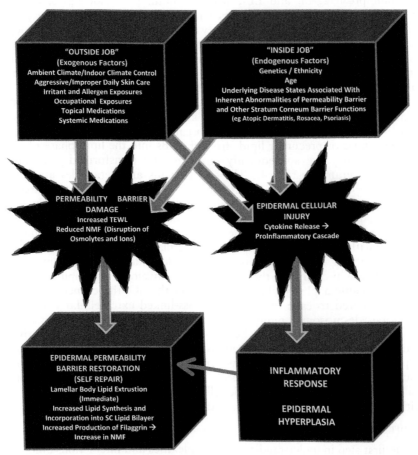

FIGURE 5.—Physiological adaptions of the stratum corneum in response to factors promoting desiccation. (e.g., increase in transepidermal water loss, decrease in natural moisturizing factor, damage or reduction in stratum corneum lipids, damage to stratum corneum proteins.) (Reprinted with permission from the Journal of Clinical and Aesthetic Dermatology.)

Once perturbed, the loss of permeability barrier function and subsequent increase in TEWL initiates multiple signaling cascades directed at restoring the permeability barrier of the SC. The major initial and quick response to an acute change in permeability barrier function is a temporary increase in LB secretion of precursor lipids into the SC where they are converted to the major lipids incorporated into the intercellular lamellar lipid membrane (lipid bilayer), and an increase in the biosynthesis of all major epidermal lipids which serves to sustain further self-repair.[22,35] The rapid response of release of LB lipids that were held in reserve can recover approximately 20 percent of the overall SC permeability barrier function.[22,35] Further repair requires additional synthesis of major SC lipids as well as other functions as discussed above.

In cases of chronic or frequently repetitive damage to SC protein and/or lipid components, more severe and more prolonged disruption of the SC permeability barrier occur simultaneously and work in concert adversely. The chronicity of this aberrant process results in an amplified signaling cascade that engages not only the desired epidermal homeostatic responses, but may also trigger the amplification of inflammatory events. In such cases, greater depth of epidermal and endothelial involvement occurs, which is more inflammatory in magnitude and can produce epidermal hyperplasia with chronic stimulation—both factors that are likely to play important roles in sustaining inflammatory dermatoses.[35,44,45] Protracted cases may be expressed clinically as severely xerotic and hyperkeratotic epidermal changes, especially on the distal fingers, distal toes, palms, soles, and heels.

THE "OVERSTRESSED" STRATUM CORNEUM: THE ADDITIVE EFFECTS OF ENDOGENOUS AND EXOGENOUS FACTORS

Endogenous factors that adversely affect the epidermal permeability barrier also diminish the capacity of the SC to physiologically adapt to exogenous factors that disrupt permeability barrier function and increase TEWL. In other words, an individual cannot change his or her genetics, ethnicity, age, or underlying disease states that are inherently associated with permeability barrier impairment. As a result, these affected individuals are at an innate disadvantage when exogenous stresses that are placed upon the structural proteins and lipids of their SC exceed its restorative abilities. In such cases, the self-repair functions of the SC are not able to keep up with the speed and/or magnitude of permeability barrier restoration needed to fully reverse the excess in TEWL. Unless corrected by proper therapeutic intervention, the clinical sequela of this scenario is initial progression to subclinical effects of SC desiccation, then to signs and symptoms of xerosis (dry skin), then to signs and symptoms of a flare of eczematous dermatitis, and finally to chronic eczematous and hyperkeratotic changes, all of which are discussed later.[3-18,22,26,32,37,38]

What endogenous characteristics have been identified that can retard the restorative capacities of the SC when exposed to exogenous stresses that disrupt the permeability barrier? Deficiencies and/or alterations in SC lipid content have been correlated with impairment of permeability barrier function, an important predisposing factor for development of xerosis.[3,5-8,22,26,38,42] A global decrease in epidermal lipid synthesis and SC lipids has been found in aged as opposed to younger skin.[38] A preliminary study, although small (N=71), has suggested that SC lipid composition and relative content may vary among different ethnicities living in the same environment.[46] With regard to underlying disease states, reduction in total SC lipid content, predominantly certain ceramide subfractions, is well documented in atopic dermatitis (AD), with the greatest decreases noted in actively eczematous skin; importantly, reductions in ceramides, although lower than in actively eczematous skin, have also been shown in xerotic and normal-appearing skin of patients with AD.[3,5-8,17,19,26,38,39,47] The inherent abnormalities of the SC permeability barrier in AD, associated with decreased SC lipid composition and content, and also in some cases filaggrin gene mutations, has been suggested as a major pathogenic factor in the development of the overall atopic diathesis, including allergic respiratory diseases and hypersensitivity (outside-in theory).[7-9,32,37,48,49]

What can be done to assist the overstressed SC in restoring the structural and functional integrity of the permeability barrier? As mentioned above, although the SC has the ability to self-repair a disrupted permeability barrier, there are many factors that can interplay to overstress the ability of the SC to fully adapt, especially when these factors are multiple, coexistent, repetitive, prolonged, and innate to other underlying medical disorders. A few active steps can be taken to optimize the health of the SC. Reducing exposure to and/or discontinuing practices that can cause damage to proteins and lipids of the SC is critical in decreasing the exogenous stress load on the permeability barrier. Such practices to avoid include overwashing; use of poorly formulated or harsh cleansers or true soaps (the latter due to alkalinity); use of cleansers with abrasives, exfoliants, or additives that are irritants; use of astringents; and use of topical medications that are not well formulated to reduce irritation potential.[4,6,40,42]

Appropriate skin care utilizing a well-formulated gentle cleanser and moisturizer, or barrier repair cream, has been shown to be beneficial in the management of disease states where the SC permeability barrier is impaired inherently by the disorder, its treatment, or both.[11-15,18,40,42,50-58] Many established moisturizers on the market today, in addition to incorporating conventional hydrating components, such as humectants, occlusives, and emollients, also include special additives or disease-specific ingredients, such as certain lipids, physiological humectants (i.e., hyaluronic acid), niacinamide, antioxidants, and amino acids.[4,15,40,50] Several of these formulations have been shown to markedly improve clinical signs and symptoms of AD and correct TEWL and corneometry parameters, thus demonstrating their ability to improve SC permeability barrier function.[51-53,55-58] Another study demonstrated improvement in recovery of the SC permeability barrier in chronically aged skin with use of a physiological lipid-based moisturizer.[56] Additional studies are warranted to further evaluate individual formulations, including attempts to differentiate properties that are relevant to clinicians and patients. Important differentiation parameters include several clinical performance measurements, regression analyses, and substantivity of effects. However, clinical differentiation does not stand alone. Proper nonbiased assessments of patient satisfaction are equally significant, including subjective feedback on therapeutic outcomes and physical formulation properties that influence adherence with continued use (i.e., texture; spreadability; ease of use; absence of malodor; product "feel" such as greasy, tacky, sticky, etc).

MORE INFORMATION ON SPECIFIC COMPONENTS OF THE STRATUM CORNEUM PERMEABILITY BARRIER

As discussed earlier, NMF is a mixture of multiple water-soluble small hygroscopic compounds that act as natural humectants. The humectant properties of NMF are essential for the activity of proteases that regulate corneocyte desquamation and moisture retention.[18,42] Free amino acids comprise approximately 40 percent of NMF and may be derived from multiple sources, including eccrine sweat, degradation of structural SC proteins, such as desmosomes and hemidesmosomes, citrulline originating from hair follicles, and degradation of filaggrin.[40,59] However, the release and degradation of filaggrin from keratohyalin granules of the stratum granulosum is believed to be the predominant source of free amino acids and PCA in the SC, with quantitative analyses showing that between 70 and 100 percent of the total free amino acids of the SC are derived from histidine-rich proteins.[59]

As stated previously, the keratohyalin granules and profilaggrin first appear in the granular layer of the epidermis. Profilaggrin in the keratohyalin granule is converted to filaggrin via enzymatic proteolysis as the cells of the granular layer transition into the SC layer. In this transition, the keratohyalin granules also intermix with keratin filaments forming the filament-matrix complex. Filaggrin is degraded into several free amino acids (histidine, glutamine, arginine), PCA, urocanic acid, ornithine, citrulline, and aspartic acid. These degradation products exhibit functions within the permeability barrier of the SC, including maintenance of hydration, pH (acidity), buffering capacity of the SC, and physiological desquamation, all of which contribute to healthy skin function and appearance.[1-3,6,22,32-34,36,37,40,42,59,60]

The clinical relevance of filaggrin and its proper degradation in helping to maintain the functional integrity of the SC permeability barrier is strongly supported by the link between filaggrin loss-of-function gene mutations and SC-impaired disorders, such as ichthyosis vulgaris (IV) and AD, both of which are chronically xerotic and associated with inherent basal cutaneous pH readings and impaired buffering capacity.[32,37,61]

WHY IS MAINTENANCE OF STRATUM CORNEUM HYDRATION SO IMPORTANT?

There are three main factors that maintain an optimal level of hydration of the epidermis and the SC.[18,22,31,40-44] The first is the formation and packaging of epidermal lipids and their organization into the intercellular lamellar lipid membrane in the SC (lipid bilayer). In the bilayer, the lipids are organized in an orthorhombic gel phase to effectively impede the passage of water through the intercellular space. Also, long-chain ceramides form a lipid layer on the surface of the cornified cell envelope. The second is the interdigitation of corneocytes within the intercellular lamellar lipid membrane, which creates an indirect and longer diffusion path for water as it attempts to traverse the SC, thus retarding TEWL. The third is the presence of NMF in the corneocytes of the SC, formed predominantly during the degradation of filaggrin.

The structural and functional integrity of the SC is highly dependent on adequate water content as many of the enzymes that catalyze vital SC functions are hydrolytic and do not function efficiently if water is present below a threshold concentration.[22,40,42] In addition to permeability characteristics, water serves to plasticize the SC as water content directly affects other physical properties, such as flexibility and pliability, resistance to shearing forces, individual desquamation of corneocytes, skin pH, and formation of the cornified cell envelope.[1,2,6,18,23,24,31,40,42-44,59,60,62]

The delicate interplay between SC water content and proper physiological SC function is further exemplified by the observation that the hydration level within the SC is not uniform under healthy physiological conditions in normal skin, ranging from approximately 15 to 25 percent at the skin surface, to approximately 40 percent at the juncture of transition between the granular layer and the SC, to about 70 percent within the lower portion of the epidermis below the SC.[20,44,62] It is believed that this water gradient is established in part by a discontinuity in the water-binding capacities between different corneocyte cell layers and may also reflect the need for different hydration levels to support specific enzymatic functions at certain depth locations within the epidermis. On electron microscopy, the corneocytes within SC levels of low water content appear less swollen than the corneocytes that have more water content at different depth points, as the swelling of corneocytes is directly proportional to skin hydration.[18]

Ultimately, in properly hydrated skin, the corneocytes shed as individual invisible cells, as the integrity of the epidermis and SC is physiologically sound from bottom to top. From a clinical standpoint, properly hydrated skin, reflected by a properly hydrated and minimally damaged SC, appears healthy, is pliable, and devoid of scaling or dryness. When the SC is desiccated, the degradation of corneodesmosomes by hydrolytic enzymes is impaired, and corneocytes tend to "clump" before shedding, thus causing roughness with visible scaling and flaking. The skin appears scaly, rough, and dull in appearance, as the features of xerotic skin emerge.[1,4,13,17,18,25,40,42,63]

WHAT IS XEROSIS (DRY SKIN)?

Regardless of the cause, dry skin, also referred to as xerosis, is the visible reaction pattern that occurs when TEWL becomes excessive and exceeds the ability of SC to adequately repair the permeability barrier. Although the term "dry skin" is commonly used by consumers, cosmeticians, scientists, researchers, physicians, and other healthcare professionals to describe one of the most common human afflictions, a clear definition

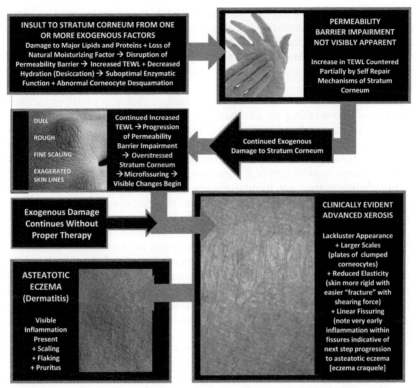

FIGURE 6.—Stepwise progression from damage to permeability barrier » xerosis » eczematous dermatitis. (Reprinted with permission from the Journal of Clinical and Aesthetic Dermatology.)

has been elusive.[63] Ultimately, dry skin is best defined clinically by its presenting signs and symptoms. Dry skin is dull in appearance, rough, scaly, flakey, and tight, often with associated pruritus, and in some cases discomfort especially in low ambient humidity.[63]

The progression from normal skin to clinically evident xerosis and subsequent eczematous changes occurs in a stepwise fashion (Fig 6). Insult to the SC, usually from one or more exogenous factors (e.g., overwashing; overbathing; use of harsh skin cleansers, astringents, or exfoliants; exposure to irritants; occupational exposures; climatic changes; low ambient humidity; certain topical medications or cosmeceuticals) causes damage and loss ("stripping") of SC lipids, damage to important SC proteins, and loss of components of NMF, leading to increased TEWL and desiccation.[4,6,40,42,63] With continued SC damage that is not countered by proper therapeutic intervention, the SC becomes "overstressed," that is, the continued insults causing disruption of the permeability barrier exceed the reparative capabilities of the SC. Over time, the clinical presentation of xerotic changes become more severe and exaggerated, and as a result of cytokine release and stimulation of an inflammatory cascade (Fig 5), can progress to eczematous dermatitis (e.g., eczema craquele, asteatotic eczema, nummular eczema, irritant hand eczema, exacerbation of AD) with associated pruritus and erythema. Epidermal hyperplasia with formation of hyperkeratotic eczema, which is associated with little or no visible inflammation, can also result from chronic damage to the permeability barrier on the hands and feet, often with associated deep fissures and pain, especially on the fingertips.

One of the most common exogenous factors that can cause epidermal damage is overwashing or overbathing, especially when combined with use of poorly formulated or harsh cleansers, especially true soaps, which are alkaline. Use of a poorly formulated, harsh, or irritant cleanser can induce deleterious effects on the SC, depending on formulation characteristics and specific ingredients (e.g., type of surfactant).[4,11-13,16,17,40,42,58,63,64] Strong cleansers that are highly efficient in removing dirt, oil, and other debris from the skin surface are also likely to produce the greatest magnitude of damage to the permeability barrier of the SC through stripping lipids and components of NMF and/or damage to SC proteins. Recognition of the importance of mild cleansers in the management of skin disease and in the maintenance of the SC permeability barrier has spurred the development of advanced mild cleanser formulations incorporating technologies and ingredients that provide a beneficial balance between gentle cleansing and efficient cleaning. These advanced cleanser systems induce negligible damage to the SC and in some cases actually deposit lipid into the SC after cleansing and rinsing.[13,40,42,58,64,65]

Certain topical products, including over-the-counter (OTC) skin care products with certain additives (e.g., alpha-hydroxy acids, astringents, abrasive granules, retinol) can induce damage to the SC leading to changes related to SC desiccation and cutaneous irritation. Topical prescription medications intended to treat specific skin disorders or cosmetic concerns may actually cause or exacerbate damage to the SC permeability barrier and possibly other epidermal functions depending on the pharmacological properties of the active ingredient(s). As will be discussed later, examples of medications that may adversely affect the SC include topical corticosteroids, topical retinoids, and benzoyl peroxide. However, the extent to which a topical formulation affects the SC permeability barrier may vary somewhat depending on the ingredients used in the vehicle. The vehicles of some products inherently induce SC damage due to specific inert ingredients used in the formulation, independent of the active ingredient(s) of the product. Other vehicles are designed to mitigate SC damage that is associated with the active ingredient(s) it contains, thus reducing potential for adverse effects related to SC desiccation. The formulation details including vehicle ingredients, information on SC-related parameters (e.g., TEWL, corneometry), and the cutaneous tolerability data of each product is important in understanding the potential effects that a product may have on the SC permeability barrier and other functions. Systemic agents that can impair the SC permeability barrier are the HMG-CoA reductase inhibitor agents used to lower serum cholesterol (e.g., simvastatin, atorvastatin, lovastatin, pravastatin). These lipid-lowering agents, commonly referred to as "the statins," interfere with cholesterol synthesis, with cholesterol being a major component of the SC intercellular lamellar lipid membrane, and may also alter the cornified cell envelope.[66]

WHAT OTHER FACTORS CAN AFFECT THE PERMEABILITY BARRIER OF THE STRATUM CORNEUM?

The pH of the SC has a significant influence on the barrier functions of the SC, with alterations in pH alone enough to cause clinically relevant changes. For example, the neutral to alkaline nature of the SC in the early neonatal period affects SC permeability and desquamation and facilitates the growth of opportunistic organisms such as *Candida albicans*, creating a milieu that is supportive of diaper dermatitis over approximately the first three months of life.[44] After that point, the SC pH develops its "sweet spot" for optimal physiological and homeostatic function and integrity, which is an acidic pH commonly referred to as the "acid mantle" of the skin.

The acidic nature of the human skin surface develops early in life, within the first few months, and is believed to be influenced by both exogenous and endogenous sources.[43,44,67,68] Exogenous sources of an acidic pH include free fatty acids produced by lipases from normal microbial flora, pilosebaceous-derived free fatty acids, and lactic acid and other eccrine-derived products.[44] Endogenous factors that produce a physiological acidic pH of the SC include cis-urocanic acid produced by degradation of histidine, free fatty acid production from phospholipids catalyzed by secretory phospholipase A2 (degradation of LB phospholipids), and via sodium-proton exchange mechanisms.[44] Acidification of skin pH has been shown to normalize SC integrity and permeability barrier recovery in neonates with neutral skin pH; expedite SC epidermal barrier recovery; optimize activity of lipid-processing enzymes and processing of LB-derived precursor lipids; and regulate corneocyte desquamation, cohesion, and integrity.[44] In addition, acidic SC pH favors growth of normal bacterial flora, as opposed to an alkaline pH, which is more supportive of the growth of pathogens such as *Staphylococcus aureus* and *C. albicans*.[67]

Other factors that can influence the functional and/or structural integrity of the SC include maintenance of a normal epidermal calcium gradient and regulation of epidermal development and SC permeability barrier homeostasis by nuclear hormone receptors and their ligands.[44]

WHAT ARE THE OTHER MAJOR "BARRIER RESPONSIBILITIES" OF THE STRATUM CORNEUM BEYOND THE PERMEABILITY BARRIER?

Although discussion of the SC permeability barrier is the focal point of this paper, there are several other "barrier responsibilities" related to specific components and functions of the SC (Table 3). A major responsibility of the SC is the antimicrobial barrier, which serves to provide protection against invasion and infection by microbial organisms, including bacteria, fungi, and viruses, but also is innately involved with some pathways of cutaneous inflammation.[28-30,69-72] The antimicrobial barrier comprises several AMPs, which are generally small, cationic polypeptides

TABLE 3.—The Stratum Corneum and Simultaneous Multitasking: Individual Epidermal Barrier Functions

Barrier Function	Major Components
Permeability Barrier	Formation of stratum corneum lipids in specific ratios from precursor lipids
	Production of lamellar bodies packaging precursor lipids and some antimicrobial peptides
	Formation of natural moisturizing factor from filaggrin (converted from profillagrin)
	Formation of cornified envelope and the corneocyte-lipid envelope
	Maintance of water gradient, calcium gradient, acid mantle (acidic pH)
	Response of primary proinflammatory cystokines to impairment of permeability barrier
Antimicrobial Barrier	Maintenance of an acidic skin pH decreases skin colonization by pathogenic bacteria and yeasts
	Antibacterial activity of stratum corneum lipids (e.g., free fatty acids, sphingosine, others)
	Genetically encoded primary antimicrobial peptides (defensins, cathelicidins, dermcidins) synthesized in SC, present in sebum and in sweat (dermicidin-derived)
	Multiple agents with antimicrobial activity as alternative function (some chemokines, some neuropeptides, others)
Antioxidant Barrier	Network of enzymatic and nonenzymatic antioxidant systems to counter oxidative stress
	Antioxidants present in epidermis (stratum corneum, skin surface lipids) and dermis
	Hydrophilic nonenzymatic antioxidants include ascorbic acid (vitamin C) and uric acid
	Major lipid-soluble nonenzymatic antioxidant is alpha-tocopherol (vitamin E)
	Co-antioxidants (ascorbic acid, ubiquinol [coenzyme Q10]) allow tocopherol regeneration
	Gradients in stratum corneum for ascorbic acid and tocopherol (lowest near surface)
	Interceptive antioxidant enzymes (catalase, superoxide dismutases, glutathione peroxidases)
	Antioxidant repair enzymes (e.g., methionine sulfoxide reductase)
	High concentration of alpha-tocopherol in sebum accounts for high levels in facial sebaceous gland stratum corneum (sebum serves as a physiological delivery pathway)
Immune Response Barrier	Dendritic cells involved in immune surveillance and antigen recognition (e.g., plasmacytoid dendritic cells, myeloid dendritic cells, Langerhans cells)
	Toll-like receptors involved in recognition of microbial pathogens and other agonists
	Antimicrobial peptides and some of their enzymatic conversion products (e.g., LL-37)
	Innate and acquired immune response pathways and balance with T regulatory cell system
Photoprotection Barrier	Epidermal melanin barrier (degree of protection related to Fitzpatrick skin type)
	Stratum corneum protein barrier
	Antioxidants within stratum corneum (protection against photo-oxidative stress)
	Optical reflective properties of the stratum corneum (stratum corneum thickness more important than epidermal thickness for protection against ultraviolet/solar radiation)

with the capacity to directly inhibit the growth of microbial organisms or indirectly mitigate microbial invasion by activating host immune response pathways. Thus, AMPs often serve as mediators of inflammation that affect epithelial and inflammatory cells, cellular proliferation, wound healing, cytokine and chemokine production, and chemotaxis.[69-72]

While cathelicidins and defensins comprise the major families of cutaneous AMPs, there are a variety of AMPs that have been identified, including some found in sebum and sweat.[28-30,69-72] While the upper stratum spinosum and stratum granulosum are the primary sites where AMPs are synthesized, these molecules are subsequently delivered into the SC where their functional activity occurs. Some AMPS, such as human beta defensin-2 (HBD-2) and cathelicidins have been shown to be localized within the LBs, which deliver these AMPs to the SC along with precursor lipids.[28,69]

In disorders where there is compromise of the SC permeability barrier and LBs are deficient, there is often associated dysfunction in the antimicrobial barrier of the SC. Examples of disorders where alterations in AMPs have been noted include AD and psoriasis.[5,6,44,73] The expression of HBD-2 and LL-37, the latter a product of cathelicidin processing, are downregulated in AD. These findings help to explain the high susceptibility of AD skin colonization and infection with *S. aureus*, and the predisposition to viral infections associated with AD, such as molluscum contagiosum and eczema herpeticum, the latter related to a decrease in the cathelicidin-derived protein LL-37 in AD.[74,75] As LL-37 exhibits antiviral properties, a decrease in LL-37 accounts at least partially for the predisposition to viral infections that often affect patients with AD. In addition, an increase in primary epidermal pro-inflammatory cytokines (e.g., tumor necrosis factor [TNF], interleukin-1 [IL-1], interleukin-6 [IL-6]) in response to epidermal insult and disruption of the SC permeability barrier is believed to assist in self-repair. However, prolonged or frequently repetitive damage to the SC can produce adverse clinical effects secondary to chronic inflammation and epidermal hyperproliferation.[76]

Other barrier functions of the SC are depicted in Table 3. Importantly, although the systems involved in each barrier function are unique and often complex, the interplay between these "functional units" of the SC is critical to the overall health and appearance of the skin. Loss of function in any one area can correlate with clinically apparent changes within the skin, and in some cases specific disease states.[6,44]

In some cases, the underlying dysfunction of the SC may be genetically programmed, such as with AD or the ichthyoses, while in other cases the underlying cause may be primarily iatrogenic, self-induced, or associated with acquired disease states. The epidermal antioxidant barrier incorporates a network of multiple nonenzymatic and enzymatic systems, which protect against oxidative changes induced by multiple exogenous causes.[77] Examples of such exogenous causes include chemical oxidants, ultraviolet radiation, air pollutants, microbial organisms including bacteria and fungi, and phagocyte-generated ROS that are directed at clearing pathogenic microbial organisms but also produce collateral damage to cutaneous tissues. Lastly, the cutaneous photoprotection barrier is provided by four potential mechanisms—the epidermal melanin barrier, the SC protein barrier, SC antioxidants, and optical reflective properties of the SC (direct correlation with SC thickness).[77]

Disease-Affected Skin and Associated Stratum Corneum Abnormalities

Atopic dermatitis. The "poster disease" that has popularized the clinical significance of "epidermal barrier dysfunction" is AD. AD is a complex cutaneous disorder associated with several operative pathogenic factors that interact to create a varied spectrum of phenotypes seen every day in clinical practice by dermatologists, allergists, and primary care physicians.[78] These multiple pathogenic factors include genetics (especially parental history); environmental influences, such as air pollutants, indoor exposures (e.g., house mite antigens, pet-related antigens), lifestyle (urban versus rural), dietary exposures, effect of antibiotic use in childhood on maturation of immunity; innate abnormalities of the epidermis including the SC permeability barrier (e.g., decrease in ceramide subfractions, filaggrin gene mutations, impaired ability to sustain SC hydration), the SC antimicrobial barrier (e.g., reduced levels of some AMPs, decrease in LL-37), and the immune response barrier; dysregulation of both innate and acquired immune response with alteration in chemokines and cytokines (e.g., Th2 imbalance, Th2-Th1 shift, increase in IgE, eosinophilia); hyper-responsive to both cutaneous allergens and irritants; role of microbial organisms (e.g., *S. aureus* colonization and superantigen production); and neurogenic and neuroimmunological factors (e.g., neuropeptides and neurotropins in epidermal nerve fibers near mast cells and Langerhans cells, increased blood levels of nerve growth factor, and substance P directly correlating with disease activity).[3,5,6-9,32,37,38,43,44,47-49,69,78] The presence of multiple pathogenetic factors in AD confounds the ability to differentiate the relative significance of each with regard to clinical presentation and therapeutic management, both in the AD population overall, and in the individual patient. Nevertheless, some of these factors are more available to clinicians as "low hanging fruit," that is, they are easier to address in the treatment of AD with what is currently available, including measures to counter the innate impairment of the SC permeability barrier and to decrease cutaneous *S. aureus* colonization.

From a clinical perspective, it is estimated that 45 percent of patients with AD present within the first six months of life, 60 percent within the first 12 months of life, and 85 percent before five years of age.[78] The extrinsic subtype of AD, which represents 60 to 90 percent of cases, is also associated with polyvalent IgE sensitization to inhalant and/or food allergens, explaining subsequent development of asthma, seasonal rhinitis, and sometimes food hypersensitivity in many patients with AD.[79] Although AD is most predominant in childhood and adolescence, and is typified by intermittent flares of eczematous skin changes and marked pruritus often involving multiple skin sites, persistence into adulthood is not uncommon, with many cases presenting as recurrent forms of eczema.[80-83] These include localized forms of eczema that are often recurrent, such as lichen simplex chronicus (LSC, "neurodermatitis"), hand eczema, eyelid dermatitis, genital pruritus (e.g., vulvar pruritus, vulvar hyperplastic dystrophy, scrotal pruritus often with LSC), asteatotic dermatitis on the legs, and sometimes diffuse forms of adult AD presenting as xerotic-pruritic skin without visible eczema, nummular eczema, and susceptibility to winter itch.

Xerosis, flares of eczematous dermatitis, and pruritus are consistent clinical features of AD.[80-84] Additionally, *S. aureus* colonization is a very common association that is often clinically silent or can present as crusted eczema ("impetiginization," infectious eczematoid dermatitis) or the actual presence of secondary staphylococcal infection.[80-85] Importantly, *S. aureus* colonization has been implicated in the pathogenesis of AD, playing a role in initiation of and/or prolongation of flares of active eczema through superantigen production and stimulation of a subsequent inflammatory cascade.[50-56,85]

SC lipids. There is a plethora of data documenting the significance of epidermal "barrier" disruptions in AD, inclusive of impairment of the SC permeability barrier, SC antimicrobial barrier, and the immune response barrier.[3,5-9,29-32,37-44,47-49,60,69-72,74,75] Abnormalities in SC lipids have been confirmed in eczematous skin, in xerotic skin, and in uninvolved skin in patients with AD.[3,5,6,8,17,26,38,39,42-44,47,48] The greatest decrease ceramide subfractions in AD patients has been shown with ceramide-1 (CER-1) in both lesional (eczematous) and nonlesional skin (visibly uninvolved without presence of eczema); however, ceramide-2 through ceramide-6 (CER-2–CER-6) were also markedly decreased in both lesional and nonlesional skin.[3,5,26,39] Decreases in CER-1 and total ceramide content were also found in the SC of AD patients with clinically xerotic skin that was otherwise devoid of visible eczematous dermatitis.[3,7] Correlation of SC ceramide content with SC permeability barrier function in patients with AD demonstrated a marked decrease in the amounts of CER-1 and CER-3, and a direct correlation of reduction in CER-3 with an increase in TEWL.[3,5,47] A three- to five-fold increase in TEWL has been observed in lesional skin of AD patients as compared to nonlesional skin.[3,5,86,87] Up to a two-fold increase in TEWL has been noted in clinically normal skin and xerotic skin (without presence of eczematous changes) in AD patients who present with active flares of eczema at other cutaneous sites.[3,5,86,87]

Filaggrin story. As discussed earlier, the role of profilaggrin production, its conversion to filaggrin, and the degradation of filaggrin to form major components of NMF are vital to physiological maintenance of SC hydration and the functional integrity of the SC permeability barrier.[6,31,32,34,37,42,88,89] Loss-of-function mutations in the filaggrin gene are collectively the strongest and most widely replicated genetic risk factor for developing AD.[88] It is estimated that as many as half of all AD cases are accounted for by a defect in at least one filaggrin gene null allele.[89] In other cases of AD, an acquired impairment of filaggrin may be present, likely the result of downregulated filaggrin protein expression induced by interleukin-4 (IL-4) and interleukin-13 (IL-13), which are increased in patients with AD.[89] Interestingly, it has been suggested that characteristics of filaggrin genes may be associated with the dry skin phenotype in the overall population, unrelated to association with specific underlying disease states such as AD. Specifically, predisposition to dry skin may be related to genetically determined "repeat copy units" in the polypeptide that is encoded for by the filaggrin gene.[88,89]

The development of filaggrin and its degradation products is a delicate balance of production, proteolysis, and inhibition of the process.[89] Every intricate step of this process needs to be functioning and in place in order to produce a healthy functional SC permeability barrier, as any alteration in the process can lead to permeability barrier dysfunction. Although loss-of-function filaggrin gene mutations are of major significance in the pathophysiology of AD, at least in many patients, a defect/deficiency in filaggrin alone may not be enough to cause AD, as suggested by a study completed in filaggrin-deficient mice, and also as some patients with filaggrin gene mutations present with ichthyosis vulgaris alone without AD.[88-90] In the murine filaggrin-deficient skin study, AD-like skin changes were induced only after intentional exposure to allergens, suggesting that antigen transfer through a defective SC permeability barrier may also be a key mechanism underlying elevated IgE allergic sensitization and initiation of cutaneous inflammation in humans with filaggrin-related atopic disease.[90]

Immune response. AD patients exhibit multiple abnormalities in their immune response barrier. A normally functioning innate immune response system recognizes pathogens and coordinates a response including anatomical and cellular mechanisms to combat invasion and infection.[6,28,30,69,71,72,75] In AD, there is both impaired microbial recognition and response.[44,69,78] Pattern recognition receptors (PRR), such as toll-like receptors (TLRs), recognize antigens and in response trigger cytokine release (e.g., IL-1, TNF), which initiates an immune response.[76,91] Unfortunately in AD, it has been shown that there are several specific TLR defects, including polymorphisms of TLR2, which may lead to a higher rate of *S. aureus* infection.[92] Another important player associated with impairment of the immune response barrier is CD14, a receptor responsible for recognizing lipopolysaccharides and other bacterial cell wall components. Low levels of CD14, similar to TLR-2 polymorphism, impair pathogen recognition and initiation of immune response in AD patients, with low CD14 levels in breast milk correlated with an increased susceptibility for development of AD in children.[93,94]

Antimicrobial peptides. Defensins, cathelicidins, and dermicidins are all AMPS that are diminished in AD.[44,69,91] As a result of reduced AMPs and other antimicrobial substances in AD, affected patients are more susceptible to bacterial colonization and infection, such as with *S. aureus*.[84,85,91,95] Additionally, levels of LL-37 and HBD-2 are lower in lesional skin of patients with AD, as compared to psoriasis lesions and normal skin, and the same has been shown with several other keratinocyte AMPs in lesional skin of AD versus psoriasis.[96,97] As noted earlier, LL-37, a product of enzymatic conversion of cathelicidins, has known antiviral activity (e.g., herpes simplex virus). Therefore, deficient levels or activity of LL-37 may explain the increased susceptibility of AD patients to certain viral infections, such as eczema herpeticum and possibly molluscum contagiosum.[98]

It has been shown that 90 percent of patients with AD exhibit colonization with *S. aureus* involving both lesional and nonlesional skin as compared to five percent of healthy controls, with up to 60 percent being toxin-producing strains of *S. aureus*.[91,99] In addition, decrease in HBD-2 and LL-37 in acute and chronic lesions of AD support susceptibility to *S. aureus*.[95] Additionally, a mutation in a TLR2 gene (R753Q) is found in increased frequency in AD, correlating with greater severity of disease, higher serum levels of IgE, and increased susceptibility to colonization with *S. aureus*.[92-100] There is evidence that *S. aureus* colonization plays a pathogenic role in AD, serving as to both trigger and prolong a flare of active eczema, through production of specific toxins called superantigens (e.g., enterotoxins A, B, and toxic shock syndrome toxin-1 [TSST-1]), which stimulate expanded populations on skin-homing T cells.[85] Evidence supporting the role of staphylococcal superantigens in AD includes the correlation of AD severity with presence of IgE antibodies to superantigens, superantigen-induced activation of infiltrating mononuclear cells augmenting allergen-induced inflammation, induction of mast cell degranulation, induction of skin- homing receptor on T cells by superantigens, and activation of Th2 cells by superantigens.[85] In addition to superantigens, staphylococci can produce nonsuperantigenic toxins, such as alpha-toxin, and compounds that can contribute to cutaneous inflammation, such as protein A and lipoteichoic acid.[100]

Topical corticosteroids. The effects of topical corticosteroids (TCS) on the SC will be discussed later under psoriasis.

Acne vulgaris. *Disease state.* There is little data confirming an innate impairment of the SC permeability barrier in acne vulgaris (AV). In one small study of patients with AV (N=36), increased TEWL, reduced SC hydration based on conductance testing, reduction in total ceramides, and reduction in free sphingosine (%) were noted in patients with AV as compared to controls.[101] Further study is needed to evaluate baseline characteristics of the SC in untreated patients with AV.

Acne therapies. Some topical acne medications are associated with signs of cutaneous irritation, such as peeling, scaling, and erythema. As a result, the association of a topical formulation or ingredient with impairment of the SC permeability barrier or other SC functions is an important consideration. Cutaneous application of benzoyl peroxide has been shown to increase TEWL, to oxidize SC antioxidants (e.g., alpha tocopherol [vitamin E]), and to cause lipid peroxidation; however, supplementation with topical vitamin E did not correct the increase in TEWL, but did reduce markers of lipid peroxidation.[102] Topical retinoids commonly induce an initial period of "retinization," characterized by peeling, flaking, and erythema ("retinoid dermatitis"), especially during the first few weeks after starting application. The use of a barrier-enhancing moisturizer prior to and during use of topical tretinoin facilitated adaptation to topical- retinoid induced signs of cutaneous irritation, decreased TEWL, and improved cutaneous hydration as measured by conductance.[103]

Rosacea. Skin sensitivity, characterized by associated signs and/or symptoms, are common in patients with the two most common clinical subtypes of rosacea, unrelated to use of any medical therapies.[10,14,68] In untreated adult patients with papulopustular rosacea (N=915) pooled from multiple studies, dryness, scaling, and edema were reported by 65 to 69 percent, 51 to 58 percent, and 32 to 38 percent of subjects, respectively.[14,103,104] In this same collective group of rosacea patients, facial skin burning, stinging, and pruritus were reported by 34 to 36 percent, 29 to 34 percent, and 49 to 52 percent of subjects, respectively.[104] According to a survey conducted by the National Rosacea Society in 1997 involving 1,023 patients with rosacea, 82 percent of these patients reported skin hyperirritability, burning, stinging, and sensitivity from commonly used skin care products.[105] Of the female responders, the three most common items reported to be irritating to facial skin included astringents/toners, soaps, and exfoliating agents. Of the male responders, the three most common causes of facial irritation included soap, cologne, and shaving lotion.

Impairment of the SC permeability barrier, as demonstrated by increased centrofacial TEWL has been documented in patients with erythematotelangiectatic rosacea (ETR), papulopustular rosacea (PPR), and also perioral dermatitis, and at least partially explains the inherent skin sensitivity that is so commonly expressed by patients with rosacea.[10] Skin sensitivity in patients with rosacea, likely related to disease-inherent SC permeability barrier impairment, is further supported by the results of lactic acid sting testing, completed in patients with ETR (n=7), PPR (n=25), and healthy skin (n=32 controls).[106] In this study, a positive sting test reaction with 5% lactic acid was found in 100 percent of ETR patients, 68 percent of PPR patients, and 19 percent of control patients.

Psoriasis. Although the pathophysiology of psoriasis is multifactorial and related to predisposing gene variants, genetic modifiers, and environmental factors, SC abnormalities have been identified that may contribute to the pathogenesis of the disease.[73,107] SC abnormalities that can translate to impairment of SC barrier functions include abnormal disposition on LBs in some phenotypes, alterations in formation of the cornified cell envelope, and decrease in filaggrin expression.[73]

Psoriasis phenotype. In both erythrodermic psoriasis and actively developing plaque psoriasis, a large number of LBs are formed. However, many of the LBs remain "entombed" in the cytosol of corneocytes, resulting in defective delivery of SC lipids to the intercellular space where the lipid bilayer is formed.[73] However, in chronic plaque psoriasis, LB contents are formed and secreted into the intercellular space of the SC, which is more consistent with nonpsoriatic healthy skin. A decrease in CER-1 has been noted from psoriatic plaques as compared to uninvolved skin and controls, with direct correlation between the CER-1 level and the increase of TEWL.[108] Interestingly, increase in TEWL noted in association with psoriasis is greatest in erythrodermic and actively developing plaque lesions, intermediate in magnitude in chronic plaque psoriasis lesions, and lowest in nonlesional skin.[109]

Differentiation markers. Markers of epidermal differentiation are also altered in psoriasis as compared to normal skin. These include an increase in keratinocyte transglutaminase type 1, which modulates an important step in the formation of the cornified cell envelope, decrease in filaggrin expression, increase in involucrin, increase in hyperproliferative keratins K6 and K16, and decrease in K1 and K10, which are markers of terminal differentiation.[73,110]

Antimicrobial barrier. In comparison to patients with AD, patients with psoriasis exhibit less susceptibility to infection. This is due to impairment of the antimicrobial barrier in AD, while an increase in AMPs has been noted in psoriasis.[95-97]

Topical corticosteroids. Application of TCS can result in visible skin abnormalities, such as atrophy, purpura, telangiectasias, and irreversible striae, which primarily result from dermal changes. In addition, microscopic and other structural changes have been associated with TCS use, many of which involve the SC and have barrier implications, such as epidermal atrophy; decreased microvasculature; decreased keratinocyte size; decreased ceramides, free fatty acids, and cholesterol; and increased TEWL.[111,112]

It has been demonstrated that as little as three days of application of topical clobetasol in both human and murine skin can induce subclinical adverse changes in the epidermis.[112] These effects include deterioration in epidermal barrier homeostasis characterized by delayed barrier recovery, abnormal SC integrity and cohesion, and the global inhibition of lipid synthesis. This study also showed improved barrier recovery and improvement in SC cohesion and integrity with the application of a physiological lipid-based moisturizer. These observations suggest that it may be prudent to use a well-formulated moisturizer as an adjunct to TCS therapy to ameliorate the adverse effects on the SC permeability barrier.

The adverse effects of TCS on the SC may be partially mitigated by the simultaneous use of a vitamin D analog based on a murine skin study. Topical calcitriol was shown to counteract the impairment of the epidermal permeability barrier and the antimicrobial barrier induced by TCS.[113] Specifically, the addition of topical calcitriol to TCS therapy significantly improved TEWL compared to TCS use alone ($p=0.024$), increased LB density compared to TCS use alone ($p=0.031$), and significantly upregulated major enzymes involved in lipid synthesis, HMG-CoA ($p=0.02$), fatty acid synthase ($p=0.02$), and serine-palmitoyl transferase ($p<0.01$). In addition, calcitriol was able to reverse the reduction of AMP expression induced by TCS, such as cathelicidin-related AMP (CRAMP) ($p<0.01$) and mouse beta-defensin 3 (mBd3) ($p<0.01$).

MANAGEMENT OF STRATUM CORNEUM PERMEABILITY BARRIER IMPAIRMENT

Maintenance of SC hydration, including assisting the SC in self-repair when conditions are adverse, is vital to sustaining healthy function and appearance of the skin. The use of a well-formulated gentle skin cleanser that produces negligible damage to the SC and a moisturizing product designed to sustain the integrity of the SC permeability barrier, with both facilitating and expediting physiological repair of the SC, is an optimal strategy for both healthy skin and disease-affected skin. Several studies have demonstrated that proper use of well-formulated skin care products augments therapeutic response to overall treatment in a variety of skin conditions, such as AD and rosacea, and/or reduces adverse effects associated with other therapies that adversely affect the SC.[4,6,11,16,18,21,22,35,40,42,50-58,64,65,103,104,105,114,115]

Importantly, moisturizing agents that incorporate quality conventional ingredients, such as humectant and occlusive agents, contain physiological lipids or ingredients that augment skin lipid synthesis, and/or include other agents that facilitate permeability barrier restoration, may be an optimal choice as these formulations are designed to target specific SC abnormalities that lead to xerotic skin changes, at least in some cases. Agents that are predominantly occlusive and/or humectant may exhibit less substantivity, may produce less overall impact on physiological barrier restoration, and are often less likely to be preferred by patients for continued use due to a greasy or sticky texture.[22,42,35,50-55] Importantly, individual formulations must be evaluated based on their own performance in both research investigations and after careful observation during clinical use. Additional research is needed to further our understanding of optimal formulations, including differentiation and use for specific disease states.

References

1. Kligman AM. A brief history of how the dead stratum corneum became alive. In: Elias PM, Feingold KR, eds. *Skin Barrier.* New York, NY: Taylor & Francis; 2006:15-24.
2. Elias PM. The epidermal permeability barrier: from Saran Wrap to biosensor. In: Elias PM, Feingold KR, eds. *Skin Barrier.* New York, NY: Taylor & Francis; 2006:25-32.
3. Proksch E, Elias PM. Epidermal barrier in atopic dermatitis. In: Bieber T, Leung DYM, eds. *Atopic Dermatitis.* New York, NY: Marcel Dekker; 2002: 123-143.
4. Del Rosso JQ. Understanding skin cleansers and moisturizers: the correlation of formulation science with the art of clinical use. *Cosmet Dermatol.* 2003;16: 19-31.
5. DiNardo A, Wertz PW. Atopic dermatitis. In: Leyden JJ, Rawlings AV, eds. *Skin Moisturization.* 1st ed. New York, NY: Marcel Dekker; 2002:165-178.
6. Harding CR. The stratum corneum: structure and function in health and disease. *Dermatol Ther.* 2004;17:6-15.
7. Yamamoto A, Serizawa S, Ito M, Sato Y. Stratum corneum lipid abnormalities in atopic dermatitis. *Arch Dermatol Res.* 1991;283:219-223.
8. Cork MJ, Danby SG, Vasilopoulos Y, et al. Epidermal barrier dysfunction in atopic dermatitis. *J Invest Dermatol.* 2009;129:1892-1908.
9. Ogawa H, Yoshiike T. A speculative view of atopic dermatitis: barrier dysfunction in pathogenesis. *J Dermatol Sci.* 1993;5:197-204.
10. Dirschka T, Tronnier H, Fölster-Holst R. Epithelial barrier function and atopic diathesis in rosacea and perioral dermatitis. *Br J Dermatol.* 2004;150: 1136-1141.
11. Del Rosso JQ, Baum EW. Comprehensive medical management of rosacea: an interim study report and literature review. *J Clin Aesthet Dermatol.* 2008;1: 20-25.
12. Draelos ZD. Concepts in skin care maintenance. *Cutis.* 2005;76:19-25.

13. Subramanyan K. Role of mild cleansing in the management of patient skin. *Dermatol Ther.* 2004;17:26-34.
14. Del Rosso JQ. The use of moisturizers as an integral component of topical therapy for rosacea: clinical results based on the assessment of skin characteristics study. *Cutis.* 2009;84:72-76.
15. Lodén M. Role of topical emollients and moisturizers in the treatment of dry skin barrier disorders. *Am J Clin Dermatol.* 2003;4:771-778.
16. Misra M, Ananthapadmanabhan KP, Hoyberg K, et al. Correlation between surfactant-induced ultrastructural changes in epidermis and transepidermal water loss. *J Soc Cosmet Chem.* 1997;48:219-234.
17. Rawlings AW, Watkinson A, Rogers J, Mayo HJ, Scott IR. Abnormalities in stratum corneum structure, lipid composition, and desmosome degradation in soap-induced winter xerosis. *J Soc Cosmet Chem.* 1994;45:203-220.
18. Rawlings AV, Scott IR, Harding CR, Bowser PA. Stratum corneum moisturization at the molecular level. *J Invest Dermatol.* 1994;103:731-740.
19. Menon GK, Norlen L. Stratum corneum ceramides and their role in skin barrier function. In: Leyden J, Rawlings A, eds. *Skin Moisturization.* New York, NY: Marcel Dekker, Inc; 2002:31-60.
20. Bouwstra JA, de Graaff A, Gooris GS, Nijsse J, Wiechers JW, van Aelst AC. Water distribution and related morphology in human stratum corneum at different hydration levels. *J Invest Dermatol.* 2003;120:750-758.
21. Kligman AM. Biology of the stratum corneum. In: Montagna W, ed. *The Epidermis.* New York, NY: Academic Press Inc; 1964.
22. Elias PM. Physiologic lipids for barrier repair in dermatology. In: Draelos ZD, ed. *Cosmeceuticals.* 1st ed. Philadelphia, PA: Elsevier-Saunders; 2005:63-70.
23. Koch PJ, Roop DR, Zhou Z. Cornified envelope and corneocyte-lipid envelope. In: Elias PM, Feingold KR, eds. *Skin Barrier.* New York, NY: Taylor & Francis; 2006:97-110.
24. Tetsuji H. Cornified envelope. In: Rawlings AV, Leyden JJ, eds. *Skin Moisturization.* 2nd ed. New York, NY: Informa Healthcare; 2009:83-97.
25. Haftek M, Simon M, Serre G. Corneodesmosomes: pivotal actors in stratum corneum adhesion and desquamation. In: Elias PM, Feingold KR, eds. *Skin Barrier.* New York, NY: Taylor & Francis; 2006:171-189.
26. Imokawa G, Abe A, Jin K, Higaki Y, Kawashima M, Hidano A. Decreased level of ceramides in stratum corneum of atopic dermatitis: an etiologic factor in atopic dry skin? *J Invest Dermatol.* 1991;96:523-526.
27. Elias PM, Feingold KR. Stratum corneum barrier function: definitions and broad concepts. In: Elias PM, Feingold KR, eds. *Skin Barrier.* New York, NY: Taylor & Francis; 2006:1-3.
28. Braff MH, Di Nardo A, Gallo RL. Keratinocytes store the antimicrobial peptide cathelicidin in lamellar bodies. *J Invest Dermatol.* 2005;124:394-400.
29. Elias PM. Stratum corneum defensive functions: an integrated view. *J Invest Dermatol.* 2005;125:183-200.
30. Schröder JM, Harder J. Antimicrobial skin peptides and proteins. *Cell Mol Life Sci.* 2006;63:469-486.
31. Elias PM, Feingold KM. Permeability barrier homeostasis. In: Elias PM, Feingold KR, eds. *Skin Barrier.* New York, NY: Taylor & Francis; 2006:337-361.
32. O'Regan GM, Irvine AD. The role of filaggrin in the atopic diathesis. *Clin Exp Allergy.* 2010;40:965-972.
33. Scott IR, Harding CR, Barrett JG. Histidine-rich protein of the keratohyalin granules. Source of the free amino acids, urocanic acid and pyrrolidone carboxylic acid in the stratum corneum. *Biochim Biophys Acta.* 1982;719:110-111.
34. Katagiri C, Sato J, Nomura J, Denda M. Changes in environmental humidity affect the water-holding property of the stratum corneum and its free amino acid content, and the expression of filaggrin in the epidermis of hairless mice. *J Dermatol Sci.* 2003;31:29-35.

35. Mao-Qiang M, Brown BE, Wu-Pong S, Feingold KR, Elias PM. Exogenous non-physiologic vs physiologic lipids. Divergent mechanisms for correction of permeability barrier dysfunction. *Arch Dermatol.* 1995;131:809-816.

36. Elias PM, Ansel JC, Woods LD, Feingold KR. Signaling networks in barrier homeostasis. The mystery widens. *Arch Dermatol.* 1996;132:1505-1506.

37. Kezic S, Kemperman PM, Koster ES, et al. Loss-of-function mutations in the filaggrin gene lead to reduced level of natural moisturizing factor in the stratum corneum. *J Invest Dermatol.* 2008;128:2117-2119.

38. Choi MJ, Maibach HI. Role of ceramides in barrier function of healthy and diseased skin. *Am J Clin Dermatol.* 2005;6:215-223.

39. Imokawa G. Ceramides as natural moisturizing factors and their efficacy in dry skin. In: Leyden JJ, Rawlings AV, eds. *Skin Moisturization.* 1st ed. New York, NY: Marcel Dekker; 2002:267-302.

40. Del Rosso JQ. Moisturizers: function, formulation, and clinical applications. In: Draelos ZD, ed. *Cosmeceuticals.* Philadelphia, PA: Saunders Elsevier; 2009: 97-102.

41. James WD, Berger TG, Elston DM. Skin: basic structure and function. In: James WD, Berger TG, Elston DM, eds. *Andrews' Diseases of the Skin.* 10th ed. Philadelphia, PA: Saunders-Elsevier; 2006:1-13.

42. Johnson AW. Cosmeceuticals: function and the skin barrier. In: Draelos ZD, ed. *Cosmeceuticals.* Philadelphia, PA: Saunders-Elsevier; 2009:7-14.

43. Cork MJ, Moustafa M, Danby S, et al. Skin barrier dysfunction in atopic dermatitis. In: Rawlings AV, Leyden JJ, eds. *Skin Moisurization.* 2nd ed. New York, NY: Informa Health; 2009:211-239.

44. Fluhr JW, Darlenski R. Skin barrier. In: Revuz J, et al. eds. *Life Threatening Dermatoses and Emergencies in Dermatology.* Heidelberg, Germany: Springer-Verlag; 2009:3-18.

45. Elias PM, Wood LC, Feingold KR. Epidermal pathogenesis of inflammatory dermatoses. *Am J Contact Dermat.* 1999;10:119-126.

46. Jungersted JM, Høgh JK, Hellgren LI, Jemec GB, Agner T. Ethnicity and stratum corneum ceramides. *Br J Dermatol.* 2010;163:1169-1173.

47. Di Nardo A, Wertz P, Giannetti A, Seidenari S. Ceramide and cholesterol composition of the skin of patients with atopic dermatitis. *Acta Derm Venereol.* 1998;78:27-30.

48. Elias PM, Hatano Y, Williams ML. Basis for the barrier abnormality in atopic dermatitis: outside-inside-outside pathogenic mechanisms. *J Allergy Clin Immunol.* 2008;121:1337-1343.

49. Leung DY. Atopic dermatitis: the skin as a window into the pathogenesis of chronic allergic diseases. *J Allergy Clin Immunol.* 1995;96:302-319.

50. Rawlings AV, Canestrari DA, Dobkowski B. Moisturizer technology versus clinical performance. *Dermatol Ther.* 2004;17:49-56.

51. Chamlin SL, Kao J, Frieden IJ, et al. Ceramide-dominant barrier repair lipids alleviate childhood atopic dermatitis: changes in barrier function provide a sensitive indicator of disease activity. *J Am Acad Dermatol.* 2002;47:198-208.

52. Lucky AW, Leach AD, Laskarzewski P, Wenck H. Use of an emollient as a steroid-sparing agent in the treatment of mild to moderate atopic dermatitis in children. *Pediatr Dermatol.* 1997;14:321-324.

53. Hanifin JM, Hebert AA, Mays SR, et al. Effects of a low-potency corticosteroid formulation plus a moisturizing regimen in the treatment of atopic dermatitis. *Curr Ther Res.* 1998;59:227-233.

54. Boguniewicz M. Conventional topical treatment of atopic dermatitis. In: Bieber T, Leung DYM, eds. *Atopic Dermatitis.* New York, NY: Marcel Dekker; 2002:453-477.

55. Draelos ZD. The effect of ceramide-containing skin care products on eczema resolution duration. *Cutis.* 2008;81:87-91.

56. Zettersten EM, Ghadially R, Feingold KR, Crumrine D, Elias PM. Optimal ratios of topical stratum corneum lipids improve barrier recovery in chronologically aged skin. *J Am Acad Dermatol.* 1997;37:403-408.

57. Frankel A, Sohn A, Patel RV, Lebwohl M. Bilateral comparison study of pimecrolimus cream 1% and a ceramide-hyaluronic acid emollient foam in the treatment of patients with atopic dermatitis. *J Drugs Dermatol.* 2011;10:666-672.

58. Levin J, Miller R. A guide to the ingredients and potential benefits of over-the-counter cleansers and moisturizers for rosacea patients. *J Clin Aesthet Dermatol.* 2011;4:31-49.

59. Levin J, Maibach H. Human buffering capacity considerations in the elderly. In: Farage M, Miller K, Maibach HI, eds. *Textbook of Aging Skin.* Berlin, Germany: Springer-Verlag; 2010:139-145.

60. Hachem JP, Man MQ, Crumrine D, et al. Sustained serine proteases activity by prolonged increase in pH leads to degradation of lipid processing enzymes and profound alterations of barrier function and stratum corneum integrity. *J Invest Dermatol.* 2005;125:510-520.

61. Levin J, Maibach HI. Human skin buffering capacity: overview. In: Zhai H, Wilhelm KP, Maibach HI, eds. *Marzulli and Maibach's Dermatotoxicology.* 7th ed. Boca Raton, FL: CRC Press, Taylor & Francis Group; 2008:971-980.

62. Caspers PJ, Lucassen GW, Carter EA, Bruining HA, Puppels GJ. *In-vivo* confocal Raman microspectroscopy of the skin: noninvasive determination of molecular concentration profiles. *J Invest Dermatol.* 2001;116:434-442.

63. Rawlings AV, et al. Dry and xerotic skin conditions. In: Leyden JJ, Rawlings AV, eds. *Skin Moisturization.* 1st ed. New York, NY: Marcel Dekker, Inc; 2002: 119-143.

64. Ananthapadmanabhan KP, Moore DJ, Subramanyan K, Misra M, Meyer F. Cleansing without compromise: the impact of cleansers on the skin barrier and the technology of mild cleansing. *Dermatol Ther.* 2004;17:16-25.

65. Ananthapadmanabhan KP, Yang L, Vincent C, et al. A new technology in mild and moisturizing cleansing liquids. *Cosmet Dermatol.* 2009;22:307-316.

66. Sparsa A, Boulinguez S, Le Brun V, Roux C, Bonnetblanc JM, Bedane C. Acquired ichthyosis with pravastatin. *J Eur Acad Dermatol Venereol.* 2007; 21:549-550.

67. Schmid-Wendtner MH, Korting HC. The pH of the skin surface and its impact on the barrier function. *Skin Pharmacol Physiol.* 2006;19:296-302.

68. Behne MJ. Epidermal pH. In: Rawlings AV, Leyden JJ, eds. *Skin Moisturization.* 2nd ed. New York, NY: Informa Healthcare; 2009:125-148;163-180.

69. DiNardo A, Gallo RL. Cutaneous barriers in defense against microbial invasion. In: Elias PM, Feingold KR, eds. *Skin Barrier.* New York, NY: Taylor & Francis; 2006:363-377.

70. Eissa A, Diamandis EP. Kallikrein-related peptidases: an emerging family of pivotal players in epidermal desquamation and barrier function. In: Rawlings AV, Leyden JJ, eds. *Skin Moisturization.* 2nd ed. New York, NY: Informa Healthcare; 2009:125-148.

71. Lee SH, Jeong SK, Ahn SK. An update of the defensive barrier function of skin. *Yonsei Med J.* 2006;47:293-306.

72. Nagy I, Kemeny L. Skin immune system. In: Revuz J, et al., eds. *Life Threatening Dermatoses and Emergencies in Dermatology.* Heidelberg, Germany: Springer-Verlag; 2009:19-28.

73. Ghadially R. Psoriasis and ichthyosis. In: Leyden JJ, Rawlings AV, eds. *Skin Moisturization.* 1st ed. New York, NY: Marcel Dekker; 2002:166-178.

74. Frohm M, Agerberth B, Ahangari G, et al. The expression of the gene coding for the antibacterial peptide LL-37 is induced in human keratinocytes during inflammatory disorders. *J Biol Chem.* 1997;272:15258-15263.

75. Schauber J, Dorschner RA, Coda AB, et al. Injury enhances TLR2 function and antimicrobial peptide expression through a vitamin D-dependent mechanism. *J Clin Invest.* 2007;117:803-811.

76. Biao L, Elias PM, Feingold KR. The role of the primary cytokines, TNK, IL-1, IL-6, in permeability barrier homeostasis. In: Elias PM, Feingold KR, eds. *Skin Barrier.* New York, NY: Taylor & Francis; 2006:305-318.

77. Thiele JJ. The epidermal antioxidant barrier. In: Elias PM, Feingold KR, eds. *Skin Barrier.* New York, NY: Taylor & Francis; 2006:379-397.

78. Bieber T, Prolss J. Atopic dermatitis. In: Gaspari AA, Tyring SK, eds. *Clinical and Basic Immunodermatology.* London, UK: Springer-Verlag; 2008:193-206.

79. Wuthrich B, Schmid-Grendelmeier P. Definition and diagnosis of intrinsic versus extrinsic atopic dermatitis. Conventional topical treatment of atopic dermatitis. In: Bieber T, Leung DYM, eds. *Atopic Dermatitis.* New York, NY: Marcel Dekker; 2002:1-20.

80. Hanifin JM, Rajka G. Diagnostic features of atopic dermatitis. *Acta Derm Venereol (Stockh).* 1980;92:44-47.

81. Diepgen TL, Fartasch M, Hornstein OP. Evaluation and relevance of atopic basic and minor features in patients with atopic dermatitis and in the general population. *Acta Derm Venereol Suppl (Stockh).* 1989;144:50-54.

82. Williams HC, Pembrokle AC, Burney PGF, et al. Community validation of the UK Working Party's diagnostic criteria for atopic dermatitis. *Br J Dermatol.* 1996;136:12-17.

83. Schultz Larsen F, Diepgen T, Svensonn A. Clinical criteria in diagnosing AD: the Lillehammer criteria 1994. *Acta Derm Venereol (Stockh).* 1996;76:115-119.

84. Leyden JJ, Marples RR, Kligman AM. *Staphylococcus aureus* in the lesions of atopic dermatitis. *Br J Dermatol.* 1974;90:525-530.

85. Leung DYM. The role of *Staphylococcus aureus* in atopic dermatitis. In: Bieber T, Leung DYM, eds. *Atopic Dermatitis.* 1st ed. New York, NY: Marcel Dekker; 2002:401-418.

86. Seidenari S, Giusti G. Objective assessment of the skin of children affected by atopic dermatitis: a study of pH, capacitance and TEWL in eczematous and clinically uninvolved skin. *Acta Derm Venereol.* 1995;75:429-433.

87. Schäfer L, Kragballe K. Abnormalities in epidermal lipid metabolism in patients with atopic dermatitis. *J Invest Dermatol.* 1991;96:10-15.

88. Irvine AD, McLean WH. Breaking the (un)sound barrier: filaggrin is a major gene for atopic dermatitis. *J Invest Dermatol.* 2006;126:1200-1202.

89. Uitto J, McGrath JA. The role of filaggrin in skin disease. In: Rawlings AV, Leyden JJ, eds. *Skin Moisturization.* 2nd ed. New York, NY: Informa Health; 2009:57-67.

90. Fallon PG, Sasaki T, Sandilands A, et al. A homozygous frameshift mutation in the mouse Flg gene facilitates enhanced percutaneous allergen priming. *Nat Genet.* 2009;41:602-608.

91. Martin DB, Gaspari AA. Toll-like receptors. In: Gaspari AA, Tyring SK, eds. *Clinical and Basic Immunodermatology.* London, UK: Springer-Verlag; 2008:67-84.

92. Ahmad-Nejad P, Mrabet-Dahbi S, Breuer K, et al. The toll-like receptor 2 R753Q polymorphism defines a subgroup of patients with atopic dermatitis having severe phenotype. *J Allergy Clin Immunol.* 2004;113:565-567.

93. Zdolsek HA, Jenmalm MC. Reduced levels of soluble CD14 in atopic children. *Clin Exp Allergy.* 2004;34:532-539.

94. Rothenbacher D, Weyermann M, Beermann C, Brenner H. Breastfeeding, soluble CD14 concentration in breast milk and risk of atopic dermatitis and asthma in early childhood: birth cohort study. *Clin Exp Allergy.* 2005;35:1014-1021.

95. Jalian HR, Kim J. Antimicrobial peptides. In: Gaspari AA, Tyring SK, eds. *Clinical and Basic Immunodermatology.* London, UK: Springer-Verlag; 2008:131-145.

96. Ong PY, Ohtake T, Brandt C, et al. Endogenous antimicrobial peptides and skin infections in atopic dermatitis. *N Engl J Med.* 2002;347:1151-1160.

97. de Jongh GJ, Zeeuwen PL, Kucharekova M, et al. High expression levels of keratinocyte antimicrobial proteins in psoriasis compared with atopic dermatitis. *J Invest Dermatol.* 2005;125:1163-1173.

98. Howell MD, Wollenberg A, Gallo RL, et al. Cathelicidin deficiency predisposes to eczema herpeticum. *J Allergy Clin Immunol.* 2006;117:836-841.

99. Leung DY. Infection in atopic dermatitis. *Curr Opin Pediatr.* 2003;15:399-404.

100. Morath S, Geyer A, Hartung T. Structure-function relationship of cytokine induction by lipoteichoic acid from *Staphylococcus aureus*. *J Exp Med*. 2001; 193:393-398.

101. Yamamoto A, Takenouchi K, Ito M. Impaired water barrier function in acne vulgaris. *Arch Dermatol Res*. 1985;287:214-218.

102. Weber SU, Thiele JJ, Han N, et al. Topical alpha-tocotrienol supplementation inhibits lipid peroxidation but fails to mitigate increased transepidermal water loss after benzoyl peroxide treatment to human skin. *Free Radic Biol Med*. 2003;34:170-176.

103. Draelos ZD, Ertel KD, Berge CA. Facilitating facial retinization through barrier improvement. *Cutis*. 2006;78:275-281.

104. Elewski BE, Fleischer AB Jr, Pariser DM. A comparison of 15% azelaic acid gel and 0.75% metronidazole gel in the topical treatment of papulopustular rosacea: results of a randomized trial. *Arch Dermatol*. 2003;139:1444-1450.

105. Torok HM. Rosacea skin care. *Cutis*. 2000;66:14-16.

106. Lonne-Rahm SB, Fischer T, Berg M. Stinging and rosacea. *Acta Derm Venereol*. 1999;79:460-461.

107. Nestle FO. Psoriasis. In: Gaspari AA, Tyring SK, eds. *Clinical and Basic Immunodermatology*. London, UK: Springer-Verlag; 2008:207-216.

108. Motta S, Monti M, Sesana S, Mellesi L, Ghidoni R, Caputo R. Abnormality of water barrier function in psoriasis. Role of ceramide fractions. *Arch Dermatol*. 1994;130:452-456.

109. Ghadially R, Reed JT, Elias PM. Stratum corneum structure and function correlates with phenotype in psoriasis. *J Invest Dermatol*. 1996;107:558-564.

110. Schroeder WT, Thacher SM, Stewart-Galetka S, et al. Type I keratinocyte transglutaminase: expression in human skin and psoriasis. *J Invest Dermatol*. 1992; 99:27-34.

111. Del Rosso J, Friedlander SF. Corticosteroids: options in the era of steroid-sparing therapy. *J Am Acad Dermatol*. 2005;53:850-858.

112. Kao JS, Fluhr JW, Man MQ, et al. Short-term glucocorticoid treatment compromises both permeability barrier homeostasis and stratum corneum integrity: inhibition of epidermal lipid synthesis accounts for functional abnormalities. *J Invest Dermatol*. 2003;120:456-464.

113. Hong SP, Oh Y, Jung M, et al. Topical calcitriol restores the impairment of epidermal permeability and antimicrobial barriers induced by corticosteroids. *Br J Dermatol*. 2010;162:1251-1260.

114. Tabata N, O'Goshi K, Zhen YX, Kligman AM, Tagami H. Biophysical assessment of persistent effects of moisturizers after their daily applications: evaluation of corneotherapy. *Dermatology*. 2000;200:308-313.

115. Johnson AW. Overview: fundamental skin care—protecting the barrier. *Dermatol Ther*. 2004;17:1-5.

Practical Evaluation and Management of Atrophic Acne Scars: Tips for the General Dermatologist

DOUGLAS FIFE, MD

Surgical Dermatology & Laser Center, Las Vegas, Nevada

ABSTRACT

Atrophic acne scarring is an unfortunate, permanent complication of acne vulgaris, which may be associated with significant psychological distress. General dermatologists are frequently presented with the challenge of evaluating and providing treatment recommendations to patients with acne scars. This article reviews a practical, step-by-step approach to evaluating the patient with atrophic acne scars. An algorithm for providing treatment options is presented, along with pitfalls to avoid. A few select procedures that may be incorporated into a general dermatology practice are reviewed in greater detail, including filler injections, skin needling, and the punch excision. (*J Clin Aesthet Dermatol.* 2011;4(8):50−57.)

Acne is a common condition that affects up to 80 percent of the adolescent population to some degree or another.[1,2] Permanent scarring from acne is an unfortunate complication of acne vulgaris. The incidence of acne scarring is not well studied, but it may occur to some degree in 95 percent of patients with acne vulgaris.[3] Studies report the incidence of acne scarring in the general population to be 1 to 11 percent.[4,5]

Having acne scars can be emotionally and psychologically distressing to patients. Along with acne, having acne scars is a risk factor for suicide[6] and also may be linked to poor self esteem, depression, anxiety, altered social interactions, body image alterations, embarrassment, anger, lowered academic performance, and unemployment.[7-9] Rather than fading with time, the appearance of scars often worsens with normal aging or photodamage.[9]

Acne scars can be classified into three different types—atrophic, hypertrophic, or keloidal. Atrophic acne scars are by far the most common type. The pathogenesis of atrophic acne scarring is not completely understood, but is most likely related to inflammatory mediators and enzymatic degradation of collagen fibers and subcutaneous fat.[10] It is not clear why some acne patients develop scars while others do not, as the degree of acne does not always correlate with the incidence or severity of scarring. The scarring process can occur at any stage of acne[10]; however, it is uniformly believed that early intervention in inflammatory and nodulocystic acne is the most effective way of preventing post-acne scarring. Once scarring has occurred, it is usually permanent.

Because of the prevalence of acne scarring and the strong negative emotions it engenders in affected patients, it is likely that dermatologists

---

Address Correspondence to: Douglas Fife, MD, 9280 W. Sunset Road, Suite 310, Las Vegas, NV 89148; E-mail: dfife@surgical-dermatology.com
Disclosure: Dr. Fife reports no relevant conflicts of interest.

will be questioned about treatment options. This article is intended to arm the general or cosmetic dermatologist with the ability to efficiently evaluate the acne scar patient, discuss the most appropriate treatment options, effectively set expectations, and decide which procedures can be done efficiently in a general dermatology clinic, and when the patient should be referred for more complicated or aggressive surgical procedures. This last item is problematic, as every dermatologist has a different skill set, comfort level performing procedures, training, and access to surgical devices or instruments. This article will not review comprehensively the literature relating to acne scars, nor will it give a step-by-step description of all techniques for treating acne scars. This article is intended to be a practical overview of the evaluation and management of the patient with acne scarring, highlighting pitfalls to avoid and discussing in more detail a few select procedures that can be most easily incorporated into a dermatology practice. This article will be limited to the evaluation and management of atrophic lesions only. Several other articles have adressed the management of keloidal acne scarring in detail.[9,11-13]

EVALUATION

Success in the management of the acne scar patient hinges on the physician's clear understanding of the patient's concerns and expectations relating to his or her scars. This management begins when the patient asks a question such as, "Doc, what can be done for my acne scars?" Before answering this question, the physician needs to attempt to find out the depth of the discussion the patient is seeking. In doing so, the physician should ask such questions as, "What bothers you about your scars?" "How distressing are the scars to you?" These types of questions should elicit this information. A history of the patient's acne and acne scars should be taken (see Table 1

TABLE 1.—Pearls for Evaluation

History

Which aspects of the patient's scarring are the most bothersome to him/her?
How distressed is the patient about his or her scars?
What are the patient's goals for treatment?
Have any prior procedures been performed to treat the scars?
Has the active acne cleared completely? How recently did the acne clear?
Was isotretinoin used? How recently was it discontinued?
Is there a history of postinflammatory hyperpigmentation (PIH)?
Is there a history of keloids or hypertrophic scars?

Physical Examination

Direct overhead lighting is optimal
Have a mirror for the patient to point out lesions
Evaluate for active acne
Define types of scars (icepick, rolling, boxcar, severely atrophic/ sclerotic)
Assess color (hypopigmentation, hyperpigmentation, purple/red discoloration)
Assess depth of the lesions
Stretch skin to see if scars disappear
Palpate for underlying fibrosis
Evaluate skin type (types III—V have increased risk of PIH with most procedures)

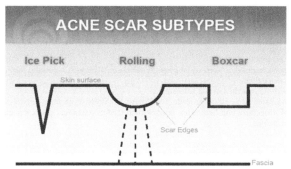

FIGURE 1.—Subtypes of atrophic acne scars. Adapted from Jacob et al.[14] (Reprinted with permission from the Journal of Clinical and Aesthetic Dermatology.)

TABLE 2.—4-Point Grading Scale for Acne Scars[15]

Grade 1: Macular
• Erythematous, hyper-, or hypopigmented marks
Grade 2: Mild Disease
• Mild atrophy, can be covered with makeup or facial hair
Grade 3: Moderate Disease
• Moderate scarring, not covered by makeup but can be flattened by manual stretching of the skin
Grade 4: Severe Disease
• Scarring not flattened with manual stretching of the skin

for a list of appropriate questions), including if and when acne cleared completely and if oral isotretinoin was utilized, as many procedures are contraindicated within six months of discontinuation of isotretinoin. It is important to ask the patient if there are specific scars, areas of scarring, or features of the scars that are most bothersome. Targeting certain scars or certain features of the scars (hyper-pigmentation, for example) may increase the chance of successful treatment and patient satisfaction.

Pearls for the physician examination are listed in Table 1. It is helpful to have overhead rather than direct lighting to accentuate the appearance of scars. Often, a handheld mirror will allow the patient to highlight specific areas and help them feel as though they are completely understood. Multiple acne scar grading classification systems of varying complexities have been introduced. The most basic, practical system divides atrophic acne scars into the following three main types: 1) icepick, 2) rolling, and 3) boxcar scars (Fig 1).[14] It is common for patients to have more than one type of scar.

A second, useful system proposed by Goodman[15] uses a four-scale grading system (Table 2). During the evaluation, scars are visually inspected, palpated, and stretched. It is important to note whether or not active inflammatory acne is present, as this may be a contraindication for treatment. In addition, improving active acne may satisfy the patient even without interventions for acne scars. The skin is stretched to distinguish between grade 3 and 4 acne scars and to determine if volumizing fillers or a facelift may minimize appearance of scars. Palpation for underlying fibrosis is important, as

---

TABLE 3.—Patient-specific issues to address in treatment planning

---

- Expectations and goals
- Financial considerations
- Are there time constraints that need to be considered? (Family photos, wedding, job interviews, presentations, sales calls)
- How much downtime can the patient tolerate?
    1) A non-ablative laser or needling procedure will have less down-time than fractional ablative laser.
    2) An excisional procedure will heal more quickly than CROSS chemical peels, dermabrasion, and ablative resurfacing
    3) A filler procedure may have less bruising and postoperative swelling than subcision
- How much discomfort is the patient willing to tolerate?

---

deeply fibrotic lesions often will only improve with excisional procedures. The patient's skin type should be noted, as patients with Fitzpatrick skin types III to VI have a higher risk of postinflammatory hyperpigmentation (PIH) with many resurfacing procedures. In addition, any discoloration is noted, including hyperpigmentation, hypopigmentation, and red/purple discoloration.

MANAGEMENT

An initial discussion with the patient to address goals, concerns, and expectations is of paramount importance. Patient-specific issues are discussed (Table 3), such as the patient's goals for treatment, ability to tolerate downtime and pain, time constraints, and financial constraints. The physician should emphasize to the patient the unpredictability of acne scar treatment, specifically, that there is usually no quick, easy, and permanent fix to this problem. While there are many effective treatments for many patients, not all improve with a specific procedure or groups of procedures. Usually, multiple procedures are required and some procedures may need to be repeated at certain intervals to maintain the improvement. The only procedures that predictably have more permanence are excisional procedures and permanent fillers, such as silicone. A mistake in the initial consultation would be to promise a certain level of improvement in acne scars or to minimize the downtime and discomfort associated with each procedure that is considered. Patients are most likely to be satisfied with their outcome (even if they have only marginal results) if the physician can help them understand the unpredictability of acne scar therapy and develop realistic expectations for improvement. In addition, side effects of each procedure planned should be discussed in detail. The risks of infection, hyperpigmentation, prolonged erythema, swelling, and poor healing/scarring are present with many procedures and should be understood by the patient.

SELECTING THE APPROPRIATE PROCEDURES

Available procedures for acne scars are listed by category in Table 4. Resurfacing procedures remove layers of skin from the top down. Injury to the dermis by resurfacing procedures is thought to cause dermal remodeling and neocollagenesis. Lifting procedures attempt to draw the base of

TABLE 4.—Acne scar procedures grouped by procedure type

Resurfacing Procedures
Chemical Peels
  • Full Face
  • CROSS Technique
Dermabrasion
Laser Resurfacing
  • Ablative/nonablative
  • Fractional
Lifting Procedures
Subcision
Fillers
  • Directly under scars
  • Volumizing
  • Autologous fat transfer
Punch evaluation
Excisional Techniques
Punch excision
Elliptical excision
Punch grafting
Other
Skin needling
Facelift
Combination techniques

TABLE 5.—Procedures to Select/Recommend by Lesion Type

Ice-Pick Scars
Punch excision
CROSS chemical peels
Rolling Scars
Subcision
Filler injections directly underneath scars
Fractional laser therapy
Skin needling
Boxcar Scars
CROSS chemical peels (for small lesions)
Punch elevation
Fractional laser therapy
Skin needling
Focal dermabrasion
Punch excision (for narrow, deep lesions)
Elliptical excision (for larger lesions)
Macular Grade 1 Scarring (Redness, Hypopigmented or Hyperpigmented)
Skin needling
Fractional ablative/nonablative laser
Nonablative laser for pigment (erythema or hyperpigmentation)
ReCell (in future)
Fibrotic OR Deep, Hypopgmented Scars
Excisional techniques

a deep scar upward towards the surface, making the skin smooth. Excisional procedures remove scars completely. Table 5 lists the most appropriate procedures to utilize for each lesion type (e.g., rolling, boxcar). If a patient has scars of varying morphologies, two or more different procedures may need to be selected (e.g., punch excisions of icepick scars and filler injections under soft, rolling scars). It is wise to do a test spot in a representative area that is in as inconspicuous of a location as possible. This may address the efficacy of a procedure and also predict the risk for side effects, such as prolonged erythema or PIH. Selecting the appropriate locations is important, as acne scars on the chest, back, and shoulders are much more resistant to treatment than scars on the face.

PROCEDURES MOST EASILY INCORPORATED INTO A GENERAL OR COSMETIC DERMATOLOGY PRACTICE

There are a few procedures that can be easily incorporated into most general dermatology practices with much less expense and training in comparison with lasers, subcision, dermabrasion, or other procedures. These procedures are soft-tissue augmentation fillers, the punch excision, and skin needling.

Soft tissue augmentation fillers. Soft-tissue fillers are effective in treating patients with rolling acne scars.[16-21] Because many dermatologists are comfortable using these materials in patients for cosmetic purposes, the transition to treatment of acne scars with these same agents is natural. Fillers for acne scarring can be utilized in two ways. First, fillers can be injected directly under individual scars for immediate improvement (Fig 2). Second, volumizing fillers, such as poly-L lactic acid or calcium hydroxylapatite, can be delivered to areas where laxity of skin or deep tissue atrophy is accentuating the appearance of acne scars (Fig 2).

Fillers injected directly under scars. Normally, cross- linked hyaluronic acid fillers are utilized for local injection under specific scars. The filler can be injected either with a cross-hatching/lattice approach or a depot injection under the scars. The optimal lesions are broad, rolling scars that are soft and distensible/stretchable. Caution should be taken if there is fibrosis under the lesion, as the deposition of filler may be uneven under the scar, resulting in extrusion of the filler material into the surrounding skin, which could possibly make the appearance worse. In addition, it is important to not deliver too much filler. It would be better to undercorrect and do touch-up treatments in the future.

Volumizing fillers. Volumizing fillers such as poly-L lactic acid (Sculptra®, Sanofi-Aventis, Paris, France) or calcium hydroxylapatite (Radiesse®, Bioform Medical Inc., Milwaukee, WI) are also widely utilized by dermatologists for volumetric replacement of deep tissue atrophy of the mid-face or for human immunodeficiency virus (HIV) lipatrophy. Atrophic acne scars in some patients are accentuated by skin laxity or loss of volume in the cheek or chin area, similar to a deflated balloon that wrinkles and has multiple depressions. These changes often worsen in appearance with age or photodamage.[9] When the skin is stretched, similar to a balloon being refilled, individual depressions and shadows are naturally minimized (Fig 3). The same techniques used to inject poly-L lactic acid and calcium hydroxylapatite for correction of HIV lipatrophy and for cosmetic augmentation of the mid-face can be used when treating acne scars. The material is placed either by periosteal depot or diffusely in the area of deep tissue atrophy to swell and lift the area as is described in other studies.[22-26]

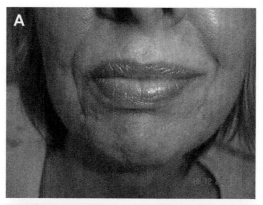

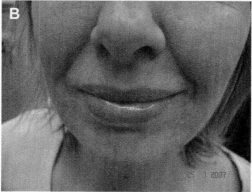

FIGURE 2.—Photos before (A) and after (B) hyaluronic acid filler injected immediately beneath rolling acne scars of the lower face. This patient was also treated with botulinum toxin to the lower face. *Photos courtesy of Greg Goodman, MD.* (Reprinted with permission from the Journal of Clinical and Aesthetic Dermatology.)

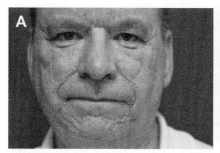 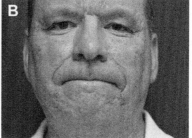

FIGURE 3.—Photos before (A) and immediately after (B) injection with poly-L lactic acid demonstrating how volumetric filling of the mid-face can improve the appearance of acne scars accentuated by underlying soft tissue loss. Although this effect is temporary, it approximates what the patient will ultimately achieve with 2 to 4 sessions of treatment. (Reprinted with permission from the Journal of Clinical and Aesthetic Dermatology.)

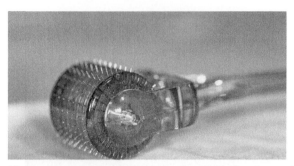

FIGURE 4.—Needling device consisting of a rolling barrel studded by 2mm-long needles. (Reprinted with permission from the Journal of Clinical and Aesthetic Dermatology.)

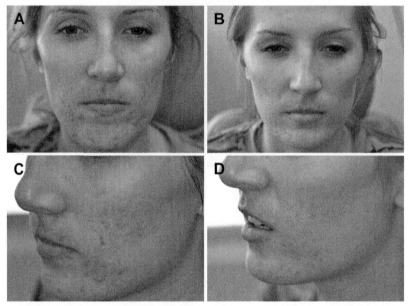

FIGURE 5.—Before (5A and 5C) and after (5B and 5D) photos after three sessions of skin needling. Although some of the improvement is from clearance of active acne, the patient also noticed improvement of her atrophic acne scars. (Reprinted with permission from the Journal of Clinical and Aesthetic Dermatology.)

Skin needling. Skin needling, also called "collagen induction therapy"[27] or "needle dermabrasion"[28] is the technique of rolling a device composed of a barrel studded with hundreds of needles, which create thousands of micropunctures in the skin to the level of the papillary to mid-dermis (Figs 4 and 5). The optimal scars to treat with skin lesion are the same as fractional laser resurfacing—rolling acne scars, superficial boxcar scars, or erythematous or hypopigmented macular (grade 1) scars. The proposed mechanism by which skin needling improves acne scars is as follows: The dermal vessels are wounded, causing a cascade of events including platelet aggregation, release of inflammatory mediators, neutrophil, monocyte, and fibroblast migration, production and modulation of extracellular matrix, collagen production, and prolonged tissue modulation.[29]

Prior to the treatment, topical anesthetic is applied for one hour. Oral anxiolytic medications, oral or intramuscular opioid analgesics, and forced cold air may also aid in patient comfort.

A sterile rolling device with needles of length 1.5 to 2.5mm is rolled across the skin with pressure in multiple directions until the area demonstrates uniform pinpoint bleeding through thousands of micropuncture sites. One study[30] describes rolling the device four times in four different directions (horizontally, vertically, and diagonally right and left) for a total of 16 passes. In the author's experience, the number of passes required to achieve uniform pinpoint bleeding of the treatment area is variable and is inversely proportional to the density of the needles on the rolling barrel. After the procedure, the area is cleansed with saline-soaked gauze and an occlusive ointment is applied. Generally, the skin oozes for less than 24 hours and then remains erythematous and edematous for 2 to 3 days. Usually, three or more treatments are required to achieve optimal clinical benefit, separated by four-week intervals.

Compared to other resurfacing procedures, this technique has many advantages. First, it is purported to be safe in all skin types and to carry the lowest risk of PIH when compared to laser resurfacing, chemical peels, or dermabrasion.[31] Second, the treatment does not result in a line of demarcation between treated and untreated skin, as usually occurs with other resurfacing procedures. This allows for specific areas of scarring to be treated without the need to treat the entire face or to "blend" or "feather" at the treatment edges. Third, the recovery period of 2 to 3 days is significantly shorter than other resurfacing procedures. Finally, needling is much less expensive to incorporate into a practice compared with a fractional laser or dermabrasion. There are no studies comparing the efficacy of skin needling to the efficacy of other resurfacing procedures.

Punch excision. Some scars that are deep or prominent are optimally removed with excisional surgical procedures. The punch excision of ice-pick acne scars or deep boxcar scars is a technique that can be easily adopted into a dermatology practice. Most dermatologists are comfortable doing punch biopsies of small pigmented nevi or of inflammatory dermatoses. The same technique is used to remove appropriate acne scars. A disposable punch biopsy instrument is selected that matches the size of the icepick or narrow boxcar scar, including the walls of the scar. These instruments come in half sizes from 1.5mm to 3.5mm. The area is infiltrated with 1% lidocaine with epinephrine (1:100,000). The scar and its walls are excised down to the subcutaneous fat layer and are carefully removed with fine forceps and iris scissors, and 6−0 polypropylene sutures are placed to close the wound, with care taken to evert the wound edges.[14] One to three sutures are placed, depending on the size of the wound created. The wound is dressed with occlusive ointment and a bandage, and the sutures are removed in seven days.

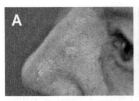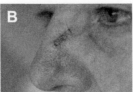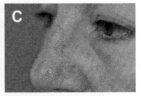

FIGURE 6.—Elliptical excision of a hypopigmented, sclerotic boxcar scar. Pretreatment (A), immediately postoperatively (B), one month postoperatively (C) showing improvement in color and contour. (Reprinted with permission from the Journal of Clinical and Aesthetic Dermatology.)

Scar spreading and suture track marks are two problems that can occur with punch excisions. Jacob et al[14] describe the value of placing a single buried suture using 6−0 Vicryl suture (Ethicon, Inc, Somerville, New Jersey) for punch holes that are 2.5mm and greater to facilitate wound healing and minimize spreading. To minimize suture track marks, it is important that the epidermal 6−0 polypropylene sutures are not tightened excessively and that they are removed no more than seven days after the procedure. A caveat to performing excisional procedures on patients with acne scars is that some of these patients have a defect in wound healing, which may explain the reason they developed acne scars in the first place, and do not heal well from excisional procedures. It may be wise to do a test spot by performing a punch excision on a scar in an inconspicuous location before performing extensive punch excisions on the same patient. Scars that are larger than 3.5mm are better excised with an elliptical excision (Fig 6). For dermatological surgeons who are comfortable operating on the face, the transition from excision of benign and malignant lesions on the face to the elliptical excision of scars is a natural process.

OTHER PROCEDURES

Other procedures that are well described for treating acne scars are subcision, punch elevation, dermabrasion, chemical reconstruction of skin scars (CROSS) chemical peels, fat transfer, permanent fillers, and ablative and nonablative fractional laser therapy. Patients can be referred to a dermatological surgeon who has the equipment and expertise to perform these procedures, or the techniques can be learned by the general dermatologist. These procedures and their indications will be briefly reviewed.

Subcision, also called "subdermal/ incisionless undermining," is indicated for the same types of scars that might be improved with fillers (i.e., rolling scars in which appearance is improved with manual stretching of the skin during examination).[13] Subcision may yield longer term results than fillers.

The CROSS technique is used for ice-pick and narrow boxcar scars.[32] A high-strength trichloroacetic acid (TCA) peel solution is placed in the base of these scars to ablate the epithelial wall and to promote dermal remodeling.

Punch elevation is a technique used to treat perfectly circular boxcar scars without underlying fibrosis.[10] A punch biopsy tool is used to incise the scar and allow it to float upward. It is then secured in place by sutures, tape, or cyanoacrylate skin glue.

Fat transfer is an alternative to the volumizing fillers for patients whose scarring is exaggerated by lax skin or soft tissue loss. Permanent fillers, such as medical-grade liquid silicone and Artefill (currently off the market in the United States), have been used in expert hands for improvement of atrophic acne scars.

Ablative and nonablative fractional lasers may be effective for all types of atrophic acne scars except for deep icepick scars. Often a combination of techniques (e.g., subcision or filler injections combined with fractional resurfacing) will yield a superior result compared to one procedure alone). In addition, nonablative large-spot lasers have been utilized effectively for treating atrophic acne scars.[33]

Pearls for management	Pitfalls to avoid
• Treat active acne before procedures for acne scars are initiated	• Failure to set appropriate expectations
• Allow red/purple macular discoloration to resolve before full evaluation and treatment of atrophic scars	• Promising a certain level of improvement
• Set appropriate expectations. Emphasize that improvement is unpredictable, often multiple procedures are required. The goal should be improvement in acne scars and not total cure.	• Failure to notice patients with unrealistic hopes or demands
• Consider excisional techniques for fibrotic, deep, or markedly hypopigmented lesions (acne excoriee)	• Inadequate questioning about history of PIH
• In older patients with lax skin or soft tissue atrophy, consider volumizing fillers (calcium hydroxylapatite or poly-L-lactic acid) or referral for facelift	• Failure to assess time constraints (patient will be unhappy if there is postprocedure erythema or hyperpigmentation for an important event)
• Globally evaluate patient's appearance (there may be more "slam dunk" procedures, such as removal of facial moles or botulinum toxin, that may have more dramatic improvement)	• Treating a large area with an aggressive procedure before doing a test spot

CONCLUSION

Due to the prevalence of acne scarring and the emotional distress it causes to those affected, dermatologists are likely to be presented with the challenge of evaluating and managing patients with atrophic acne scars. Having an approach to efficiently evaluate and develop an appropriate treatment plan for these patients will increase the chances for patient satisfaction. Setting the appropriate expectations and goals for improvement is imperative during the initial consultation. Prior to the initiation of any procedures, it is of utmost importance to frankly discuss the unpredictability of results in acne scar therapy and the possible need for multiple procedures over a period of time. Selecting the most appropriate procedures for each lesion type will increase the chance of success. For the treatment of atrophic acne scars, the punch excision, injection of dermal and volumizing fillers, and skin needling are procedures that can be easily incorporated into a dermatology practice, providing the general dermatologist with a valuable opportunity not only to improve a patient's acne scarring but also to enhance self esteem so often impacted by the long-lasting effects of acne scarring.

References

1. Kranning KK, Odland GF. Prevalence, morbidity, and cost of dermatological diseases. *J Invest Dermatol.* 1979;73:395-401.
2. Johnson MT, Roberts J. Skin conditions and related need for medical care among persons 1-74 years. United States, 1971-1974. *Vital Health Stat 11.* 1978;(212): i-v. 1–72.
3. Layton AM, Henderson CA, Cunliffe WJ. A clinical evaluation of acne scarring and its incidence. *Clin Exp Dermatol.* 1994;19:303-308.
4. Cunliffe WJ, Gould DJ. Prevalence of facial acne vulgaris in late adolescence and in adults. *Br Med J.* 1979;1:1109-1110.
5. Goulden V, Stables GI, Cunliffe WJ. Prevalence of facial acne in adults. *J Am Acad Dermatol.* 1999;41:577-580.
6. Cotterill JA, Cunliffe WJ. Suicide in dermatological patients. *Br J Dermatol.* 1997;137:246-250.
7. Koo JY, Smith LL. Psychologic aspects of acne. *Pediatr Dermatol.* 1991;8: 185-188.
8. Koo J. The psychosocial impact of acne: patients' perceptions. *J Am Acad Dermatol.* 1995;32:S26-S30.
9. Rivera AE. Acne scarring: a review and current treatment modalities. *J Am Acad Dermatol.* 2008;59:659-676.
10. Goodman GJ, Baron JA. The management of postacne scarring. *Dermatol Surg.* 2007;33:1175-1188.
11. Miteva M, Romanelli P. Hypertrophic and keloidal scars. In: Tosti A, Pie De Padova M, Beer K, eds. *Acne Scars: Classification and Treatment.* London, UK: Informa Healthcare; 2010:11-19.
12. Shockman S, Paghdal KV, Cohen G. Medical and surgical management of keloids: a review. *J Drugs Dermatol.* 2010;9:1249-1257.
13. Tsao SS, Dover JS, Arndt KA, Kaminer MS. Scar management: keloid, hypertrophic, atrophic, and acne scars. *Semin Cutan Med Surg.* 2002;21:46-75.
14. Jacob CI, Dover JS, Kaminer MS. Acne scarring: a classification system and review of treatment options. *J Am Acad Dermatol.* 2001;45:109-117.
15. Goodman GJ, Baron JA. Postacne scarring: a qualitative global scarring grading system. *Dermatol Surg.* 2006;32:1458-1466.
16. Barnett JG, Barnett CR. Treatment of acne scars with liquid silicone injections: 30-year perspective. *Dermatol Surg.* 2005;31:1542-1549.
17. Beer K. A single-center, open-label study on the use of injectable poly-L-lactic acid for the treatment of moderate to severe scarring from acne or varicella. *Dermatol Surg.* 2007;33:S159-S167.
18. Epstein RE, Spencer JM. Correction of atrophic scars with artefill: an open-label pilot study. *J Drugs Dermatol.* 2010;9:1062-1064.
19. Goldberg DJ, Amin S, Hussain M. Acne scar correction using calcium hydroxylapatite in a carrier-based gel. *J Cosmet Laser Ther.* 2006;8:134-136.
20. Sadove R. Injectable poly-L-lactic acid: a novel sculpting agent for the treatment of dermal fat atrophy after severe acne. *Aesthetic Plast Surg.* 2009;33:113-116.
21. Sadick NS, Palmisano L. Case study involving use of injectable poly-L-lactic acid (PLLA) for acne scars. *J Dermatolog Treat.* 2009;20:302-307.
22. Beer K, Yohn M, Cohen JL. Evaluation of injectable CaHA for the treatment of mid-face volume loss. *J Drugs Dermatol.* 2008;7:359-366.
23. Carruthers A, Carruthers J. Evaluation of injectable calcium hydroxylapatite for the treatment of facial lipoatrophy associated with human immunodeficiency virus. *Dermatol Surg.* 2008;34:1486-1499.
24. Fitzgerald R, Vleggaar D. Using poly-L-lactic acid (PLLA) to mimic volume in multiple tissue layers. *J Drugs Dermatol.* 2009;8:s5-s14.
25. Lizzul PF, Narurkar VA. The role of calcium hydroxylapatite (Radiesse) in nonsurgical aesthetic rejuvenation. *J Drugs Dermatol.* 2010;9:446-450.

26. Schierle CF, Casas LA. Nonsurgical rejuvenation of the aging face with injectable poly-L-lactic acid for restoration of soft tissue volume. *Aesthet Surg J.* 2011;31: 95-109.
27. Aust MC, Fernandes D, Kolokythas P, Kaplan HM, Vogt PM. Percutaneous collagen induction therapy: an alternative treatment for scars, wrinkles, and skin laxity. *Plast Reconstr Surg.* 2008;121:1421-1429.
28. Camirand A, Doucet J. Needle dermabrasion. *Aesthetic Plast Surg.* 1997;21: 48-51.
29. Fabbrocini G, Fardella N, Monfrecola A. Needling. In: Tosti A, Pie De Padova M, Beer K, eds. *Acne Scars: Classification and Treatment.* London, UK: Informa Healthcare; 2010:57-66.
30. Fabbrocini G, Fardella N, Monfrecola A, Proietti I, Innocenzi D. Acne scarring treatment using skin needling. *Clin Exp Dermatol.* 2009;34:874-879.
31. Fabbrocini G, Annunziata MC, D'Arco V, et al. Acne scars: pathogenesis, classification and treatment. *Dermatol Res Pract.* 2010;2010:893080.
32. Lee JB, Chung WG, Kwahck H, Lee KH. Focal treatment of acne scars with trichloroacetic acid: chemical reconstruction of skin scars method. *Dermatol Surg.* 2002;28:1017-1021.
33. Keller R, Belda Júnior W, Valente NY, Rodrigues CJ. Nonablative 1,064-nm Nd: YAG laser for treating atrophic facial acne scars: histologic and clinical analysis. *Dermatol Surg.* 2007;33:1470-1476.

Antiperspirant and Deodorant Allergy: Diagnosis and Management

Matthew J. Zirwas, MD, and Jessica Moennich, MD

CASE

A 42-year-old man presented with a recurrent axillary dermatitis that had been ongoing for several years (Fig 1). The dermatitis was intensely itchy when present. He had been patch tested twice with the Thin-Layer Rapid Use Epicutaneous (T.R.U.E.) Test and no positive reactions had been found, leading to a diagnosis of irritant dermatitis and treatment with topical steroids on an as needed basis.

Due to continued outbreaks, the patient referred himself to a contact dermatitis center where expanded patch testing was undertaken. He was found to have 1+ reactions to fragrance mix 1 and balsam of Peru, and 2 to 3+ patch-test reactions to fragrance mix 2, compositae mix, ylang-ylang oil, lyral, tea tree oil, Arnica montana, lichen acid mix, and Lavender Absolute. He was patch-test negative to his current deodorant, but wished to use an antiperspirant/deodorant combination product. Fragrance-free antiperspirant/deodorant products were recommended and the patient's eruption has not recurred.

INTRODUCTION

Deodorants and antiperspirants are two of the most commonly used cosmetic products, with millions of consumers applying these products to their axilla every day. Deodorants are used to mask odor; whereas, antiperspirants are used to reduce the amount of sweat produced. These two activities are often combined into single products. While deodorants are considered cosmetic products because they do not change the function of the skin, antiperspirants are classified as drugs and are therefore subject to rules and regulations set forth by the Food and Drug Administration (FDA). The active ingredient in antiperspirants is usually aluminum based, which reduces sweat by causing obstruction of the eccrine glands.[1] Deodorants work by two different mechanisms—antimicrobial agents decrease the number of bacteria that produce volatile odoriferous substances and

---

Clinical Contact Dermatitis is a new Special Section dedicated to featuring all types of contact dermatitis and providing information on prevention, diagnosis, and treatment of these skin disorders. If you would like to contribute to this section, please contact Matthew J. Zirwas, MD; E-mail: Matt.zirwas@osumc.edu

Authors: Dr. Matthew J. Zirwas, MD, is Assistant Professor of Dermatology, The Ohio State University. Jessica Moennich is a Medical Student, The Ohio State University, Columbus, Ohio. The authors report no relevant conflicts of interest.

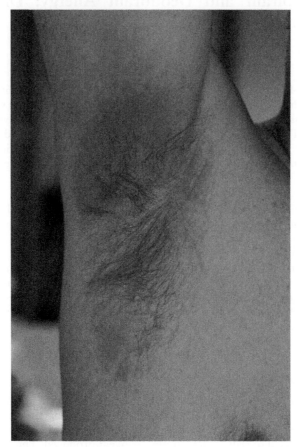

FIGURE 1.—A 42-year-old man with axillary dermatitis. (Reprinted with permission from the Journal of Clinical and Aesthetic Dermatology.)

fragrances cover any odors that are produced.[1] Recently, naturally occurring zeolite minerals, in the form of potassium alum or ammonium alum crystals, have been marketed as all-natural alternatives to deodorants and antiperspirants. These products are sold in solid crystal form. The consumer is instructed to wet the crystal and apply the product to the underarm area to prevent odor. Although no research has been published evaluating the mechanism of action of these products, the company that markets them, Crystal Body Deodorant (French Transit, Ltd., Burlingame, California), claims that the mineral salts create an environment in which bacteria cannot survive.

Antiperspirants and deodorants are generally very safe products. However, these products have received much attention as the possible cause of increasing rates of breast cancer, with most hypotheses indicating the estrogenic properties of parabens as the main contributing factor. Numerous studies supporting[2] and discrediting[3] this claim have been published, but recently the FDA and the National Cancer Institute have stated that antiperspirants and deodorants are not linked to cancer. In addition to these concerns, aluminum exposure from deodorant use has been blamed for the rising incidence of Alzheimer's Disease (AD). A recent review of 46 studies looking at aluminum exposure and risk of developing AD concluded that aluminum is, in fact, a risk factor for the development of disease.[4] However, this review evaluated oral, topical, and environmental exposure. There has been only one study specifically assessing the risk of developing AD with the use of aluminum-containing deodorants. This study looked at 130 matched pairs of cases and controls and concluded that the odds ratio for the use of aluminum containing deodorants and the development of AD was 1.6, with higher risk associated with more frequent use.[5] However, these results were inconclusive due to the use of surrogate respondents and the length of time over which exposure may have occurred. Therefore, this topic remains controversial, although authors of the article review suggest that avoidance of general aluminum exposure may decrease the risk of developing AD.[4] Rare side effects from the use of antiperspirants and deodorants, such as the development of cutaneous granulomas,[6] have been reported, but the most frequently experienced adverse events are nonspecific irritant reactions and sensitization to compounds contained within the product resulting in the development of allergic contact dermatitis (ACD).

Cosmetic allergy is a common and frustrating problem. A recent survey in the United Kingdom found that 23 percent of female subjects and 13.8 percent of male subjects will experience an adverse reaction to a personal-care product in the course of a year.[7] Although not all of these reactions are allergic in nature, approximately 10 percent of patients patch tested will test positive for allergy to cosmetics.[7] Deodorants and antiperspirants are among the most common products causing cosmetic allergy, thus these products and their constituents are frequently used when patch testing individuals with ACD. In fact, in a review of patch-testing results from 1998 to 2002, the Information Network of Departments of Dermatology (IVDK) found that deodorants are the most frequently tested personal-care products.[8]

The axillary area may be predisposed to ACD, although this has not been conclusively demonstrated. Several factors may contribute to susceptibility to sensitization to products applied to the axilla, including differences in axillary skin phenotype[9] and prolonged occlusion in the area.[10]

Following a positive patch test, finding deodorants or antiperspirants that are free of the detected allergens can be problematic for patients due to the widespread use of a number of common allergens. We sought to systematically evaluate the potentially allergenic ingredients in products that are widely available to consumers in the United States. This information should be helpful to clinicians who detect allergy to ingredients that are potentially present by allowing them to better assess the likelihood of past, present, and future exposure to these allergens via antiperspirants and deodorants.

METHODS

We utilized a recently published database of all deodorants and antiperspi-rants available on the shelves at Walgreens Pharmacies (Chicago, Illinois).[11] For each product, this database lists all allergens from the North American Contact Dermatitis Group (NACDG) screening panel that are present. The information in the database was collected and extracted by a dermatol-ogist with specific expertise in ACD. Using this database, we entered each deodorant or antiperspirant and the allergens in that product into a Micro-soft Excel (Seattle, Washington) spreadsheet. Using filters, we then analyzed the number of deodorants or antiperspirants containing each allergen.

RESULTS

One hundred seven deodorants and antiperspirants were included in the database. Of the 107 products, 97 contained fragrance, making it the most commonly present allergen (Table 1). Of the 10 products that did not contain fragrance, two contained potential allergens that are fragrance related—essential oils and biological additives. Thus, there were eight products in the database that were truly fragrance free and definitely safe for patients with fragrance allergy.

The second most commonly present allergen was propylene glycol (PG), a water-soluble vehicle ingredient, with 51 of the 107 deodorants or anti-perspirants containing the solvent. The third most common allergens were essential oils and biological derivatives, which were found in 11 of the 107 products.

Parabens and Vitamin E (tocopherol) were each found in two of the 107 products. Parabens are frequently used preservatives, and vitamin E is commonly added to cosmetic products due to the belief that it has antiox-idant properties. The final allergen found in the database was lanolin, which was present in one product.

Several products are free of the most important allergens and can, there-fore, often be empirically recommended in cases of suspected antiperspi-rant or deodorant allergy prior to patch testing. These products are listed in Table 2.

DISCUSSION

The most commonly occurring allergen found in our search was fragrance, which was present in 90 percent of the deodorants contained

TABLE 1.—Common Allergens Found in 107 Deodorants and Antiperspirants

Allergen	Number of Products Containing Allergen	Percent of Products Containing Allergen
Fragrance	97/107	90%
Propylene glycol	51/107	47%
Essential oils and biological additives	11/107	10%
Parabens	2/107	2%
Vitamin E	2/107	2%
Lanolin	1/107	1%

TABLE 2.—Low Allergenicity Deodorants and Antiperspirants

Product	Antiperspirant or Deodorant
Almay Hypo-Allergenic Fragrance Free Roll On	Antiperspirant/deodorant
Certain Dri®	Antiperspirant
Crystal Roll-On Body Deodorant for Sensitive Skin	Deodorant
Crystal Stick Body Deodorant for Sensitive Skin	Deodorant
Mitchum Roll-On Unscented	Antiperspirant/deodorant
Secret Soft Solid Platinum Deodorant Unscented	Deodorant
Stiefel B-Drier	Antiperspirant/deodorant

in the Walgreens database. Fragrance is added to deodorants not only to increase marketability, but also to enhance their function by counteracting underarm odor. Axillary dermatitis has been shown to be overrepresented in individuals with known fragrance allergies. In fact, history of a rash due to the use of a scented deodorant increases the risk of fragrance allergy by a factor of 2.4.[12] Also of note, a study performed by Johansen et al[13] demonstrated the ability of deodorants to elicit clinically significant allergic reactions in fragrance-sensitive individuals. In this study, which looked at 20 deodorants applied to the axilla and forearm of 14 patients, 60 percent of the deodorants tested resulted in a positive reaction, and the elicitation potential of each of these deodorants was related to the concentration of the allergen contained and not simply its presence in the product.[13] In general, ACD due to fragrance is a frequently encountered and frustrating clinical problem. Approximately 1 to 4 percent of the general population and 10 percent of the patch-test clinic population will experience ACD when exposed to fragrance.[11,14] This percentage is trending upward, possibly due to the increased use of fragrance-containing products.[15] About 3,000 compounds are used in the perfume industry, and individual products may contain anywhere from 10 to 300 of these,[16] making diagnosis and avoidance of the offending agent extremely difficult. Standard patch testing for fragrance allergy employs two allergens: fragrance mix and balsam of Peru. The most frequently encountered compounds responsible for ACD found in deodorants are geraniol, eugenol, and hydroxycitronellal, all of which are present in the fragrance mix.

Unfortunately, due to the evolving nature of the fragrances used by the perfume industry, the sensitivity of the fragrance mix and balsam of Peru is decreasing, and they are currently estimated to identify only 60 to 70 percent of individuals with fragrance allergy.[11] Therefore, when patients present with axillary dermatitis and a high clinical suspicion of ACD, it may be beneficial to use the patients' own products for patch testing in order to decrease the incidence of false-negative results.[17] In addition, strong consideration should also be given to testing with additional allergens, such as balsam of Tolu, fragrance mix 2, botanicals, and lichen acid mix, which may identify patients whose fragrance allergy would otherwise not be detected by standard fragrance allergens.

Propylene glycol, a solvent with moisturizing, antiseptic, and preservative properties, was the second most commonly present allergen and was present in 47 percent of the deodorants contained in the Walgreens database. It is used in a wide range of products, including cosmetics, food, toothpaste, and mouthwash, and functions in deodorants to stabilize the aqueous phase of the product. There is some controversy surrounding the allergic potential of PG. The NACDG found that 4.2 percent of patients referred for patch testing have a positive patch test to PG, but other studies have reported an incidence of positive reactions ranging from 0.1 to 3.8 percent.[18] This large variability may be due to the fact that PG is a strong irritant (the Material Safety Data Sheet advises avoidance at concentrations over 50 percent[11]); therefore, patch testing may yield false-positive reactions. This irritant property of PG is particularly relevant to antiperspirants and deodorants, where long-term occlusion in the underarm area may contribute to the induction of irritant dermatitis.[10] Currently, the NACDG uses 30 percent PG in water for patch testing, a concentration that has significant potential for skin irritation.[19] At times, this irritation may be misinterpreted as contact dermatitis, leading to questionable data regarding true allergic potential of the product. To verify positive patch-test results, Funk et al suggest repeated patch test with serial dilutions, biopsies of affected skin, and oral challenge tests,[19] but these methods are rarely used in the clinical setting. Propylene glycol is commonly found in deodorants at a concentration of 2 to 5 percent of product weight.[20] This relatively low concentration may be below the elicitation threshold for some patients with PG allergy, but since it is difficult, if not impossible, to prospectively identify PG allergic patients who will tolerate PG-containing products and because their elicitation threshold may change over time, it is prudent to recommend that all patients with a positive patch test to PG avoid antiperspirants and deodorants containing this allergen.

Essential oils were present in 10 percent of the antiperspirants and deodorants analyzed in our search. Essential oils, naturally occurring mixtures of substances derived from plants, are frequently used fragrance ingredients. They have a highly variable composition of many different compounds and are known sensitizers. A recent study analyzed seven essential oils using the local lymph node assay for individual hazard assessment. This study looked at the seven essential oils used most commonly in fragrances and found basil oil to have the lowest concentration needed to elicit a positive response.[21] The same study also found that the three major components of essential oils—citral, eugenol, and geraniol—had similar elicitation potentials as their parent compound. Another found that ylang-ylang oil and lemongrass oil have significant abilities to induce sensitization.[22] These and other studies indicate that essential oils and their components are important allergens to consider when evaluating a patient with ACD.

Parabens were found in only two, or 1.8 percent, deodorants analyzed in the Walgreens database. Parabens, including methyl paraben, ethyl paraben, butyl paraben, and propyl paraben, are preservatives used for their antibacterial and antifungal properties. They are generally efficacious, inexpensive, and safe. Although widely used, parabens can cause ACD in sensitized individuals. Paraben allergy is a relatively uncommon entity with rates of sensitization cited at 0 to 3.5 percent of the population. One study assessing cosmetic allergy in 1,937 patients found that only 0.3 percent reacted to patch testing with parabens.[23] In addition, the *paraben paradox*, a term coined by Fisher, implies that individuals who are allergic to parabens will often only have a reaction when the compound is applied to already inflamed skin and will not experience any reaction when it is applied to normal, nonirritated skin.[24,25] Parabens are frequently used in cosmetic products and perhaps the low frequency at which they were used in the deodorants we analyzed reflects a public perception that they may be related to the increasing incidence of breast cancer.[26] Although this concern may have led manufacturers to avoid the use of parabens in antiperspirants and deodorants, it is important to note that this hypothesis linking parabens and breast cancer has not been proven and has been refuted by multiple studies.[3]

Vitamin E, or tocopherol, was found in two, or 1.8 percent, of the deodorants contained in our search. It is used as an inexpensive and natural preservative and at times is also added to beauty products due to the belief that it functions as an antioxidant and moisturizer. Vitamin E's antioxidant properties have been attributed to its ability to remove free radicals and inhibit lipid peroxidation in cell membranes.[27] It has also been hypothesized to play a role in antiproliferative cell signaling events.[28] Although tocopherol is generally believed to be a benign addition to many beauty products, it can occasionally cause allergic dermatitis. In fact, the NACDG reported that 1.1 percent of those patch tested with dl-alpha-tocopherol experienced positive reactions, and there are several case reports of axillary dermatitis specifically related to tocopherol found in deodorant.[28,29] Although these infrequent cases illustrate the rarity of tocopherol-induced dermatitis, it is important to note that tocopherol may be responsible for more cases of ACD than recognized. For example, one large-scale outbreak of papular and follicular dermatitis occurred in Switzerland following the use of a new cosmetics line.[30] Perrenoud et al patch tested 77 of these patients and found that the agent responsible for the outbreak was tocopherol linoleate.[30] With this data in mind, they concluded that oxidized vitamin-E derivatives may be responsible for irritation to many cosmetic products.

Lanolin was present in one deodorant contained in the Walgreens database. Lanolin is a mixture of cholesterol and several fatty acid esters that are derived from the secretions of sheep sebaceous glands. Although the exact allergens are unknown, it has been proposed that wool alcohols are the main sensitizers present in lanolin.[31] Currently, 30-percent wool alcohol is recommended for patch testing patients with suspected lanolin allergy.[32] In the past, lanolin has been considered a significant source of allergy, and many products on the market are listed as lanolin-free. Recently these statistics have come into question. Wakelin et al proposed that the stated frequency of allergy is falsely elevated due to the fact that lanolin sensitivity was previously assessed in those individuals at high risk.[33] In a chart review of 24,449 patients patch tested with 30-percent wool alcohol, annual rates of sensitization of 1 to 7 percent were demonstrated, with an overall incidence of less than two percent in the patch-test population. Wakelin et al also commented on potential risk factors that might indicate future lanolin allergy, including female sex, increased age, lower leg venous stasis, and the presence of anogenital dermatitis. Several other studies have supported the suggestion that the true incidence of sensitivity to lanolin is quite low.[34-36] The NACDG reported an incidence of positive patch tests to lanolin of 2.2 percent in their 2001–2002 sample of patients. The rarity at which we found lanolin to be used in antiperspirants and deodorants, coupled with the rarity of sensitization to lanolin in the general population, suggests that ACD due to lanolin in deodorants is an infrequently encountered clinical problem.

CONCLUSION

Antiperspirants and deodorants are widely used cosmetic products and are frequently the cause of axillary dermatitis. Compounds contained in these products have the potential to cause irritant and allergic reactions in many consumers, making it important for doctors to be aware of the ingredients most likely to blame for these adverse reactions. Our search of the Walgreens database found that fragrance, PG, essential oils and biological additives, parabens, vitamin E, and lanolin were the most commonly used potential allergens in antiperspirants and deodorants. While it is important to keep these compounds in mind when assessing a patient with an underarm rash, it is often difficult to determine exactly which ingredient is to blame. Therefore, empirically recommending low allergenicity products, such as those contained in Table 2, may be beneficial for these patients. Also of note, new crystal products, which claim to be all natural and free of any additives, may also be useful in these patients. Unfortunately, axillary dermatitis is difficult to manage, and the problem may persist despite avoidance of common allergens. In these cases, further work-up with patch testing or biopsy may be warranted.

References

1. Benohanian A. Antiperspirants and deodorants. *Clin Dermatol.* 2001;19:398-405.
2. McGrath KG. An earlier age of breast cancer diagnosis related to more frequent use of antiperspirants/deodorants and underarm shaving. *Eur J Cancer Prev.* 2003;12:479-485.
3. Mirick DK, Davis S, Thomas DB. Antiperspirant use and the risk of breast cancer. *J Natl Cancer Inst.* 2002;94:1578-1580.
4. Ferreira PC, Piai Kde A, Takayanagui AM, Segura-Muñoz SI. Aluminum as a risk factor for Alzheimer's disease. *Rev Lat Am Enfermagem.* 2008;16:151-157.
5. Graves AB, White E, Koepsell TD, Reifler BV, van Belle G, Larson EB. The association between aluminum-containing products and Alzheimer's disease. *J Clin Epidemiol.* 1990;43:35-44.
6. Montemarano AD, Sau P, Johnson FB, James WD. Cutaneous granulomas caused by an aluminum-zirconium complex: an ingredient of antiperspirants. *J Am Acad Dermatol.* 1997;37:496-498.
7. Orton DI, Wilkinson JD. Cosmetic allergy: incidence, diagnosis, and management. *Am J Clin Dermatol.* 2004;5:327-337.

8. Uter W, Geier J, Schnuch A, Frosch PJ. Patch test results with patients' own perfumes, deodorants and shaving lotions: results of the IVDK 1998-2002. *J Eur Acad Dermatol Venereol.* 2007;21:374-379.

9. Watkinson A, Lee RS, Moore AE, et al. Is the axilla distinct skin phenotype? *Int J Cosmet Sci.* 2007;29:60.

10. Agren-Jonsson S, Magnusson B. Sensitization to propantheline bromide, trichlorocarbanilide and propylene glycol in an antiperspirant. *Contact Dermatitis.* 1976;2:79-80.

11. Scheman A, Jacob S, Zirwas M, et al. Contact allergy: alternatives for the 2007 North American contact dermatitis group (NACDG) Standard Screening Tray. *Dis Mon.* 2008;54:7-156.

12. Johansen JD. Fragrance contact allergy: a clinical review. *Am J Clin Dermatol.* 2003;4:789-798.

13. Johansen JD, Rastogi SC, Bruze M, et al. Deodorants: a clinical provocation study in fragrance-sensitive individuals. *Contact Dermatitis.* 1998;39:161-165.

14. Gerberick GF, Robinson MK, Felter SP, White IR, Basketter DA. Understanding fragrance allergy using an exposure-based risk assessment approach. *Contact Dermatitis.* 2001;45:333-340.

15. Lunder T, Kansky A. Increase in contact allergy to fragrances: patch-test results 1989-1998. *Contact Dermatitis.* 2000;43:107-109.

16. Kieć-Swierczyńska M, Krecisz B, Swierczyńska-Machura D. Allergy to cosmetics. I. Fragrances. *Med Pr.* 2004;55:203-206.

17. Daecke CM, Schaller J, Goos M. Value of the patient's own test substances in epicutaneous testing. *Hautarzt.* 1994;45:292-298.

18. Lessmann H, Schnuch A, Geier J, Uter W. Skin-sensitizing and irritant properties of propylene glycol. *Contact Dermatitis.* 2005;53:247-259.

19. Funk JO, Maibach HI. Propylene glycol dermatitis: re-evaluation of an old problem. *Contact Dermatitis.* 1994;31:236-241.

20. World Intellectual Property Organization website. http://www.wipo.int/pctdb/en/wo.jsp?IA=EP2005004828&wo=2005112879&DISPLAY=STATUS. Accessed August 30, 2008.

21. Lalko J, Api AM. Investigation of the dermal sensitization potential of various essential oils in the local lymph node assay. *Food Chem Toxicol.* 2006;44:739-746.

22. Frosch PJ, Johansen JD, Menné T, et al. Further important sensitizers in patients sensitive to fragrances. *Contact Dermatitis.* 2002;47:279-287.

23. Kieć-Swierczyńska M, Krecisz B, Swierczyńska-Machura D. Contact allergy to preservatives contained in cosmetics. *Med Pr.* 2006;57:245-249.

24. Fisher AA. Esoteric contact dermatitis. Part I: the paraben paradox. *Cutis.* 1996;57:65-66.

25. Fisher AA. Esoteric contact dermatitis. Part II: the paraben paradox. *Cutis.* 1996;57:135-138.

26. Darbre PD, Aljarrah A, Miller WR, Coldham NG, Sauer MJ, Pope GS. Concentrations of parabens in human breast tumours. *J Appl Toxicol.* 2004;24:5-13.

27. Packer L, Weber SU, Rimbach G. Molecular aspects of alpha-tocotrienol antioxidant action and cell signalling. *J Nutr.* 2001;131:369S-373S.

28. Minkin W, Cohen HJ, Frank SB. Contact dermatitis from deodorants. *Arch Dermatol.* 1973;107:774-775.

29. Aeling JL, Panagotacos PJ, Andreozzi RJ. Letter: allergic contact dermatitis to vitamin E aerosol deodorant. *Arch Dermatol.* 1973;108:579-580.

30. Perrenoud D, Homberger HP, Auderset PC, et al. An epidemic outbreak of papular and follicular contact dermatitis to tocopheryl linoleate in cosmetics. Swiss Contact Dermatitis Research Group. *Dermatology.* 1994;189:225-233.

31. Oleffe JA, Blondeel A, Boschmans S. Patch testing with lanolin. *Contact Dermatitis.* 1978;4:233-247.

32. Hjorth N, Trolle-Larsen C. Skin Reactions to Ointment Bases. *Trans St Johns Hosp Dermatol Soc.* 1963;49:127-140.

33. Wakelin SH, Smith H, White IR, Rycroft RJ, McFadden JP. A retrospective analysis of contact allergy to lanolin. *Br J Dermatol*. 2001;145:28-31.
34. Epstein E. The detection of lanolin allergy. *Arch Dermatol*. 1972;106:678-681.
35. Holness DL, Nethercott JR, Adams RM, et al. Concomitant positive patch test results with standard screening tray in North America 1985–1989. *Contact Dermatitis*. 1995;32:289-292.
36. Christophersen J, Menné T, Tanghøj P, et al. Clinical patch test data evaluated by multivariate analysis. Danish Contact Dermatitis Group. *Contact Dermatitis*. 1989;21:291-299.

Statistics of Interest to the Dermatologist

Marin A. Weinstock, MD, PhD, and Margaret M. Boyle, BS
Brown University Dermatoepidemiology Unit, Providence, Rhode Island

Morbidity and Mortality

Table   1 Reportable Infectious Diseases, United States
Table   2 HIV/AIDS: Geographic Distribution
Table   3 AIDS: Cumulative Cases, United States
Table   4 Deaths from Selected Causes, United States
Table   5 Cancer Incidence, United States
Table   6 Melanoma: Incidence and Mortality, United States
Table   7 Melanoma: Five-Year Relative Survival
Table   8 Contact Dermatitis, Belgium

Health Care Delivery in the United States

Table   9 Dermatology Trainees
Table   10 Diplomates of the American Board of Dermatology
Table   11 Physicians Certified in Dermatologic Subspecialties
Table   12 Dermatologic Outpatient Care
Table   13 Health Insurance Coverage
Table   14 Health Insurance Coverage by Family Income
Table   15 National Health Expenditures
Table   16 Expenditure for Consumer Advertising of Prescription Products, United States

Miscellaneous

Table   17 American Academy of Dermatology Skin Cancer Screening Program
Table   18 Leading Dermatology Journals

TABLE 1.—New Cases of Selected Reportable Infectious Diseases in the United States

	1940	1950	1960	1970	1980	1990	2000	2010	2011*
AIDS	***	***	***	***	***	41,595	40,758	34,247	33,015**
Anthrax	76	49	23	2	1	0	1	0	1
Congenital Rubella	***	***	***	77	50	11	9	0	0
Congenital Syphilis	***	***	***	***	***	3,865	529	213	240
Diphtheria	15,536	5,796	918	435	3	4	1	0	0
Gonorrhea	175,841	286,746	258,933	600,072	1,004,029	690,169	358,995	280,555	301,968
Hansen's Disease	***	44	54	129	223	198	91	57	50
Lyme Disease	0	***	***	***	***	***	17,730	27,895	23,974
Measles	291,162	319,124	441,703	47,351	13,506	27,786	86	61	212
Plague	1	3	2	13	18	2	6	2	2
Rocky Mountain Spotted Fever	457	464	204	390	1,163	651	495	155	204
Syphilis (primary and secondary)	***	23,939	16,145	21,982	27,204	50,223	5,979	12,164	12,803
Toxic-Shock Syndrome	***	***	***	***	***	322	135	###	###
Toxic-Shock Syndrome (staphylococcal)	***	***	***	***	***	***	***	73	71
Toxic-Shock Syndrome (streptococcal)	***	***	***	***	***	***	***	155	114
Tuberculosis#	102,984##	121,742##	55,494	37,137	27,749	25,701	16,377	11,181	10,521
U.S. Population (millions)	132	151	179	203	227	249	281	309	313

Sources:

Centers for Disease Control and Prevention: Summary of Provisional Cases of Notifiable Diseases, United States, 2011. *Morbidity and Mortality Weekly Report* 60(51):1762-1775, 2012.

Centers for Disease Control and Prevention: *HIV Surveillance Report, 2010*, Vol. 22. Atlanta: U.S. Department of Health and Human Services, Centers for Disease Control and Prevention, Division of HIV/AIDS Prevention, National Center for HIV/AIDS, Viral Hepatitis, STD, and TB Prevention. March, 2012. http://www.cdc.gov/hiv/topics/surveillance/resources/reports/.

Centers for Disease Control and Prevention: Trends in Tuberculosis, United States, 2011. *Morbidity and Mortality Weekly Report* 61(11):181-185, 2012.

U.S. Census Bureau, Population Division: Table 1. Monthly Population Estimates for the United States: April 1, 2010 to March 1, 2012 (NA-EST2011-01-0312). Release Date: April, 2012.

Centers for Disease Control and Prevention: Summary of Notifiable Diseases, United States, 2000. *Morbidity and Mortality Weekly Report* 49(518&52):1167-1174, 2001.

Centers for Disease Control and Prevention: Annual Summary 1994:Reported morbidity and mortality. *Morbidity and Mortality Weekly Report* 1994;43(53):[70-71].

Centers for Disease Control and Prevention: Annual Summary 1984:Reported morbidity and mortality. *Morbidity and Mortality Weekly Report* 33:124-129, 1986.

Key:

*For 52 weeks ending December 31, 2011. Case counts for reporting year 2011 are provisional and subject to change.

**Estimated numbers resulted from statistical adjustment that accounted for reporting delays and missing risk-factor information, but not for incomplete reporting. U.S. subtotal (not dependent areas).

***Data not available.

#Reporting criteria changed in 1975.

##Data include newly reported active and inactive cases.

###Toxic-Shock Syndrome now subdivided into staphylococcal and streptococcal.

TABLE 2.—Estimates of HIV/AIDS, 2010

Region	Adults and Children Living with HIV	Adults and Children Newly Infected with HIV	Adult Prevalence of HIV Infection %	AIDS-Related Deaths Among Adults and Children
Sub-Saharan Africa	21.6-24.1 million	1.7-2.1 million	4.7-5.2	1.1-1.4 million
Middle East and North Africa	350,000-570,000	40,000-73,000	0.2-0.3	25,000-42,000
South and South-East Asia	3.6-4.5 million	230,00-340,000	0.3-0.3	210,000-280,000
East Asia	580,000-1.1 million	48,000-160,000	0.1-0.1	40,000-76,000
Oceania	48,000-62,000	2,400-4,200	0.2-0.3	1,200-2,000
Central and South America	1.2-1.7 million	73,000-140,000	0.3-0.5	45,000-92,000
Caribbean	170,000-220,000	9,400-17,000	0.8-1.0	6,900-12,000
Eastern Europe and Central Asia	1.3-1.7 million	110,000-200,000	0.8-1.1	74,000-110,000
Western and Central Europe	770,000-930,000	22,000-39,000	0.2-0.2	8,900-11,000
North America	1.0-1.9 million	24,000-130,000	0.5-0.9	16,000-27,000
Total	34 million	2.7 million	0.8	1.8 million
	31.6-35.2 million	2.4-2.9. million	0.8-0.8	1.6-1.9 million

Source:
Global HIV/AIDS Response: Epidemic update and health sector progress towards Universal Access: Progress Report 2011. Joint United Nations Programme on HIV/AIDS (UNAIDS) World Health Organization (WHO), 2011.

TABLE 3.—AIDS Cases by Age Group and Exposure Category, and Cumulative Totals Through 2010, United States

	2010 Estimated** No.	Cumulative* Estimated** No.
Male adult or adolescent exposure category		
Male-to-male sexual contact	16,796	541,330
Injection drug use	2,745	186,122
Male-to-male sexual contact and injection drug use	1,446	79,048
Heterosexual contact***	3,629	74,708
Other****	133	11,851
SUBTOTAL	24,749	893,058
Pediatric exposure category (<13 years at diagnosis)		
Perinatal	18	8,617
Other*****	4	859
SUBTOTAL	23	9,475
TOTAL#	33,015	1,129,127

Source:
Centers for Disease Control and Prevention: *HIV Surveillance Report, 2010,* Vol. 22. Atlanta: U.S. Department of Health and Human Services, Centers for Disease Control and Prevention, Division of HIV/AIDS Prevention, National Center For HIV/AIDS, Viral Hepatitis, STD, and TB Prevention. March, 2012. http://www.cdc.gov/hiv/topics/surveillance/resources/reports/.

Key:
*From the beginning of the epidemic through 2010.
**Estimated numbers resulted from statistical adjustment that accounted for reporting delays, and missing risk-factor information, but not for incomplete reporting.
***Heterosexual contact with a person known to have, or to be at high risk for HIV infection.
****Includes hemophilia, blood transfusion, perinatal exposure, and risk factor not reported or identified.
*****Includes hemophilia, blood transfusion, and risk factor not reported or not identified.
#Because column totals for estimated numbers were calculated independently of the values for the subpopulations, the values in each column may not sum to the column total.

TABLE 4.—Selected Causes of Death, United States, 1999 and 2009

	Number of Deaths	
Causes of Death	1999	2009
Malignant Melanoma	7,215	9,199
Infections of the skin	983	1,969
Motor vehicle traffic accidents	40,965	34,485
Accident involving animal being ridden	110	118
Accidental drowning and submersion	3,529	3,517
Victim of lightning	64	31
Homicide and legal intervention	17,287	17,194
All cancer	549,838	567,628
All causes	2,391,399	2,437,163

Source:
Centers for Disease Control and Prevention, National Center for Health Statistics. Underlying Causes of Death 1999-2009 on CDC WONDER Online Database, released 2012. Data for year 2009 are compiled from the Multiple Cause of Death File 2009, Series 20, No. 20, 2012.
Data for Years 1999 - 2004 are compiled from Multiple Cause of Death File 1999-2004, Series 20, No. 2J, 2007. Available from http://wonder.cdc.gov/ucd-icd10.html.

TABLE 5.—Annual Percent Change in Cancer Incidence in the United States

| Top 20 Highest Incidence Sites | Annual Percent Change | |
	1992-2009	1975-1991
Thyroid	5.8	0.8
Liver and Intrahepatic Bile Duct	3.6	3.0
Melanoma of the skin	2.6	3.7
Kidney and Renal Pelvis	2.4	2.4
Pancreas	0.8	−0.2
Non-Hodgkin Lymphoma	0.5	3.6
Hodgkin Lymphoma	0.3	0.4
Myeloma	0.2	1.2
Corpus Uteri	0.2	−2.1
Esophagus	0.1	0.7
Urinary Bladder	0.0	0.6
Leukemia	−0.1	0.1
Brain and Other Nervous System	−0.2	1.2
Breast (female)	−0.4	2.2
Oral Cavity and Pharynx	−0.7	−0.6
Lung and Bronchus	−0.8	1.5
Ovary	−1.1	0.0
Stomach	−1.4	−1.5
Prostate	−1.5	4.9
Colon and Rectum	−1.6	−0.1
All sites	−0.3	1.3

Note:
SEER 9 registries.
Rates are per 100,000 and age-adjusted to the 2000 US Standard Population (19 age groups–Census P25-1130) standard.
Rates are for invasive cancers only.
Source:
Surveillance Research Program, National Cancer Institute SEER*Stat Software (www.seer.cancer.gov/seerstat) version 7.0.9.
Surveillance, Epidemiology, and End-Results (SEER) Program, (www.seer.cancer.gov) SEER*Stat Database: Incidence-SEER 9 Pops (1973-2009) <Katrina/Rita Population Adjustment> Linked to County Attributes–Total U.S.,1969-2010 Counties, National Cancer Institute DCCPS, Surveillance Research Program, Surveillance Systems Branch, released April, 2012 based on the November 2011 submission.
Howlader N, Noone AM, Krapcho M, Neyman N, Aminou R, Altekruse SF, Kosary CL, Ruhl J, Tatalovich Z, Cho H, Mariotto A, Eisner MP, Lewis DR, Chen HS, Feuer EJ, Cronin KA, (eds). *SEER Cancer Statistics Review, 1975-2009 (Vintage 2009 Populations)*, National Cancer Institute. Bethesda, MD, http://seer.cancer.gov/csr/1975-2009 pops09/, based on November 2011 SEER data submission, posted to the SEER web site, April 2012.

TABLE 6.—Melanoma Incidence and Mortality Rates, United States

Year	Incidence*	Mortality**
1973	6.8	1.9
1974	7.2	2.1
1975	7.9	2.1
1976	8.2	2.2
1977	8.9	2.3
1978	9.0	2.3
1979	9.5	2.4
1980	10.5	2.3
1981	11.1	2.4
1982	11.2	2.5
1983	11.1	2.5
1984	11.4	2.5
1985	12.8	2.6
1986	13.3	2.6
1987	13.7	2.6
1988	12.9	2.6
1989	13.7	2.7
1990	13.9	2.8
1991	14.6	2.7
1992	14.8	2.7
1993	14.6	2.7
1994	15.6	2.7
1995	16.4	2.7
1996	17.3	2.8
1997	17.7	2.7
1998	17.9	2.8
1999	18.3	2.6
2000	18.9	2.7
2001	19.6	2.7
2002	19.2	2.6
2003	19.5	2.7
2004	20.5	2.7
2005	22.3	2.8
2006	21.9	2.7
2007	21.5	2.7
2008	22.8	2.7
2009	22.6	2.8

Estimated new cases of melanoma in 2012: 76,250; estimated deaths: 9,180.
Source:
Surveillance Research Program, National Cancer Institute SEER*stat Software (www.seer.cancer.gov/seerstat) version 7.0.9.
Surveillance, Epidemiology, and End-Results (SEER) Program, (www.seer.cancer.gov) SEER*Stat Database: Incidence-SEER 9 Pops (1973-2009) <Katrina/Rita Population Adjustment> Linked to County Attributes–Total U.S., 1969-2010 Counties, National Cancer Institute DCCPS, Surveillance Research Program, Surveillance Systems Branch, released April 2012 based on the November 2011 submission.
Surveillance, Epidemiology, and End-Results (SEER) Program, SEER* Stat Database: Mortality-All COD, Total US (1969-2009) <Katrina/Rita Population Adjustment> Linked to County Attributes–Total U.S., 1969-2010 Counties, National Cancer Institute DCCPS, Surveillance Research Program, Surveillance Systems Branch, released April, 2012. Underlying mortality data provided by the National Center for Health Statistics (www.cdc.gov/nchs).
Howlader N, Noone AM, Krapcho M, Neyman N, Aminou R, Altekruse SF, Kosary CL, Ruhl J, Tatalovich Z, Cho H, Mariotto A, Eisner MP, Lewis DR, Chen HS, Feuer EJ, Cronin KA, (eds). *SEER Cancer Statistics Review: 1975-2009 (Vintage 2009 Populations),* National Cancer Institute. Bethesda, MD, http://seer.cancer.gov/csr/1975-2009 pops09/, based on November 2011 SEER data submission, posted to the SEER website, April 2012.
Estimated New Cancer Causes and Deaths by Sex, US, 2012, *Cancer Facts & Figures 2012,* Atlanta: American Cancer Society, 2012.
Key:
*SEER 9 areas. Rates are per 100,000 and are age-adjusted to the 2000 US Standard population (19 age groups–Census P25-1130) standard.
**National Center for Health Statistics public use data file for the total US. Rates per 100,000 and age-adjusted to the 2000 U.S. standard population. (19 age groups–Census P25-1130) standard.

TABLE 7.—Melanoma Five-Year Relative Survival

Year	Whites	Blacks
By Year at Diagnosis		
1960-63*	60%	—
1970-73*	68%	—
1975-77[+]	82%	57%
1978-80[+]	83%	60%
1981-83[+]	83%	62%
1984-86[+]	86%	70%
1987-89[+]	88%	79%
1990-92[+]	89%	62%
1993-95[+]	90%	70%
1996-98[+]	91%	74%
1999-2001[+]	92%	75%
2002-2008[+]	93%	70%
By Stage at Diagnosis (2002-2008)**		
Local	98%	92%
Regional	63%	50%
Distant	15%	27%

Notes:

Relative survival is the observed survival divided by the survival expected in a demographically similar subgroup of the general population.

Survival estimates among blacks are imprecise due to small numbers of cases observed.

Source:

Howlader N, Noone AM, Krapcho M, Neyman N, Aminou R, Altekruse SF, Kosary CL, Ruhl J, Tatalovich Z, Cho H, Mariotto A, Eisner MP, Lewis DR, Chen HS, Feuer EJ, Cronin KA, (eds). *SEER Cancer Statistics Review: 1975-2009 (Vintage 2009 Populations)*, National Cancer Institute. Bethesda, MD, http://seer.cancer.gov/csr/1975-2009 pops09/, based on November 2011 SEER data submission, posted to the SEER website, April 2012.

Key:

— Insufficient data

*Rates are based on the End Results data from a series of hospital registries and one population-based registry.

[+]Rates are from the SEER 9 registries. Rates are based on follow-up of patients into 2009.

**Rates are from the SEER 18 registries. Rates are based on follow-up of patients into 2009.

TABLE 8.—Contact Dermatitis in Belgium: Proportion of Positive Patch Tests to Standard Chemicals in 256 Patients With at Least 1 Positive Reaction (Among 498 Patients Tested in 2011)

1	Nickel sulphate	34.5 %
2	Fragrance mix I	18.2 %
3	Paraphenylenediamine	14.0 %
4	Balsam of Peru	13.1 %
5	Potassium dichromate	11.2 %
6	Cobalt chloride	11.1 %
7	Fragrance mix II	7.9 %
8	Methyl(chloro)isothiazolinone	5.2 %
9	Formaldehyde	4.0 %
10	Benzocaine	3.6 %
11	Colophonium	3.6 %
12	Thiuram mix	3.6 %
13	Wool alcohols	3.2 %
14	Hydroxyisohexyl-3-cyclohexene carboxaldehyde	2.8 %
15	Isopropyl-phenylparaphenylenediamine	2.8 %
16	Paratertiarybutylphenol-formaldehyde resin	2.8 %
17	Methyldibromo glutaronitrile	2.4 %
18	Sesquiterpene lactone mix	2.0 %
19	Budesonide	1.6 %
20	Epoxy resin	1.6 %
21	Mercapto mix	1.6 %
22	Neomycin sulphate	1.6 %
23	Quaternium-15	1.6 %
24	Mercaptobenzothiazole	1.2 %
25	Paraben mix	0.8 %
26	Primin	0.8 %
27	Tixocortol pivalate	0.8 %
28	Clioquinol	0.0 %

(From Goossens A., University Hospital, Katholieke Universiteit Leuven, Belgium, personal communication, February 2012.)

TABLE 9.—Dermatology Trainees in the United States

Year Residency to be Completed	Male Residents	Female Residents	Unknown	Total
MD Programs				
2012	150	257	0	407
2013	156	250	0	406
2014	158	271	0	429
2015	5	8	0	13
2016	3	0	0	3
DO Programs				
2012	13	2	2	17
2013	13	26	0	39
2014	14	14	9	37

Source:
American Academy of Dermatology, personal communication, February, 2012.

TABLE 10.—Diplomates Certified by the American Board of Dermatology from 1933–2011

Decade Totals (Inclusive Dates)	Average Number Certified per Year
1933-1940	69
1941-1950	74
1951-1960	76
1961-1970	112
1971-1980	247
1981-1990	271
1991-2000	295
2001-2010	340
TOTAL 1933 through 2010	14,719

Individual Year Totals	Actual Number Certified
1999	286
2000	283
2001	305
2002	309
2003	307
2004	329
2005	352
2006	319
2007	342
2008	377
2009	385
2010	379
2011	376

Source:
The American Board of Dermatology, Inc., personal communication, February, 2012.

TABLE 11.—Physicians Certified in Dermatologic Subspecialties

A. Physicians Certified for Special Qualification in Dermatopathology, 1974-2011

| Year | Average Number Certified Per Year | | |
	Dermatologists	Pathologists	Total
1974-75	108	44	302
1976-80	54	49	515
1981-85	37	34	351
1986-90	11	14	125
1991-95	20	20	196
1996-00	14	32	227
2001-05	15	46	306
2006-10	31	49	403
Actual Number Certified			
2006	32	37	69
2007	26	50	76
2008	27	54	81
2009	28	51	79
2010	41	57	98
2011	34	48	82
Total Number Certified 1974 through 2011	1158	1352	2510

B. Dermatologists Certified for Special Qualification in Clinical and Laboratory Dermatological Immunology, 1985-2011

Year	Number Certified
1985	52
1987	16
1989	22
1991	15
1993	5
1997	5
2001	6
Total 1985 through 2011	121

C. Dermatologists Certified for Special Qualification in Pediatric Dermatology

Year	Number Certified
2004	90
2006	41
2008	31
2010	33
Total 2004 through 2010	195

Note:
No special qualification examination for Dermatopathology was administered in 1992, 1994, and 1996.
No special qualification examination in Clinical and Laboratory Dermatological Immunology was administered in 1986, 1988, 1990, 1992, 1994, 1995, 1996, 1998, 1999, 2000, or since 2002.
Special qualification in Pediatric Dermatology began in 2004. No special qualification examination in Pediatric Dermatology was administered in 2005, 2007, 2009 or 2011.
Source:
American Board of Dermatology and American Board of Pathology, personal communication, February, 2012.

TABLE 12.—Visits to Non-Federal Office-Based Physicians in the United States, 2009

	Type of Physician					
	Dermatologist		Other		All Physicians	
	Number of		Number of		Number of	
Diagnosis	Visits (1000's)	Percent	Visits (1000's)	Percent	Visits (1000's)	Percent
Acne vulgaris	3,473	10.2	*	*	4,018	0.4
Eczematous dermatitis	2,593	7.6	5,749	0.6	8,342	0.8
Warts	1,543	4.5	1,811	0.2	3,354	0.3
Skin cancer	2,517	7.4	1,434	0.1	3,950	0.4
Psoriasis	1,210	3.6	*	*	1,413	0.1
Fungal infections	*	*	1,416	0.1	2,076	0.2
Hair disorders	*	*	*	*	1,427	0.1
Actinic keratosis	3,216	9.5	*	*	3,757	0.4
Benign neoplasm of the skin	2,639	7.8	1,226	0.1	3,865	0.4
All disorders	34,024	100.0	1,003,773	100.0	1,037,796	100.0

Figures may not add to totals because of rounding.
Source:
Centers for Disease Control and Prevention, National Center for Health Statistics, 2009 National Ambulatory Medical Care Survey, personal communication, February, 2012.
*Figure suppressed due to small sample size.

TABLE 13.—Health Insurance Coverage of the United States Population, 2010

	Children 1-17 Years	Adults 18-64 Years	Adults 65 Years and Over
Individually Purchased Insurance	6%	7%	29%
Employment-based-Coverage	55%	59%	33%
Public Insurance, All types	38%	22%	94%
Medicaid	35%	17%	9%
No Health Insurance	10%	19%	2%

Note:
Some individuals have both public and private insurance, so the numbers will not add to 100%.
Source:
Fronstin P, "Sources of Health Insurance and Characteristics of the Uninsured: Analysis of the March 2011 Current Population Survey." *EBRI Issue Brief,* No. 362. Employee Benefit Research Institute, Washington DC, September, 2011.
DeNavas-Walt, Carmen, Bernadette D. Proctor, and Jessica C. Smith, U.S. Census Bureau, Current Population Reports, P60-239, *Income, Poverty, and Health Insurance Coverage in the United States: 2010.* U.S. Government Printing Office, Washington, DC, 2011.

TABLE 14.—Selected Sources of Health Insurance, Children and Adults under Age 65, by Family Income, 2010

Yearly Family Income Level	Employment-Based Coverage %	Individually Purchased %	Public %	Uninsured %	Total %
under $10,000	11	5	50	35	100
$10,000-$19,999	18	5	45	34	100
$20,000-$29,999	33	6	34	31	100
$30,000-$39,999	49	7	26	25	100
$40,000-$49,999	59	7	21	20	100
$50,000-$74,000	71	8	14	14	100
$75,000 and over	85	8	8	7	100
Total	59	7	22	19	100

Note:
Details may not add to totals because individuals may receive coverage from more than one source.
Source:
Fronstin P, "Sources of Health Insurance and Characteristics of the Uninsured: Analysis of the March 2011 Current Population Survey." *EBRI Issue Brief,* No. 362. Employee Benefit Research Institute, Washington DC, September, 2011.

TABLE 15.—National Health Expenditure Amounts: Selected Calendar Years

Spending Category	1980	1990	2000	2009	2020*
Total National Health Expenditures	246	696	1,310	2,486	4,638
Health Services and Supplies	234	670	1,262	2,330	4,338
Personal Health Care	215	609	1,138	2,090	3,841
Hospital Care	102	254	417	759	1,410
Professional Services	67	217	425	675	1,164
Physician and Clinical Services	47	158	289	506	868
Other Professional Services	4	18	39	67	129
Dental Services	13	32	61	102	168
Other Personal Health Care	3	10	37	123	272
Nursing Home and Home Health	20	65	126		
Home Health Care	2	13	32	68	136
Nursing Home Care	18	53	94		
Nursing Care Facilities and Continuing Care Residential Communities				137	218
Retail Outlet Sale of Medical Products	26	73	171	328	640
Prescription Drugs	12	40	122	250	513
Other Medical Products	14	33	49	78	127
Durable Medical Equipment	4	11	18	35	55
Other Non-Durable Medical Products	10	23	31	43	72
Program Administration and Net Cost of Private Health Insurance	12	40	81	163	343
Government Public Health Activities	7	20	44	77	154
Investment	12	26	48	156	301
Research**	6	13	29	45	93
Structures and Equipment	7	14	19	111	208

Note:
Numbers may not add to totals because of rounding.
Source:
Centers for Medicare and Medicaid Services, Office of the Actuary, April, 2012.
Key:
*Projected values. The health spending projections were based on the National Health Expenditures released in January, 2011. The projections include impacts from the Affordable Care Act.
**Research and development of expenditures of drug companies and other manufacturers and providers of medical equipment and supplies are excluded from research expenditures. These research expenditures are implicitly included in the expenditure class in which the product falls, in that they are covered by the payment received for that product.

TABLE 16.—Spending on Consumer Advertising of Prescription Products, United States

Year	(Annual Dollars in Millions)
2011	4,039
2010	4,174
2009	4,571
2008	4,412
2007	4,905
2006	4,745
2005	4,132
2004	4,084
2003	3,082
2002	2,514
2001	2,479
2000	2,150*
1999	1,590
1998	1,173
1997	844
1996	595
1995	313
1994	242
1993	165
1992	156
1991	56
1990	48
1989	12

Source:
Kantar Media, Copyright 2012. Magazine Publishers of America, Inc. personal communication, April, 2012.
*Estimated

TABLE 17.—Results of the American Academy of Dermatology Skin Cancer Screening Program 1985-2011

Year	Number Screened	Basal Cell Carcinoma	Suspected Diagnosis Squamous Cell Carcinoma	Malignant Melanoma
1985	32000	1056	163	97
1986	41486	3049	398	262
1987	41649	2798	302	257
1988	67124	4457	474	435
1989	78486	6266	761	593
1990	98060	7959	1069	872
1991	102485	8110	1193	1062
1992	98440	8403	1280	1054
1993	97553	7067	1068	2465*
1994	86895	6908	1235	1010
1995	88934	7503	1317	1353
1996	94363	8713	1656	1399
1997	99554	8730	1685	1469
1998	89536	6687	1308	1078
1999	89916	5790	1136	635
2000	65854	5074	1053	653
2001	70562	5192	1102	642
2002	64492	4733	1009	692
2003	70692	4481	1032	489
2004	71243	4891	1165	760
2005	82532	5659	1411	794
2006	85272	6354	1649	876
2007	90484	6193	1852	883
2008	88249	5746	1739	749
2009	92977	6179	1928	906
2010	92996	6329	2152	957
2011	127875	7181	2631	937
Total	2,209,709	161508	33768	23379

Source:
American Academy of Dermatology: *2011 Skin Cancer Screening Statistics*, March, 2012.
Key:
*Number of cases included melanoma, "rule out melanoma," and lentigo maligna.

TABLE 18.—Leading Dermatology Journals

Journal	Total Citations in 2010	Number of Articles Published in 2010	Impact Factor
Journal of Investigative Dermatology	22854	250	6.3
Journal of the American Academy of Dermatology	19751	219	4.3
British Journal of Dermatology	19577	346	4.4
Archives of Dermatology	13298	126	4.2
Dermatologic Surgery	6152	296	2.3
Contact Dermatitis	5392	93	3.7
International Journal of Dermatology	5111	226	1.3
Dermatology	4961	128	2.7
Burns	4141	177	1.7
Acta Dermato-Venereologica	3998	72	2.8
Journal of the European Academy of Dermatology	3781	228	3.3
Clinical and Experimental Dermatology	3771	235	1.3
Journal of Cutaneous Pathology	3281	208	1.7
Experimental Dermatology	3197	189	4.2
Wound Repair and Regeneration	2888	80	3.4
Archives of Dermatological Research	2588	93	2.0
American Journal of Dermatopathology	2576	145	1.3
Pediatric Dermatology	2497	180	1.1
Pigment Cell Melanoma Research	2492	63	4.8
Journal of Dermatological Science	2475	89	3.7
Clinical Dermatology	2221	88	2.4
Mycoses	2118	99	1.7
European Journal of Dermatology	2105	113	2.4
Journal of Dermatology	2028	128	1.4
Cutis	1949	84	1.0

Source:
Journal Citation Reports Web Version 2010:JCR, Science Edition, June, 2011, Philadelphia: Thomson Reuters. February, 2012.

CLINICAL DERMATOLOGY

1 Urticarial and Eczematous Disorders

Allergic contact stomatitis caused by a polyether dental impression material

Batchelor JM, Todd PM (Addenbrooke's NHS Hosp Foundation Trust, Cambridge, UK)
Contact Dermatitis 63:296-297, 2010

A case of allergic contact stomatitis caused by a dental impression material is described. Adverse reactions had been reported to an older version of the material, but none since the manufacturer changed the catalyst. This is the first reported case of a patient reacting to the new catalyst, the sulfonium salt (2-cyano-1-methylethyl)dodecylethylsulfoniumtetrafluoroborate(1-).

▶ A variety of oral lesions can be seen following dental procedures. These include aphthae caused by trauma, lichenoid lesions, and allergic stomatitis, among others. Metals, especially mercury and gold, have been most often implicated in exogenous production of oral lesions by local factors, with acrylates also reported to cause allergic stomatitis and lichenoid lesions. Dental impression materials are an unusual cause. This case report reminds us that the materials used to make an impression with which to construct crowns or dentures may sometimes cause allergy. It also shows that when standard patch testing is negative, testing with suspected materials is often necessary. Index of suspicion is important once one looks beyond the usual suspects.

J. F. Fowler, MD

---

p-Phenylenediamine sensitization and occupation

Malvestio A, Bovenzi M, Hoteit M, et al (Univ of Trieste, Italy; et al)
Contact Dermatitis 64:37-42, 2011

Background.—p-Phenylenediamine (PPD) is an extreme delayed-type skin sensitizer, and is relevant in both occupational and non-occupational exposures.

Objectives.—To estimate the prevalence of PPD sensitization in a population of consecutive patients with suspected allergic contact dermatitis who attended units of dermatology or occupational medicine in north-eastern

Italy and to investigate the association between their PPD sensitization and occupation.

Patients/Materials/Methods.—A total of 14 464 patients (67.6% women and 32.4% men) with suspected allergic dermatitis underwent patch testing. The associations between patch test results and occupations were studied by multivariate logistic regression analysis.

Results.—In both sexes, PPD sensitization was significantly associated with hairdressing and beauty occupation [women, odds ratio (OR) 6.58, 95% confidence interval (CI) 3.76–11.50; men, OR 22.3, 95% CI 4.18–119]. In the female group, PPD sensitization was also significantly higher in professional drivers (OR 5.31, 95% CI 1.76–16.1), barmaids (OR 1.89, 95% CI 1.04–3.44), and cleaners (OR 1.82, 95% CI 1.24–2.68). In the male group, PPD sensitization was significantly higher in bakers and waiters (OR 13.0, 95% CI 1.38–123), household workers (OR 8.46, 95% CI 1.68–42.8), and printers (OR 5.68, 95% CI 1.50–21.5).

Conclusions.—Our study showed that workers in several occupations may be at higher risk of developing sensitization to PPD. It is of importance to reduce possible exposure to PPD-crossreacting substances in these occupations.

▶ The article discusses the prevalence of p-paraphenylenediamine (PPD) contact dermatitis in a large cohort of occupational dermatitis patients from northern Italy. The diagnosis was supported by patch testing and its incidence calculated separately by sex, occupation, and age groups with thorough methodology. This comprehensive epidemiological study reinforces what most of us have learned about PPD contact and occupational dermatitis. More specifically, PPD dermatitis is a highly prevalent cause of hand dermatitis in hairdressers. The authors also list the incidence of PPD contact dermatitis in hair-dye users. What is useful for clinicians in this article is the listing of all other occupations that put patients at high risk for PPD contact dermatitis. Many of these affected occupations, such as drivers, barmaids, and bakers, are far removed from the typical beauty and hair-styling industry. Nevertheless, these other workers are still put at risk for PPD contact dermatitis because of the presence of PPD in the materials that these workers contact regularly on the job. This listing can help clinicians keep in mind these other professions that can put patients at risk for PPD dermatitis. The article also points out the related facial dermatitis that many PPD dermatitis patients concomitantly encounter, since PPD is used in hair dyes that can come in contact with the face. The one career the study did not list was tattoo artists because PPD use in Europe is banned from reinforcing colorful henna tattoos. In the United States, PPD is still allowed in these tattoos, which are commonly painted on Indian wedding participants. Hence, American clinicians must consider this use of PPD when we try to detect the cause of contact dermatitis of the hand in our patients.

K. Nguyen, MD

A prospective multicenter study evaluating skin tolerance to standard hand hygiene techniques

Chamorey E, Marcy P-Y, Dandine M, et al (Antoine Lacassagne Cancer Ctr, Nice, France; Cannes General Hosp, France; et al)
Am J Infect Control 39:6-13, 2011

We performed a prospective multicenter study to assess the dryness and irritation of the hands in health care facilities, and to evaluate whether that disinfection with an alcohol-based hand rub (ABHR) is better tolerated than classic handwashing with mild soap and water. Our study was conducted in 9 sites in the summer and winter. A team of investigators evaluated dryness and irritation. This study takes into account most of the individual and environmental risk factors (age, sex, use of a protective agent, constitutional factors, personal factors, external factors, institution, function, and number of consecutive working days). The results from the 1932 assessments collected show that traditional handwashing is a risk factor for dryness and irritation, whereas the use of ABHR causes no skin deterioration and might have a protective effect, particularly in intensive use. These results provide a strong argument to counter the rear-guard resistance to the use of ABHRs.

▶ There have been 2 major techniques for hand hygiene: hand washing with antimicrobial soaps and disinfection with an alcohol-based hand rub (ABHR). Some patients have the notion that ABHR are harsher on the skin, although microbiologic studies have shown that ABHR often exhibit an advantage over traditional hand washing. This multicenter prospective study compared ABHR and hand washing. Participants were surveyed and assessed during their day-to-day work environment in both winter and summer months. Variables included were sex, risk factors (allergy, atopy, skin disease), self-inflicted injuries, external factors, and use of protective agents. Investigators evaluated for dryness and irritation. Approximately 80% of patients were health care workers (HCWs) and 20% were non-HCW staff, and approximately 33% of patients had constitutional risk factors such as allergy, atopy, or skin disease. Half of the staff used a protective agent such as a cream or an ointment. In a univariate analysis, the frequency of hand washing with mild soap appears to increase the risk of skin dryness ($P < 10^{-6}$). The frequency of disinfection with an ABHR was not associated with dryness of hands. Cold season also augmented skin dryness of the hands. In a multivariate analysis, the frequency of disinfection with ABHR was still not associated with skin dryness and was a protective factor ($P = 4.10^{-3}$). In the univariate and multivariate analyses, the frequency of hand washing with soap remained significantly related to irritation of the hands. Irritation was not associated with the frequency of disinfection with ABHR in either univariate or multivariate analyses. This study may be helpful for those with drying skin conditions who frequently have to disinfect themselves as an occupation. The most surprising element of this study was the protective factor of ABHR after multiple uses. A study examining the stratum corneum on a microscopic level may help in explaining this phenomenon. Furthermore, more controlled prospective studies are needed on this subject to confirm the findings of this report. Considering how common hand eczema is in clinical practice and how difficult it is to treat when the chronicity of hyperkeratosis sets in, more research in this area is an unmet need.

G. K. Kim, DO

J. Q. Del Rosso, DO

A comparative trial comparing the efficacy of tacrolimus 0.1% ointment with aquaphor ointment for the treatment of keratosis pilaris
Breithaupt AD, Alio A, Friedlander SF (Univ of California at San Diego)
Pediatr Dermatol 28:459-460, 2011

Keratosis pilaris is common, but little information exists regarding effective therapy for this sometimes clinically and often cosmetically troublesome disorder. This small pilot study compared the efficacy of Aquaphor ointment with tacrolimus ointment 0.1% and found that both were effective and well tolerated by patients.

▶ Keratosis pilaris (KP) is a common chronic disorder characterized by focal follicular hyperkeratosis, with or without visible perifollicular inflammation. Even in cases that are not very apparent visibly, KP exhibits the palpable texture of semifine to rough sandpaper and most often involves the posterior-lateral arms. The face, anterior thighs, and/or buttocks may also be involved. KP is observed in both children and adults and is most often encountered in patients who have atopic dermatitis, even when the latter is quiescent clinically. This article presents a double-blinded, bilateral, paired-comparison study assessing the effectiveness and safety of topical tacrolimus ointment 0.1% (Tac-Oint) and a well-established, branded, nonmedicated ointment, Aquaphor (Aq-Oint), in the treatment of KP in 30 patients (60 limbs) aged 2 to 16 years. The patients were alternately assigned to consistently apply Aq-Oint twice a day or Tac-Oint twice a day to a designated limb on the right or left side, respectively, to allow for bilateral comparison. The duration of treatment was 4 weeks, with 27 patients completing the study (assessment of 54 limb sides).

Statistically significant improvements in the overall assessment of KP relative to baseline scores were found on both the Tac-Oint—treated sides ($P < .001$) and the Aq-Oint—treated sides ($P < .005$). Improvements were determined on the basis of multiple efficacy parameters with the use of an investigator global assessment (IGA) scale. The efficacy parameters included erythema, pustules, hyperkeratosis, and follicular prominence. Tac-Oint exhibited better improvement overall; however, the number of study participants was too small to draw definitive conclusions regardless of statistical analyses. Reduction in IGA score after 4 weeks was noted in 81% of Tac-Oint—treated sites and in 78% of Aq-Oint—treated sites. This study found that Tac-Oint was more likely to lead to a $> 75\%$ reduction in cutaneous parameters of KP; however, these observations were not statistically significant. This short study has some definite weaknesses, including the short duration of therapy (4 weeks), a very short follow-up period after treatment was stopped (2 weeks), the absence of an untreated control group with KP, and the lack of severity grading. Tolerability reactions at application sites did occur with both agents, with minor pruritus and mild transient skin burning noted with 26% and 15% of Tac-Oint—treated sites, respectively, and with 15% and 4% of Aq-Oint—treated sites, respectively. Nevertheless, from the perspective of the treated subjects, all reported that both treatments improved their KP and that they would use either agent again to treat their KP.

Although the authors concluded that "it is reassuring to have confirmatory evidence" that a relatively inexpensive, over-the-counter, nonmedicated ointment (Aq-Oint) can produce results comparable to those obtained by topical tacrolimus ointment for KP, we agree that larger comparative studies are needed over a longer duration to confirm these results. As this study was too small, there were too many limitations in design, and there was oversight with lack of data capture of some important parameters; confirmatory evidence is not an appropriate description of what the data from this study truly tell the clinician. However, the potential for efficacy in some patients is an acceptable conclusion based on the data provided by this small study. Well-designed and properly powered clinical trials with other agents used to treat KP are also needed. It is important to recognize that the optimal protocol design to evaluate KP has not yet been determined with reasonable consensus to date. This fact emphasizes the need for leaders in dermatologic research to focus on KP as a disease state and, in concert, to develop the best research methodologies and protocols to assess therapeutic outcomes with different agents. Many patients who present to dermatology practices are specifically troubled by KP. Finding therapies that are both effective and safe for KP is a major unmet need in dermatology.

J. Q. Del Rosso, DO

G. K. Kim, DO

The EU Nickel Directive revisited — future steps towards better protection against nickel allergy
Thyssen JP, Uter W, McFadden J, et al (Copenhagen Univ Hosp Gentofte, Hellerup, Denmark; Friedrich Alexander Univ, Erlangen, Germany; St Thomas' Hosp, London, UK; et al)
Contact Dermatitis 64:121-125, 2011

In July 2001, the EU Nickel Directive came into full force to protect European citizens against nickel allergy and dermatitis. Prior to this intervention, Northern European governments had already begun to regulate consumer nickel exposure. According to part 2 of the EU Nickel Directive and the Danish nickel regulation, consumer items intended to be in direct and prolonged contact with the skin were not allowed to release more than 0.5 µg nickel/cm2/week. It was considered unlikely that nickel allergy would disappear altogether as a proportion of individuals reacted below the level defined by the EU Nickel Directive. Despite this, the EU Nickel Directive part 2 was expected to work as an operational limit that would sufficiently protect European consumers against nickel allergy and dermatitis. This review presents the accumulation of epidemiological studies that evaluated the possible effect of this major public health intervention. Also, it evaluates recent exposure assessment studies that have been performed using the dimethyl glyoxime test. It is concluded that the EU Nickel Directive has started to change the epidemiology of nickel allergy in Europe but it should be revisited to better protect consumers and workers since nickel allergy and dermatitis remain very frequent.

▶ This is a review article that examines the efficacy of public policy established in the European Union in July 2001 banning certain nickel-containing products sold to consumers. Specifically, it summarizes the results of research published since July 2001 on the frequency of nickel-containing products sold to consumers in the European Union, and it records the rates of nickel-induced contact dermatitis seen thereafter. While some believe that consumer products are a major cause of nickel-induced contact dermatitis, others show that environmental exposure to nickel may actually reduce rates of nickel sensitivity.[1]

A discussion of the burden of nickel-induced contact dermatitis to society would enhance this article. Hand eczema is likely the most debilitating manifestation of nickel-induced contact dermatitis in that it prevents individuals from working, is costly and difficult to treat because of its chronic nature, and is painful and unsightly. Hand eczema due to nickel is caused either by direct contact with a nickel allergen (consumer product, occupational exposure) or through systemic absorption of ingested nickel through food and water. Policies eliminating products with high nickel content may not affect the rate of nickel sensitization, debilitating hand eczema, or cost to society because ingestion of nickel will remain.

P. Saitta, DO

Reference

1. Smith-Sivertsen T, Tchachtchine V, Lund E. Environmental nickel pollution: does it protect against nickel allergy? *J Am Acad Dermatol.* 2002;46:460-462.

Clinically relevant contact allergy to formaldehyde may be missed by testing with formaldehyde 1·0%
Hauksson I, Pontén A, Gruvberger B, et al (Lund Univ, Malmö, Sweden)
Br J Dermatol 164:568-572, 2011

Background.—It has been found that patch testing with 15 μL formaldehyde 2·0% aq. detects twice as many allergies as by testing with 1·0%. The clinical relevance of positive patch test reactions is often difficult to determine. Repeated open application tests are simple to do and help to evaluate the significance of patch test results.

Objectives.—To study the clinical relevance of contact allergy to formaldehyde detected by 2·0% formaldehyde (0·60 mg cm^{-2}) but not by 1·0%.

Methods.—Eighteen patients positive to formaldehyde 2·0% but negative to 1·0%, and a control group of 19 patients with dermatitis but without allergy to parabens, formaldehyde and formaldehyde releasers were included in the study. Formaldehyde 2000 p.p.m., the maximum concentration permitted in leave-on cosmetics according to the EU Cosmetics Directive, was added to a batch of moisturizer preserved with parabens. The same batch without formaldehyde served as a control. The study was double-blinded and randomized. The patients were provided with both moisturizers and instructed to apply one of them twice a day on a marked-out 5 × 5-cm area on the inside of one upper arm and the other moisturizer on the other arm. Reading of the test sites was done once a week for a maximum of 4 weeks.

Results.—In the control group there were no allergic reactions to either of the moisturizers. Nine of 17 formaldehyde-allergic patients reacted with an allergic reaction to the moisturizer which contained formaldehyde ($P < 0·001$). No positive reactions were observed to the moisturizer without formaldehyde.

Conclusions.—Our results demonstrate that contact allergy to formaldehyde 2·0% may be clinically relevant.

▶ Selection of patch test (PT) allergens often requires a balance between using an allergen at a concentration that will maximize detection of allergic contact dermatitis (ACD) and using it at a concentration that may lead to unacceptable irritant PT responses. Formaldehyde is a good example. It is a very important allergen, ranking around one of the top 5 most common allergens in most reports from around the world. Therefore, accurate detection of formaldehyde allergy is necessary. Most centers routinely test formaldehyde at a concentration of 1%. I have routinely added formaldehyde at 2% to virtually all patients I test. Anecdotally, I have found that some patients with clinically relevant formaldehyde allergy will react only to the 2% concentration. This report confirms that finding. The authors carefully assessed a series of individuals who were PT negative to 1% formaldehyde but positive at 2%. These patients performed a repeated open application test with a formaldehyde-containing moisturizer. Half of them developed ACD at the test site. This is a significant number with this type of testing. While some patients with a positive PT to 2% formaldehyde may be showing an irritant response that is not clinically relevant, a good number of them are truly allergic and would have been missed if they had been tested with only a 1% concentration.

J. F. Fowler, MD

"Car Seat Dermatitis": A Newly Described Form of Contact Dermatitis
Ghali FE (Univ of Texas Southwestern, Dallas)
Pediatr Dermatol 28:321-326, 2011

Over the last several years, our clinic has documented an increasing trend of contact dermatitis presenting in areas that are in direct contact with certain types of car seats composed of a shiny, nylon-like material. Our practice has encountered these cases in both atopic and nonatopic infants, with a seasonal predilection for the warmer months. This brief report highlights some of the key features of this condition and alerts the clinician to this newly described form of contact dermatitis.

▶ Car seat dermatitis (CSD) in infants has been increasing in prevalence over the past few years. It presents as a strikingly uniform eruption that occurs symmetrically and bilaterally, affecting the elbows, upper posterior thighs, lower legs, and occipital scalp. This is a case report series of patients with CSD (N = 21) with information on atopic history, location, treatment, and response. It may be theorized that the propensity to develop this contact dermatitis (CD) may be greater in patients with atopic dermatitis (AD), seen in 12 of 21 atopic patients (57%) in this small series, compared with 9 of 21 without an atopic background (43%). The size of the overall group is too small to conclude definitely; however, this reminds us that patients with AD can often develop allergic CD, evidenced also by the common development of periumbilical pruritic papules related to contact with nickel in snaps or buckles on pants. In this case series, it appears that CDS was an exacerbating factor in AD patients. Treatment of these patients included barrier protection (thick padding between car seat and infant), manufacturer replacement of the seat pad, or entire replacement of the car seat with a entirely different material. Follow-up was obtained in 19 of 21 patients, with atopic patients showing remarkable improvement in the contact areas but continuing to have persistent AD in other ares. Secondary infection was noted in 4 of 21 patients (19%). It was also noted that the incidence of CSD was higher in warmer months as seen during the late spring through fall: 17 of 21 (81%). This may be explained by less area of skin coverage by clothing during the warmer season. In addition, the researchers observed that in this case series all the car seats were composed of a shiny, nylon-like fabric material. The majority of these car seats contain a foam with expanded polystyrene, also known as EPS, which may have been the allergenic culprit. Another complaint from many of the parents of affected children was that the infants were known to be "sweaty" in this material, which may have contributed to the leaching out and release of irritants or allergens. One weakness in this report is a lack of patch testing to confirm a true allergy, because it was assumed that EPS was the most likely cause of the CD. Also, a longer follow-up period may reveal that those labeled as nonatopic may become atopic later on in life. Nevertheless, CSD is an entity recognized as a cause of CD that seems to respond quickly to discontinuation of exposure (ie, barrier protection, change of material) and topical corticosteroid therapy (ie, mid-potency agent). A symmetric and uniform CD accentuated at the sites of predilection mentioned earlier suggests that this entity be placed high on the differential diagnosis list in infants and young children using car seats.

G. K. Kim, DO
J. Q. Del Rosso, DO

Age-related sensitization to *p*-phenylenediamine

Almeida PJ, Borrego L, Limiñana JM (Hospital Universitario Insular de Gran Canaria, Spain)

Contact Dermatitis 64:158-184, 2011

Background.—Hairdressers are occupationally exposed to *p*-phenylene-diamine (PPD), which is a potent contact allergen. The prevalence of PPD sensitization varies worldwide, perhaps reflecting cultural differences in hair fashions and hair care. New sources of sensitization include henna tattoos. Patients living in Gran Canaria were patch tested to determine if they had PPD sensitization.

Methods.—A total of 456 consecutive patients suspected to have contact dermatitis underwent patch testing using the TRUE test with PPD 0.09 mg/cm^2. The test readings were obtained for D2 and D4. The sources of PPD sensitization were divided into consumer hair dye exposures, occupational hair dye exposures, henna tattoo exposures, and unknown exposures.

Results.—Thirty-nine patients demonstrated PPD sensitivity. About 50% were either hairdressers or users of consumer hair dyes. Approximately 20% developed sensitivity after contact with black henna tattoos. For 28% of patients the exposure was unknown. Analysis indicated a clinical correlation between patient age and origin of sensitization, forming three distinct subgroups. The youngest group comprised children who were usually sensitized by exposure to henna tattoos. The next age group included hairdressers, who were usually in the fourth decade of life. The oldest subgroup was composed of consumer hair dye users and those whose sensitization was of unknown origin. Many had a dermatitis unrelated to PPD. The group with unknown exposure included patients who may have had no history of PPD exposure but developed contact dermatitis as well as patients sensitized to PPD by cross-reaction with structurally related compounds.

Conclusions.—These results are not based on a large patient sample but demonstrate an age-related pattern of sensitization to PPD. Further epidemiological study is needed to confirm this pattern.

▶ Exposure to certain allergens that cause allergic contact dermatitis (ACD) may differ on the basis of age, sex, ethnicity, and other factors. Because greater exposure is likely to lead to greater incidence of ACD, understanding these differences may help us identify likely allergens in different groups. This report nicely shows that the source of exposure to paraphenylenediamine (PPDA) varies significantly with age. It also points out that so-called henna tattoos usually contain high levels of PPDA. Those who were sensitized with tattoos were about 10 to 20 years old, hairdressers were around 35 years old, and clients dyeing their hair were around 45 years of age.

J. F. Fowler, MD

A half of schoolchildren with 'ISAAC eczema' are ill with allergic contact dermatitis
Czarnobilska E, Obtulowicz K, Dyga W, et al (Jagiellonian Univ Med College, Krakow, Poland)
J Eur Acad Dermatol Venereol 25:1104-1107, 2011

Background.—Similarity in clinical symptoms between atopic eczema (AE) and allergic contact dermatitis (ACD) may lead to misdiagnoses in both clinical practice and epidemiological studies. As patch testing for contact allergy does not seem popular among paediatric allergists, the resulting bias leads mainly to under diagnosing of ACD and over diagnosing of AE in children and adolescents.

Objectives.—To assess the frequency of AE and ACD among children and adolescents who answered affirmatively the eczema module of ISAAC questionnaire.

Methods.—Of 9320 schoolchildren involved in an allergy screening programme, 143 consecutive participants were recruited for the present study. The inclusion criterion was affirmative answers to questions from the eczema module of the International Study of Asthma and Allergies in Childhood (ISAAC) questionnaire. The children were examined by two allergists: a paediatrician and a dermatologist, and the children underwent patch testing.

Results.—We diagnosed AE in 46 (55.4%) children and 18 (30.0%) adolescents, whereas 32 (38.6%) children and 31 (51.7%) adolescents were diagnosed with ACD, with a considerable overlap of both diseases. Nine of 46 (19.6%) children and 13 of 25 (52.0%) adolescents with affirmative answers to the question about flexural eczema were diagnosed with ACD, while lacking features sufficient for the diagnosis of AE according to Hanifin and Rajka. Based on the indices from the whole population tested (9320 pupils), a rough estimate of the general ACD prevalence was 5.8% for adolescents, and 8.5% for children, which is close to the figure of 7.2% observed previously in Danish schoolchildren.

Conclusions.—Our data demonstrate that 'ISAAC eczema' is an epidemiological entity that embraces comparable portions of cases of atopic eczema and allergic contact dermatitis, and possibly also other less frequent pruritic dermatoses. Each case of chronic recurrent dermatitis in children requires differential diagnosis aimed at allergic contact dermatitis and inflammatory dermatoses other than atopic eczema, even when predominantly localized in flexural areas.

▶ The International Study of Asthma and Allergies in Childhood (ISAAC) questionnaire was intended for studying the epidemiology of atopic eczema (AE). However, the authors of this study noticed that the number of children with allergic contact dermatitis (ACD) also fulfilled the ISAAC criteria. The authors wanted to assess the frequency of AE and ACD in children and adolescents during the ISAAC-based allergy screening program. There were 9320 schoolchildren involved in the program, and 143 consecutive participants recruited.

There was a comparable proportion of AE and ACD in this study, which may demonstrate that contact sensitization can coexist with the atopic tendency. In this study, 55.4% (n = 46) of children and 30.0% (n = 18) of adolescents were diagnosed with AE. In contrast, 38.6% (n = 32) of children and 51.7% (n = 31) of adolescents were diagnosed with ACD. There was also a tendency toward decreasing AE and increasing ACD frequency with age. Nine of 46 (19.6%) children and 13 of 25 (52.0%) adolescents with flexural eczema were diagnosed with ACD. Clinical differentiation between ACD and AE may be difficult, especially if made on morphological appearance alone, and obtaining thorough medical and family histories must be mandated to determine atopic background. This study revealed that among children and adolescents who affirmatively answer the ISAAC eczema questions, the frequencies of ACD and AE were comparable. The ISAAC questionnaire, considered an epidemiological indicator of AE, seems to be nonspecific for AE, ACD, and possibly also other eczematous dermatoses in children. The ISAAC questions should not be regarded as an epidemiological substitute for the diagnosis of atopic eczema because half of the cases may in fact be allergic contact dermatitis.

G. K. Kim, DO

J. Q. Del Rosso, DO

Allergens responsible for allergic contact dermatitis among children: a systematic review and meta-analysis
Bonitsis NG, Tatsioni A, Bassioukas K, et al (Univ of Ioannina Med School, Greece; Univ of Ioannina School of Medicine, Greece)
Contact Dermatitis 64:245-257, 2011

Background.—Multiple studies have evaluated diverse allergens in paediatric populations. Consensus is still lacking on which allergens are most commonly implicated in allergic contact dermatitis.

Objectives.—To evaluate the proportion of positive reactions for allergens tested in children and to identify allergens with positive reactions in at least 1% of them.

Methods.—This was a systematic review of studies in PubMed (1966–2010) investigating allergens in at least 100 enrolled children. Proportions of positive reactions for each allergen were combined with random effects models across studies.

Results.—We included 49 studies with available data on 170 allergens. Each study tested a median of two allergens. Among the 94 allergens evaluated by at least two studies, 58 had estimates of positive reactions of at least 1% by random effects calculations, and for 21 of them the 95% confidence interval ensured that the proportion of positive reactions was at least 1%. The top five allergens tested by at least two studies included nickel sulfate, ammonium persulfate, gold sodium thiosulfate, thimerosal, and toluene-2,5-diamine (*p*-toluenediamine). For most allergens, the proportion of positive reactions was higher in studies published after 1995 than in earlier studies ($p = 0.0065$).

Conclusions.—This meta-analysis offers guidance on which allergens are most prevalent in the paediatric population and should have priority for inclusion in standardized allergen series.

▶ Recent reports have suggested that rates of allergic contact sensitization in children have increased. Many studies have assessed diverse allergens in the pediatric population with small sample sizes. This is a systematic review and meta-analysis of studies in PubMed investigating allergens in at least 100 enrolled children. Only studies that evaluated allergic contact dermatitis using patch testing were included. There were 49 studies that were included in this analysis; only 2 were from the United States, and 170 allergens were tested. The top 5 allergens tested were nickel sulfate, ammonium persulfate, gold sodium thiosulfate, thimerosal, and toluene-2,5-diamine. For most allergens, the positive reactions were higher in studies published after 1995 than in earlier studies ($P = .0065$). For 140 allergens, the 95% upper confidence interval (CI) could not exclude the possibility of a 1% positivity rate. Although a few allergens were consistently included in most of the studies, most allergens were tested in a limited number of investigations, and most of the studies were performed in Europe. This analysis also revealed that for most allergens, the positive reaction rates have increased in the last 15 years compared with earlier studies. One weakness of this review was that, ideally, a pediatric series should include allergens with the highest proportion of positive patch test reactions in children coupled with relevant contact sensitization. However, this was not possible on the basis of the data provided. Positive reaction rates may vary on the basis of exposure to allergens in the target population. In addition, most of the studies were performed in the European population, and it may be useful to obtain more evidence on different populations from other continents as well. Also, the age group of the patients was variable in these studies, and they may be subject to different allergens. These groups should ideally be separated for analysis. For studies like this, the quality of data reporting is the main limitation, and registries may be necessary for recording protocols of all studies on testing allergens.

G. K. Kim, DO

J. Q. Del Rosso, DO

Advances in allergic skin disease, anaphylaxis, and hypersensitivity reactions to foods, drugs, and insects in 2010
Sicherer SH, Leung DYM (Mount Sinai School of Medicine, NY; Natl Jewish Health, Denver, CO)
J Allergy Clin Immunol 127:326-335, 2011

This review highlights some of the research advances in anaphylaxis; hypersensitivity reactions to foods, drugs, and insects; and allergic skin disease that were reported in the *Journal* in 2010. Key epidemiologic observations include an apparent increase in peanut allergy, with more than 1% of children affected, and increasing evidence that early food allergen exposure, rather than avoidance, might improve allergy outcomes. Advances in food allergy diagnosis include improved insights into prognosis and estimation of severity through component-resolved diagnostics and characterization of IgE binding to specific epitopes. Regarding treatment, oral and epicutaneous immunotherapy show promise. Studies of drug allergies show insights into pathophysiology, and studies on insect hypersensitivity reveal improved diagnostic methods. Genetic and functional studies have revealed the important role of epidermal differentiation products in the pathogenesis of atopic dermatitis. Cross-talk between the atopic immune response with the innate immune response have also been found to predispose to infection in patients with atopic dermatitis. New therapeutic approaches to control chronic urticaria have also been identified during the past year.

▶ There have been recent advances in hypersensitivity reactions to foods, drugs, and insects. This is a review highlighting some of the advances that have been reported. Recent research has found that maternal ingestion of peanuts during pregnancy was associated with increased risk of sensitization in atopic infants. Also, oral immunotherapy shows promise for the treatment of peanut allergy. Epidemiologic studies have shown in a database of >1 million person-years, an increased risk for anaphylaxis among people with asthma. Researchers have found that the risk of side effects during vespid venom immunotherapy was related to baseline tryptase levels. Studies are also indicating that the identification of plasmacytoid dendritic cells plays a role in drug reactions with eosinophilia and systemic symptoms (DRESS). For atopic patients, studies have found that some filaggrin breakdown products are antimicrobial. This may at least partially explain why patients with atopic dermatitis and associated filaggrin gene mutations exhibit increased skin colonization with *Staphylococcus aureus*, crusted eczema, and bacterial pyoderma. Also discussed in this article is familial atypical cold urticaria, which has been identified as a new variant of cold urticaria. These are a few of the advances that have been made in our understanding of the mechanisms and treatment of allergic skin disease and will help to improve patient care in the future.

G. K. Kim, DO

J. Q. Del Rosso, DO

Eczema across the World: The Missing Piece of the Jigsaw Revealed
Williams HC (Univ Hosps NHS Trust, Nottingham, UK)
J Invest Dermatol 131:12-14, 2011

Cleverly using records obtained from the 2003 National Survey of Children's Health (NSCH), Shaw *et al.* provide a pioneering glimpse into the burden of eczema across the United States. Using parental reports of a doctor's diagnosis of eczema in the past 12 months, the authors show that eczema affects around 9—18% of children age 17 and under. The study confirms reported associations such as living in metropolitan areas, higher household education level, and black ethnicity. Novel findings include the demonstration of higher eczema prevalence along the East Coast. The study correlates well with previous reports and may help point to environmental factors that contribute to the development of eczema.

▶ Since the United States opted out of participating in the International Study of Asthma and Allergies in Childhood, Shaw et al[1] took it upon themselves to assess the prevalence of eczema in the United States by looking at a subset of surveys sent to parents in 2003 aimed at assessing childhood health. They focused on a question in the survey asking if their child had ever been given a diagnosis of "eczema or any kind of skin allergy?" Their compiled data led to the conclusions described above.

I agree with the author's assessment that the wording used in the survey given to parents is rather vague as it relates to childhood eczema. The wording could lead to potential misinterpretation by the parent of not only the doctor's assessment of the purported skin condition but by the parents' understanding of what they believe a skin allergy to be, leading to many more false-positive results. In spite of this, the data relating elevated prevalence of childhood eczema in blacks and the higher educated and urban populations is consistent with those of previous studies. Still, these data only describe a rudimentary snapshot of the epidemiology of the disease. We still lack even minimal details about these ethnic/education groups and environmental factors that might explain the link between them and the disease itself. So the data are laudable in their reinforcement of a greater understanding of this disease, which consumes so much of a nation's health care resources, but clearly much greater detail is needed to draw useful conclusions that may eventuate into benefits for patients and the economy.

Hopefully, in the wake of the relatively disappointing health care benefits most are experiencing with electronic medical records, the compilation of data for studies such as these will be much easier to come by in the near future, especially if the diagnosis codes for "eczema" and "dermatitis" are further subdivided in the upcoming new ICD-9 coding lists. However, there are still issues related to accuracy when using diagnosis coding to obtain data. Furthermore, if the current climate of health care continues on its current course and health care dollars become more and more scarce, data such as these may aid certain states, or regions within states, in fighting for more funding for particularly prevalent diseases.

J. M. Suchniak, MD

Reference

1. Shaw TE, Currie GP, Koudelka CW, Simpson EL. Eczema prevalence in the United States: data from the 2003 National Survey of Children's Health. *J Invest Dermatol.* 2011;131:67-73.

Leucoderma after Chinese sofa dermatitis

Vives R, Ana V, Hervella M, et al (Hosp de Navarra, Pamplona, Spain)
Contact Dermatitis 64:58-62, 2011

Background.—Dimethylfumarate is a potent contact sensitizer with antimicrobial and mold-preventing effects. Sofa dermatitis has affected hundreds of patients who are exposed to dimethylfumarate in sachets designed to prevent mold in furniture being stored or transported. A case of allergic contact dermatitis developed in a man who came into contact with dimethylfumarate in a leather sofa.

> *Case Report.*—Man, 49, had widespread pruritic erythematous dermatitis of 2 weeks' duration that had begun on his thighs but now extended to the back, buttocks, and arms. The affected skin sites had been in contact with a sofa purchased 6 months previously, so a diagnosis of allergic contact dermatitis was made. Oral prednisone and avoidance of contact with the sofa resulted in healing of the dermatitis, but in 4 weeks the patient developed hyperpigmented areas at the resolved dermatitis sites. Biopsy of the sites showed no melanocytes. Patch tests with the baseline Spanish contact dermatitis research group series, textile dyes, and footwear series yielded a nonrelevant positive result for wood alcohols. A positive result was obtained from patch testing with dimethylfumarate. However, the patch test site did not develop depigmentation. After 2 years of follow-up, the depigmented areas remained. The patient reported no personal or family history of vitiligo or other autoimmune disease. Depigmentation after contact eczema has been reported in various settings, such as occupationally or after the private use of sensitizing agents such as phenol and cathecol derivatives or sulfhydryl compounds. The lack of vitiligo history makes this less likely, but the repeated exposure to dimethylfumarate for 6 months, the location of the acquired depigmented areas at sites where contact dermatitis had been, and the temporal association suggested leukoderma after dimethylfumarate dermatitis.

Conclusions.—Contact leukoderma is characterized by the loss of pigment after exposure to chemicals that produce specific, selective melanocytopenia. Either allergic dermatitis or toxic depigmenting effects can precede contact leukoderma. The exact mechanism by which the pigmentary change occurs is unknown. It may result from a melanocytotoxic effect independent of its sensitizing potential. Genetic susceptibility and the nature of the chemical contribute to the severity of the lesions. Dimethylfumarate should be added to the list of substances that can cause depigmentation.

▶ Allergic contact dermatitis (ACD) to dimethylfumarate has reached epidemic proportions in Europe, primarily because of exposure from furniture imported from China. Occasionally, hypopigmentation can result from ACD, especially from more severe eruptions. Phenolic chemicals used in disinfectants and in plastics manufacture are the most commonly reported causative agents and can sometimes cause hypopigmentation even in the absence of clinically obvious ACD. This report reminds us that a rare complication of ACD is hypopigmentation.

J. F. Fowler, MD

Deodorants are the leading cause of allergic contact dermatitis to fragrance ingredients
Heisterberg MV, Menné T, Andersen KE, et al (Univ of Copenhagen, Hellerup, Denmark; Odense Univ Hosp, Denmark; et al)
Contact Dermatitis 64:258-264, 2011

Background.—Fragrances frequently cause contact allergy, and cosmetic products are the main causes of fragrance contact allergy. As the various products have distinctive forms of application and composition of ingredients, some product groups are potentially more likely to play a part in allergic reactions than others.

Aim.—To determine which cosmetic product groups cause fragrance allergy among Danish eczema patients.

Method.—This was a retrospective study based on data collected by members of the Danish Contact Dermatitis Group. Participants ($N = 17716$) were consecutively patch tested with fragrance markers from the European baseline series (2005–2009).

Results.—Of the participants, 10.1% had fragrance allergy, of which 42.1% was caused by a cosmetic product: deodorants accounted for 25%, and scented lotions 24.4%. A sex difference was apparent, as deodorants were significantly more likely to be listed as the cause of fragrance allergy in men (odds ratio 2.2) than in women. Correlation was observed between deodorants listed as the cause of allergy and allergy detected with fragrance mix II (FM II) and hydroxyisohexyl 3-cyclohexene carboxaldehyde.

Conclusion.—Deodorants were the leading causes of fragrance allergy, especially among men. Seemingly, deodorants have an 'unhealthy' composition of the fragrance chemicals present in FM II.

▶ Cosmetic products are a significant source of allergic contact dermatitis. This is a study determining the distribution of cosmetic product groups as the cause of fragrance allergy-related allergic contact dermatitis (ACD) among Danish eczema patients. The authors also examined the gender differences and evaluated whether there was an association between the cosmetic product listed as having caused a fragrance allergy and the different fragrance markers detecting an allergy. ACD from 1 or more of the fragrance markers was found in 1790 patients (10.1%). Cosmetic products were the cause of fragrance-induced ACD in 753, comprising 42.1% of those with fragrance allergy. The most common source of ACD were deodorants (25.3%), scented lotions (24.2%), fine fragrances (16.0%), shampoos (13.0%), liquid soaps (10.8%), aftershaves

(2.7%), lipsticks (1.9%), and others (1%). Deodorants played a large role in men, accounting for 37.9% of the 145 products listed as causing ACD from fragrances (P < .001). Scented lotions and fine fragrances played the largest role in women accounting for 28.5% and 19.7%, respectively, of the products listed with a gender difference that was significant (P < .001). Also the deodorants that caused ACD contained 1.3- to 8.9-fold higher concentrations of allergenic fragrance substances than those that did not. In this study, the authors found that the use of deodorants are associated with an increased risk of ACD from fragrances in eczema-prone patients. In the general population, deodorants were the leading cause of allergic and irritant contact dermatitis. Certain factors may explain why deodorants are associated with a high risk of developing fragrance-induced ACD. The environment in the axillary region is moist and occluded, and the presence of hair follicles can increase the penetration of certain allergens. Shaving also has been known to increase the penetration of certain allergens. Because deodorants are used in a sensitive occlusive area, it is important to recognize this as an important sensitizing agent; fragrances may need to be fully avoided or used in lower concentrations than in other products used in different body locations.

G. K. Kim, DO

J. Q. Del Rosso, DO

A Prospective Study of Filaggrin Null Mutations in Keratoconus Patients with or without Atopic Disorders

Droitcourt C, Touboul D, Ged C, et al (Natl Reference Centre for Rare Skin Disorders, Bordeaux, France; Natl Reference Centre for Keratoconus, Bordeaux, France; Univ of Bordeaux, France)
Dermatology 222:336-341, 2011

Background.—Atopic dermatitis (AD) is significantly associated with keratoconus (KC). An inherited component for KC has been suggested. Filaggrin (*FLG*) mutations are a strong genetic risk factor for AD. Since filaggrin is also expressed in the corneal epithelium, we hypothesized a common aetiology for ichthyosis vulgaris (IV), AD and KC.

Objectives.—We examined the prevalence of AD and IV in a KC population. We also studied the expression of filaggrin in normal and KC cornea and analysed 2 prevalent loss-of-function *FLG* alleles (R501X and 2282del4) in a KC population. Finally we examined whether the population with KC and *FLG* mutations had specific clinical characteristics.

Results.—Of 89 KC patients, 38 had current or a history of AD and/or IV. Five patients were carriers of at least 1 *FLG* mutant allele and had a clinical diagnosis of AD and IV with a severer KC.

Conclusion.—The low frequency of *FLG* mutations is surprising since 42.7% of our KC population had AD associated or not with IV; the expected frequency would have been 12—15%, based on our previous studies. Further studies are required to look at other possible *FLG* mutations or other candidate genes.

▶ Keratoconus (KC) has been linked with atopic dermatitis (AD) in the literature. KC, observable as a conical shape to the cornea on side-view examination, is a condition with corneal dystrophy, thinning, and ectasia, which can lead to loss of visual acuity. Studies have postulated an association between AD and altered expression of epithelial barrier proteins, such as filaggrin (FLG) in the cornea, which is present in both central and peripheral corneal epithelium. The authors in this study hypothesized that FLG gene mutations are a source of common dysfunction in both the corneal epithelium in KC and the stratum corneum in patients with AD. Eighty-nine patients were diagnosed with KC and 38 with a history of AD. Among these patients, 19 had ichthyosis vulgaris (IV). In this study, there was a weak presence of FLG in the corneal protein extracts. Also, it was surprising to find that there was a lower mutated allele frequency (6.8%) than expected. Within the KC population, there were 42.7% with a history of AD, with or without IV. The authors estimated the frequency of FLG gene mutations in KC to be 12% to 15% based on other previous studies. However, the limitations to this study were that not all FLG gene mutations were tested, and results may vary with less-common mutations that were not tested for in this study. Further studies with a larger population of patients evaluating FLG gene mutations and other genetic abnormalities may be needed to answer if there is a true link between KC and AD and if the presence of concurrent IV is a contributing factor.

G. K. Kim, DO
J. Q. Del Rosso, DO

Effectiveness of prevention programmes for hand dermatitis: a systematic review of the literature
van Gils RF, Boot CRL, van Gils PF, et al (VU Univ Med Centre, Amsterdam, The Netherlands; Natl Inst for Public Health and the Environment, Bilthoven, The Netherlands; et al)
Contact Dermatitis 64:63-72, 2011

Hand dermatitis is a prevalent disease with an episodic, chronic character. The use of medical resources is high and is often related to reduced (work) functioning. The burden is therefore high for patients and society. Management of hand dermatitis is often unsatisfactory, and for this reason prevention is important. The effectiveness of prevention programmes is, however, unknown. This study evaluates if comprehensive prevention programmes for hand dermatitis, that include worker education as an element, are effective on occurrence, adherence to preventive measures, clinical outcomes and costs compared to usual care or no intervention. The literature was systematically searched using PubMed and Embase, from the earliest to January 2010 for relevant citations. The methodological quality was assessed by two reviewers using the Cochrane criteria. The GRADE approach was used to determine the level of evidence. After reading the full text articles, 7 publications met our inclusion criteria. We found that there is moderate evidence for the effect of prevention programmes on lowering occurrence and improving adherence to preventive measures, and low evidence for the effect on improving clinical outcomes and self-reported outcomes. No studies reporting on costs were found. It can be concluded that there is moderate evidence for the effectiveness of prevention programmes of hand dermatitis versus usual care or no intervention. However, more high quality studies including cost-effectiveness are needed.

▶ Hand dermatitis is a rather common condition that can impact individuals not only on a physical level, such as in work functioning, but also psychosocially. Medical treatment may not always be the only effective option. Expanding management considerations to include prevention programs may help in reducing the emergence and chronicity of hand dermatitis and recurrences after effective treatment. To this end, a systematic review of the literature was performed by van Gils et al to determine the effectiveness of prevention programs, including worker education, for hand dermatitis. Evaluation of prevention programs looked at their effectiveness related to occurrence, adherence to preventative measures, clinical outcomes, and costs. The benefit of this review is the conclusion that there is moderate evidence for the effectiveness of both skin-protective measures and skin care education to help reduce occurrence and to increase adherence with management recommendations. Unfortunately, there was only low-level evidence for improvement on clinical outcomes, and no information was available on its effect on cost. Ultimately, there is evidence that prevention programs are an important consideration. Additionally, the article even advises skin care education and skin protection measures as part of worker training for those involved in wet work or high-risk occupations. From a practical management perspective, this article helps reiterate the importance of good skin care education as well as taking the time to review appropriate skin protection options for individuals either with or at risk for hand dermatitis. Overall, the article provides useful considerations and suggestions for the management of hand dermatitis.

B. D. Michaels, DO

J. Q. Del Rosso, DO

Genetic variations in toll-like receptor pathway genes influence asthma and atopy

Tesse R, Pandey RC, Kabesch M (Hannover Med School, Germany)
Allergy 66:307-316, 2011

Innate immunity is a pivotal defence system of higher organisms. Based on a limited number of receptors, it is capable of recognizing pathogens and to initiate immune responses. Major components of these innate immunity pathogen recognition receptors are the toll-like receptors (TLRs), a family of 11 in humans. They are all membrane bound and through dimerization and complex downstream signaling, TLRs elicit a variety of specific and profound effects. In recent years, the role of TLRs signaling was not only investigated in infection and inflammation but also in allergy. Fuelled by the hygiene hypothesis, which suggests that allergies develop because of a change in microbial exposure and associated immune signals early in life, it had been speculated that alterations in TLRs signaling could influence allergy development. Thus, TLR genes, genetic variations of these genes, and their association with asthma and other atopic diseases were investigated in recent years. This review provides an overview of TLR genetics in allergic diseases.

▶ The article starts with a comprehensive summary about the current knowledge on toll-like receptor (TLR) signaling pathways in humans. The authors review the function, modulation, regulation, and downstream activation by TLRs of adapter molecules, which are responsible for the variety of innate immune responses against multiple organisms through recognition of molecular patterns common to groups of pathogens, instead of recognizing individual pathogens, which make these receptors so "great" ("toll" in German). Recent studies have related the innate immune system to initial responses to environment factors in allergy development through disruptions in the function of the different barrier surfaces and/or genetic variation in components of the immune system including TLRs. CD14 is a receptor expressed on the surface of macrophages and monocytes that lacks a transmembrane domain and uses TLR4 to transmit downstream signals. Genetic variations in CD14 and TLR4 have been related to the development of atopy and allergic reactions. Significant TLR polymorphisms associated with atopic asthma have been found in TLRs 1, 2, 4, 6, and 10. One interesting finding represents the relationship between TLR2 mutations and susceptibility to *Streptococcus aureus*, one of the most common pathogens associated with atopic dermatitis exacerbations. Studies showing TLR9 polymorphisms associated with atopic eczema have obtained mixed results, so further evaluation is warranted to define its role in atopic dermatitis. TLRs 7, 8, and 10 have shown associations with asthma and allergy, but it is too soon to draw any conclusions. Genetic variations in TLR pathways, including MyD88-dependent pathway genes, such as IL1RL1, MD2, and MAP3K7IP1, have also been associated with atopy and asthma. In addition, polymorphisms in the IL1RL1 gene have been significantly related with eosinophils and immunoglobulin (Ig)E levels in asthma. Variations in genes IL18R1 and IL18RAP are also associated with IgE levels and asthma. Polymorphisms in the NFKB1 gene were not significantly associated with atopic dermatitis. Other genes such as TOLLIP and IRAK-M need further evaluation. Finally, the authors discuss the crucial role of the CD14 gene in the gene-environment interaction in atopic conditions. CD14 promoter polymorphism C159T was able to modify IgE levels depending on the level of exposure of domestic endotoxin exposure through mechanisms not well understood. This is still a developing field, and the authors hope that technological advances in genetics will help in elucidating the gene-environment interaction that appears to be, if not critical, at least of high importance in the development, susceptibility, and perpetuation of allergic conditions.

B. Berman, MD, PhD

S. Amini, MD

Efficacious and safe management of moderate to severe scalp seborrhoeic dermatitis using clobetasol propionate shampoo 0.05% combined with ketoconazole shampoo 2%: a randomized, controlled study
Ortonne J-P, Nikkels AF, Reich K, et al (Hôpital de l'Archet 2, Nice Cedex, France; ULG Liège, Belgium; SCIDerm GmbH, Hamburg, Germany; et al)
Br J Dermatol 165:171-176, 2011

Background.—Topical antifungals and corticosteroids are the mainstay of treatment for seborrhoeic dermatitis. The short-contact clobetasol propionate 0.05% shampoo (CP) is an efficacious and safe once-daily treatment for scalp psoriasis.

Objectives.—To evaluate the efficacy and safety of CP alone and combined with ketoconazole shampoo 2% (KC) in the treatment of moderate to severe scalp seborrhoeic dermatitis.

Methods.—This randomized and investigator-blinded study consisted of three phases, each lasting 4 weeks. During the treatment phase, subjects were randomized to receive KC twice weekly (K2), CP twice weekly (C2), CP twice weekly alternating with KC twice weekly (C2 + K2) or CP four times weekly alternating with KC twice weekly (C4 + K2). All subjects received KC once weekly during the maintenance phase and were untreated during the follow-up phase.

Results.—At the end of the treatment phase, all three CP-containing regimens were significantly more efficacious than K2 in decreasing the overall disease severity ($P < 0.05$). Both combination regimens were also significantly more efficacious than K2 in decreasing each individual sign of the disease ($P < 0.05$). While the C2 and C4 + K2 groups experienced slight worsening during the maintenance phase, the efficacy of C2 + K2 was sustained and remained the highest among all groups. All regimens were well tolerated without inducing any skin atrophy. Similarly low incidences of telangiectasia, burning and adverse events were observed among the four groups.

Conclusions.—The combination therapy of twice-weekly CP alternating with twice-weekly KC provided significantly greater efficacy than KC alone and a sustained effect in the treatment of moderate to severe scalp seborrhoeic dermatitis.

▶ Seborrheic dermatitis is an inflammatory condition often involving the scalp as well as other skin sites such as the paranasal region, eyebrows, periauricular region, central chest, and genital region. Commensal yeast proliferation (*Malassezia* spp) has been implicated in this disease, and antifungal agents and corticosteroids have led to improvement of lesions. The investigators evaluated clobetasol propionate shampoo 0.005% (CP) and ketoconazole shampoo 2% (KC), both as monotherapy and in combination regimens, for severe exacerbations of seborrheic dermatitis, followed by maintenance with once-weekly KC treatment. A total of 326 subjects were randomized into the investigator-blinded multiphase study. The first phase consisted of 80 subjects receiving KC twice weekly (K2), 82 subjects receiving CP twice weekly (C2), 82 subjects receiving CP twice weekly alternating with KC twice weekly (C2 + K2), and 82 subjects receiving CP 4 times weekly alternating with KC twice weekly (C4 + K2). At week 4, the subjects receiving C2 had a significantly greater reduction from baseline in total sum score (TSS: sum of erythema, scaling, and pruritus) compared with the subjects receiving K2 ($P < .05$). The subjects receiving the 2 combination therapies, C2 + K2 or C4 + K2, had significantly greater reductions from baseline to week 4 in TSS than the subjects receiving K2 ($P < .05$). Both combination therapies were significantly more efficacious than the KC monotherapy in decreasing the severity of scaling and pruritus at week 4 ($P < .05$ for scaling, $P < .05$ for pruritus). More subjects in the C2, C2 + K2 and C4 + K2 groups reported being satisfied with the overall treatment compared with the K2 group ($P < .05$). After 4 weeks, KC was used once a week as maintenance therapy in all 4 study groups. The regimen associated with the highest efficacy during the maintenance phase was the group originally treated over the first 4 weeks with C2 + K2, suggesting therapeutic value is suppressing the inflammation of seborrheic dermatitis with twice-weekly intermittent use of CP and concurrently suppressing growth of *Malassezia* spp with KC twice weekly. This approach to therapy appears to be effective and safe in moderate to severe seborrheic dermatitis of the scalp and reduces the disease rebound that can occur with topical corticosteroid monotherapy or frequent topical corticosteroid use.

G. K. Kim, DO
J. Q. Del Rosso, DO

Occupational hand eczema caused by nickel and evaluated by quantitative exposure assessment
Jensen P, Thyssen JP, Johansen JD, et al (Copenhagen Univ Hosp Gentofte, Hellerup, Denmark; et al)
Contact Dermatitis 64:32-36, 2011

Background.—EU legislation has reduced the epidemic of nickel contact allergy affecting the consumer, and shifted the focus towards occupational exposure. The acid wipe sampling technique was developed to quantitatively determine skin exposure to metals.

Objectives.—To assess the clinical usefulness of the acid wipe sampling technique as part of the diagnostic investigation for occupational nickel allergy-associated hand dermatitis.

Patients and Methods.—Six patients with vesicular dermatitis on the hands were included. Acid wipe sampling of skin and patch testing with a nickel sulfate dilution series were performed.

Results.—Nickel was detected in all samples from the hands. In all patients, the nickel content on the hands was higher than on the non-exposed control area.

Conclusions.—Occupational exposure to nickel-releasing items raised the nickel content on exposed skin as compared with a non-exposed control site. Nickel-reducing measures led to complete symptom relief in all cases. In cases of a positive nickel patch test reaction and hand eczema, patients should perform the dimethylglyoxime (DMG) test on metallic items at home and at work. The acid wipe sampling technique is useful for the diagnosis of occupational hand eczema following screening with the inexpensive DMG test.

▶ Hand dermatitis is one of the most challenging disease entities we as practitioners have to treat. Deductive reasoning or patch testing can narrow the diagnosis down to allergic contact dermatitis to nickel, but once the sources of the offending agents are recognized, it may still be hard to know which objects are creating the most trouble and to what degree. The dimethyl glyoxime test can be used to identify potential items that may release nickel, but the magnitude of allergen exposure and its cumulative effects in an affected patient cannot be known for a given object with this test alone. The authors here have proposed a method to quantify the amount of nickel exposure one accumulates at a given point during work activity. All patients in the study showed higher levels of nickel exposure on the volar index finger, followed by the palm, and the least amount on an unexposed arm, as would be expected. This information, if creatively used, could help patients decide which items in the workplace need to be adjusted, replaced, or avoided to manage their exposure.

The test would seem most practical in the workplace, where one would expect to encounter the same items under the same conditions in a predictable way. However, it may be more difficult to see how this test would be as useful in a nonoccupational setting where some household items may be more transiently encountered, such as with food containers, clothing, and tools used intermittently.

Additionally, it is not clear just how practical it may be to perform this test in a clinical setting. In this study, the authors had to dissolve the collection wipes in a beaker of nitric acid and then put them on a vibrating table for 30 minutes prior to sending them off to be analyzed. It is not likely an outsourced laboratory would handle something like this, and the collection procedure would need to be done by the practitioner, which may be challenging. If a simplified system could be developed, this may prove to be a useful tool in helping patients with allergies to nickel and other metal allergies such as cobalt and chromium.

J. M. Suchniak, MD

The relevance of chlorhexidine contact allergy

Liippo J, Kousa P, Lammintausta K (Turku Univ Hosp, Finland; The Helsinki Asthma and Allergy Association in Finland)
Contact Dermatitis 64:229-234, 2011

Background.—Chlorhexidine is used for disinfection of skin and mucosae in medicine and dentistry. Prolonged exposure may lead to contact sensitization and allergic contact dermatitis or stomatitis.

Objectives.—The purpose of this study was to analyse the sources of chlorhexidine exposure and sensitization, and to obtain data on the prevalence of sensitization and chlorhexidine-related contact allergy.

Patients and Methods.—From 1999, patch testing was performed with chlorhexidine digluconate (0.5% aq.) on 7610 general dermatology patients with suspected contact allergy at the Turku University Hospital Dermatology Department. The medical records were reviewed concerning the patients' exposure to chlorhexidine.

Results.—A positive patch reaction to chlorhexidine was seen in 36 patients (0.47%). Current dermatitis or stomatitis caused by chlorhexidine-containing topical medicaments was seen in 5 patients. Chlorhexidine sensitization contributed to the current dermatitis in 11 patients. A history of earlier exposure to chlorhexidine-containing products was recalled by only 16 sensitized patients, whereas no exposure was revealed in 4 cases.

Conclusions.—Chlorhexidine-containing corticosteroid creams, skin disinfectants and oral hygiene products are principal sources of chlorhexidine contact sensitization. Exposure to chlorhexidine in cosmetics may lead to delayed improvement of eczema in sensitized patients, emphasizing the importance of identifying the potential cosmetic sources.

▶ Chlorhexidine is a topically applied antimicrobial agent active against gram-positive and gram-negative bacteria and is commonly used as a perioperative antiseptic or for suppression of skin colonization with bacteria such as *Staphylococcus aureus*. Concern has been raised about contact allergy related to the use of chlorhexidine. Chlorhexidine is found in hand disinfectants used for general antiseptic hand washing and oral hygiene products and in some topical corticosteroid creams in Finland. This is a study of 7610 patients suspected of contact allergy to chlorhexidine in which patch testing to chlorhexidine digluconate (0.5% aqueous solution) was performed. Results revealed that positive patch test reactions to chlorhexidine gluconate were seen in 36 patients (0.47%) aged 13 to 84 years. The primary diagnosis was atopic dermatitis in 8 patients and chronic nummular dermatitis in 6 patients. Allergic contact dermatitis was diagnosed in 14 of 36 patients. These 14 patients also had multiple other contact sensitivities, and, for 5 patients, chlorhexidine appeared to be the major causative agent. Healing or improvement of the current dermatitis or stomatitis was seen when these patients avoided chlorhexidine. Also, cosmetic products containing chlorhexidine were suspected of having caused worsening of skin symptoms in 7 of 36 patients. Chlorhexidine-containing topical medicines that are used to treat inflamed or injured skin were considered to be a principal source of sensitization in this study. Hand disinfectants were the principal source of chlorhexidine sensitization in 4 patients with hand dermatitis, but multiple other factors also contributed. Limitations were that multiple contact allergens were also identified and the possibility of "angry back" or irritant reactions may have revealed false-positive results in some cases. Also, testing with 0.25% compared with 0.125% chlorhexidine solutions may have revealed more true-positive results. This study suggests that chlorhexidine-containing topical corticosteroid creams, skin disinfectants, and oral hygiene products may be sources of sensitization to chlorhexidine.

G. K. Kim, DO
J. Q. Del Rosso, DO

Importance of treatment of skin xerosis in diabetes

Seité S, Khemis A, Rougier A, et al (Hôpital L'Archet 2, Nice, France)
J Eur Acad Dermatol Venereol 25:607-609, 2011

Background.—Cutaneous complications are common in diabetes patients and previous studies have shown that diabetes can affect some biophysical skin characteristics. However, the interest of emollients in diabetes has never been clearly demonstrated; i.e. whether they are able to limit skin complications in diabetes patients.

Objective.—The aim of this study was to evaluate the tolerance and the effect of an emollient on patient with diabetes.

Method.—Forty patients with diabetes applied the emollient twice daily for 1 month on one arm and one leg, in normal conditions.

Results.—A 1-month treatment with an emollient allows a similar skin hydration rate in diabetics to that in healthy people. This dry skin improvement is accompanied by a significant reduction in pruritus and desquamation, and a significant improvement in the skin barrier function.

Conclusion.—Emollient treatment can be useful in the management of diabetes by limiting skin complications associated with elevated blood sugar.

▶ Diabetic patients are obviously at risk for certain systemic changes, and attention to these changes is of primary concern. However, changes in functional and mechanical properties of the skin and their implications, such as xerosis and pruritus, may occur in diabetic patients similar to other endocrine disorders, but preventative measures can often be overlooked. Even more important is that xerosis may lead to cracking in the skin and increase the potential for skin infections and subsequent consequences, especially in the lower extremities. Noting that studies on emollients for improvement of skin changes in diabetic patients is lacking, Seité et al sought to determine if the use of emollients is effective in diabetic skin. According to their study of 40 patients (most had type 1 diabetes), patients treated with an emollient twice a day for 1 month had a significant increase in skin hydration, which was correlated with a reduction in both transepidermal water loss and the desquamation index. The hydration rate at the end of treatment in diabetic patients was similar to that in healthy patients. The emollients were also well tolerated. In addition, the study results showed that an emollient can improve xerosis within 1 month, as well as desquamation and pruritus. Given these results, management of all diabetic patients should include a suggestion of the use of an emollient not only for the treatment of skin xerosis, desquamation, and pruritus, but also for preventative measures and avoidance of these potential complications of fissured and/or excoriated skin.

B. D. Michaels, DO

J. Q. Del Rosso, DO

Folic Acid Use in Pregnancy and the Development of Atopy, Asthma, and Lung Function in Childhood

Magdelijns FJH, Mommers M, Penders J, et al (Maastricht Univ, The Netherlands)
Pediatrics 128:e135-e144, 2011

Background.—Recently, folic acid supplementation during pregnancy was implicated as a potential risk factor for atopic diseases in childhood.

Objective.—To investigate whether folic acid supplementation and higher intracellular folic acid (ICF) levels during pregnancy increase the risk of childhood atopic diseases.

Methods.—In the KOALA Birth Cohort Study ($N = 2834$), data on eczema and wheeze were collected by using repeated questionnaires at 3, 7, 12, and 24 months, 4 to 5 years, and 6 to 7 years after delivery. Atopic dermatitis and total and specific immunoglobulin E levels were determined at age 2 years and asthma and lung function at age 6 to 7 years. We defined folic acid use as stand-alone and/or multivitamin supplements according to the period of use before and/or during pregnancy. ICF levels were determined in blood samples taken at ~35 weeks of pregnancy ($n = 837$). Multivariable logistic and linear regression analyses were conducted, with generalized estimating equation models for repeated outcomes.

Results.—Maternal folic acid supplement use during pregnancy was not associated with increased risk of wheeze, lung function, asthma, or related atopic outcomes in the offspring. Maternal ICF level in late pregnancy was inversely associated with asthma risk at age 6 to 7 years in a dose-dependent manner (P for trend $= .05$).

Conclusions.—Our results do not confirm any meaningful association between folic acid supplement use during pregnancy and atopic diseases in the offspring. Higher ICF levels in pregnancy tended, at most, toward a small decreased risk for developing asthma.

▶ Folic acid supplementation before and during the first trimester of pregnancy has been linked to a decrease in the risk of congenital malformations. However, recent studies have demonstrated a possible increased risk of asthma with increased levels of folic acid. This is a study conducted within the prospective

KOALA Birth Cohort Study in the Netherlands with the goal of investigating early life risk factors for atopy and asthma. Healthy pregnant women were recruited in weeks 10 to 14 of their pregnancy from an ongoing prospective cohort study. Venous blood samples were taken at approximately 35 weeks of pregnancy to determine the intracellular folic levels (ICF). During the home visit, at age 2 years (n = 842), manifestations of atopic dermatitis were assessed and blood samples were taken for determining total and specific IgE levels. There were no major differences observed in the distribution of characteristics of the cohort at birth, at 2 years, and after 6 to 7 years of follow-up. Folic acid use during pregnancy was not associated with increased risk of developing eczematous dermatitis or atopic dermatitis, high total IgE levels, allergic sensitization, or asthma in the child. High serum total IgE level at 2 years was inversely associated with folic acid use at some point during pregnancy but was not statistically significant after adjustment for confounders. Higher ICF levels in late pregnancy revealed a small decreased risk for developing asthma. Although this study did not find a correlation between ICF and atopy, there may be different mechanisms at play during pregnancy rather than after birth. Also, the authors did not consider other sources of folic acid such as dietary intake of leafy greens and how they could affect ICF levels. More studies on folic acid use and ICF levels during pregnancy are needed before definitive conclusions can be made.

G. K. Kim, DO

J. Q. Del Rosso, DO

The effects of pajama fabrics' water absorption properties on the stratum corneum under mildly cold conditions

Yao L, Li Y, Gohel MDI, et al (The Hong Kong Polytechnic Univ, Hung Hom, Kowloon)

J Am Acad Dermatol 64:e29-e36, 2011

Background.—The interaction of textiles with the skin is a fertile area for research.

Objective.—The aim of this study was to investigate the effects of clothing fabric on the stratum corneum (SC) under mildly cold conditions.

Methods.—A longitudinal controlled parallel study was designed to investigate the effects of the liquid/moisture absorption properties of pajama fabrics on the SC water content, transepidermal water loss, skin surface acidity (pH), and sebum.

Results.—The hygroscopicity of pajama fabrics had significant associations with the SC water content and transepidermal water loss on the skin of the volunteers' backs. Sebum in the hydrophilic cotton group was slightly lower than in the polyester groups and hydrophobic cotton groups. Subjects felt warmer in the hydrophobic groups than in the hydrophilic groups. The hydrophilicity of the fabric also showed an association with overnight urinary free catecholamines.

Limitations.—In this study, detailed components of sebum were not analyzed.

Conclusions.—The hygroscopicity of the fabric may be a key factor influencing SC hydration during daily wear under mildly cold conditions.

▶ Sauna suits and gloves are often recommended to patients to occlude the skin and to enhance penetration of a topical corticosteroid. This occlusion is reported to result in improved moisturization and increased penetration of topical agents. Therefore, it makes perfect sense that certain pajama fabrics may have a similar effect and improve skin moisturization and affect other skin properties that can affect treatment outcomes.

The objective of this study was to investigate how 4 different pajama fabrics interact with the stratum corneum (SC) and if the hygroscopic properties of pajama fabric would influence skin hydration, acidity, sebum, subjective sensations, including perception of temperature, sleep quality, and the production of urinary catecholamines. The results of this study were determined by corneometer, tewameter, sebumeter, skin pH meter, and high-performance liquid chromatography with electrochemical detection of overnight urinary adrenaline.

The results showed differences in transepidermal water loss (TEWL) and the stratum corneum water content (SCWC) in response to wearing different pajamas. The TEWL in the hydrophobic cotton was higher than in the hydrophilic cotton and polyester groups. SCWC was lower in the hydrophilic polyester group than the hydrophobic and hydrophilic cotton groups. However, it was also determined that there was no significant difference in SCWC and TEWL between the hydrophilic and hydrophobic cotton groups. No significant changes were seen in sebum production, skin acidity, urine catecholamines, or any subjective factors tested except for skin warmth. Subjects felt warmer in the hydrophobic fabrics.

Their conclusion stated simply is that hygroscopic fabrics such as cotton, silk, and wool may possibly help manage dry or atopic skin in the wintertime. This is likely due to an increased water vapor microclimate above the skin secondary to the water-absorbing properties of the pajama fabric. Even though such hygroscopic fabrics appear to be associated with more water loss from the skin, the water absorbed in the microclimate of the skin and pajama fabric allows the constant reabsorption of water by the SC and hence an increased SCWC. If the results of this study hold true, perhaps a new recommendation in the management of atopic dermatitis and xerotic skin will involve wearing hygroscopic fabrics.

Overall, the reporting of the results in this article was confusing. Within the abstract, the results are reported as if they are significant; however, only in the article is it specified that many of the results reported in the abstract are nonsignificant findings. Also, the results of this study were based on an interindividual comparison of skin properties relative to different pajama fabrics. Given the interindividual variation in skin properties from person to person, perhaps a more accurate comparison of pajama fabrics could be made using individual subjects and different fabrics over a series of nights, assessing results with each individual and not among different individuals.

J. Levin, DO

J. Q. Del Rosso, DO

Preventing eczema flares with topical corticosteroids or tacrolimus: which is best?
Williams HC (Queen's Med Centre Univ Hosp NHS Trust, Nottingham, UK)
Br J Dermatol 164:231-233, 2011

Background.—The two treatment approaches currently used for eczema are a reactive mode, in which medication is given as needed during exacerbations in patients with mild disease, and a proactive mode, in which the patient with moderate to severe eczema receives medication to induce a remission, then regular treatments to maintain control. The two medication families used are topical corticosteroids and topical tacrolimus. The effectiveness of these medications in these two modes was the topic of systematic reviews.

Methods.—Four randomized controlled trials (RCTs) comparing topical fluticasone and vehicle were combined in a meta-analysis. A similar RCT investigated topical methylprednisolone aceponate. Three studies of topical tacrolimus versus vehicle were also combined.

Results.—The risk of a future flare was half as much with the topical fluticasone as with the vehicle. The methylprednisolone aceponate was able to reduce the risk of subsequent flares slightly better than the fluticasone did. The combined results for the topical tacrolimus showed that the overall relative reduction in flare risk was less than for the corticosteroids. In addition, there is more clinical experience with corticosteroids than with tacrolimus, and the size of the benefit appears to be greater for the steroids. As yet, tacrolimus does not offer any clinical advantage over corticosteroids for the treatment of eczema, whether in a reactive or a proactive mode of application.

Conclusions.—It is useful to have options for treatment, and tacrolimus offers one the ability to help persons who have not responded to corticosteroids and those who might suffer an adverse reaction to long-term corticosteroid use. The two treatment modes need to be compared directly to yield a better understanding of their merits. This comparison should also address cost-effectiveness and adverse effects for each treatment.

▶ This editorial attempts to answer the question, "What is best for treating flares in patients with atopic eczema, topical corticosteroids (CS) or tacrolimus?" Perhaps the standard of care in treating eczema flares is gentle cleansers, topical CS, emollients, and adjunctive therapies to achieve remission. This would be followed by intermittent topical CS use and/or topical calcineurin inhibitor use for maintenance. Taking into consideration costs, adverse events (short and long term), and effectiveness of treatment, it appears that topical CS therapy with or without intermittent use of topical tacrolimus provides the best chance for obtaining remission.

J. L. Smith, MD

The role of epigenetics in the developmental origins of allergic disease

North ML, Ellis AK (Queen's Univ, Kingston, Ontario, Canada)
Ann Allergy Asthma Immunol 106:355-361, 2011

Objective.—To review current research findings in the field of epigenetics pertaining to the developmental origins of allergic disease.

Data Sources.—We examined original research and review articles identified from MEDLINE, OVID, and PubMed that addressed the topic of interest, using the search terms *atopy, allergy, asthma, development, IgE, origins,* and *cord blood* paired with *epigenetic(s).* Relevant references from each article were also procured for review.

Study Selection.—Articles were selected based on their relevance to the contributory role of epigenetic modifications in asthma and other atopic diseases.

Results.—There is increasing evidence pointing to the influence of prenatal and early life exposures on the development of allergic disease. A growing body of literature supports the theory that transient environmental pressures can have permanent effects on gene regulation and expression through epigenetic mechanisms. Histone modifications have been associated with degree of bronchial hyperresponsiveness and corticosteroid resistance in asthma. Epigenetic mechanisms can operate independently in various cell types; recent studies have suggested a role in the differentiation of human T cells. Murine studies have revealed that a maternal diet rich in methyl donors can enhance susceptibility to allergic inflammation in the offspring, mediated through increased DNA methylation. Murine studies have also implicated epigenetically modified dendritic cells in the transmission of allergic risk from mothers to offspring.

Conclusion.—The current literature offers exciting data to support a role for epigenetics in the development and persistence of asthma and allergic rhinitis. However, further human studies are necessary to explore these mechanisms and assess future clinical applicability.

▶ Past research has shown that allergic diseases and asthma have been associated with a genetic predisposition and environmental triggers. Epigenetics is an emerging field of study that has started to play a role in explaining key gene-environment interactions. This is a literature review of the various roles that epigenetics play in fetal development. The epigenetic code is established during development, and changes that occur in specific cell types in response to the environment play a role in the emergence of allergies and asthma. An example of epigenetics is the imprinting process by which a gene from one parent is suppressed through DNA methylation and histone alterations. Epigenetics has been demonstrated in mouse models, where maternal nutrition significantly shifts the phenotypes of offspring. Authors also suggest that there is likely a window of vulnerability during the prenatal period when environmental influences lead to changes to the epigenetic code. Also, studies have revealed a potential risk for routine folic acid supplementation and the increased risk of allergic airway disease. Although there are many studies demonstrating the effects of epigenetics in animal models, evidence in humans is limited at present. However, to date, there is evidence demonstrating histone acetylation/deacetylation and its role in asthma and COPD. Further studies are clearly needed to determine the specific disease processes mediated by epigenetic modifications.

G. K. Kim, DO

J. Q. Del Rosso, DO

Utility of routine laboratory testing in management of chronic urticaria/ angioedema

Tarbox JA, Gutta RC, Radojicic C, et al (Cleveland Clinic Foundation, OH)
Ann Allergy Asthma Immunol 107:239-243, 2011

Background.—Laboratory tests are routinely ordered to identify or rule out a cause in patients with chronic urticaria/angioedema (CUA). The results of these tests are usually within normal limits or unremarkable.

Objective.—To investigate the proportion of abnormal test results in patients with CUA leading to a change in management and in outcomes of care.

Methods.—Retrospective analysis of a random sample of adult patients with CUA from 2001–2009.

Results.—Cases totaled 356:166 with urticaria and angioedema (AE), 187 with urticaria, and 3 with only AE. Patients were predominately women (69.1%) and white (75.6%), with a mean age of 48 ± 15 years. Abnormalities were commonly seen in complete blood counts (34%) and in complete metabolic panels (9.4%). Among the 1,872 tests that were ordered, results of 319 (17%) were abnormal. Of 356 patients, 30 underwent further testing because of abnormalities in laboratory work. This represented 30 of 1,872 tests (1.60%). Only 1 patient benefited from a subsequent change in management.

Conclusions.—Laboratory testing in CUA patients referred for an allergy and immunology evaluation rarely lead to changes in management resulting in improved outcomes of care.

▶ Trying to find the etiology of chronic urticaria/angioedema (CU/AE) is usually a fruitless effort. In most cases, the cause is not determined even with laboratory evaluation. This study evaluated the utility of routine laboratory testing in patients with CU/AE. There were 356 patients evaluated with CU and/or AE, 166 with CU/AE, 187 with CU, and 3 with AE. Among these patients, 1872 laboratory tests were obtained. There was a 17% rate of abnormal laboratory test results, but this finding was not necessarily relevant and did not lead to any changes in management or beneficial outcome. There was only 1 case in which laboratory findings lead to improved outcome. The authors in this study advocate reassuring the patient and limiting laboratory evaluation to a more cost-effective strategy, unless the history or physical examination directs the need for specific tests. The authors also recommend prescribing up to 4 times the conventional dose of a second-generation agent for at least 4 weeks as a reasonable treatment approach because not all patients with CU respond to conventional doses. Among the 30 patients who required additional workup for laboratory abnormalities, 29 were able to achieve control of their symptoms on H1 and H2 antihistamines. There were some limitations related to this study. Patients with C1-inhibitor deficiency syndrome were excluded. Patients whose laboratory testing was performed before being consulted were excluded from this study, and results may therefore be biased. Also, laboratory tests were limited in that only selected tests were performed and an unknown underlying systemic condition may have been missed. However, researchers concluded that routine laboratory exams are of low yield and a more cost-effective way is to reassure patients that the majority of CU/AE cases are unrelated to an underlying condition.

G. K. Kim, DO
J. Q. Del Rosso, DO

2 Psoriasis and Other Papulosquamous Disorders

Adalimumab for moderate to severe chronic plaque psoriasis: efficacy and safety of retreatment and disease recurrence following withdrawal from therapy
Papp K, Crowley J, Ortonne J-P, et al (Probity Med Res, Waterloo, Ontario, Canada; Bakersfield Dermatology, CA; Nice Univ Hosp, France; et al)
Br J Dermatol 164:434-441, 2011

Background.—Adalimumab is effective for moderate to severe chronic plaque psoriasis; however, data regarding retreatment following withdrawal and subsequent relapse are limited.

Objectives.—To evaluate the efficacy and safety of adalimumab if interrupted and then resumed in patients with moderate to severe psoriasis.

Methods.—Patients in a long-term adalimumab open-label extension study (NCT00195676) who achieved a Physician's Global Assessment (PGA) score of 'Mild' (2), 'Minimal' (1) or 'Clear' (0) were withdrawn from adalimumab and monitored for relapse to PGA of 'Moderate' (3) or worse. The subgroup of interest had stable psoriasis control, defined as PGA of 0/1 for ≥12 weeks on every other week (eow) dosing before withdrawal. Relapsing patients were retreated with adalimumab (80 mg at week 0 and 40 mg eow starting at week 1). PGA, Psoriasis Area and Severity Index responses, fatigue, pharmacokinetics and immunogenicity were assessed.

Results.—In total, 525 patients were withdrawn from adalimumab; the subgroup with stable psoriasis control comprised 285 patients. Of these, 178 relapsed (median = 141 days) before treatment reinitiation and 107 did not relapse. Patients without relapse by 40 weeks off therapy reinitiated adalimumab. Rates of PGA 0/1 after 16 weeks of adalimumab retreatment were 89% for patients without relapse and 69% for patients who relapsed. Relapsers experienced significantly less fatigue after retreatment. Nine patients (3%) had serious adverse events (two were infections). No rebound or allergic reactions occurred.

Conclusions.—Adalimumab-treated patients who discontinued therapy and subsequently relapsed had a good likelihood of regaining clinical efficacy following adalimumab reinitiation.

▶ We generally regard continuous therapy as the paradigm for the use of biological therapies. However, patients on these agents for psoriasis often discontinue therapy for multiple reasons. These include the occurrence of infections, voluntary drug holidays, or changes in insurance coverage. Patients may stop therapies for short periods or extended amounts of time. Therefore, it is important for clinicians to know whether retreatment with the same biological agent will be effective after such a withdrawal from therapy. For adalimumab, this study demonstrates that most patients are able to recapture efficacy in this setting. For patients without relapse, rates of Physician's Global Assessment (PGA) 0/1 after 16 weeks of adalimumab retreatment were 89%; rates of PGA 0/1 were 69% for individuals who experienced relapse. In addition, relapsers experienced significantly less fatigue after retreatment. These data provide important insight into the appropriate management of patients on adalimumab.

J. Weinberg, MD

The Impact of Methodological Approaches for Presenting Long-Term Clinical Data on Estimates of Efficacy in Psoriasis Illustrated by Three-Year Treatment Data on Infliximab
Papoutsaki M, Talamonti M, Giunta A, et al (A. Sygros Hosp, Athens, Greece; Univ of Rome Tor Vergata, Italy)
Dermatology 221:43-47, 2010

Background.—Psoriasis affects about 2–3% of the Caucasian population. Biologics such as infliximab, etanercept, adalimumab and ustekinumab are efficacious treatments of plaque-type psoriasis. Critical to monitoring drug efficacy and safety is availability of long-term data. Despite the chronic nature of psoriasis, to date limited long-term clinical data have been available, as challenges are inherent in conducting a long-term analysis. With increasing time, it is more likely that the number of patients discontinuing treatment will also increase, due to loss of efficacy, adverse events or loss to follow-up. Interpretation of these data becomes confounded when one must consider missing data. Several approaches to analysing long-term data exist, and each accounts for missing data differently.

Objective.—To demonstrate that the choice of a particular analysis method to account for missing data has great impact on the assessed response rate.

Methods.—We used data from an open-label study over 3 years of continuous treatment with infliximab in patients with plaque-type psoriasis. These data were analysed by three methods—last observation carried forward, observed values and non-responder imputation—to account for missing data.

Results.—The 3-year PASI 75 responses varied from 41 to 75%, depending on the method of analysis; this shows that the response rate can almost double when a more liberal analytical approach is used.

Conclusions.—While it is clear that the need for long-term data on biologics in psoriasis is great, considering the analysis undertaken is important when designing long-term studies and interpreting the resulting data. When analysis methods such as observed values only or last observation carried forward are used, the results of the more conservative nonresponder imputation should also be presented to give a fair overview of the long-term efficacy of a treatment for plaque-type psoriasis.

▶ The authors of this article used data from a 3-year, open-label trial of infliximab for psoriasis to demonstrate how variable the results are when different methods are used to analyze response rates. Three methods were used: (1) nonresponder imputation assumes that subjects who have dropped out of the study or have been lost to follow-up are nonresponders; (2) observed values analysis only includes those subjects who remain in the study, ignoring those who have discontinued; and (3) last observation carried forward assigns the same improvement scores as occurred at the last observed visit or patients who are lost to follow-up. The nonresponder imputation is the most conservative method because even patients who have left the study for reasons other than nonresponse (such as subjects who moved away from the study center) are considered treatment failures. The observed values analysis is much more favorable to the study drug because individuals who may have discontinued the study because of inadequate response or who dropped out because of side effects simply won't be counted. The last observation carried forward analysis can be the most liberal of all because a patient who responded at one point and then didn't return because of inadequate response would be incorrectly counted as a responder.

Using the 3 methods of analysis, the Psoriasis Area Severity Index-75 response rate at 3 years was 41.2% using a nonresponder imputation analysis, 65.6% using last observation carried forward analysis, and 75.0% using the observed values analysis. Given the variability in these results, the authors advocate that the more conservative nonresponder imputation data be presented when results using the other analyses are given.

The findings presented in this article are not surprising. The educational value of looking at studies critically using different analytical methods cannot be overemphasized.

M. Lebwohl, MD

Efficacy and safety of ABT-874, a monoclonal anti–interleukin 12/23 antibody, for the treatment of chronic plaque psoriasis: 36-week observation/ retreatment and 60-week open-label extension phases of a randomized phase II trial

Kimball AB, Gordon KB, Langley RG, et al (Massachusetts General Hosp, Boston; NorthShore Univ HealthSystem and the Univ of Chicago, IL; Dalhousie Univ, Halifax, Nova Scotia, Canada; et al)
J Am Acad Dermatol 64:263-274, 2011

Background.—ABT-874, an anti–interleukin-12 and -23 antibody, was previously shown to be significantly more effective compared with placebo during a 12-week phase II study of psoriasis. We report here safety and efficacy data of ABT-874 during subsequent phases of this study.

Objective.—We sought to examine the preliminary efficacy and safety of ABT-874 for moderate to severe psoriasis beyond 12 weeks.

Methods.—Patients with chronic plaque psoriasis who responded to ABT-874 during the initial randomized, placebo-controlled, 12-week study phase were eligible for a 36-week observation/retreatment phase. During the subsequent 60-week, open-label extension phase, eligible patients were retreated with one of two ABT-874 dosages. Efficacy was measured using Psoriasis Area and Severity Index and physician global assessment scores; safety was monitored by adverse events (AEs), laboratory parameters, and vital signs.

Results.—During the observation/retreatment phase, 130 of 180 patients were eligible for retreatment. After 12-week retreatment with ABT-874, 55% to 94% of retreated patients (n = 58) achieved a 75% or greater reduction in Psoriasis Area and Severity Index score. Among patients receiving ABT-874 through the first 48 weeks, there were no deaths and 4 patients with serious AEs; one patient discontinued because of an AE. During the open-label extension (N = 105), there were no deaths or serious infections, and 3 serious AEs.

Limitations.—Lack of placebo or active comparator groups limited statistical analysis in later study phases. Dosing differences existed between groups, and only week-12 responders were eligible for retreatment.

Conclusion.—ABT-874 continued to show good efficacy and safety during withdrawal and reinitiation of therapy.

▶ Interleukin (IL)-23 has recently emerged as a key cytokine in the development of psoriasis. Antibodies directed against the p40 subunit of IL-12 and IL-23 have been used successfully to treat chronic plaque psoriasis (CPP). Ustekinumab is currently marketed for the treatment of CPP, and a second drug, briakinumab, has also demonstrated efficacy. In an initial 12-week placebo-controlled trial of ABT-874 (now called briakinumab) with dose-ranging evaluation, the drug was found to be dramatically effective for the treatment of plaque psoriasis. Of the 180 patients initially treated in that study, 130 who achieved at least Psoriasis Area and Severity Index score (PASI) 75 were entered into a 36-week observation/retreatment phase. Fifty-eight of 130 patients lost their PASI 50 response and were retreated. Of the 120 patients who lost their PASI 75 response, the time to loss of response ranged from 57 to 184 days. Among the retreated patients, the percentage of patients who achieved PASI 75 responses at 12 weeks ranged from 54.5% for those who received a single 200 mg dose up to 93.8% for those who were retreated with 100 mg every other week. One hundred five of the patients achieved PASI 75 and were eligible to enter a 60-week open-label extension phase of this study. In that phase, patients were retreated upon loss of response below PASI 50. Ninety-six of the 105 patients were retreated from 1 to 5 times, and only 9 patients never lost PASI 50 response and therefore did not require retreatment. The proportion of patients who achieved PASI 75 with the first and second retreatment was approximately 50% but fell with subsequent treatments. With the third retreatment, only approximately 25% of patients achieved PASI 75. There was also an increase in patients with anti-ABT-874 antibodies after repeated treatments.

In summary, a high proportion of patients responded to initial treatment with ABT-874 and responses were sustained. With 1 or 2 retreatments, there continued to be good responses, but the proportion of patients who achieved PASI 75 diminished with subsequent retreatments.

M. Lebwohl, MD

Adalimumab for Treatment of Moderate to Severe Chronic Plaque Psoriasis of the Hands and Feet: Efficacy and Safety Results From REACH, a Randomized, Placebo-Controlled, Double-Blind Trial
Leonardi C, Langley RG, Papp K, et al (Central Dermatology, St Louis, MO; Dalhousie Univ, Halifax, Nova Scotia, Canada; Probity Med Res, Waterloo, Ontario, Canada; et al)
Arch Dermatol 147:429-436, 2011

Objective.—To determine the efficacy, safety, and sustainability of response to adalimumab therapy for moderate to severe chronic plaque psoriasis involving hands and/or feet.

Design.—Sixteen-week, randomized, double-blind, placebo-controlled evaluation of adalimumab therapy for moderate to severe chronic plaque psoriasis involving the hands and/or feet with a 12-week open-label extension (Randomized Controlled Evaluation of Adalimumab in Treatment of Chronic Plaque Psoriasis of the Hands and Feet [REACH]).

Setting.—Multicenter outpatient study in the United States and Canada.

Participants.—Patients with chronic plaque psoriasis on the hands and/or feet with a Physician's Global Assessment of hands and/or feet (hfPGA) score of "moderate" or above.

Intervention.—Patients were randomized 2:1 to adalimumab (80 mg at week 0, then 40 mg every other week starting at week 1) or to matching placebo.

Main Outcome Measure.—Percentage of patients achieving an hfPGA score of "clear" or "almost clear" at week 16.

Results.—Seventy-two patients (adalimumab [n = 49]; placebo [n = 23]) were evaluated. Baseline percentages of patients with moderate and severe hfPGA scores were 76% and 24%, respectively, for the adalimumab group and 74% and 26%, respectively, for the placebo group. At week 16, 31% and 4% of patients randomized to adalimumab and placebo, respectively, achieved an hfPGA score of clear or almost clear ($P = .01$). At week 28, 80% of the hfPGA clear or almost clear response was maintained from week 16 (25% for patients randomized to adalimumab). Adverse events in both groups were generally mild to moderate. In both periods combined, nasopharyngitis (27% and 13% for adalimumab- and placebo-treated patients, respectively) was most frequently reported.

Conclusion.—Adalimumab is efficacious and well tolerated for treatment of chronic plaque psoriasis of hands and/or feet, with efficacy largely maintained to 28 weeks.

Trial Registration.—clinicaltrials.gov Identifier: NCT00735787.

▶ Chronic plaque psoriasis of the hands and feet can certainly be a problematic disease state for patients in multiple ways, including its effect on quality of life, function, and in terms of the available treatment options, as many are often unsatisfactory. In this recent article, Leonardi et al report the results of a multicenter outpatient REACH trial (Randomized controlled Evaluation of Adalimumab in treatment of Chronic plaque psoriasis of the Hands and feet). The trial sought not only to determine the efficacy and safety of adalimumab therapy in the treating moderate to severe chronic plaque psoriasis of the hands and feet, but also if this therapy could obtain a sustained response. The study was divided into 2 parts: (1) a placebo-controlled period for weeks 0 through 16 that included 72 patients, 49 that were randomly assigned to adalimumab (of which 41 completed) and 23 randomly assigned to placebo (of which 18 of these patients completed) and (2) an extension period (weeks 17–28), of which 40 of the patients in the adalimumab group completed, and 13 of the patients in the placebo group completed. Thus, one limitation of the study was that 19 of the patients did not complete the entire trial, resulting in a relatively small number of study participants. Despite this limitation, the results of the study were reasonably encouraging. Of the patients with moderate to severe chronic plaque psoriasis of the hands and feet, 31% were found to have achieved a Physician's Global Assessment score of clear to almost clear at week 16 (vs 4% in the placebo group). And of these patients, 80% maintained this response of clear to almost clear at week 28. Study exclusion criteria included psoralen and ultraviolet A (UVA) phototherapy within 4 weeks, use of topical therapies (except class VI and VII topical corticosteroids), and UVB phototherapy and excessive sun tanning or tanning bed use within 2 weeks of the study.

It is arguable that concomitant use of these additional therapies may have improved the efficacy results. Beyond efficacy and a sustainable response, the majority of adverse effects reported were mild to moderate in severity, with nasopharyngitis the most commonly reported event. As noted in the article, there were no reported cases of death, serious infection, demyelinating disease, lupus-like syndrome, lymphoma, or nonmelanoma skin cancer. Thus, based on the findings in this study, adalimumab was shown to be a useful alternative agent in the treatment of moderate to severe chronic plaque psoriasis of the hands and feet and one that should at least be considered in the treatment armamentarium for those patients who are deemed appropriate for systemic therapy.

B. D. Michaels, DO

J. Q. Del Rosso, DO

Acute respiratory distress syndrome complicating generalized pustular psoriasis (psoriasis-associated aseptic pneumonitis)

Kluger N, Bessis D, Guillot B, et al (Hôpital Saint-Eloi, Montpellier, France)
J Am Acad Dermatol 64:1154-1158, 2011

Generalized pustular and/or erythrodermic psoriasis may have severe or even lethal complications. A peculiar noninfectious acute respiratory distress syndrome (so-called "sterile pneumonitis") has been described in generalized pustular psoriasis and/or erythrodermic psoriasis. We report a new case in a 14-year-old girl with a long history of pustular psoriasis and review the published work on this complication. The girl developed sterile pneumonitis during a disease flare-up, and high-dose corticosteroid therapy was quickly initiated. Within a few days, her clinical and radiological status was dramatically improved. The pathogenesis of aseptic pneumonitis is unknown, but various proinflammatory cytokines have been implicated, especially tumor necrosis factor-alpha, which could play a role in the recruitment of leukocytes to the lung. This complication has rarely been reported but should be more widely known as the differential diagnoses include congestive heart failure, acute lung infection related or unrelated to immunosuppressive therapy, and drug hypersensitivity reaction. Early recognition would avoid delays in the correct management of this potentially lethal complication, which requires high-dose systemic corticosteroid therapy.

▶ "Sterile pneumonitis," an unusual noninfectious form of acute respiratory distress syndrome (ARDS), has been described in generalized pustular psoriasis and erythrodermic psoriasis. Early diagnosis can ensure that this potentially lethal complication is correctly managed. This is a case report of a 14-year-old girl who was admitted with an exacerbation of pustular psoriasis and erythroderma. She had a previous history of generalized pustular psoriasis triggered by oropharyngeal or ear infections. The patient was hospitalized in June 2009 for hyperthermia with painful extensive pustular plaques. She developed deterioration of pulmonary function with polypnea and arterial hypoxia in the context of apyrexia. Chest x-ray and computerized tomographic (CT) scanning showed bilateral alveolar condensation of the upper lobes and mild right-sided pleurisy as well as enlarged axillary and mediastinal lymph nodes. Skin, blood, and pharynx cultures were all negative for bacteria or viral infection. Sputum culture was not performed because of absence of a productive cough. The patient was treated with intravenous pulsed corticosteroid therapy with a combination of antibiotics. The diagnosis of ARDS was made. Drug-induced hypersensitivity was also considered in the diagnosis. Methotrexate hypersensitivity was considered, but no circulating eosinophilia was observed. This case report illustrates marked improvement with intravenous corticosteroid therapy with a follow-up chest CT showing disappearance of alveolar condensation within 72 hours of initiation of therapy. The pathophysiology of this disease is unknown, and more research is needed to provide appropriate guidelines on diagnosis and treatment of this potentially lethal complication of psoriasis. Diagnostic accuracy is especially important, as use of systemic corticosteroid therapy in psoriasis is fraught with the potential for a diffuse pustular eruption.

G. K. Kim, DO

J. Q. Del Rosso, DO

Efficacy of psoralen plus ultraviolet A therapy vs. biologics in moderate to severe chronic plaque psoriasis: retrospective data analysis of a patient registry

Inzinger M, Heschl B, Weger W, et al (Med Univ of Graz, Austria)
Br J Dermatol 165:640-645, 2011

Background.—Few studies have directly compared the clinical efficacy of psoralen plus ultraviolet A (PUVA) vs. biologics in the treatment of psoriasis.

Objectives.—To compare the clinical efficacy of PUVA and biologic therapies for psoriasis under daily life conditions.

Methods.—Data from a psoriasis registry (http://www.psoriasis-therapie register.at) of 172 adult patients with moderate to severe chronic plaque psoriasis treated between 2003 and 2010 were analysed retrospectively. These patients had received oral PUVA [118 treatment courses including 5-methoxypsoralen (5-MOP; $n = 32$) and 8-methoxypsoralen (8-MOP; $n = 86$)] and/or biologic agents [130 treatment courses including adalimumab ($n = 18$), alefacept ($n = 32$), efalizumab ($n = 17$), etanercept ($n = 38$), infliximab ($n = 7$) and ustekinumab ($n = 18$)]. Treatment responses were analysed in terms of Psoriasis Area and Severity Index (PASI) improvement, including complete remission (CR) and reduction of PASI by at least 90% (PASI 90) or 75% (PASI 75), at treatment completion for PUVA (median time 10·3 and 9·2 weeks, for 8-MOP and 5-MOP, respectively) and at week 12 for biologics.

Results.—Intention-to-treat—as observed CR, PASI 90 and PASI 75 rate was 22%, 69% and 86% for PUVA compared with 6%, 22% and 56% for adalimumab ($P = 0·0034$ by adapted Wilcoxon test), 3%, 3% and 25% for alefacept ($P = 0·000000002$), 6%, 6% and 59% for efalizumab ($P = 0·000053$), 6%, 29% and 39% for etanercept ($P = 0·0000086$), 29%, 71% and 100% for infliximab ($P = 0·36$) and 6%, 39% and 67% for ustekinumab ($P = 0·028$). When applying a more conservative *post-hoc* modified worst-case scenario analysis, with CR of 15%, PASI 90 of

58% and PASI 75 of 69%, PUVA was superior only to alefacept $(P = 0 \cdot 000013)$, efalizumab $(P = 0 \cdot 015)$ and etanercept $(P = 0 \cdot 0037)$. There were no statistically significant differences in PASI reduction rates between PUVA and infliximab.

Conclusions.—Retrospective analysis of registry data revealed that the primary efficacy of PUVA was superior to that of certain biologics. Prospective head-to-head studies of PUVA and biologics are warranted to confirm these observations.

▶ After 30 years of performing phototherapy, I have found that psoralen + ultraviolet A light (PUVA), and especially oral retinoid + PUVA (re-PUVA) is far superior to the current array of biologics for the treatment of psoriasis vulgaris. Clinical studies in independent centers have corroborated this observation. Those with fair skin types I and II experience more of the side effects of therapy than do those with skin types III, IV, and V. Perhaps it would be better to consider restricting PUVA therapy to individuals with the darker skin types. Even under these circumstances, this therapy should be limited when the skin shows signs of being compromised. It is also important to remember that PUVA is a potential carcinogen in all patients. Likewise, there are risks to taking biologics. Many of these risks are clear, but many of these agents are relatively new and lacking long-term side effect data. This article is a good reminder that PUVA, and especially re-PUVA, has a place in the treatment of patients with severe psoriasis.

E. A. Tanghetti, MD

Guidelines of care for the management of psoriasis and psoriatic arthritis: Section 6. Guidelines of care for the treatment of psoriasis and psoriatic arthritis: Case-based presentations and evidence-based conclusions
Menter A, Korman NJ, Elmets CA, et al (Baylor Univ Med Ctr, Dallas; Univ Hosps Case Med Ctr, Cleveland, OH; Univ of Alabama at Birmingham; et al)
J Am Acad Dermatol 65:137-174, 2011

Psoriasis is a common, chronic, inflammatory, multisystem disease with predominantly skin and joint manifestations affecting approximately 2% of the population. In the first 5 parts of the American Academy of Dermatology Psoriasis Guidelines of Care, we have presented evidence supporting the use of topical treatments, phototherapy, traditional systemic agents, and biological therapies for patients with psoriasis and psoriatic arthritis. In this sixth and final section of the Psoriasis Guidelines of Care, we will present cases to illustrate how to practically use these guidelines in specific clinical scenarios. We will describe the approach to treating patients with psoriasis across the entire spectrum of this fascinating disease from mild to moderate to severe, with and without psoriatic arthritis, based on the 5 prior published guidelines. Although specific therapeutic recommendations are given for each of the cases presented, it is important that treatment be tailored to meet individual patients' needs. In addition, we will update the prior 5 guidelines and address gaps in research and care that currently exist, while making suggestions for further studies that could be performed to help address these limitations in our knowledge base.

▶ Psoriasis is a chronic disease with multiple modalities of treatment depending on the extent and involvement. The American Academy of Dermatology has previously published 5 parts of the *Psoriasis Guidelines of Care*, and this review is its sixth and final section. This current guideline section is a thorough evaluation of psoriasis treatment applications that is particularly useful for practitioners. Namely, it provides a comprehensive approach to treatment based on the level of psoriatic disease involvement—from the treatment of limited disease to moderate and severe disease, as well as for patients who present with psoriatic arthritis. In addition, it provides specific clinical case scenarios for help in understanding the appropriate treatment applications for a particular patient. For example, clinical case scenarios are presented followed by a thorough discussion regarding the pros and cons and considerations of a particular treatment for each patient that is presented. Treatment algorithms are also provided throughout the text that can be of further benefit to the practitioner. Given the breadth of information in the article and its particular attention to the clinical application of the information, this guideline section (number 6 of 6 total sections) provides essential material for review by all practitioners who treat psoriasis and psoriatic arthritis in addition to being a great resource tool for clinicians.

B. D. Michaels, DO
J. Q. Del Rosso, DO

Long-term etanercept in pediatric patients with plaque psoriasis
Paller AS, Siegfried EC, Eichenfield LF, et al (Northwestern Univ Med School, Chicago, IL; Saint Louis Univ, MO; Univ of California, San Diego; et al)
J Am Acad Dermatol 63:762-768, 2010

Background.—No systemic therapies are approved by the US Food and Drug Administration for the treatment of psoriasis in children and adolescents.

Objective.—We sought to evaluate the long-term safety and efficacy of etanercept in pediatric patients (aged 4-17 years) with moderate to severe plaque psoriasis.

Methods.—Patients who completed or received substantial treatment benefit in a 48-week, randomized, double-blind, placebo-controlled study (N = 211) evaluating the efficacy and safety of once-weekly etanercept (0.8 mg/kg) were enrolled in this 264-week open-label extension study. The primary end point was the occurrence of adverse events. Secondary end points included Psoriasis Area and Severity Index 50%, 75%, and 90% responses compared with baseline; static Physician Global Assessment;

and clear and clear/almost clear static Physician Global Assessment status. Results from a 96-week interim analysis are presented.

Results.—Of 182 enrolled patients, 181 received treatment and 140 (76.9%) completed week 96. A total of 145 patients (80.1%) reported adverse events; 5 serious adverse events occurred in 3 patients, none of which were treatment related. Observed Psoriasis Area and Severity Index 50% (89%), 75% (61%), and 90% (30%) responses compared with baseline at week 96 were similar to those observed in the double-blind trial. The static Physician Global Assessment was maintained through week 96, when 47% of patients achieved clear/almost clear status.

Limitations.—This is an interim analysis from an open-label study.

Conclusion.—Extended treatment with etanercept in pediatric patients with moderate to severe plaque psoriasis was generally well tolerated, and efficacy was maintained through 96 weeks.

▶ In 2008, Paller et al published the results of a double-blind, placebo-controlled trial of etanercept in the treatment of plaque psoriasis in pediatric patients.[1] A 5-year, open-label extension study was continued, and the data presented in this article represents the 96-week interim analysis.

In the original trial, patients ages 4 to 17 years were treated with weekly etanercept at a dose of 0.8 mg/kg with a maximum dose of 50 mg weekly. Psoriasis Area Severity Index (PASI) 50, 75, and 90 responses were reported using observed case analysis, last observation carried forward imputation for missing values, and treatment failure imputation for missing values. Of 182 enrolled patients, 181 were treated and 140 completed through week 96. Using observed case analysis, PASI 50, 75, and 90 response rates at week 96 were 89%, 61%, and 30%, respectively. Using last observation carried forward imputation, the response rates were 85%, 58%, and 29%. And using treatment failure imputation, the corresponding PASI response rates were 68%, 46%, and 23%. Static Physician Global Assessments (SPGA) were also performed, and by the 3 analysis methods, 47%, 48%, and 36% of patients were clear or almost clear at week 96 using last observation carried forward imputation, and treatment failure imputation, respectively. There were 5 serious adverse events in 3 patients, and none were attributed to treatment.

Despite these impressive 2-year results and the recommendation of a US Food and Drug Administration Panel to approve etanercept for the treatment of psoriasis in pediatric patients, the FDA requested so much additional information from the makers of etanercept that the sponsor withdrew the application for approval. Unfortunately, it is unlikely we will ever see the approval of etanercept for psoriasis in pediatric patients, and this is likely to have a negative affect on any pharmaceutical company's attempt to pursue a biologic therapy for psoriasis in children.

M. Lebwohl, MD

Reference

1. Paller AS, Siegfried EC, Langley RG, et al. Etanercept treatment for children and adolescents with plaque psoriasis. *N Engl J Med.* 2008;358:241-251.

Intermittent etanercept therapy in pediatric patients with psoriasis

Siegfried EC, Eichenfield LF, Paller AS, et al (Cardinal Glennon Children's Hosp and Saint Louis Univ, MO; Rady Children's Hosp and Univ of California, San Diego; Children's Memorial Hosp and Northwestern Univ Med School, Chicago, IL; et al)
J Am Acad Dermatol 63:769-774, 2010

Background.—Stopping and restarting etanercept is well tolerated in adult psoriasis, but little is known about intermittent use in pediatric psoriasis.

Objective.—We sought to assess safety and efficacy of etanercept administered intermittently in children with psoriasis.

Methods.—At study entry, patients were 4 to 17 years old with moderate to severe stable plaque psoriasis (Psoriasis Area and Severity Index [PASI] score $\geq$ 12). After an initial 12-week, double-blind period and a 24-week, open-label period, eligible patients (ie, achieved 75% improvement in PASI response from baseline [PASI 75]) were re-randomized to a 12-week, double-blind withdrawal-retreatment period: patients received placebo (withdrawal) or etanercept as long as they maintained PASI 75; otherwise, they were retreated with open-label etanercept (retreatment).

Results.—The 138 patients who entered the withdrawal-retreatment period were re-randomized equally between placebo and etanercept. In the group treated with blinded or open-label etanercept, 52 of 65 (80%; observed data) patients maintained or regained PASI 75 at the end of the 12-week period. In all, 45 of 64 (70%) patients on blinded etanercept maintained PASI 75 at every study visit during the 12-week period, compared with 35 of 65 (54%) patients who did so on blinded placebo. No patient had a serious adverse event, serious infection, or withdrew from study because of an adverse event.

Limitations.—Small study and short observation period are limitations.

Conclusion.—During the final 12-week withdrawal-retreatment period of this 48-week study, intermittent etanercept therapy appeared safe, with no patients experiencing a serious adverse event or serious infection, and effective, with 80% of patients on etanercept maintaining or regaining PASI 75 at the end of the 12-week period.

▶ Psoriasis is commonly a chronic disease that requires continuous treatment. However, for some patients, it is characterized by more extended periods of remission and intermittent relapse. In the clinical setting, interruption of therapy may occur for reasons such as disease remission, discontinuation of insurance coverage, cost-effectiveness, concurrent disease, intercurrent illness, or preparation for surgery. The risks involved in stopping and restarting therapy are relapse, rebound, or tachyphylaxis and inability to regain efficacy.

Etanercept is a soluble tumor necrosis factor (TNF) receptor fusion protein that is an antagonist of endogenous TNF. It is FDA approved to treat adults with moderate to severe plaque psoriasis and children aged 4 years and more with polyarticular juvenile rheumatoid arthritis. Etanercept administered once weekly has been reported previously in a randomized, double-blinded, placebo-controlled trial to be safe and to significantly reduce disease severity in children and adolescents with moderate to severe plaque psoriasis. Stopping and restarting etanercept therapy in adults has been demonstrated to be well tolerated, and this study is the first to report on the stopping and restarting of etanercept in pediatric patients with psoriasis.

In this study, patients who initially responded to etanercept therapy were then rerandomized to a new study in which half received a placebo (withdrawal phase) and half received the active drug for 12 weeks. In 85% of the patients during the withdrawal phase, Psoriasis Area and Severity Index 75 (PASI 75) was maintained with no occurrence of rebound past baseline disease. This demonstrates that a majority of pediatric patients in whom etanercept is stopped may experience continued control of psoriasis and that stopping therapy is not associated with severe flares or conversion of psoriasis morphology. Of the patients who stopped therapy and required retreatment, 36% regained PASI 75 within 4 to 8 weeks. This rate is similar to that seen in the initial treatment phase of the study, showing that reinitiation of therapy regains control of the disease without tachyphylaxis or the inability to regain efficacy. Of the patients rerandomized to etanercept, 80% had maintained or achieved PASI 75 at week 48, demonstrating that etanercept can remain efficacious for at least up to 1 year. In addition, no patient discontinued the study because of an adverse event or infection, and no serious adverse effects were reported during this period.

Although the study's limitations include a small number of subjects and a short observation period, it demonstrates that intermittent therapy with etanercept in pediatric patients with moderate to severe plaque psoriasis is safe, well tolerated, and efficacious. This may prove to be a cost-effective therapeutic option compared with nonsystemic therapy for the group of patients with moderate to severe plaque psoriasis.

M. Caglia, MD

S. Friedlander, MD

Psoriasis and melanocytic naevi: does the first confer a protective role against melanocyte progression to naevi?
Balato N, Di Costanzo L, Balato A, et al (Università di Napoli Federico II, Naples, Italy)
Br J Dermatol 164:1262-1270, 2011

Background.—Some of the cytokines that have effects on melanogenesis are also reported to be involved in psoriasis.

Objectives.—We therefore studied the relationship between psoriasis and melanocytic naevi. In particular, the aim of our study was to investigate the number of melanocytic naevi in patients with psoriasis vs. controls.

Methods.—We performed a prospective case–control study, analysing 93 adult patients with psoriasis and 174 adult aged-matched controls. For each participant a questionnaire was completed to establish personal data, personal medical history, and personal and familial history of skin cancer and psoriasis. We analysed interleukin (IL)-1α, IL-6 and tumour necrosis factor (TNF)-α gene expression at the peripheral blood mononuclear cell level in patients with psoriasis and in controls.

Results.—In our study, patients with psoriasis presented a lower number of areas with naevi in comparison with controls ($P < 0.0001$). Nobody had ever had squamous cell carcinoma or melanoma in the psoriatic group; moreover, there was a significant difference in familial history of melanoma between the two groups (none in the psoriatic group vs. 8% in the control group; $P < 0.05$). IL-1α, IL-6 and TNF-α expression levels were higher in patients with psoriasis.

Conclusions.—People with psoriasis had fewer melanocytic naevi. This suggests that the proinflammatory cytokine network in psoriasis skin might inhibit melanogenesis, melanocyte growth and/or progression to naevi.

▶ Psoriasis is a disease that results in an inflammatory mediator soup including cytokines, chemokines, and growth factors. The authors in this study prospectively examined inflammatory cytokines may be linked to a decrease in nevi. This study analyzed the frequency and the distribution of nevi in 93 adult patients with psoriasis and 174 age-matched controls. The psoriasis group had a lower number of areas with nevi in comparison with the control group ($P < .0001$). Ten of 93 patients (11%) with psoriasis had at least 1 lesion clinically diagnosed as a congenital nevus compared with 28 of 174 (16%) in the control group ($P < .01$). In addition, the prevalence of atypical nevi was lower in the psoriasis group (3%) compared with controls (11.5%), and there was a family history of melanoma of 8% in controls as compared with 0% among those with psoriasis. Expression levels of IL-1α, IL-6, and TNF-α in the psoriasis group were higher than in controls. These cytokines are upregulated and involved in keratinocyte proliferation in psoriasis and were tested to examine whether cytokines found in patients with psoriasis led to the inhibition of melanogenesis and melanocytic growth because of the inhibitory effects on tyrosinase activity. To conclude, the authors found fewer melanocytic nevi in subjects with psoriasis, which may be associated with the proinflammatory cytokines that inhibit melanogenesis and melanocyte growth. Further data are needed before a definitive statement can be made that is clinically relevant.

G. K. Kim, DO
J. Q. Del Rosso, DO

3 Bacterial and Fungal Infections

Treatment of subcutaneous phaeohyphomycosis and prospective follow-up of 17 kidney transplant recipients
Ogawa MM, Galante NZ, Godoy P, et al (Federal Univ of São Paulo, Brazil)
J Am Acad Dermatol 61:977-985, 2009

Background.—Subcutaneous phaeohyphomycosis in solid organ recipients may have an adverse outcome.

Objective.—We sought to describe the disease course, treatment, and outcome of allograft function in kidney transplant recipients with phaeohyphomycosis.

Methods.—Seventeen patients were followed for a mean period of 25.4 months to analyze the clinical response to treatment.

Results.—There was no treatment failure or relapsing disease among 12 patients who completed treatment. Two patients were still in treatment with disease remission. One patient discontinued the study during treatment with partial remission, one died after finishing treatment with disease remission, and one was dropped from the study because contact was lost. Immunosuppressive regimens were not changed. Two of 17 patients had a significant reduction in allograft function.

Limitations.—The follow-up time was short and the number of patients was small.

Conclusions.—The outcome of phaeohyphomycosis in kidney transplant recipients was favorable with minimal impact on renal allograft function.

▶ Phaeohyphomycotic infections are caused by melanin-producing fungi (dematiaceous fungi) that exist in tissue as pleomorphic and admixed hyphal and yeast-like forms. Although the disorder can be caused by different species, the disease as a whole is considered to be an opportunistic infection. Organ transplant recipients are at particular risk because of the immunosuppressive medications used to prevent rejection. The prevalence of this disease among renal transplant recipients is not known with certainty, but it has been estimated to be less than 1% in 1 large cohort.[1]

In this case series, the authors detailed the characteristics, treatment, and outcome of 17 kidney transplant patients with subcutaneous phaeohyphomycosis. Interestingly, all patients presented with either 1 (71%) or multiple (29%) subcutaneous cysts/abscesses. The distal lower limb was most often affected, as were men (71%), and both these observations comport to the assumed mechanism of localized tissue inoculation.

Diagnosis was made via direct histologic observation or tissue culture. Treatment consisted of surgery, with or without systemic antifungal medications. Complete surgical extirpation was achieved in 71% of patients, with partial extirpation achieved in 24%. One patient experienced spontaneous remission after fine-needle aspiration.

Systemic antifungal medication, most often itraconazole (100-800 mg/d), was used in 70% of patients because of (1) the presence of multiple lesions, (2) known incomplete surgical extirpation, or (3) documented fungal neurotropism. Other triazole-based antifungal drugs, including voriconazole, have been reported to be successful.[2,3] Antifungal management was continued for at least 6 months. Although the follow-up period was relatively short (mean, 25.4 months), the overall results were favorable, with no disseminated disease and minimal impact on renal allograft function (77% of patients had stable serum creatinine levels).

A systemic calcineurin inhibitor, such as cyclosporin and tacrolimus, was used in the immunosuppressive regimen of all the patients, and the authors speculated that the antifungal properties of these drugs may have been partially protective against life-threatening systemic disease.

Anecdotally, I have seen only 2 phaeohyphomycotic infections in renal transplant patients in my practice at a larger tertiary-care facility, but both cases involved men, and both infections were on the lower extremity. Therefore, it is important for a dermatologist to be familiar with the cystic presentation of this disease process in this setting, particularly because histologic examination and tissue culture are important in rendering a final diagnosis and commencing appropriate surgical and/or pharmacologic care.

W. A. High, MD, JD, MEng

References

1. Mesa A, Henao J, Gil M, Durango G. Phaeohyphomycosis in kidney transplant patients. *Clin Transplant.* 1999;13:273-276.
2. Vermeire SE, de Jonge H, Lagrou K, Kuypers DR. Cutaneous phaeohyphomycosis in renal allograft recipients: report of 2 cases and review of the literature. *Diagn Microbiol Infect Dis.* 2010;68:177-180.
3. Larsen CG, Arendrup MC, Krarup E, Pedersen M, Thybo S, Larsen FG. Subcutaneous phaeohyphomycosis in a renal transplant recipient successfully treated with voriconazole. *Acta Derm Venereol.* 2009;89:657-658.

Severe Refractory Erythema Nodosum Leprosum Successfully Treated with the Tumor Necrosis Factor Inhibitor Etanercept

Ramien ML, Wong A, Keystone JS (Univ of Ottawa, Canada; Univ of Alberta, Edmonton, Canada; Univ of Toronto, Ontario, Canada)
Clin Infect Dis 52:e133-e135, 2011

Erythema nodosum leprosum (ENL), or type II reaction, is a common complication of lepromatous leprosy that can cause significant patient debility. First-line therapy includes prednisone and thalidomide, with clofazimine reserved for patients who do not respond to first-line treatment. We present the case of a 33-year-old woman with ENL that failed to respond adequately to conventional therapy over a 6-year period. Because of the severe nature of her disease and the adverse effects of therapy that she experienced, a trial of etanercept was undertaken, which led to full resolution of her ENL. The rationale behind our choice of therapy and its future implications are discussed.

▶ Erythema nodosum leprosum (ENL), or type II reaction, is associated with lepromatous leprosy. It can occur before, during, or following therapy for leprosy and represents a major cause of morbidity in this patient population. ENL is a complex immune-mediated phenomenon secondary to the presence of the leprosy bacillus. The condition presents clinically as tender erythematous subcutaneous nodules, in association with a variable degree of systemic involvement. Fever, arthritis, lymphadenitis, neuritis, iridocyclitis, and nephritis may also be part of the clinical presentation. Mild cases of ENL can be treated successfully with antiinflammatory agents. More severe cases may require systemic therapy. In this setting, prednisone and thalidomide have been traditionally used in the treatment of ENL in the absence of contraindications, with clofazimine reserved as a second-line agent. There are various toxicities associated with all of these options. This case report is encouraging, with an impressive response to etanercept. Although studies are necessary to further elucidate the use of etanercept, this case provides a new therapeutic option in the treatment of this difficult condition.

J. Weinberg, MD

Methicillin-Resistant Coagulase-Negative Staphylococci in the Community: High Homology of SCCmec IVa between *Staphylococcus epidermidis* and Major Clones of Methicillin-Resistant *Staphylococcus aureus*

Barbier F, Ruppé E, Hernandez D, et al (Bacteriology Unit and Natl Reference Ctr for Emergence of Resistance in Commensal Flora, Paris, France; Univ of Geneva Hosps, Geneva, Switzerland; et al)
J Infect Dis 202:270-281, 2010

Background.—Data on community spread of methicillin-resistant coagulase-negative staphylococci (MR-CoNS) are scarce. We assessed their potential role as a reservoir of staphylococcal cassette chromosome mec (SCCmec) IVa, the leading SCCmec subtype in community-acquired methicillin-resistant *Staphylococcus aureus* (CA-MRSA).

Methods.—Nasal carriage of MR-CoNS was prospectively investigated in 291 adults at hospital admission. MR-CoNS were characterized by SCCmec typing, long-range polymerase chain reaction (PCR) for SCCmec IV, and multiple-locus variable-number tandem repeat analysis (MLVA) for *Staphylococcus epidermidis* (MRSE) strains. Three SCCmec IVa elements were fully sequenced.

Results.—The carriage rate of MR-CoNS was 19.2% (25.9% and 16.5% in patients with and patients without previous exposure to the health care system, respectively; $P = .09$). MR-CoNS strains ($n = 83$, including 58 MRSE strains with highly heterogeneous MLVA patterns) carried SCCmec type IVa ($n = 9$, all MRSE), other SCCmec IV subtypes ($n = 9$, including 7 MRSE), other SCCmec types ($n = 15$), and nontypeable SCCmec ($n = 50$). Long-range PCR indicated structural homology between SCCmec IV in MRSE and that in MRSA. Complete sequences of SCCmec IVa from 3 MRSE strains were highly homologous to those available for CA-MRSA, including major clones USA300 and USA400.

Conclusions.—MR-CoNS are probably disseminated in the community, notably in subjects without previous exposure to the health care system. MRSE, the most prevalent species, may act as a reservoir of SCCmec IVa for CA-MRSA.

▶ Two key facts emerge from the data in this article. One is the confirmation that there exist strains of *Staphylococcus epidermidis* in the French community that are methicillin resistant even in individuals without prior hospital exposure. These bacteria contain staphylococcal cassette chromosome mec (SCCmec) material that is incredibly heterogenous and which may seemingly evolve between patients without underlying health risk factors and without antibiotic pressure. The next is that the data help support the suspicion that methicillin-resistant coagulase-negative staphylococci may be somehow transferring their SCCmec material to strains of methicillin-sensitive species of *Staphylococcus aureus*, either in the community or in the hospital. This combination of diversity in the SCCmec genetic material and subsequent transfer to other staphylococcal subtypes reveals a set of circumstances that could potentially lead to an evolving resistance mechanism for bacterial resistance. Easy transferability of such a wide array of antibiotic-resistant genes could conceivably outpace our ability to develop antibiotics to fight them, as seems to be happening now in various parts of the world.

The extensive laboratory work undertaken by the authors in this article to provide good data detailing cross-transmission of resistance genes between species of staphylococcus, underscores how important methicillin-resistant strains of bacteria are becoming in the worldwide community. As practitioners, we need to remain acutely cognizant of this fact and take every opportunity to prescribe antibiotics appropriately and educate the public about the importance of proper hygiene.

J. M. Suchniak, MD

Effect of filaggrin breakdown products on growth of and protein expression by *Staphylococcus aureus*
Miajlovic H, Fallon PG, Irvine AD, et al (Trinity College, Dublin, Ireland)
J Allergy Clin Immunol 126:1184-1190, 2010

Background.—Colonization of the skin by *Staphylococcus aureus* in individuals with atopic dermatitis exacerbates inflammation. Atopic dermatitis is associated with loss-of-function mutations in the *filaggrin (FLG)* gene, accompanied by reduced levels of filaggrin breakdown products on the skin.

Objective.—To assess the affect of growth in the presence of the filaggrin breakdown products urocanic acid (UCA) and pyrrolidone carboxylic acid (PCA) on fitness of and protein expression by *S aureus*.

Methods.—*S aureus* was grown for 24 hours in the presence of UCA and PCA, and the density of the cultures was monitored by recording OD_{600} values. Cell wall extracts and secreted proteins of *S aureus* were isolated and analyzed by SDS-PAGE. Cell wall—associated proteins known to be involved in colonization and immune evasion including clumping factor B, fibronectin binding proteins, protein A, iron-regulated surface determinant A, and the serine-aspartate repeat proteins were examined by Western immunoblotting.

Results.—Acidification of growth media caused by the presence of UCA and PCA resulted in reduced growth rates and reduced final cell density of *S aureus*. At the lower pH, reduced expression of secreted and cell wall—associated proteins, including proteins involved in colonization (clumping factor B, fibronectin binding protein A) and immune evasion (protein A), was observed. Decreased expression of iron-regulated surface determinant A due to growth with filaggrin breakdown products appeared to be independent of the decreased pH.

Conclusion.—*S aureus* grown under mildly acidic conditions such as those observed on healthy skin expresses reduced levels of proteins that are known to be involved in immune evasion.

▶ The understanding of how *Staphylococcus aureus* has impacted atopic dermatitis has clearly evolved. Many dermatologists were trained that it was a superinfecting agent, and we used antibiotics to control its impact. Then we learned about protein A and its ability to switch steroid receptors on lymphocytes to make them bind steroids when in an alpha mode to beta mode. As our ability to survey for protein balances increased, improving understanding of how filaggrin affects transepidermal water loss and the integrity of the epidermis, our potential of controlling the impact of *S aureus* can increase without the unnecessary exposure to antibiotics while still modifying the defects inherent to the skin of atopic patients.[1,2]

We are now in an era of research in which links between structure and function are now better understood. As the article states, there are some important cycles that escalate the progression of atopic dermatitis. Initially, the article shows that the T_H2 inflammatory cascade, especially interleukin (IL)-4 and IL-13, involved in atopic dermatitis are closely influenced by expression of fibronectin. In addition, the predisposition to infection by *S aureus* is related to alkaline pH levels. Eventually, we see that the predisposed mutations to filaggrin gene products can result in reduction of important acids that modulate the pH and contribute to natural moisturizing factor, which helps the cycle of susceptibility to infection and, with the activity of some of the same interleukins, there is reduction of filaggrin all over again.

By taking into account the impact of these mechanisms and replacing the inherent defect, such as ceramides, physiologic lipids, and in this case filaggrin, the cycles that affect the balance between structure and function can be modulated. As the advance of therapeutics continues with that mindset, so does the potential for controlling the disease as opposed to just treating symptoms.

N. Bhatia, MD

References

1. Gómez MI, O'Seaghdha M, Magargee M, Foster TJ, Prince AS. *Staphylococcus aureus* protein A activates TNFR1 signaling through conserved IgG binding domains. *J Biol Chem.* 2006;281:20190-20196.
2. Forsgren A, Svedjelund A, Wigzell H. Lymphocyte stimulation by protein A of *Staphylococcus aureus. Eur J Immunol.* 1976;6:207-213.

Cellulitis: diagnosis and management
Bailey E, Kroshinsky D (Columbia Univ College of Physicians and Surgeons, NY; Massachusetts General Hosp, Boston)
Dermatol Ther 24:229-239, 2011

Cellulitis is an acute infection of the dermal and subcutaneous layers of the skin, often occurring after a local skin trauma. It is a common diagnosis in both inpatient and outpatient dermatology, as well as in the primary care setting. Cellulitis classically presents with erythema, swelling, warmth, and tenderness over the affected area. There are many other dermatologic diseases, which can present with similar findings, highlighting the need to consider a broad differential diagnosis. Some of the most common mimics of cellulitis include venous stasis dermatitis, contact dermatitis, deep vein thrombosis, and panniculitis. History, local characteristics of the affected area, systemic signs, laboratory tests, and, in some cases, skin biopsy can be helpful in confirming the correct diagnosis. Most patients can be treated as an outpatient with oral antibiotics, with dicloxacillin or cephalexin being the oral therapy of choice when methicillin-resistant *Staphylococcus aureus* is not a concern.

▶ Cellulitis is an acute infection of the dermis and subcutaneous tissue. However, cases misdiagnosed as cellulitis may represent other dermatologic or systemic conditions. This is a review of differential diagnosis, treatment, and management of cellulitis. Trauma to the skin is an important risk factor for the development of cellulitis. Potential sources include intravenous drug use, human bites, intentional piercings, and self-induced skin trauma. The differential diagnosis of cellulitis includes stasis dermatitis, contact dermatitis, thrombophlebitis, panniculitis, and erythema migrans. Cultures of bullae, pustules, or ulcers should be performed. A skin biopsy is not routinely performed in many cases, especially on initial evaluation. Imaging techniques can sometimes help to distinguish cellulitis from more severe infections or causes of tissue infiltration warranting radiologic consultation to choose the optimal technique based on the clinical presentation and objectives of the clinician wanting the radiologic test. Simple cellulitis without underlying abscess is usually caused by pathogenic streptococci. *Staphylococcus aureus*, both methicillin-sensitive (MSSA) and methicillin-resistant (MRSA), is a possible culprit if there is an underlying abscess, history of penetrating trauma, or multiple lesions suggestive of MRSA infection. Therapeutic options include penicillinase-resistant penicillins, amoxicillin with clavulanate, some oral cephalosporins (cephalexin, cefdinir), clindamycin, or some newer macrolides. When an abscess or pustular lesions are observed, obtaining bacterial culture and sensitive testing before initiating therapy is suggested. If patients are systemically ill or unable to tolerate oral therapy, intravenous antibiotic therapy may be indicated depending on the severity of presentation and its progression. For patients with immunodeficiency syndromes, atypical mycobacteria, fungi, and viruses should be considered. Most cases of simple cellulitis without systemic symptoms, underlying abscess formation, or signs of deeper tissue penetration can be treated successfully with oral antibiotic therapy in the outpatient setting with proper follow-up. Most cases typically resolve without need for further therapy.

G. K. Kim, DO

J. Q. Del Rosso, DO

Comparative Effectiveness of Antibiotic Treatment Strategies for Pediatric Skin and Soft-Tissue Infections
Williams DJ, Cooper WO, Kaltenbach LA, et al (Vanderbilt Univ, Nashville, TN; et al)
Pediatrics 128:e479-e487, 2011

Objective.—To compare the effectiveness of clindamycin, trimethoprim-sulfamethoxazole, and β-lactams for the treatment of pediatric skin and soft-tissue infections (SSTIs).

Methods.—A retrospective cohort of children 0 to 17 years of age who were enrolled in Tennessee Medicaid, experienced an incident SSTI between 2004 and 2007, and received treatment with clindamycin (reference), trimethoprim-sulfamethoxazole, or a β-lactam was created. Outcomes included treatment failure and recurrence, defined as an SSTI within 14 days and between 15 and 365 days after the incident SSTI, respectively. Adjusted models stratified according to drainage status were used to estimate the risk of treatment failure and time to recurrence.

Results.—Among the 6407 children who underwent drainage, there were 568 treatment failures (8.9%) and 994 recurrences (22.8%). The adjusted odds ratios for treatment failure were 1.92 (95% confidence interval [CI]: 1.49–2.47) for trimethoprim-sulfamethoxazole and 2.23 (95% CI: 1.71–2.90) for β-lactams. The adjusted hazard ratios for recurrence were 1.26 (95% CI: 1.06–1.49) for trimethoprim-sulfamethoxazole and 1.42 (95% CI: 1.19–1.69) for β-lactams. Among the 41 094 children without a drainage procedure, there were 2435 treatment failures (5.9%) and 5436 recurrences (18.2%). The adjusted odds ratios for treatment failure were 1.67 (95% CI: 1.44–1.95) for trimethoprim-sulfamethoxazole and 1.22 (95% CI: 1.06–1.41) for β-lactams; the adjusted hazard ratios for recurrence were 1.30 (95% CI: 1.18–1.44) for trimethoprim-sulfamethoxazole and 1.08 (95% CI: 0.99–1.18) for β-lactams.

Conclusions.—Compared with clindamycin, use of trimethoprim-sulfamethoxazole or β-lactams was associated with increased risks of treatment failure and recurrence. Associations were stronger for those with a drainage procedure.

▶ Appropriate selection of antibiotics is an important concern in treating pediatric skin and soft tissue infections (SSTIs), especially with the growing burden of community-associated methicillin-resistant *Staphylococcus aureus*. To help address this concern, Williams, et al conducted a large retrospective cohort study of children who experienced an SSTI and were treated with 1 of 3 antibiotics: trimethoprim-sulfamethoxazole, clindamycin, or a β-lactam antibiotic. The results of the study were both noteworthy and useful. According to their study, children who had a drainage procedure for their SSTI and received 1 of the 3 types of antibiotics, either trimethoprim-sulfamethoxazole or a β-lactam antibiotic, doubled their odds for treatment failure compared with the use of clindamycin. Not only was there a decrease in treatment failure with clindamycin, but the risk of recurrence was also higher when either trimethoprim-sulfamethoxazole or a beta-lactam antibiotic was used. Based on the results of this large study, the authors appropriately questioned the routine use of trimethoprim-sulfamethoxazole for purulent SSTIs. For children who did not have a drainage procedure for their SSTI, the risk of treatment failure was also higher for trimethoprim-sulfamethoxazole and beta-lactam antibiotics than for clindamycin. The risk of recurrence was also higher for nondrained SSTIs if trimethoprim-sulfamethoxazole was used, but there was no increased risk of recurrence with β-lactam agents versus clindamycin. Given these data, the authors noted that β-lactam antibiotics may still be effective for nonpurulent SSTIs. Ultimately, the authors provided important information to support the finding that for the acute treatment of SSTIs, especially purulent SSTIs undergoing drainage, clindamycin was superior to both trimethoprim-sulfamethoxazole and β-lactam antibiotics. To this end, the authors meet their objectives and provide relevant useful data to any practitioner treating pediatric SSTIs; however, results may differ among other patient populations of geographic communities.

B. D. Michaels, DO

J. Q. Del Rosso, DO

Enterococcus faecalis Complicating Dermal Filler Injection: A Case of Virulent Facial Abscesses
Rousso JJ, Pitman MJ (New York Eye and Ear Infirmary)
Dermatol Surg 36:1638-1641, 2010

Background.—Dermal filler injections are often used to augment soft tissues. Hyaluronic acid (HA) products are among the best choices for this because of a low immunogenicity, isovolemic degradation, and low incidence of complications. Infection after soft tissue augmentation injection is generally an adverse event related to improper technique. Early infections resemble a typical inflammatory response, but late onset is decidedly infectious and should alert the health care provider to the need for care. However, it is not uncommon for poorly trained personnel to perform cosmetic procedures, which increases the risk of infection. A healthy young woman developed an infection after soft tissue augmentation for her "congenitally deep nasolabial folds."

> *Case Report.*—Woman, 21, came for emergency treatment of severe right-sided maxillary and infraorbital facial pain and edema. She had had symptoms for 2 months, but they worsened 5 days previously. Initial complaints began 2 days after having dermal filler injections to the lips and nasolabial folds with a high-concentration HA-lidocaine product at an oculoplastic surgeon's office. She suffered erythema and local injection site induration during the first week post-injection. After a month, she developed a subcutaneous infectious reaction that required hospitalization for 48 hours and use of intravenous (IV) ampicillin-sulbactam to provide broad coverage of Gram-positive aerobes. She was prescribed a 10-day course of oral cephalexin on discharge, and symptoms improved but then recurred and worsened over the next month. An oral surgeon aspirated 3 mL of purulent fluid from the maxillary abscesses and restarted oral cephalexin 2 days previously but the patient's symptoms worsened and she came to the emergency department. She had noticeable facial asymmetry and a 5-cm area of soft tissue edema and erythema from the right maxillary region to the preseptal area of the right orbit. Lesser inflammation involved the left maxillary area. Bilateral palpation revealed several areas of induration in the upper lip.
>
> Computed tomography (CT) of the face and orbits showed extensive soft tissue stranding over the maxilla bilaterally and inferiorly to the level of the mandibular body and superiorly to the right lower eyelid. Multiple abscesses were seen bilaterally along the nasolabial folds.
>
> At surgery, bilateral gingivolabial incisions revealed multiple abscesses of the nasolabial folds, which were opened using blunt dissection to drain large amounts of purulent discharge. Copious bacitracin irrigation was performed over the surgical field. The drainage sites were packed with quarter-inch gauze. Lip abscesses were drained via stab incisions on the gingival surface plus blunt dissection.
>
> The patient was given an empiric IV antibiotic regimen of vancomycin and ampicillin-sulbactam to cover possible methicillin-resistant *Staphylococcus aureus* while in the hospital. Packing

was removed gradually to prevent the abscesses from recurring. Cultures of the discharge yielded *Enterococcus faecalis* sensitive to trimethoprim-sulfamethoxazole, prompting a change in antibiotics. Seven days after surgery the patient was discharged with oral antibiotics. One month later all the signs and symptoms of infection had resolved.

Conclusions.—HA filler injections are relatively safe for treating wrinkles and deep nasolabial folds, but severe complications can occur. It is important to cleanse the skin meticulously before the procedure and maintain clean technique throughout the injection. Complications should be recognized early and treated to prevent exacerbation of the situation and the need for aggressive management.

▶ "Risks, benefits, and alternatives" are 3 of the most important words in medicine, and as cosmetic procedures are part of the practice of medicine, those words should be understood by everyone who is involved with patients undergoing such procedures. At the same time, "do no harm," which are 3 words of equal importance, implies that understanding the consequences of a procedure is just as critical as technical performance. As the practice of cosmetic surgery expands its definitions and boundaries, and as the qualifications for being able to perform these procedures continue to expand, the ability to manage consequences and adverse outcomes needs to expand as well, especially with those directly involved with performance of or assistance with such procedures.

The discussion section reminds us about 2 simple components to preparation: adequate cleansing of the treatment field and removal of cosmetics and makeup. Outpatient procedures often take place on the spot, and patients are even told that they can return to their normal day after treatment, so removal of makeup can be a nuisance for some patients. However, incomplete surgical cleansing and removal of makeup, as discussed here, was believed to be the source of the infection, and not the hyaluronic acid filler or the brand chosen. The entire case took several weeks to evolve after the initial procedure, so the history was pivotal to the discovery of the source of infection. We are reminded that the skin was compromised with the insertion of the needle, allowing the opportunity for infection. Moreover, as in any wound infection, proper surgical technique requires more than performing the procedure, and the results here confirm that. Unfortunately, the entire case could add contempt for the practice of cosmetic surgery on the part of qualified practitioners who do not want to deal with significant adverse consequences. Even the title of the article, "*Enterococcus faecalis* Complicating Dermal Filler Injection," could reinforce hesitation of the institution of these procedures in one's practice, creating the potential for conclusions that "fillers are bad." Many of our colleagues already fear the liability as well as the maintenance involved in cosmetic surgery, so if the source of *E faecalis* is minimized, so is the risk of infection, therefore improving the benefits of the procedure. The story states that the patient was given the treatment free of charge and alternatives were not given consideration. Three important concepts referred to earlier were not emphasized. As clearly stated in the article, "The growing population of poorly trained personnel performing cosmetic procedures increases the risk of infection," which, roughly translated, should remind us that this population is not trained to clean up their own mess.

N. Bhatia, MD

Randomized Controlled Trial of Cephalexin Versus Clindamycin for Uncomplicated Pediatric Skin Infections
Chen AE, Carroll KC, Diener-West M, et al (Johns Hopkins Med Institutions, Baltimore, MD; Johns Hopkins Bloomberg School of Public Health, Baltimore, MD; et al)
Pediatrics 127:e573-e580, 2011

Objective.—To compare clindamycin and cephalexin for treatment of uncomplicated skin and soft tissue infections (SSTIs) caused predominantly by community-associated (CA) methicillin-resistant *Staphylococcus aureus* (MRSA). We hypothesized that clindamycin would be superior to cephalexin (an antibiotic without MRSA activity) for treatment of these infections.

Patients and Methods.—Patients aged 6 months to 18 years with uncomplicated SSTIs not requiring hospitalization were enrolled September 2006 through May 2009. Eligible patients were randomly assigned to 7 days of cephalexin or clindamycin; primary and secondary outcomes were clinical improvement at 48 to 72 hours and resolution at 7 days. Cultures were obtained and tested for antimicrobial susceptibilities, pulsed-field gel electrophoresis type, and Panton-Valentine leukocidin status.

Results.—Of 200 enrolled patients, 69% had MRSA cultured from wounds. Most MRSA were USA300 or subtypes, positive for Panton-Valentine leukocidin, and clindamycin susceptible, consistent with CA-MRSA. Spontaneous drainage occurred or a drainage procedure was performed in 97% of subjects. By 48 to 72 hours, 94% of subjects in the cephalexin arm and 97% in the clindamycin arm were improved ($P = .50$). By 7 days, all subjects were improved, with complete resolution in 97% in the cephalexin arm and 94% in the clindamycin arm ($P = .33$). Fevers and age less than 1 year, but not initial erythema > 5 cm, were associated with early treatment failures, regardless of antibiotic used.

Conclusions.—There is no significant difference between cephalexin and clindamycin for treatment of uncomplicated pediatric SSTIs caused predominantly by CA-MRSA. Close follow-up and fastidious wound care of appropriately drained, uncomplicated SSTIs are likely more important than initial antibiotic choice.

▶ This is a randomized controlled study comparing clindamycin and cephalexin for the treatment of uncomplicated skin and soft tissue infections (SSTIs) caused predominately by community-associated methicillin-resistant *Staphylococcus aureus* (CA-MRSA). Eligible subjects included patients aged 6 months to

18 months who presented to pediatric centers (outpatient treatment). There were 200 subjects who were equally randomized to receive oral cephalexin (40 mg/kg/d, administered 3 times a day) or oral clindamycin (20 mg/kg/d, 3 times a day). Subjects were followed up after 48 to 72 hours for re-evaluation. There were 100 patients in the cephalexin arm and 100 patients in the clindamycin arm. Four subjects were hospitalized. There was no difference in clinical outcomes after 2 to 3 days or at 7 days between those children who received cephalexin and those who received clindamycin. Adverse events included hospitalization from treatment failure, which was uncommon and equal in the 2 study arms. Also, one patient in the clindamycin arm did develop colitis from *Clostridium difficile*, but the infection resolved without treatment. This may be one of the many reasons for avoiding clindamycin for the clinician. There are several limitations to this study. First, not all infections were attributable to MRSA and not all MRSA species were susceptible in vitro to clindamycin. Second, in clinical practice, most clinicians treat empirically without waiting for the results of culture and susceptibility testing, and, currently, incision and drainage has been shown to be needed and effective in many cases of abscess-type lesions. However, it may have been beneficial to add an incision and drainage arm, alone and with each antibiotic for comparison for matching clinical presentations (ie, lesions types, lesion numbers, extent of involvement). In conclusion, overall the authors found no difference in patients treated with clindamycin and cephalexin in SSTIs in the pediatric population; however, concerns regarding regional differences in CA-MRSA susceptibility to clindamycin remain based on available literature. For older pediatric patients who can use a tetracycline agent, oral doxycycline may be a preferred choice, as it generally provides in vitro susceptibility coverage against *S aureus* with very good therapeutic activity, including for CA-MRSA.

G. K. Kim, DO
J. Q. Del Rosso, DO

4 Viral Infections (Excluding HIV Infection)

Intradermal injection of PPD as a novel approach of immunotherapy in anogenital warts in pregnant women
Eassa BI, Abou-Bakr AA, El-Khalawany MA (Al-Azhar Univ, Tanta, Egypt; Cairo Univ, Egypt)
Dermatol Ther 24:137-143, 2011

Immunotherapy for treatment of recalcitrant warts was used through different modalities including intralesional injection of purified protein derivative (PPD), which is an extract of *Mycobacterium tuberculosis*, used for testing exposure to tuberculin protein, either from a previous vaccination or from the environment. This method is used to evaluate the efficacy of a new approach of intradermal injection of PPD in the treatment of anogenital warts in pregnant women. A total of 40 pregnant women, aged 20–35 years, and presenting with anogenital warts were enrolled in this study. Human papillomavirus (HPV) typing was done using the GP5+/GP6+PCR assay. The patients were treated with weekly injections of PPD given intradermally in the forearms, and evaluated for the response regularly. HPV type-6 was the predominant genotype (67.5%). Overall, the improvement in this study was 85% and was related to the extent of tuberculin reactivity. Nineteen (47.5%) patients demonstrated complete clearance, 15 (37.5%) had partial response, and three (7.5%) had minimal response. Three (7.5%) cases did not respond to treatment. Side effects were minimal and insignificant. Treatment of anogenital warts in pregnant women with intradermal injection of PPD was found to be a unique, safe, and effective modality of immunotherapy.

▶ Many compliments to the authors for constructing a study protocol that involved a group of patients with unique treatment needs. Performing the necessary subtyping of the warts to determine whether they were potentially malignant (6 and 11 vs 16 and 18) was essential to inclusion in the study but also represents an important screening step in the prognosis for these patients. Many clinicians do not have experience with immunotherapy because the mechanisms of action may not be clear to them, but as we see here, the selection of the agent used and its known safety in pregnancy, in addition to the low side effect and pain potential, creates a new option.

The correlation between the amount of induration at the injection site and the percentage of clearance of warts should also be emphasized in reviewing the data. As explained in the discussion, there are many potential explanations of how immunotherapy would be effective against the activity of human papillomavirus (HPV). The last one listed, "HPV may elude host recognition," is an inherent component in the pathogenesis of warts: the virus-infected epithelial cells begin replicating at the basal layer and essentially hide from the immune system because there is not a clear antigen presentation. In contrast, herpes simplex infections are characterized by ballooning degeneration of epithelial cells that rupture and create a brisk inflammatory response. This is complicated by the concept that pregnancy itself is a relative state of immunosuppression because of the effects of estrogen and progesterone on the hypothalamic-pituitary-adrenal axis.

After reading the data presented here, it makes sense to incorporate this modality into practice for the pregnant patient who usually has few options that are either tolerable or successful.

N. Bhatia, MD

Intralesional Immunotherapy with *Candida* Antigen for the Treatment of Molluscum Contagiosum in Children
Enns LL, Evans MS (Univ of Arkansas for Med Sciences and Arkansas Children's Hosp)
Pediatr Dermatol 28:254-258, 2011

Intralesional injection of *Candida* and other antigens is an established and useful therapy for warts; a cutaneous immune response can induce improvement and or clearance of warts, often with response in anatomically distinct lesions other than those injected. Molluscum contagiosum virus is a common cutaneous infection seen primarily in pediatric dermatology clinics. Treatment is often unsatisfactory, painful, and time consuming. A retrospective chart review was conducted to examine the efficacy of intralesional injection of *Candida* antigen into a maximum of three individual molluscum lesions. Twenty-nine patients were treated with this therapy; 55% had complete resolution. In addition, 37.9% experienced partial resolution, yielding an overall response rate of 93%. Only two patients failed to respond (6.9%). In addition, only four patients reported a single adverse effect of pain with injection. No other adverse effects were reported or noted clinically. Scarring was absent. No recurrences were reported at the time of publication. This report establishes the efficacy of intralesional injection of *Candida* for molluscum contagiosum.

▶ This retrospective chart review looks at the success rates of treating molluscum contagiosum (MC) with intralesional Candida antigen. Additionally, the authors detail the procedure with photographs of the treatment protocol. In 29 children aged 2 to 17 years, 1 to 3 lesions were treated with approximately 0.3 mL of Candida antigen for each session. On average, the patients had MC for 11.9 months before onset of treatment and had failed previous standard therapies. The number of treatment sessions ranged from 1 to 6, with an average of 2.4 treatments. Time between treatments averaged 47.5 days. A complete response was seen in 16 patients (55.2%), a partial response in 11 (37.9%), and no response in 2 patients (6.9%).

In a disorder that resolves spontaneously, the question is whether the treatment resulted in improvement or if the infection ran its course. Unfortunately that question cannot be answered without a placebo group. Nonetheless, options for treating children with numerous MC lesions are limited. Destructive methods, such as curettage, cantharidin, and cryotherapy, are most effective in patients with a handful of lesions but are not good options for extensive infection.[1,2] Use of intralesional Candida antigen remains an alternative treatment for select patients with MC.

A. Zaenglein, MD

References

1. Cathcart S, Coloe J, Morrell DS. Parental satisfaction, efficacy, and adverse events in 54 patients treated with cantharidin for molluscum contagiosum infection. *Clin Pediatr (Phila)*. 2009;48:161-165.
2. Hanna D, Hatami A, Powell J, et al. A prospective randomized trial comparing the efficacy and adverse effects of four recognized treatments of molluscum contagiosum in children. *Pediatr Dermatol*. 2006;23:574-579.

Incidence of Postherpetic Neuralgia After Combination Treatment With Gabapentin and Valacyclovir in Patients With Acute Herpes Zoster: Open-label Study

Lapolla W, DiGiorgio C, Haitz K, et al (Ctr for Clinical Studies, Houston, TX; et al)

Arch Dermatol 147:901-907, 2011

Objective.—To evaluate the efficacy of treatment with gabapentin plus valacyclovir hydrochloride for the prevention of postherpetic neuralgia in patients with acute herpes zoster.

Design.—Uncontrolled, open-label study.

Setting.—A private dermatology clinic.

Participants.—Consecutive immunocompetent adults (age, ≥50 years) who presented with herpes zoster within 72 hours of vesicle formation with moderate to severe pain (≥4 on the 10-point Likert scale) were recruited for study participation.

Intervention.—The patients received 1000 mg of valacyclovir hydrochloride 3 times a day for 7 days plus gabapentin at an initial dose of 300 mg/d, titrated up to a maximum of 3600 mg/d, side effects permitting.

Main Outcome Measures.—Proportion of patients with zoster pain (pain>0) at 3, 4, and 6 months as well as average pain severity, the proportion of patients with sleep disturbance, and quality-of-life measures (determined by the Medical Outcome Study Short Form 36-Item Health Survey).

Results.—A total of 133 patients (mean age, 64.6 years) were enrolled in the study. The overall incidence of zoster pain at 6 months was 9.8%.

Conclusion.—The combination of gabapentin and valacyclovir administered acutely in patients with herpes zoster reduces the incidence of postherpetic neuralgia.

Trial Registration.—clinicaltrials.gov Identifier: NCT01250561.

▶ Postherpetic neuralgia (PHN) is a painful consequence of acute herpes zoster infection that affects selected individuals, usually among the older population. Once established as chronic and past the clearance of the acute herpes zoster episode, the pain of PHN can often be severe and difficult to manage. Treatment aimed at prevention of this concerning sequelae is therefore a major goal. Accordingly, Lapolla et al sought to determine the effectiveness of adding gabapentin to valacyclovir and to determine ultimately whether this would aid in decreasing the incidence of PHN. The results of their study were promising. Based on their findings in 133 patients, there was an overall decrease in the 6-month pain prevalence and incidence of PHN when the combination therapy was administered in the acute stages (within 72 hours of vesicle formation) in patients with herpes zoster infection with moderate to severe pain. The percentage of patients reporting pain at the 6-month time point was 9.8%, and the incidence of PHN for the study participants as a whole was 6.8%. These decreased levels of reported PHN-associated pain with this combination were lower than any other reported therapies based on available data, although comparisons among studies are problematic. One limitation of this study is that this study did not include a comparison with a placebo agent, as this is hard to carry out with a disorder that is painful. Another is the open-label design. Thus, there is no definitive way to confirm that the results were exclusively because of the addition of gabapentin to valacyclovir based on this trial. However, it should be noted that the prevalence of post-zoster pain at 6 months was lower than other included trials that just used valacyclovir alone without gabapentin. Based on this comparison, there appears to be reasonably good evidence that lower levels of reported pain can be attained at 6 months when gabapentin is added to valacyclovir. Given this data, this study meets its objective, and the use of gabapentin should be considered by dermatologists when treating patients with herpes zoster infection, especially those at greater risk for PHN. Importantly, dermatologists who consider adding gabapentin to their armamentarium need to familiarize themselves with potential adverse effects and possible drug interactions.

B. D. Michaels, DO
J. Q. Del Rosso, DO

Human Papillomavirus–Induced Lesions on Tattoos May Show Features of Seborrheic Keratosis
Valeròn-Almazán P, Bastida J, Rivero P, et al (University Hospital Dr Negrín, Canary Islands, Spain; et al)
Arch Dermatol 147:370, 2011

Background.—Reports indicate that persons may be inoculated with human papillomavirus (HPV) when undergoing tattoo placement. Three cases were identified.

> *Case Reports.*—Woman, 29, and two men, 24 and 26, had rapidly enlarging lesions after tattooing. Several brown papules were located on tattoos of the shoulder, arm, and flank during clinical examination. The two men had generalized "fat fingers" as well. Histopathologic evaluation demonstrated a basaloid cell proliferation with hyperkeratosis and acanthosis of varying degrees. A cellular infiltrate with macrophages that contained inorganic pigment was noted around dermal vessels. HPV DNA was identified in lesions on the woman and one man, specifically, HPV-57 and HPV-2.

Conclusions.—Only one case of seborrheic keratosis on a tattoo was reported previously. HPV may cause some cases of nongenital seborrheic keratosis.

▶ Human papillomavirus (HPV) is a causative agent in many epidermal tumors, both benign and malignant. As in actinic keratosis (AK) or squamous cell carcinoma (SCC), injuries to the epidermis such as photodamage or sunburns can promote HPV as a trigger of atypical proliferation. This mechanism is often linked to the E6 and E7 late proteins that inactivate the p53 tumor suppressor gene to counter intrinsic apoptosis as well as impairing DNA repair. If we consider tattoo placement as a traumatic injury, the potential for activation of virus-induced acanthosis increases. As demonstrated in this case report, the injury may have served as a promoter for HPV, resulting in the histological variant of the verrucous papules. Clinically, the differential diagnosis may include warts, but as the authors report, the development of seborrheic keratosis is also linked to HPV, which should alert the clinician to the possibility after tattoo placement.

N. Bhatia, MD

A study on the association with hepatitis B and hepatitis C in 1557 patients with lichen planus
Birkenfeld S, Dreiher J, Weitzman D, et al (Ben-Gurion Univ of the Negev, Beer-Sheva, Israel)
J Eur Acad Dermatol Venereol 25:436-440, 2011

Background.—Previous reports have demonstrated contradicting results on the association between lichen planus and hepatitis.

Objectives.—The aim of this study was to investigate the association between lichen planus and viral hepatitis.

Methods.—Patients with lichen planus were compared with controls regarding the prevalence of viral hepatitis in a case-control study using logistic multivariate regression models. The study was performed utilizing the medical database of Clalit Health Services.

Results.—The study included 1557 lichen planus patients over the age of 20 years and 3115 age- and gender-matched controls. The prevalence of hepatitis C in patients with lichen planus was higher than that in the control group (1.9%, 0.4% respectively, $P < 0.001$). In a multivariate analysis, lichen planus was associated with hepatitis C (OR 4.19, 95% CI 2.21; 7.93). The prevalence of hepatitis B in patients with lichen planus was similar to that in the control group (0.9%, 0.5% respectively, $P = 0.12$). A multivariate analysis revealed that lichen planus was not associated with hepatitis B (OR 1.69, 95% CI 0.82; 3.47).

Conclusion.—Lichen planus is associated with hepatitis C but not with hepatitis B. Physicians who care for patients with lichen planus should consider screening patients with lichen planus for hepatitis C.

▶ This is a retrospective analysis of a large database that associates lichen planus (LP) with hepatitis C. The study included 1557 patients with LP and 3115 age frequency—matched and gender frequency—matched controls. The prevalence of hepatitis C in patients with LP was higher than in the control group ($P < .001$), and in a multivariate analysis, hepatitis C was associated with LP (odds ratio, 4.19) after controlling for age, gender, smoking status, and socioeconomic status. Previous studies of this relationship showed inconsistent results but, importantly, had much smaller sample sizes. The large sample size in this study gives much more weight to the association of hepatitis C and LP.

S. M. Purcell, DO

Herpes Zoster Vaccine in Older Adults and the Risk of Subsequent Herpes Zoster Disease

Tseng HF, Smith N, Harpaz R, et al (Southern California Kaiser Permanente, Pasadena, CA; Ctrs for Disease Control and Prevention, Atlanta, GA)
JAMA 305:160-166, 2011

Context.—Approximately 1 million episodes of herpes zoster occur annually in the United States. Although prelicensure data provided evidence that herpes zoster vaccine works in a select study population under idealized circumstances, the vaccine needs to be evaluated in field conditions.

Objective.—To evaluate risk of herpes zoster after receipt of herpes zoster vaccine among individuals in general practice settings.

Design, Setting, and Participants.—A retrospective cohort study from January 1, 2007, through December 31, 2009, of individuals enrolled in the Kaiser Permanente Southern California health plan. Participants were immunocompetent community-dwelling adults aged 60 years or older.

The 75 761 members in the vaccinated cohort were age matched (1:3) to 227 283 unvaccinated members.

Main Outcome Measure.—Incidence of herpes zoster.

Results.—Herpes zoster vaccine recipients were more likely to be white, women, with more outpatient visits, and fewer chronic diseases. The number of herpes zoster cases among vaccinated individuals was 828 in 130 415 person-years (6.4 per 1000 person-years; 95% confidence interval [CI], 5.9-6.8), and for unvaccinated individuals it was 4606 in 355 659 person-years (13.0 per 1000 person-years; 95% CI, 12.6-13.3). In adjusted analysis, vaccination was associated with a reduced risk of herpes zoster (hazard ratio [HR], 0.45; 95% CI, 0.42-0.48); this reduction occurred in all age strata and among individuals with chronic diseases. Risk of herpes zoster differed by vaccination status to a greater magnitude than the risk of unrelated acute medical conditions, suggesting results for herpes zoster were not due to bias. Ophthalmic herpes zoster (HR, 0.37; 95% CI, 0.23-0.61) and hospitalizations coded as herpes zoster (HR, 0.35; 95% CI, 0.24-0.51) were less likely among vaccine recipients.

Conclusions.—Among immunocompetent community-dwelling adults aged 60 years or older, receipt of the herpes zoster vaccine was associated with a lower incidence of herpes zoster. The risk was reduced among all age strata and among individuals with chronic diseases.

▶ Herpes zoster vaccine is a live attenuated varicella zoster virus (VZV) vaccine initially licensed in 2006 for adults age 60 years and older and was recently approved to include the 50- to 59-year-old group. The vaccine is administered as a single 0.65-mL dose subcutaneously in the deltoid region of the arm. Contraindications include immunocompromised patients and those with gelatin or neomycin allergies, with allergies to any other vaccine components, or who are pregnant. Most common adverse reactions reported are headache and injection-site reaction. The current retrospective cohort study found that those who received the VZV vaccine had 55% reduced risk of herpes zoster regardless of age, race, and presence of chronic diseases. These results confirm previous reports from the Shingles Prevention Study. Some limitations as noted by authors are that the average length of follow-up was relatively short (<2 years), and follow-up information was passively obtained through health care encounters and electronic health records, which may lead to misclassification of vaccination or herpes zoster status or incomplete confirmation of actual events that transpired.

S. Bellew, DO

J. Q. Del Rosso, DO

Efficacy, safety and tolerability of green tea catechins in the treatment of external anogenital warts: a systematic review and meta-analysis

Tzellos TG, Sardeli C, Lallas A, et al (Aristotle Univ of Thessaloniki, Greece; Hosp of Venereal and Skin Diseases of Thessaloniki, Greece)
J Eur Acad Dermatol Venereol 25:345-353, 2011

Background.—External anogenital warts (EGWs) are non-malignant skin tumours caused by human papillomavirus. They are one of the fastest growing sexually transmitted diseases. Current treatments are unsatisfactory. Green tea sinecatechin Polyphenon E ointment is a botanical extract from green tea leaves exhibiting anti-oxidant, anti-viral and anti-tumour properties.

Objective.—The aim of this study was to integrate valid information and provide basis for rational decision making regarding efficacy and safety of green tea extracts in the treatment of EGWs.

Methods.—A systematic search in electronic databases was conducted using specific key terms. Main search was performed independently by two reviewers. The accumulated relevant literature was subsequently systematically reviewed and a meta-analysis was conducted.

Results.—Three randomized, double-blind, placebo-controlled studies evaluating efficacy and safety of Polyphenon E 15% and 10% in the treatment of warts were included in the systematic review and meta-analysis. A total of 660 men and 587 women were enrolled. Regarding primary outcome, both Polyphenon E 15% and 10% demonstrated significantly higher likelihood of complete clearance of baseline and baseline and new warts compared with controls. No significant heterogeneity was detected. Recurrence rates were very low. Commonest local skin sign was erythema and local skin symptom was itching.

Conclusions.—Efficacy of Polyphenon 15% and 10%, at least for the primary endpoint, is clearly indicated. Polyphenon E treatment exhibits very low recurrence rates and appears to have a rather favourable safety and tolerability profile. Recommendations for future studies should include evaluation of the efficacy of green tea catechins in the treatment of internal anogenital warts and direct comparison with its principal comparator, imiquimod.

▶ Treatment for external anogenital warts (EGW) is often not satisfactory. Current treatment options include such therapies as cryotherapy, laser ablation, curettage, topical imiquimod, topical trichloroacetic acid, and topical podophyllin. Many of these treatment options can cause pain and have the potential for unwanted skin reactions or even scarring. Other than imiquimod, most ablate treated tissue without any substantial effect on subclinical viral load in surrounding tissue. Tzellos et al present a review and meta-analysis on a potential alternative treatment option for EGW: green tea sinecatechin Polyphenon E ointment, an extract from green tea leaves. Polyphenon E has 10% and 15% formulations. Based on their review of 3 qualifying studies, it was determined that both formulations had clearly demonstrated effectiveness in the treatment of EGW with regard to lesion reduction over time. However, reasonable clearance of lesions may require up to 16 weeks of application, unlike for other treatment modalities, which have shorter durations of therapy or are immediate procedures. Despite this, all 3 studies found that the onset of clearance for Polyphenon E started at 2 weeks of treatment, and at endpoint, clearance rates were much better than in the control group. In addition, this therapy is well tolerated, with most local skin reactions rated as mild, including erythema and pruritus—both of which peaked after 2 to 4 weeks of treatment. Local skin reactions, however, were considered an important indicator for achieving clinical response. Unfortunately, there were no head-to-head trials versus other treatment options as a basis for comparison, but based on the review, both formulations of Polyphenon E ointment were suggested to be superior in terms of recurrence rates. This may not be a valid conclusion because all 3 studies included treatment follow-up periods of only 12 weeks for complete responders. A potential drawback of the medication is the recommended frequency of 3 applications a day. Ultimately, based on the available studies, Polyphenon E ointment currently appears to be a safe, well-tolerated, and effective therapy and one that deserves consideration as a potential treatment alternative for EGW.

B. D. Michaels, DO

J. Q. Del Rosso, DO

Herpes Zoster in the Distribution of the Trigeminal Nerve After Nonablative Fractional Photothermolysis of the Face: Report of 3 Cases
Firoz BF, Katz TM, Goldberg LH, et al (DermSurgery Associates, Houston, TX; Laser and Skin Surgery Ctr of New York; et al)
Dermatol Surg 37:249-252, 2011

Background.—After either a primary infection with the varicella zoster virus (VZV) or vaccination, the virus remains latent in the dorsal root ganglion until reactivated to produce herpes zoster. Reactivation usually occurs in older adults or immunocompromised patients. The presentation of herpes zoster lesions is along a dermatomal distribution, following the pathways of the involved nerves. Unilateral dermatomal pain and clustered vesicle outbreaks are characteristic in immunocompetent individuals. Mechanical trauma has been indicated as a possible risk factor for developing herpes zoster. Among the possible precipitating events are liposuction, face lift, soft tissue augmentation with calcium hydroxylapatite, pulsed dye laser treatments, and head and neck reconstruction. Three cases of herpes zoster on the face after fractional photothermolysis (FP) treatment were reported.

    Case Reports.—Case 1: Woman, 51, underwent FP for facial rhytides and enlarged pores. She was taking 20 mg of prednisone daily for an asthma flare and antibiotics for resolving pneumonia at the time of her second treatment. She had no family history of herpes zoster. She was given a topical triple anesthetic cream 1 hour before treatment and ketorolac 30 mg for pain prophylaxis. A week after treatment she developed a painful, burning vesicular eruption in the V3 distribution of the trigeminal nerve. Viral culture confirmed VZV. She was successfully treated with valacyclovir 1000 mg 3 times a day for 1 week.

Case 2: Woman, 54, was being treated for rhytides, enlarged pores, and photoaging on the face. She was taking levothyroxine and had a history of nonmelanoma skin cancer, but no family history of herpes zoster. At her second treatment she received ibuprofen 600 mg and triple anesthetic numbing cream for 1 hour before FP. Two weeks later she developed a painful, burning vesicular eruption across the upper left forehead and left eyebrow in the V1 distribution of the trigeminal nerve. Viral culture confirmed VZV. Acyclovir 800 mg 5 times a day for 7 days resolved the eruption.

Case 3: Woman, 53, was being treated for acne scarring. Three days after her second laser treatment she developed a vesicular eruption in the V1 distribution of the trigeminal nerve with ophthalmic involvement. Antiviral eye drops and valacyclovir 1000 mg 3 times a day for 7 days led to a resolution of her symptoms.

Conclusions.—The exact mechanisms by which VZV becomes reactivated is not understood, but various stimuli have been identified. These include emotional stress, ultraviolet or ionizing radiation, and chemical substances. All three of the patients reported were in their sixth decade. The VZV vaccine is only approved for patients age 60 or older because they are at higher risk for developing herpes zoster. None of these patients had a family history of herpes zoster. Each patient developed eruptions in the distribution of the trigeminal nerve, a facial nerve, after FP treatment to the face. Thus mechanical trauma or stimulation of sensory nerve fibers may have contributed to the reactivation of the virus.

▶ This report of 3 cases of facial herpes zoster brings to light a newly reported complication following nonablative fractional photothermolysis. All 3 cases occurred in zoster-naïve patients and developed within 2 weeks after treatment. It is interesting to note this complication because it is extremely unexpected given the noninvasive nature of this nonablative laser treatment. Outbreaks of herpes zoster have been reported after cosmetic treatments that ablate or disrupt the skin barrier. Most recently, outbreaks of herpes zoster have been described following treatment with botulinum toxin.[1] In the present article, the authors recommend that patients with a family history of herpes zoster receive zoster prophylaxis before undergoing fractional photothermolysis. However, they do not suggest prophylaxis for patients with a personal history of zoster given that recurrence is rare. Their recommendations can be questioned because this may not be a worthwhile practice given that it is exposure to or previous "chickenpox" that predisposes patients to herpes zoster and not necessarily a family history. For instance, it would be helpful to know how many patients were treated with nonablative fractional photothermolysis over the time period that these 3 cases developed to determine the incidence of herpes zoster after fractional photothermolysis. It would also be interesting to know the number of patients undergoing fractional photothermolysis with a family history of herpes zoster. Further investigation is warranted before firm recommendations on herpes zoster prophylaxis can be made.

E. Graber, MD

Reference

1. Graber EM, Dover JS, Arndt KA. Two cases of herpes zoster appearing after botulinum toxin type a injections. *J Clin Aesthet Dermatol.* 2011;4:49-51.

Photodynamic therapy of condyloma acuminatum in a child

Chen M, Xie J, Han J (Sun Yat-Sen Univ, Guangzhou, Guangdong, China)
Pediatr Dermatol 27:542-544, 2010

Conventional therapies for condyloma acuminatum in children are often associated with unsatisfactory response and high recurrence rate. Here, we present a 9-year-old girl with vulvar condyloma acuminatum successfully treated with topical 5-aminolaevulinic acid mediated photodynamic therapy. 5-aminolaevulinic acid mediated photodynamic therapy is a promising therapy for condylomata acuminata in children.

▶ The successful use of aminolevulinic acid (ALA) photodynamic therapy (PDT) to treat condyloma located in the vulvar area of a child provides us with a successful treatment option for this challenging problem. Traditional procedural therapies for condyloma are often painful and can result in scarring. Topical therapies are associated with prolonged treatment and often significant side effects. Given the age of the patient and the delicate location of the lesion where scarring needed to be absolutely minimized, the use of ALA PDT provided an excellent solution in this case. The use of PDT to successfully treat condyloma in 12 men was reported as early as 2003.[1] PDT also proved to be highly successful in treating urethral lesions in 164 subjects.[2] Sustained clearance of condyloma following PDT is generally greater than 90% during follow-up evaluations (> 6 months). Comparative studies in condyloma using CO_2 laser ablation have shown that PDT is associated with a lower recurrence rate and fewer adverse affects.[3] The authors of the case report did not mention which form of anesthesia was used on the child or the amount of red light delivered during each treatment. Generally, red light dosing for condyloma is in the 70- to 100-J/cm^2 range.

G. Martin, MD

References

1. Stefanaki IM, Georgiou S, Themelis GC, Vazgiouraki EM, Tosca AD. In vivo fluorescence kinetics and photodynamic therapy in condylomata acuminata. *Br J Dermatol.* 2003;149:972-976.

2. Wang XL, Wang HW, Wang HS, Xu SZ, Liao KH, Hillemanns P. Topical 5-amino-laevulinic acid-photodynamic therapy for the treatment of urethral condylomata acuminata. *Br J Dermatol*. 2004;151:880-885.
3. Chen K, Chang BZ, Ju M, Zhang XH, Gu H. Comparative study of photodynamic therapy vs CO2 laser vaporization in treatment of condylomata acuminata: a randomized clinical trial. *Br J Dermatol*. 2007;156:516-520.

5   HIV Infection

Skin disorders in Korean patients infected with human immunodeficiency virus and their association with a CD4 lymphocyte count: a preliminary study
Kim T-G, Lee K-H, Oh S-H (Yonsei Univ College of Medicine, Seoul, Korea)
J Eur Acad Dermatol Venereol 24:1476-1480, 2010

Background.—Dermatological disorders are quite common in human immunodeficiency virus (HIV)-infected patients. However, cutaneous findings in Korean HIV-infected patients have not been properly investigated.

Objective.—To investigate the spectrum of dermatological disorders in Korean HIV-infected individuals according to a CD4 lymphocyte count.

Methods.—A retrospective clinical study was carried out from June 2002 to January 2008. We comprehensively collected information regarding HIV-associated skin problems, laboratory data and the history of highly active antiretroviral therapy (HAART).

Results.—Ninety-nine HIV-seropositive patients (mean age: 39.6 ± 11.3 years, males: 94.9%) were included in this study. Of them, 55 patients (55.6%) presented with at least one skin problem. The four most common dermatological disorders were eosinophilic pustular folliculitis (18.6%), symptomatic syphilis (comprising of primary and secondary syphilis) (17.1%), seborrhoeic dermatitis (17.1%) and condyloma acuminatum (12.8%). The group with a CD4 lymphocyte count $< 200 \times 10^6$ cells/L showed a significantly higher prevalence of Kaposi sarcoma compared with the group with a CD4 lymphocyte count $> 200 \times 10^6$ cells/L ($P = 0.014$). Condyloma was more prevalent in the group with a CD4 count $> 200 \times 10^6$ cells/L ($P = 0.022$). The patients treated with HAART had a lower prevalence of neurosyphilis compared with the non-treated group ($P = 0.018$).

Conclusions.—Diverse dermatological conditions were demonstrated in Korean HIV-infected patients. Kaposi sarcoma was associated with a low CD4 lymphocyte count, but condyloma was associated with a high CD4 lymphocyte count. The prevalence of syphilis in our study was higher than that of Western countries. HAART seemed to be associated with the low prevalence of neurosyphilis.

▶ Patients infected with human immunodeficiency virus (HIV) can have various skin conditions throughout the course of their illness, some of which may occur in greater frequency or with greater severity in this population. Although there have been many studies in the Western population, there are few studies completed in the Asian population. This is a retrospective study from 2002 to 2008 of 99 patients diagnosed with HIV, with 78 of these patients on highly active antiretroviral therapy (HAART). Fifty-five patients presented with at least 1 skin problem, and the total number of cases of skin disease was 70. The most common skin disorders were eosinophilic pustular folliculitis (18.6%), symptomatic syphilis (17.1%), seborrheic dermatitis (17.1%), and condyloma accuminatum (12.8%). The group with a CD4 lymphocyte count less than 200×10^6 cells per liter showed significantly higher prevalence of Kaposi sarcoma ($P = .014$) compared with the group having greater than 200×10^6 CD4 cells per liter. The prevalence of dermatologic diseases was not associated with HAART, but those on HAART had lower prevalence of neurosyphilis compared with the nontreated group ($P = .018$). This is the largest study that investigates HIV-associated skin disease in a Korean population. Although in Western countries, homosexual contact and intravenous drug use are the most common methods of HIV transmission, most Korean HIV infections are from heterosexual contact. Another finding of this study was that skin disorders in HIV-positive Korean patients were different in that there were fewer opportunistic infections compared with Western countries. One limitation to this study was that it was a small retrospective study. Larger studies are needed to confirm these results. In conclusion, Korean HIV-positive patients had more symptomatic syphilis and Kaposi sarcoma associated with a low CD4 lymphocyte count compared with patients in Western countries; however, the study population was too small to draw any definitive conclusions concerning disease-specific susceptibilities based on ethnicity or demographics.

G. K. Kim, DO

J. Q. Del Rosso, DO

6 Disorders of the Pilosebaceous Apparatus

A prospective trial of the effects of isotretinoin on quality of life and depressive symptoms

McGrath EJ, Lovell CR, Gillison F, et al (Royal United Hosp, Bath, UK; Univ of Bath, UK)

Br J Dermatol 163:1323-1329, 2010

Background.—Isotretinoin is an efficacious treatment for acne, but has been controversially linked with depression.

Objectives.—This study aimed to examine the effects of isotretinoin on quality of life (QoL) and depression using a prospective design.

Methods.—The WHOQOL-BREF QoL measure and Centre for Epidemiological Studies Depression Scale were administered to consecutive outpatients with acne who were prescribed either isotretinoin ($n = 65$) or antibiotic treatment ($n = 31$). Patients and physicians rated acne severity independently. Groups were compared at baseline with a matched community sample ($n = 94$) and measurements repeated at 3 months for treatment groups.

Results.—There were no differences between the three groups at baseline in terms of age, gender, depression or overall QoL. Acne was more severe in the treatment groups ($P < 0.001$). Depression was negatively correlated with QoL ($P < 0.001$) and hence was included as a covariate in repeated-measures analyses of QoL. Acne improved over time in both treatment groups ($F = 48.2$, $P < 0.001$). There was no detectable deterioration in depression score in either group ($F = 1.1$, not significant). QoL in the physical and social domains improved ($P < 0.001$) while psychological and environmental QoL was unchanged over time. The improvement in social QoL was greater in the isotretinoin group ($P < 0.05$). Those patients with higher baseline depression scores showed greater improvements in physical, psychological and social QoL ($P < 0.001$).

Conclusions.—Treatment of acne improves QoL, particularly in those with more depressive symptoms at the outset. Mood deterioration was not detected, but the possibility of subtle or rare mood effects of isotretinoin cannot be ruled out.

▶ The goal of this study was to compare the quality of life (QoL) in acne patients before and after treatment with either isotretinoin (n = 65) or antibiotics (n = 31) with comparison to a matched sample of subjects from the community (n = 94). A QoL questionnaire and depression scale were administered at baseline and every 3 months of treatment, and then acne was assessed by a physician. The study showed that there was no deterioration in the depression score and QoL in the physical and social domains improved in treatment groups. There have been many efforts to address the issue of depression and isotretinoin in several similar studies. Little new information is provided by this study. Larger epidemiological studies have not supported an association, but as mentioned by the authors, there remains the possibility that in certain cases, there may be a link between depression and isotretinoin therapy.

D. Thiboutot, MD

---

5 mg/day finasteride treatment for normoandrogenic Asian women with female pattern hair loss
Yeon JH, Jung JY, Choi JW, et al (Seoul Natl Univ College of Medicine and Seoul Natl Univ Bundang Hosp, Korea; et al)
J Eur Acad Dermatol Venereol 25:211-214, 2011

Background.—Various treatments have been attempted for female pattern hair loss (FPHL), including topical minoxidil, oral antiandrogen and finasteride. But, there is no consensus on the standard treatment options. Clinical efficacy of finasteride in treating FPHL is still in controversy, but there is a tendency to high dose finasteride, which is more effective than lower dose.

Objectives.—The purpose of this study was to evaluate the clinical efficacy of high dose (5 mg/day) oral finasteride in normoandrogenic Asian women with FPHL.

Methods.—Total of 87 normoandrogenic, pre and post-menopausal women with FPHL were enrolled in this study. They were treated with oral finasteride (Proscar®), 5 mg daily for 12 months. Efficacy was evaluated with hair density and thickness changes assessed by phototrichogram and global photographs using 7-point scale.

Results.—Eighty-six patients completed 12 months of finasteride treatment schedule. One patient (1.1%) withdrew due to headache. At initial visits, mean hair density was $90 \pm 22/cm^2$ and mean hair thickness was 64 ± 11 μm. After 12 months of finasteride treatment, hair density was significantly increased to $107 \pm 23/cm^2$ (P < 0.001), and hair thickness was also significantly increased to 70 ± 9 μm (P = 0.02). In global photographs, 70 (81.4%) of the 86 patients were improved (57 were slightly, 10 were moderately and four were greatly improved). Patients without any changes were 13 (15.1%) and 3 (3.5%) patients reported slightly aggravated.

Four patients (4.6%) reported adverse events (headache, menstrual irregularity, dizziness and increased body hair growth). However, these adverse events were mild and disappeared soon.

Conclusions.—Oral finasteride, 5 mg/day, may be an effective and safe treatment for normoandrogenic women with FPHL.

▶ Female pattern hair loss (FPHL) is the most common cause of hair loss in women and is seen in higher incidences with advanced aging. Finasteride has been used in male pattern androgenic alopecia but is still considered controversial in women. This is a study evaluating the efficacy of high-dose (5 mg/d) of oral finasteride in normoandrogenic Asian women with FPHL. There were 87 women (range 21-69 years old) with FPHL enrolled with normal androgen levels, thyroid, iron, and ferritin levels. Patients were treated with oral finasteride 5-mg dose daily for 12 months with no other topical or oral treatment. Evaluation was performed with photographic assessment and phototrichogram for hair density and thickness; global photographic assessments were also performed. After finasteride treatment, hair density was significantly increased to $107 \pm 23/cm^2$ ($P < 0.001$), and hair thickness was significantly increased to 70 ± 9 μm ($P = 0.02$) in both pre- and postmenopausal groups. Mean global photographic assessment score after finasteride treatment was 0.98. Phototrichogram demonstrated an 18.9% mean increment of hair density and 9.4% mean increment of hair thickness. Only 4 patients (4.6%) experienced mild side effects including headache, menstrual irregularity, dizziness, and increased body hair. Results for this study with hair density is similar to 2% topical minoxidil solution. One limitation is that it was not randomized but an open-label clinical trial. A comparative study with a placebo control group is necessary in future studies. In conclusion, finasteride may be an option for normoandrogenic women who are experiencing FPHL.

G. K. Kim, DO

J. Q. Del Rosso, DO

Acne fulminans: explosive systemic form of acne
Zaba R, Schwartz RA, Jarmuda S, et al (Poznan Univ School of Med Sciences, Poland; New Jersey Med School, Newark)
J Eur Acad Dermatol Venereol 25:501-507, 2011

Acne fulminans (AF) is a rare severe form of acne vulgaris associated with systemic symptoms. It primarily affects male adolescents. Although the aetiology of AF remains unknown, many theories have been advanced to explain it. There have been reported associations with increased androgens, autoimmune complex disease and genetic pre-disposition. The disease is destructive, with the acute onset of painful, ulcerative nodules on the face, chest and back. The associated systemic manifestations such as fever, weight loss and musculoskeletal pain are usually present at the onset. The patients are febrile, with leucocytosis and an increased erythrocyte sedimentation rate. They may require several weeks of hospitalization. The treatment of

AF has been challenging; the response to traditional acne therapies is poor. The recommended treatment is aggressive and consists of a combination of oral steroids and isotretinoin. To avoid the relapses, duration of such treatment should not be less than 3-5 months. Although the prognosis for patients treated appropriately is good, these acute inflammatory nodules often heal with residual scarring.

▶ Acne fulminans (AF) is not only a rare and severe form of acne vulgaris, but it is a form that can be clinically challenging in regard to its manifestations and treatment. The etiology of acne fulminans also remains uncertain. This article provides a nice review of the major aspects of the disease state, including its pathogenesis, cutaneous and systemic features, and appropriate treatment. In the article, Zaba et al include succinct tables on the main features of AF for review and the recommended treatment options. Important follow-up commentary is also provided on treatment options, including potential sequelae of delayed treatment and early discontinuation of treatment. For those interested, this article provides a summation of the current theories that have been proposed for its pathophysiology, including genetic, infectious, and immunological causes. Although no one theory is definitive, some proffered causes include intense immune-mediated type III and type IV hypersensitivity reactions to *Propionibacterium acnes*, elevated blood levels of testosterone, a postulation that AF is an autoimmune complex disease, a viral infectious etiology, genetic and hereditary factors, and even isotretinoin (especially too high a dose initially) as a precipitator of AF, although ironically, oral isotretinoin is one of the treatments for it, albeit at a different dosing regimen and in combination with oral corticosteroid therapy (ie, prednisone). Overall, in this article, Zaba et al present an insightful and thorough review of AF and one that is clinically relevant for use by dermatologists in the management of AF.

B. D. Michaels, DO
J. Q. Del Rosso, DO

A pilot methodology study for the photographic assessment of post-inflammatory hyperpigmentation in patients treated with tretinoin

Rossi AB, Leyden JJ, Pappert AS, et al (J&J Group of Consumer Companies, Paris, France; Skin Study Ctr, Broomall, PA; Univ of Medicine and Dentistry of New Jersey-Robert Wood Johnson Univ Hosp, Brunswick, NJ; et al)
J Eur Acad Dermatol Venereol 25:398-402, 2011

Background.—Post-inflammatory hyperpigmentation (PIH) is a common occurrence in patients with acne vulgaris, particularly in those with skin of colour.

Aims.—A previous study has demonstrated the benefit of tretinoin (retinoic acid) in the treatment of PIH; however, there is currently no standard protocol to evaluate change in PIH following treatment. Based on these findings, we performed a pilot, exploratory, blinded, intraindividual-controlled methodology study that consisted of a photographic assessment protocol with facial mapping.

Materials and Methods.—The study was based on a secondary analysis of a phase 4, community-based trial of 544 acne patients who were treated with tretinoin gel microsphere 0.04% or 0.1%. Only patients with Fitzpatrick types III–V (skin of colour) were included in the study; subjects with Fitzpatrick skin type VI were excluded because the photographic assessment did not allow for proper evaluation.

Results.—Despite the small number of subjects evaluated ($n = 25$), the results revealed consistent assessment of improvement in PIH between two independent graders (weighted $\kappa = 0.84$).

Conclusion.—Further study with a larger population is recommended to validate the accuracy of this method.

▶ Postinflammatory hyperpigmentation (PIH) is a common sequela of resolved acne vulgaris (AV) lesions and is problematic because of both its persistence and the multitude of pigmented macules present on the face, especially in people with Fitzpatrick skin types III to VI (darker skin color). Topical retinoids have been shown to help resolve both inflammatory and comedonal AV lesions and to hasten the resolution of PIH. This blinded, randomized, intraindividual controlled study evaluated tretinoin microsphere gel (0.04% and 0.1%) used once daily for 12 weeks specifically in patients with AV who were more prone to PIH (Fitzpatrick types III-V). The study was a subanalysis of 25 patients who were part of a larger community-based trial (N = 544) that included a broader variety of skin types. Patients with Fitzpatrick skin type VI were excluded because of the limitations of photographic assessment. The 25 patients included in the study were treated with either tretinoin 0.04% (n = 21) or tretinoin 0.1% (n = 4). Digital photographs were taken of each patient during all 4 study visits with the use of standardized equipment and methodology. The results were analyzed with facial mapping techniques that included 3 angles to view the face. The investigators decided to use a target lesion evaluation rather than an overall facial evaluation because PIH can appear anywhere on facial skin in patients with facial AV. Using the PIH severity scale designed as part of the protocol, 2 independent blinded graders rated improvements in PIH that ranged from 77% to 100% over the study course, with evaluations based on photographs taken at baseline and at weeks 4, 8, and 12. Assessments of the degree of improvement in PIH between the 2 independent graders were analyzed and determined to be valid ($\kappa = 0.84$). The limitations of this study were that it was not performed prospectively, not all skin types were included, and other confounding factors such as sunlight exposure were not controlled for. Because of the limited number of subjects, the uneven distribution between the tretinoin strengths used, and the lack of breakdown among the 3 Fitzpatrick skin types (III, IV, and V) that were included in the subanalysis, a comparison of results between the 0.04% and 0.1% strengths of tretinoin microsphere gel could not be completed. Interestingly, the authors also commented that the primary objective of this pilot study was to evaluate the development of methodology to measure improvement in PIH that would be clinically relevant and that this study was not intended to evaluate definitively the therapeutic benefit of tretinoin therapy. A larger study with proper controls, study size, and protocol design is needed to validate the accuracy of this method.

J. Q. Del Rosso, DO

G. K. Kim, DO

Comparison of tretinoin 0.05% cream and 3% alcohol-based salicylic acid preparation in the treatment of acne vulgaris

Babayeva L, Akarsu S, Fetil E, et al (Dokuz Eylul Univ, Izmir, Turkey)
J Eur Acad Dermatol Venereol 25:328-333, 2011

Background.—No single effective topical treatment is available for treating all pathogenic factors causing acne vulgaris (AV). Salicylic acid (SA), tretinoin (all-TRA) and clindamycin phosphate (CDP) are known to to be effective agents depending on their comedolytic and anti-inflammatory properties.

Objective.—To compare the efficacy and tolerability of SA and CDP combination (SA + CDP) with all-TRA and CDP (all-TRA + CDP) in patients with mild to moderate facial AV.

Methods.—Forty-six patients aged between 18 and 35 years were enrolled in a 12-week prospective, single-blind, randomized and comparative clinical study. Efficacy was assessed by lesion counts, global improvement, quality of life index and measurement of skin barrier functions. Local side effects were also evaluated.

Results.—Both combinations were effective in reducing total lesion (TL), inflammatory lesion (IL) and non-inflammatory lesion (NIL) counts and showed significant global improvement as evaluated by the investigator. At the end of the study, there was no significant difference between the two groups in terms of all lesion counts. In addition, TL counts decreased faster in the all-TRA + CDP group compared with those in the SA + CDP group, with a significant difference between the two groups occurring as early as 2 weeks. Safety evaluations demonstrated that the incidence of mild to moderate side effects generally peaked at week 2 and declined gradually thereafter. Both combinations did not have an effect on stratum corneum hydration, although skin sebum values decreased with SA + CDP treatment.

Conclusions.—Combination of SA + CDP and all-TRA + CDP was effective in decreasing lesion counts and well tolerated with minimal local cutaneous reactions in patients with mild to moderate AV.

▶ The pathogenesis of acne vulgaris (AV) is multifactorial with 4 primary factors including excess sebum production, *Propionibacterium acnes* colonization, follicular hyperkeratinization, and release of inflammatory mediators into the skin. Therefore, treatment regimens tend to include combinations that best attack more than 1 mechanism. Salicylic acid is a desmolytic agent commonly found in over-the-counter topical acne medications. It promotes desquamation and combats hyperkeratinization found early in acne-affected follicles. Clindamycin, a topical antibiotic, acts by direct killing of P acnes. All transretinoic acid, tretinoin (all-TRA) is a derivative of vitamin A; it has the benefit of being a topical come-dolytic and exhibits direct antiinflammatory effects as well. This current prospective, single-blind, randomized comparative study found that both combinations, salicylic acid + clindamycin and all-TRA + clindamycin, effectively reduced inflammatory and comedonal lesion counts. Both combinations were well tolerated without significant side effects. Limitations of the study include small sample size (N = 46) and that the investigator was not blinded to treatments. These findings echo a previous study that showed no significant difference between these combinations but found combination treatments had significant benefits compared with clindamycin alone.[1]

S. Kim, DO

Reference

1. NilFroushzadeh MA, Siadat AH, Baradaran EH, Moradi S. Clindamycin lotion alone versus combination lotion of clindamycin phosphate plus tretinoin versus combination lotion of clindamycin phosphate plus salicylic acid in the topical treatment of mild to moderate acne vulgaris: a randomized control trial. *Indian J Dermatol Venereol Leprol.* 2009;75:279-382.

Antibiotics, Acne, and *Staphylococcus aureus* Colonization
Fanelli M, Kupperman E, Lautenbach E, et al (Univ of Pennsylvania School of Medicine, Philadelphia)
Arch Dermatol 147:917-921, 2011

Objectives.—To determine the frequency of *Staphylococcus aureus* colonization among patients with acne and to compare the susceptibility patterns between the patients who are using antibiotics and those who are not using antibiotics.

Design.—Survey (cross-sectional) study of patients treated for acne.

Setting.—Dermatology outpatient office practice.

Participants.—The study included 83 patients who were undergoing treatment and evaluation for acne.

Main Outcome Measure.—Colonization of the nose or throat with *S aureus.*

Results.—A total of 36 of the 83 participants (43%) were colonized with *S aureus.* Two of the 36 patients (6%) had methicillin-resistant *S aureus*; 20 (56%) had *S aureus* solely in their throat; 9 (25%) had *S aureus* solely in their nose; and 7 (19%) had *S aureus* in both their nose and their throat. When patients with acne who were antibiotic users were compared with nonusers, the prevalence odds ratio for the colonization of *S aureus* was 0.16 (95% confidence interval [CI], 0.08-1.37) after 1 to 2 months of exposure and increased to 0.52 (95% CI, 0.12-2.17) after 2 months of exposure ($P = .31$). Many of the *S aureus* isolates were resistant to treatment with clindamycin and erythromycin (40% and 44%, respectively), particularly the nasal isolates. Very few showed resistance rates (<10%) to treatment with tetracycline antibiotics.

Conclusion.—Unlike current dogma about the long-term use of antimicrobial agents, the prolonged use of tetracycline antibiotics commonly used to treat acne lowered the prevalence of colonization by *S aureus* and did not increase resistance to the tetracycline antibiotics.

▶ Methicillin-resistant *Staphylococcus aureus* (MRSA) is responsible for both uncomplicated and complicated cutaneous infections, as well as systemic infections that are often life-threatening. MRSA colonization, commonly of nares, perineum, axillae, and pharynx, is a common source of potential reinfection. Patients with acne vulgaris (AV) are often exposed to oral and topical antibiotics for extended periods of time. Interestingly, the tetracycline class of antibiotics, commonly used for AV, has also been used as initial antibiotic therapy to eradicate cutaneous MRSA infections. This has become a growing concern to the dermatology community because of the possibility of resistance to MRSA. This article discusses a cross-sectional survey-based study including 83 acne patients evaluating the colonization of *S aureus* and antibiotic-resistant rates. All patients had oropharyngeal and nasal swabs for *S aureus* and were tested for resistance to clindamycin, erythromycin, trimethoprim-sulfamethoxazole, ciprofloxacin, tetracycline, doxycycline, and minocycline. Thirty-six of the 83 participants (43%) were colonized with *S aureus* and 2 of the 36 (6%) with MRSA. Twenty of the participants (56%) had *S aureus* solely in their nose, and 7 (19%) had *S aureus* in both their nose and throat. Overall, the use of antibiotics (oral or topical) to treat AV was associated with a decreased risk of *S aureus* colonization. Fewer than 10% of the isolates of *S aureus* were resistant to tetracyclines. However, this study did have some limitations. First, the authors could not conclude that they identified all patients colonized with *S aureus* because only the oropharynx and anterior nares were swabbed. Also, authors did not examine patients at all points in time before and after antibiotic therapy. It was unknown whether patients were chronic carriers of *S aureus* prior to inclusion, an important consideration since staphylococcal carriage is not uncommon in the general population. In addition, the etiology of colonization with *S aureus* was unknown, and it was difficult to conclude without doubt whether antibiotic therapy used to treat AV was the sole reason for resistance. A prospective study evaluating colonization before the onset of antibiotics with continuous cultures is needed to determine the true *S aureus* colonization rates and presence of antibiotic resistance to agents such as tetracyclines. In conclusion, this study demonstrated that the use of tetracycline antibiotics does not increase the prevalence of and resistance to *S aureus* as previously thought. Nevertheless, the study was small and preliminary in design and evaluated a relatively short duration of use. Although this study is an important first step and challenges the assumption that chronic antibiotic use may select for or induce development of MRSA, additional well-designed and large-scale studies are needed.

G. K. Kim, DO
J. Q. Del Rosso, DO

A Case of Acne Fulminans in a Patient with Ulcerative Colitis Successfully Treated with Prednisolone and Diaminodiphenylsulfone: A Literature Review of Acne Fulminans, Rosacea Fulminans and Neutrophilic Dermatoses Occurring in the Setting of Inflammatory Bowel Disease
Wakabayashi M, Fujimoto N, Uenishi T, et al (Shiga Univ of Med Science, Otsu, Japan)
Dermatology 222:231-235, 2011

A 19-year-old Japanese man had been treated for ulcerative colitis for 2 years. He was admitted to our hospital with nodulocystic inflammatory papules and pustules on his face and chest, high-grade fever, arthralgia and general malaise. A biopsy specimen from a pustule showed prominent infiltration of neutrophils in the epidermis and dermis, particularly around hair follicles. We made a diagnosis of acne fulminans. The systemic administration of prednisolone at 30 mg daily for 1 week immediately improved his skin lesions and other symptoms; however, during tapering of prednisolone at 20 mg daily, skin lesions flared up. The addition of oral diaminodiphenylsulfone improved the skin lesions. Although there have been a few reports of acne fulminans associated with Crohn's disease, this is the first case report of acne fulminans in a patient with ulcerative colitis. It is noteworthy that the addition of diaminodiphenylsulfone was effective for treating the relapse of acne fulminans in this case.

▶ Acne fulminans is a devastating but fortunately rare form of acne. It mainly occurs following institution of oral isotretinoin therapy. This drug-related form usually lacks systemic symptoms. The spontaneous form of acne fulminans is more severe and rarer than cases associated with starting oral isotretinoin. Research is lacking on the disease, probably due as much to its rarity as to our inability to leave it untreated for study. The coincidence of Crohn disease with acne fulminans is tantalizing. As every dermatologist is aware, isotretinoin has been blamed as a cause of inflammatory bowel disease (IBD) on the basis of retrospective studies. I have long suspected that this is not the case. Rather, severe acne and IBD share a predisposing defect in the regulation of inflammation. This case would support that hypothesis.

G. Webster, MD, PhD

Cortexolone 17α-propionate 1% cream, a new potent antiandrogen for topical treatment of acne vulgaris. A pilot randomized, double-blind comparative study vs. placebo and tretinoin 0·05% cream
Trifu V, Tiplica G-S, Naumescu E, et al (Central Emergency Clinical Military Hosp 'Dr Carol Davila', Bucharest, Romania; Clinical Hosp Colentina, Bucharest, Romania; Clinical Hosp of Dermato-Venerology 'Prof. Dr Scarlat Longhin', Bucharest, Romania; et al)
Br J Dermatol 165:177-183, 2011

Background.—Acne vulgaris is a disorder of the pilosebaceous unit in which the androgens contribute to its onset and persistence. The use of antiandrogens is therefore potentially effective; however, antiandrogens for topical use are not available on the market. Cortexolone 17α-propionate (CB-03-01; Cosmo S.p.A, Lainate, Italy) is a new potent topical antiandrogen potentially useful in acne vulgaris.

Objectives.—To evaluate the safety and the topical efficacy of CB-03-01 1% cream in acne vulgaris as compared with placebo and with tretinoin 0·05% cream (Retin-A®; Janssen-Cilag).

Methods.—Seventy-seven men with facial acne scored 2−3 according to Investigator's Global Assessment (IGA) were randomized to receive placebo cream ($n = 15$), or CB-03-01 1% cream ($n = 30$), or tretinoin 0·05% cream ($n = 32$) once a day at bedtime for 8 weeks. Clinical efficacy was evaluated every 2 weeks including total lesion count (TLC), inflammatory lesion count (ILC), acne severity index (ASI) and IGA. Safety assessment included local irritancy score, laboratory tests, physical examination, vital signs and recording of adverse events.

Results.—CB-03-01 1% cream was very well tolerated, and was significantly better than placebo regarding TLC ($P = 0·0017$), ILC ($P = 0·0134$) and ASI ($P = 0·0090$), and also clinically more effective than comparator. The product also induced a faster attainment of 50% improvement in all the above parameters.

Conclusions.—This pilot study supports the rationale for the use of topical antiandrogens in the treatment of acne vulgaris. CB-03-01 1% cream seems to fit with the profile of an ideal antiandrogen for topical use.

▶ This is the first study of repeated application of a new topical antiandrogen, cortexolone 17α-propionate 1% cream (CB-03-01) in human subjects with acne. CB-03-01 is a nonsteroidal antiandrogen that blocks the androgen receptor and is rapidly inactivated in the skin. Seventy-seven men with mild to moderate acne vulgaris (AV) were randomly assigned to receive once-daily treatment with the CB-03-01 1% cream (n = 30), tretinoin cream 0.05% (n = 32), or placebo (n = 15) for 8 weeks. Efficacy variables included percentage of changes in total lesions, inflammatory lesions, "success" based on Investigator's Global Assessment (IGA), and a calculated acne severity index. Safety was assessed by use of an irritancy score, laboratory monitoring, and assessment of adverse events. The antiandrogen was significantly better than placebo in terms of lesion counts and the calculated acne severity index but not better based on the IGA. No differences between tretinoin 0.05% cream and CB-03-01 1% cream were noted with the exception of inflammatory lesion counts at week 6. Of note is that this is a pilot study conducted in men with approximately half having mild AV. In clinical practice, AV in women appears to be more hormonally driven. These preliminary findings are somewhat encouraging, and moving forward, therapeutic outcomes will need to be substantiated in appropriately designed clinical trials.

D. Thiboutot, MD

Alopecia areata: Clinical presentation, diagnosis, and unusual cases

Finner AM (Trichomed Hair Clinic, Berlin, Germany)
Dermatol Ther 24:348-354, 2011

Alopecia areata (AA) is a nonscarring hair loss disorder with a 2% lifetime risk. Most patients are below 30 years old. Clinical types include patchy AA, AA reticularis, diffuse AA, AA ophiasis, AA sisiapho, and perinevoid AA. Besides scalp and body hair, the eyebrows, eyelashes, and nails can be affected. The disorder may be circumscribed, total (scalp hair loss), and universal (loss of all hairs). Atopy, autoimmune thyroid disease, and vitiligo are more commonly associated. The course of the disease is unpredictable. However, early, long-lasting, and severe cases have a less favorable prognosis. The clinical diagnosis is made by the aspect of hairless patches with a normal skin and preserved follicular ostia. Exclamations mark hairs and a positive pull test signal activity. Dermoscopy may reveal yellow dots. White hairs may be spared; initial regrowth may also be nonpigmented. The differential diagnosis includes trichotillomania, scarring alopecia, and other nonscarring hair loss disorders such as tinea capitis and syphilis.

▶ Alopecia areata (AA) is commonly seen in the dermatologic setting and affects men, women, and children. AA usually presents with 1 or more nonscarring focal hairless patches. This article discusses clinical presentation, diagnosis, and unusual cases of AA. Patchy AA is the most common form, occurring in up to 75% of patients. A specific band-like pattern of AA along the occipital hairline extending toward the temples is called ophiasis. The ophiasis pattern is reported to be a predictor of a poor prognosis for hair regrowth. Dermoscopy can reveal yellow dots or keratotic plugs in the follicular ostia that are suggestive of but not specific for AA. Exclamation-mark hairs are another sign of acute disease. Nail changes can be seen in alopecia patients, such as small pits, red-spotted lunula, and trachyonychia. AA can also be associated with autoimmune thyroid disease, vitiligo, Down syndrome, and sickle cell anemia. Many conditions can mimic AA, such as telogen effluvium, trichotillomania, and noninflammatory tinea capitis. In up to 50% of patients, AA spontaneously regrows within 12 months. In alopecia totalis and universalis, the chances of full recovery is < 10%. A positive family history, duration of > 12 months without regrowth, > 50% of scalp involvement, atopy, and other associated changes are negative prognostic factors. For many of these patients, the initial presentation will predict the disease course.

G. K. Kim, DO
J. Q. Del Rosso, DO

Rosacea — global diversity and optimized outcome: proposed international consensus from the Rosacea International Expert Group

Elewski BE, Draelos Z, Dréno B, et al (Univ of Alabama, Birmingham; Dermatology Consulting Services, Highpoint, NC; Nantes Univ Hosp, Nantes Cedex, France; et al)
J Eur Acad Dermatol Venereol 25:188-200, 2011

Background.—The absence of specific histological or serological markers, the gaps in understanding the aetiology and pathophysiology of rosacea, and the broad diversity in its clinical manifestations has made it difficult to reach international consensus on therapy guidelines.

Objective.—The main objective was to highlight the global diversity in current thinking about rosacea pathophysiology, classification and medical features, under particular consideration of the relevance of the findings to optimization of therapy.

Methods.—The article presents findings, proposals and conclusions reached by the ROSacea International Expert group (ROSIE), comprising European and US rosacea experts.

Results.—New findings on pathogenesis provide a rationale for the development of novel therapies. Thus, recent findings suggest a central role of the antimicrobial peptide cathelicidin and its activator kallikrein-5 by eliciting an exacerbated response of the innate immune system. Cathelicidin/kallikrein-5 also provide a rationale for the effect of tetracyclines and azelaic acid against rosacea. Clinically, the ROSIE group emphasized the need for a comprehensive therapy strategy — the triad of rosacea care — that integrates patient education including psychological and social aspects, skin care with dermo-cosmetics as well as drug- and physical therapies. Classification of rosacea into stages or subgroups, with or without progression, remained controversial. However, the ROSIE group proposed that therapy decision making should be in accordance with a treatment algorithm based on the signs and symptoms of rosacea rather than on a prior classification.

Conclusion.—The ROSIE group reviewed rosacea pathophysiology and medical features and the impact on patients and treatment options. The group suggested a rational, evidence-based approach to treatment for the various symptoms of the condition. In daily practice this approach might be more easily handled than prior subtype classification, in particular since patients often may show clinical features of more than one subtype at the same time.

▶ This article provides an overview of the pathogenesis and treatment of rosacea by the members of an international consensus group. Their main objective was to have a dialogue regarding international variations in diagnosis and treatment of rosacea to propose international treatment guidelines. The article is a thorough review of the subject and proposes that physicians should follow a triad of rosacea care, including patient education, skin care, and treatment based on symptoms and signs. The need for additional research into the pathophysiology of rosacea as a means for improvements in therapy is emphasized.

D. Thiboutot, MD

A 6-month maintenance therapy with adapalene-benzoyl peroxide gel prevents relapse and continuously improves efficacy among patients with severe acne vulgaris: results of a randomized controlled trial

Poulin Y, Sanchez NP, Bucko A, et al (Centre de Recherche Dermatologique du Québec Metropolitan, Canada; Sanchez Dermatology, Aibonito, Puerto Rico; Academic Dermatology Associates, Albuquerque, NM; et al)
Br J Dermatol 164:1376-1382, 2011

Background.—Acne vulgaris is a chronic and frequently recurring disease. A fixed-dose adapalene-benzoyl peroxide (adapalene-BPO) gel is an efficacious and safe acne treatment.

Objectives.—To assess the long-term effect of adapalene-BPO on relapse prevention among patients with severe acne after successful initial treatments.

Methods.—This is a multicentre, double-blind, randomized and controlled study. In total, 243 subjects who had severe acne vulgaris and at least 50% global improvement after a previous 12-week treatment were randomized into the present study to receive adapalene-BPO gel or its vehicle once daily for 24 weeks.

Results.—At week 24, compared with vehicle, adapalene-BPO resulted in significantly higher lesion maintenance success rate (defined as having at least 50% improvement in lesion counts achieved in initial treatment) for all types of lesions (total lesions: $78 \cdot 9\%$ vs. $45 \cdot 8\%$; inflammatory lesions: $78 \cdot 0\%$ vs. $48 \cdot 3\%$; noninflammatory lesions: $78 \cdot 0\%$ vs. $43 \cdot 3\%$; all $P < 0 \cdot 001$). Significantly more subjects with adapalene-BPO than with vehicle had the same or better Investigator's Global Assessment score at week 24 than at baseline ($70 \cdot 7\%$ vs. $34 \cdot 2\%$; $P < 0 \cdot 001$). The time when 25% of subjects relapsed was 175 days with adapalene-BPO and 56 days with vehicle (17 weeks earlier; $P < 0 \cdot 0001$). Adapalene-BPO led to further decrease of lesion counts during the study and $45 \cdot 7\%$ of subjects were 'clear' or 'almost clear' at week 24. It was also safe and well tolerated in the study.

Conclusions.—Adapalene-BPO not only prevents the occurrence of relapse among patients with severe acne, but also continues to reduce disease symptoms during 6 months.

▶ This is a randomized, double-blind, vehicle-controlled study evaluating adapalene-benzoyl peroxide (A/BPO) maintenance therapy over 6 months after initial combination treatment with doxycycline, 100 mg daily, compared with vehicle alone used for maintenance therapy in patients with severe acne vulgaris at the outset of the initial treatment. Inflammatory and noninflammatory lesion counts with Investigator Global Assessment were also performed. There were

123 patients treated with A/BPO and 120 treated with vehicle. After 24 weeks of treatment, subjects receiving A/BPO had a significantly superior decrease in inflammatory and noninflammatory lesions ($P < .001$). Significant differences at week 4 were observed in favor of A/BPO for total lesion counts ($P < .05$) and noninflammatory lesions ($P < .01$) and week 8 for inflammatory lesion ($P < .01$). To add, 70.7% of subjects on the A/BPO group remained stable over the course of the study once peak effect of the therapy was achieved. BPO and a topical retinoid are both suitable for long-term use, especially as these medications do not cause or promote the emergence of bacterial resistance. The authors concluded that this study showed the benefit of A/BPO for long-term therapy. It is also safe, well tolerated, and efficacious in many patients in preventing relapse with continued reduction in acne lesions over time.

G. K. Kim, DO

J. Q. Del Rosso, DO

A microbial aetiology of acne: what is the evidence?

Shaheen B, Gonzalez M (Cardiff Univ School of Medicine, UK)
Br J Dermatol 165:474-485, 2011

A microbial aetiology of acne has been suggested since the beginning of the last century. There is considerable evidence, circumstantial at best, which suggests that micro-organisms, particularly *Propionibacterium acnes*, are important in the pathogenesis of acne vulgaris. However, it is still unclear whether *P. acnes* is actually a causal agent in the development of noninflamed or inflamed acne lesions. Based on a review of the microbiological data on normal and acne-affected skin, we propose that *P. acnes* neither initiates comedogenesis nor has a role in the initiation of inflammation in inflamed acne lesions.

▶ Many believe that *Propionibacterium acnes* is important in the pathogenesis of acne. However, the exact pathogenesis involving *P acnes* is still unclear, with these authors challenging its role because it is part of the normal flora of the skin. This article reviews the microbiological data on normal and acne-prone skin to evaluate the role of *P acnes* in the pathogenesis of acne vulgaris. *P acnes* was found to be highest in the oily regions of the body such as the face and upper trunk. The authors found that the microflora of normal or acne-affected pilosebaceous follicles (inflamed and noninflamed) consists of 3 major genera of micro-organisms (*Propionibacterium* spp, *Staphylococcus* spp, and *Malassezia* spp). They also commented that from their review of literature that *P acnes* is not a requirement for comedogenesis. However, the authors did recognize that after colonization of the pilosebaceous follicles with *P acnes*, the organism can aggravate and intensify abnormal desquamation by releasing lipases, but presence of *P acnes* is not required for the initiation of an acne lesion. It was also proposed that the *P acnes* biofilm may act as a biological glue in causing adhesiveness of keratinocytes and aggravating comedogenesis. Also

P acnes may play a role in the intensification of the inflammatory process by its enzymatic, antigenic, chemoattractant, and complement activation activities. Induction of toll-like receptors 2 and 4 may be another mechanism in which *P acnes* contributes to acne lesions. However, according to these authors, other microorganisms such as *Staphylococcus* spp and *Malassezia* spp may also be the culprit. The authors concluded from studies that *P acnes* does not initiate comedogenesis and is not the sole source of inflammation in acne vulgaris. However, patients with severe acne have increased levels of antibodies to *P acnes*. In conclusion, the authors advocated that *P acnes* may act primarily as a bystander, and other factors such as androgens, abnormalities of sebaceous lipids, and cytokines may play a more active and direct role in the initiation of acne vulgaris. Importantly, it is recognized that *P acnes* does not appear to initiate acne vulgaris; however, it does play an important role in promoting inflammation through several potential pathways.[1]

G. K. Kim, DO
J. Q. Del Rosso, DO

Reference

1. Bellew S, Thiboutot D, Del Rosso JQ. Pathogenesis of acne vulgaris: what's new, what's interesting and what may be clinically relevant. *J Drugs Dermatol.* 2011; 10:582-585.

Does isotretinoin have effect on vitamin D physiology and bone metabolism in acne patients?
Ertugrul DT, Karadag AS, Tutal E, et al (Ankara Kecioren Res and Training Hosp, Turkey)
Dermatol Ther 24:291-295, 2011

Isotretinoin is an effective therapy for severe nodulocystic acne. Several experimental studies suggest that it may have an effect on vitamin D physiology. In the present study, the authors aimed to investigate the effect of isotretinoin treatment on the metabolism of vitamin D in acne patients. A prospective analysis of 50 consecutive acne patients who were treated with isotretinoin for 3 months was done. Before and after 3 months of treatment, 25 hydroxy vitamin D, 1,25 dihydroxy vitamin D, and bone alkaline phosphatase, calcium, phosphate, and parathormone levels were measured. The 25 hydroxy vitamin D and serum calcium levels decreased significantly ($p < 0.0001$, $p < 0.05$, respectively), whereas 1,25 dihydroxy vitamin D, parathormone, and bone alkaline phosphatase levels increased significantly after 3 months of isotretinoin treatment ($p < 0.005$, $p < 0.005$, $p < 0.0001$, respectively). Aspartate aminotransferase, total cholesterol, low-density lipoprotein cholesterol, and triglyceride levels also increased significantly after isotretinoin treatment. This prospective clinical study showed that isotretinoin has an effect on vitamin D metabolism. Further clinical studies with longer periods of follow-up are needed to understand the effect of isotretinoin on vitamin D and bone metabolism.

▶ Oral isotretinoin has been known to cause both osteoporosis and hyperostotic changes of the bone, especially with longer courses of therapy. However, it has been suggested that even 1 month of oral isotretinoin exposure could decrease bone mineral density (BMD) and negatively affect bone metabolism. This is a prospective study of 50 patients with moderate to severe nodulocystic acne vulgaris (AV) on oral isotretinoin therapy initiated at 0.5 to 0.75 mg/kg body weight daily and then adjusted to 0.80 mg/kg/day as maintenance dosage after 1 month, and continued for at least 5 months. Laboratory examinations of 25 hydroxyvitamin D (25-HVD), 1,25 dihydroxy vitamin D (1,25-DHVD), bone alkaline phosphatase (BAP), calcium, phosphate and parathyroid hormone (PTH) levels were measured. The 25-HVD and serum calcium levels decreased significantly ($P < .0001$, $P < .05$, respectively). The levels of 1,25-DHVD, PTH and BAP levels increased significantly after 3 months of therapy ($P < .005$, $P < .005$, $P < .0001$, respectively). No patients dropped out of this study because of medication side effects. It was found that during the study, calcium and 25-HVD levels decreased significantly, whereas BAP, PTH, and 1,25(OH) 2D levels increased significantly after 3 months of treatment with oral isotretinoin for AV. The stimulation of CYP24A1 by isotretinoin was suggested as an explanation for the fall in the 25HVD levels, although analysis of this pathway was not explored. The CYP24 gene may be of interest in the future to determine whether certain individuals are more susceptible to bone changes with isotretinoin therapy. Also, this study did not evaluate BMD, which would be of major interest. In summary, this study revealed that oral isotretinoin decreases 25-HVD levels, ultimately leading to decrease in serum calcium and increase in serum PTH and BAP levels. One limitation was that there were no controls, and concurrent medications that may have affected laboratory values were unknown. The authors suggest that the decrease in BMD with isotretinoin treatment that has been shown in some studies may be due to osteomalacia rather than osteoporosis.

G. K. Kim, DO

J. Q. Del Rosso, DO

Comparison of the epidemiology of acne vulgaris among Caucasian, Asian, Continental Indian and African American women
Perkins AC, Cheng CE, Hillebrand GG, et al (Massachusetts General Hosp, Boston; Procter & Gamble, Cincinnati, OH)
J Eur Acad Dermatol Venereol 25:1054-1060, 2011

Background.—Acne vulgaris is a common skin disease with a large quality of life impact, characterized by comedones, inflammatory lesions, secondary dyspigmentation and scarring. There are few large objective studies comparing acne epidemiology between racial and ethnic groups.

Objective.—This study aimed to define the prevalence and subtypes of acne in women of different racial groups from four ethnicities.

Methods.—The sample consisted of 2895 (384 African American, 520 Asian, 1295 Caucasian, 258 Hispanic and 438 Continental Indian) women ranging in age from 10 to 70 years. Photographs of subjects were graded for acne lesions, scars, dyspigmentation, and measurements taken of sebum excretion and pore size.

Results.—Clinical acne was more prevalent in African American and Hispanic women (37%, 32% respectively) than in Continental Indian, Caucasian and Asian (23%, 24%, 30% respectively) women. All racial groups displayed equal prevalence of both subtypes of acne with the exception of Asians, for whom inflammatory acne was more prevalent than comedonal (20% vs. 10%) acne, and in Caucasians, for whom comedonal acne was more prevalent than inflammatory (14% vs. 10%) acne. Hyperpigmentation was more prevalent in African American and Hispanic (65%, 48% respectively) than in Asian, Continental Indian and Caucasian (18%, 10%, 25% respectively) women. Dyspigmentation and atrophic scarring were more common in African American and Hispanic women than in all other ethnicities. There was a negative correlation between pore size and skin lightness for all ethnicities. Sebum production was positively correlated with acne severity in African American, Asian and Hispanic women, and pore size was positively correlated with acne in African American, Asian and Continental Indian women, (for all above results, $P < 0.05$).

Limitations.—Only female participants were recruited. Data collection was restricted to four cities, with some ethnicities from single cities. Acne was evaluated only on the left side of the face and the two-dimensional nature of photography may not capture all skin surface changes.

Conclusion.—Acne prevalence and sequelae were more common in those with darker skin types, suggesting that acne is a more heterogeneous condition than previously described and highlighting the importance of skin-colour tailored treatment.

▶ Acne vulgaris (AV) is a common inflammatory skin disorder worldwide. In the past, AV has been treated as a homogenous disease. However, recent data suggest that AV may differ among various racial and ethnic groups. This is a study of 2895 women (44% Caucasian, 19% Asian, 15% Continental Indian, 13% Asian American, and 9% Hispanic) evaluating acne severity, scars, dyspigmentation, pore size, and sebum secretion. Asians had a higher prevalence of inflammatory lesions (20%) compared with other ethnicities. In addition, Caucasians had a higher incidence of comedonal acne (14%) compared with other ethnicities. Hyperpigmentation was most prevalent in African Americans and Hispanics (65% and 48%). AV was most prevalent clinically in African Americans (37%; $P < .01$). When Asian women were broken down by ethnicity and location, Asian women from Los Angeles (Chinese, Korean, and Japanese) had the highest prevalence of acne at 41%. Sebum secretion was considerably higher in patients with clinical AV ($P < .01$) than those without AV. Also, there was no correlation between pore size and AV. Additionally, there was a negative correlation between pore size and skin lightness (P < .001). The authors found that African Americans had the highest rates of secondary hyperpigmentation and scarring. They suggest that this may be due to deeper inflammation, as found in recent studies in African American individuals with AV. Treatment for this darker skin group may include more antiinflammatory-based therapies. The authors also found that Asians living in Los Angeles compared with those living in Japan had higher prevalences of AV, which may suggest an environmental factor or dietary influence. Because the Japanese diet is lower in sugar and total fat, the authors speculated that it may be due to diet. The limitations of this study are that it included only women, and there was no separation in Asians and Hispanics according to specific regions of origin. Also, photographic images present a limitation because of technique and variability. In conclusion, the authors demonstrated in this study that AV is a heterogenous condition, and racial consideration is important when considering targeted therapy for AV.

G. K. Kim, DO

J. Q. Del Rosso, DO

Cicatricial alopecia
Berlin JM, Wang AL, McDuffie BC, et al
J Am Acad Dermatol 63:547-548, 2010

Background.—The histologic characteristics of discoid lupus erythematosus include superficial and deep perivascular and peri-adnexal lymphocytic infiltrate that can continue down into the follicular infundibulum along with a thickened basement membrane zone. A case was reported in a woman with progressive hair loss.

Case Report.—Woman, 56, had patchy areas of hair loss that had increased progressively over the previous 2 years and had not significantly responded to nizoral shampoo. Her medical history included idiopathic thrombocytopenic purpura. Physical examination demonstrated discrete patches of scarring alopecia with central hypopigmentation and erythema. The possible diagnoses included discoid lupus erythematosus, folliculiltis decalvens, lichen planopilaris, and classic pseudopelade or Brocq alopecia. The most likely diagnosis was discoid lupus erythematosus, which is seen as round or discoid lesions with follicular plugging and scale. Erythema can be present, usually seen more prominently in the center of the alopecic patch rather than peripherally. Atrophic, sclerotic plaques can develop. Most patients complain of pruritus or pain, but the lesions can be asymptomatic. Diagnosis can be facilitated by a skin biopsy and the morphology of the eruption. Direct immunofluorescence is positive in up to 70% of cases. Often there is a linear granular deposition of immunoglobulin G and C3 at the dermoepidermal junction. Initially cases are treated with intralesional and topical corticosteroids. Systemic retinoids, methyltrexate, and antimalarial agents are the second line of treatment, with isotretinoin and thalidomide used for severe and refractory cases.

Conclusions.—The management of discoid lupus erythematosus begins with a differentiation between scarring and nonscarring alopecia. In scarring or cicatricial alopecia, connective tissue replaces the follicular epithelium. A punch biopsy specimen can help confirm the diagnosis. Treatment depends on the severity and persistence of the lesions.

▶ This brief article summarizes the findings associated with discoid lupus erythematosus (DLE), a type of cicatricial or scarring alopecia. Cicatricial alopecia refers to destruction of the hair follicle and replacement of the follicular epithelium with connective tissue, which may lead to permanent hair loss. Differential diagnosis includes DLE, lichen planopilaris, acne keloidalis, folliculitis decalvans, pseudopelade of Brocq, and alopecia mucinosa. In DLE, patients may present with history of patchy hair loss, erythema, atrophy, follicular plugging, and hypo- or hyperpigmentation. Diagnosis can be aided by a 4-mm punch biopsy, which may show superficial and deep perivascular and periadnexal lymphocytic infiltrate, dermal mucin, thickening of basement membrane, vacuolar interface, and follicular plugging. Direct immunofluorescence shows linear granular deposition of IgG and C3 at the dermoepidermal junction in 70% of cases. Initial retreatment options include intralesional and topical corticosteroids (of adequate potency), if lesions are caught early in the inflammatory stage before cicatricial changes occur. As the pathologic process is perifollicular, response to topical corticosteroids needs to be rapid; otherwise, intralesional injection should be utilized to assure therapy is administered to the depth of involvement of the disease. Antimalarial agents (ie, hydroxychloroquine), systemic retinoids, or methotrexate are sometimes helpful. Use of thalidomide has also been reported in refractory DLE. Once cicatricial changes are fully developed, therapeutic agents are of limited benefit.

S. Bellew, DO

J. Q. Del Rosso, DO

Central hair loss in African American women: Incidence and potential risk factors
Olsen EA, Callender V, McMichael A, et al (Duke Univ Med Ctr, Durham, NC; Howard Univ, Mitchellville, MD; Wake Forest Univ, Winston-Salem, NC; et al)
J Am Acad Dermatol 64:245-252, 2011

Background.—Although central scalp hair loss is a common problem in African American women, data on etiology or incidence are limited.

Objective.—We sought to determine the frequency of various patterns and degree of central scalp hair loss in African American women and to correlate this with information on hair care practices, family history of hair loss, and medical history.

Methods.—Five hundred twenty-nine subjects at six different workshops held at four different sites in the central and/or southeast United States participated in this study. The subjects' patterns and degree of central scalp hair loss were independently assessed by both subject and investigator using a standardized photographic scale. Subjects also completed a detailed questionnaire and had standardized photographs taken. Statistical analysis was performed evaluating answers to the questionnaire relative to pattern of central hair loss.

Results.—Extensive central scalp hair loss was seen in 5.6% of subjects. There was no obvious association of extensive hair loss with relaxer or hot comb use, history of seborrheic dermatitis or reaction to a hair care product, bacterial infection, or male pattern hair loss in fathers of subjects; however, there was an association with a history of tinea capitis.

Limitations.—There was no scalp biopsy correlation with clinical pattern of hair loss and further information on specifics of hair care practices is needed.

Conclusions.—This central scalp photographic scale and questionnaire provide a valid template by which to further explore potential etiologic factors and relationships to central scalp hair loss in African American women.

▶ Central centrifugal cicatricial alopecia (CCCA) has been clinically recognized in the female African American population for years. Originally described as "hot comb alopecia," the exact etiology of CCCA has yet to be elucidated. In a recently reported population-based study of CCCA, researchers found a high prevalence of central hair loss in African American women with significant association with diabetes mellitus type 2 ($P = .01$), bacterial scalp infections ($P = .045$), and hairstyles that incorporate traction ($P = .02$).[1] In contrast, the current study of 529 African American women found the only statistically significant association was with a personal history of tinea capitis. More specifically, the report finds a more significant association between tinea capitis and a more advanced pattern graded as 3 through 5 hair loss versus patterns 0 through 2 ($P = .0009$). Limitations as stated by authors include no biopsy confirmation, data collected based on memory of distant events subject to recall bias, and no information on whether a particular hair-care process would be more problematic or safer if used in a specific way. For clinicians, efforts should be made to identify treatable inflammatory conditions at an earlier stage to prevent this type of hair loss.

S. Bellew, DO

J. Q. Del Rosso, DO

Reference

1. Kyei A, Bergfeld WF, Piliang M, Summers P. Medical and environmental risk factors for the development of central centrifugal cicatricial alopecia: a population study. *Arch Dermatol.* 2011;147:909-914.

Acne-associated syndromes: models for better understanding of acne pathogenesis

Chen W, Obermayer-Pietsch B, Hong J-B, et al (Technische Universitaet Muenchen, Munich, Germany; Medizinische Universitaet Graz, Austria; Natl Taiwan Univ Hosp and Yun-Lin Branch, Taipei; et al)

J Eur Acad Dermatol Venereol 25:637-646, 2011

Acne, one of the most common skin disorders, is also a cardinal component of many systemic diseases or syndromes. Their association illustrates the nature of these diseases and is indicative of the pathogenesis of acne. Congenital adrenal hyperplasia (CAH) and seborrhoea-acne-hirsutism-androgenetic alopecia (SAHA) syndrome highlight the role of androgen steroids, while polycystic ovary (PCO) and hyperandrogenism-insulin resistance-acanthosis nigricans (HAIR-AN) syndromes indicate insulin resistance in acne. Apert syndrome with increased fibroblast growth factor receptor 2 (*FGFR2*) signalling results in follicular hyperkeratinization and sebaceous gland hypertrophy in acne. Synovitis-acne-pustulosis-hyperostosis-osteitis (SAPHO) and pyogenic arthritis-pyoderma gangrenosum-acne (PAPA) syndromes highlight the attributes of inflammation to acne formation. Advances in the understanding of the manifestation and molecular mechanisms of these syndromes will help to clarify acne pathogenesis and develop novel therapeutic modalities.

▶ Acne vulgaris is the most common skin condition observed in the dermatologic setting. It is also a disease that can have other associated systemic diseases and syndromes. This is a review of recent findings, clinical manifestations, molecular changes, and therapeutic advancements with acne-associated diseases. Congenital adrenal hyperplasia (CAH) is a disease characterized by excess secretion of adrenocorticotropic hormone (ACTH) and overstimulation of the adrenal glands. Acne and hirsutism are the main cutaneous manifestations of CAH seen in adolescence. Treatments for CAH include cautious oral glucocorticoid therapy and monitoring of serum dehydroepiandrosterone (DHEA) levels. The concurrent presence of seborrhea, acne, hirsutism and androgenetic alopecia (SAHA) indicates androgen excess in women. SAHA syndrome is due to an increased sensitivity to normal androgen levels. This syndrome is treated symptomatically with lifestyle modification, oral contraceptives, and antiandrogen medications. Polycystic ovarian syndrome (PCOS) is a complex endocrine disorder that presents in women with findings that include infertility, hirsutism, acne, and alopecia. Lifestyle modification, insulin sensitizers, and oral contraceptives are the most common therapeutic approaches for PCOS. Hyperandrogenism-insulin resistance-acanthosis nigricans (HAIR-AN) syndrome is another acne-related syndrome that is considered a unique subtype of PCOS. The current management resembles that of SAHA and PCOS. Synovitis-acne-pustulosis-hyperostosis-osteitis syndrome is a rare condition associated with inflammatory bowel disease. This condition can be treated with immunotherapeutic agents and is characterized by intermittent exacerbations. Pyogenic arthritis-pyoderma gangrenosum-acne syndrome (PAPA syndrome) is considered an autoinflammatory disease, with sterile arthritis, pyoderma gangrenosum (PG), and acne conglobata (AC) being characteristic clinical features. Dapsone has been used in PAPA syndrome because of its antineutrophilic effect, with efficacy noted for both PG and AC. Alpert syndrome, also known as acrocephalosyndactyly, is an inherited syndrome characterized by synostoses of extremities, vertebrae, and skull, with syndactyly of fingers and toes. These patients have acne in an unusual distribution with lesions extending to the surface areas of the forearms. Acne can be a clue to an underlying syndrome of which the clinician may be unaware. Further studies evaluating syndromes associated with acne may help investigators to better understand acne pathogenesis and ultimately find novel therapeutic treatments.

G. K. Kim, DO

J. Q. Del Rosso, DO

Frontal fibrosing alopecia: a clinical review of 36 patients

Samrao A, Chew A-L, Price V (Univ of California San Francisco; Guy's and St Thomas' NHS Foundation Trust, London, UK)
Br J Dermatol 163:1296-1300, 2010

Background.—Frontal fibrosing alopecia (FFA) is a primary lymphocytic cicatricial alopecia with a distinctive clinical pattern of progressive fronto-temporal hairline recession. Currently, there are no evidence-based studies to guide treatment for patients with FFA; thus, treatment options vary among clinicians.

Objectives.—We report clinical findings and treatment outcomes of 36 patients with FFA, the largest cohort to date. Further, we report the first evidence-based study of the efficacy of hydroxychloroquine in FFA using a quantitative clinical score, the Lichen Planopilaris Activity Index (LPPAI).

Methods.—A retrospective case note review was performed of 36 adult patients with FFA. Data were collected on demographics and clinical findings. Treatment responses to hydroxychloroquine, doxycycline and mycophenolate mofetil were assessed using the LPPAI. Adverse events were monitored.

Results.—Most patients in our cohort were female (97%), white (92%) and postmenopausal (83%). Apart from hairline recession, 75% also reported eyebrow loss. Scalp pruritus (67%) and perifollicular erythema (86%) were the most common presenting symptom and sign, respectively. A statistically significant reduction in signs and symptoms in subjects treated with hydroxychloroquine ($P < 0.05$) was found at both 6- and 12-month follow up.

Conclusions.—In FFA, hairline recession, scalp pruritus, perifollicular erythema and eyebrow loss are common at presentation. Despite the limitations of a retrospective review, our data reveal that hydroxychloroquine is significantly effective in reducing signs and symptoms of FFA after both 6 and 12 months of treatment. However, the lack of a significant reduction in signs and symptoms between 6 and 12 months indicates that the maximal benefits of hydroxychloroquine are evident within the first 6 months of use.

▶ Frontal fibrosing alopecia (FFA) is a cicatricial form of hair loss with progressive recession of the frontotemporal hairline, occurring in postmenopausal women. The histologic findings seen in FFA are similar to those in lichen planopilaris (LPP). This is a retrospective review of medical records and histopathology reports of 36 patients with FFA. Medical records were examined for data on demographics (age, sex, and menopausal status), duration and extent of the disease, clinical findings (symptoms and signs of the disease), anagen pull test results, concurrent scalp diagnoses, biopsy results, and treatment responses (hydroxychloroquine, doxycycline, and mycophenolate mofetil). Sixteen of the 25 evaluable treatment courses (64%) were with hydroxychloroquine, 4 (16%) with doxycycline, and 5 (20%) with mycophenolate mofetil. The differences between the Lichen Planopilaris Activity Index (LPPAI) scores across all time periods were statistically significant ($P = .003$) for hydroxychloroquine. The difference between the LPPAI at 0 and 6 months and between the LPPAI at 0 and 12 months was also significant ($P = .0045$ and $.0196$, respectively). The 4 patients on doxycycline were treated for a median of 18 months with 2 patients having a reduction in signs and symptoms at 6 months. For mycophenolate mofetil, at the 6 month follow up, 3 (60%) patients had responded to treatment. In this study, perifollicular erythema and loss of eyebrows were frequently seen at the time of initial presentation (86% and 75%, respectively). Seven of 36 patients (19%) also reported hair loss on their upper and lower limbs. No associated laboratory or hormonal abnormalities have been identified of FFA. This retrospective study revealed the efficacy of each therapeutic agent as it pertains to FFA, with hydroxychloroquine being significantly effective in reducing signs and symptoms in patients with FFA, especially within the first 6 months of treatment.

G. K. Kim, DO

J. Q. Del Rosso, DO

Combination therapy with adapalene—benzoyl peroxide and oral lymecycline in the treatment of moderate to severe acne vulgaris: a multicentre, randomized, double-blind controlled study
Dréno B, Kaufmann R, Talarico S, et al (Hôpital Hotel Dieu, France; Goethe-Univ Hosp, Germany; UNIFESP—Universidade Federal de São Paulo, Brazil; et al)
Br J Dermatol 165:383-390, 2011

Background.—Oral antibiotics in association with a topical retinoid with or without benzoyl peroxide (BPO) are the recommended first-line option in the treatment of moderate to severe acne vulgaris.

Objectives.—To evaluate the efficacy and safety of oral lymecycline 300 mg with adapalene $0 \cdot 1\%$—BPO $2 \cdot 5\%$ (A/BPO) fixed-dose gel in comparison with oral lymecycline 300 mg with a vehicle gel in subjects with moderate to severe acne vulgaris.

Methods.—A total of 378 subjects were randomized in a double-blind, controlled trial to receive once-daily lymecycline with either A/BPO or vehicle for 12 weeks. Evaluations included percentage changes from baseline in lesion counts, success rate (subjects 'clear' or 'almost clear'), skin tolerability, adverse events and patients' satisfaction.

Results.—The median percentage reduction from baseline in total lesion counts at week 12 was significantly higher ($P < 0·001$) in the lymecycline with A/BPO group ($-74·1\%$) than in the lymecycline with vehicle group ($-56·8\%$). The success rate was significantly higher ($47·6\%$ vs. $33·7\%$, $P = 0·002$) in subjects treated with lymecycline and A/BPO. Both inflammatory and noninflammatory lesions were significantly reduced at week 12 (both $P < 0·001$) with a rapid onset of action from week 2 for noninflammatory lesions ($P < 0·001$) and week 4 for inflammatory lesions ($P = 0·005$). The A/BPO and lymecycline combination was well tolerated. The proportion of satisfied and very satisfied subjects was similar in both groups, but the number in the A/BPO group who were 'very satisfied' was significantly greater ($P = 0·031$).

Conclusion.—These results demonstrate the clinical benefit of combining A/BPO with lymecycline in the treatment of moderate to severe acne vulgaris.

▶ Combination therapy with benzoyl peroxide (BP), a topical retinoid, and an oral antibiotic has been recommended for first-line treatment of moderate to severe acne vulgaris (AV). To add, oral isotretinoin remains the treatment of choice for severe inflammatory acne, but there are those who cannot or do not wish to start oral isotretinoin, and the refractory nature of AV is considered by some to be a prerequisite to the use of oral isotretinoin. This is a randomized, double-blind, vehicle-controlled, 12-week study of 378 subjects that received once-daily oral lymecycline 300 mg with either adapalene 0.1%-benzoyl peroxide 2.5% (A/BP) gel or vehicle gel in subjects with moderate to severe AV. Oral lymecycline has been found to be similar to immediate-release minocycline with fewer treatment-related adverse events. At each visit and at week 12, total lesion counts were statistically significant between the 2 groups, with the A/BP gel group showing a faster onset of action from week 2 and greater efficacy thereafter compared with the vehicle group ($P < .001$). The incidence of side effects was comparable between the 2 groups: 8.4% in the combination group and 8.0% in the vehicle group. Results of this study showed that A/BP gel and lymecycline significantly improve both inflammatory and noninflammatory lesions in moderate to severe AV. Also, there have been no reports of hyperpigmentation with lymecycline, and it has been shown to be less phototoxic compared with doxycycline. This combination topical and oral treatment was shown to be an effective option for those with moderate to severe AV, offering the convenience of a single topical product and a single oral product, both used once daily.

G. K. Kim, DO

J. Q. Del Rosso, DO

Expert Opinion: Efficacy of superficial chemical peels in active acne management—what can we learn from the literature today? Evidence-based recommendations

Dréno B, Fischer TC, Perosino E, et al (Univ Hosp Ctr, Nantes, France; Skin and Laser Ctr, Potsdam, Germany; Practice for Dermatology and Aesthetic Medicine, Rome, Italy; et al)

J Eur Acad Dermatol Venereol 25:695-704, 2011

Background.—Superficial chemical peels offer therapeutic results in a convenient, affordable treatment. Many clinicians use these peels in the treatment of acne and acne-prone oily skin.

Objectives.—This article examines the evidence base that supports the widespread use of superficial peels in this setting.

Methods.—A search of the English language medical literature was performed to identify clinical trials that formally evaluated the use of chemical peeling in active acne.

Results.—Search of the literature revealed very few clinical trials of peels in acne (N = 13); a majority of these trials included small numbers of patients, were not controlled and were open label. The evidence that is available does support the use of chemical peels in acne as all trials had generally favourable results despite differences in assessments, treatment regimens and patient populations. Notably, no studies of chemical peels have used an acne medication as a comparator. As not every publication specified whether or not concomitant acne medications were allowed, it is hard to evaluate clearly how many of the studies evaluated the effect of peeling alone. This may be appropriate, however, given that few clinicians would use superficial chemical peels as the sole treatment for acne except in rare instances where a patient could not tolerate other treatment modalities.

Conclusions.—In the future, further study is needed to determine the best use of chemical peels in this indication.

▶ Superficial chemical peels have become increasingly popular for the management of active lesions of acne vulgaris (AV) and for maintenance therapy. Superficial peels using agents such as glycolic acid (GA) and salicylic acid (SA) serve to promote exfoliation. Currently, there are few strong evidence-based studies for the use of superficial peels for AV. This is a review of the literature evaluating the efficacy of superficial peels for the management of AV. There was a total of 32 articles found on AV and chemical peels (ie, with GA and SA). Thirteen studies were identified that used chemical peels for AV lesions. Chemical peels have a comedolytic effect, which may be observed immediately after the procedure. A mean reduction of approximately 50% of lesions has been observed in studies overall. Superficial inflammatory lesions have been shown to decrease during treatment with chemical peels, with a greater effect correlating with the number of sessions performed. There was only one report of chemical peels with nodulocystic lesions requiring up to 9 treatments to achieve a decrease in 50% of these lesions. Studies of superficial chemical peels for AV were limited by study design and population size. Also, the majority of studies did not control for topical medication, and therefore it was difficult to evaluate the efficacy of the peels alone. Although the evidence for superficial chemical peels is not strong, they may serve as an adjunct to other topical therapies in some cases of AV. Currently there are no head-to-head studies of superficial chemical peels compared with topical acne medications for AV.

G. K. Kim, DO

J. Q. Del Rosso, DO

Topical and intralesional therapies for alopecia areata

Alkhalifah A (Riyadh Military Hosp, Saudi Arabia)
Dermatol Ther 24:355-363, 2011

Alopecia areata is a common form of nonscarring alopecia. It affects males and females equally and has no racial predilection. It usually affects the scalp, but any hair-bearing area can be involved. It presents as patchy hair loss, loss of hair on the entire scalp (alopecia totalis), or the whole body (alopecia universalis). The histopathology varies according to the disease stage, but usually a perifollicular lymphocytic infiltrate is seen. The course of the disease and response to treatment are unpredictable. Various therapeutic modalities are used including topical, intralesional, and systemic agents, although none are curative or preventive. This article will review the available topical and intralesional agents that are used in the treatment of alopecia areata and suggest a management approach based on the age of the patient and extent of the disease.

▶ Alopecia areata (AA) is a common inflammatory nonscarring alopecia seen in both children and adults. AA can be associated with nail changes (ie, pitting) and sometimes autoimmune disease, although most cases exhibit no clinically significant systemic associations. There have been many therapeutic options used by the dermatologist, but none are curative. To add, there is a lack of objective parameters to measure treatment response. This is a review of topical and intralesional treatments for AA with an emphasis on age-based management. Intralesional corticosteroid (ILC) injections, despite their wide use, are not supported by randomized controlled trials to demonstrate efficacy in patients with AA. The mechanism of action of topical minoxidil in promoting hair growth, although not fully understood, may be through vasodilation, angiogenesis, and/or enhanced cell proliferation, with inconsistent response noted in AA. Anthralin has been shown to decrease the expression of tumor necrosis factor α and can be used as a short contact therapy, although it is messy and discolors skin where applied. Randomized controlled trails for phototherapy with oral or topical psoralen plus UVA light are also lacking. Topical tacrolimus and pimecrolimus have been used in the clinical setting, but the results have not been encouraging, likely because of penetration that is too superficial to access around the follicular bulb. Photodynamic therapy was also shown to be ineffective in the treatment of patients with AA. The authors emphasize that a medical history should be taken and all hair-nail-bearing areas should be examined before treatment. No routine testing is required for patients with AA. The age of the patient needs to be factored in when selecting treatment, as does the extent of the disease. The authors suggest a combination of minoxidil 5% with a midpotency topical corticosteroid as first-line treatment for patients younger than 10 years. For patients older than 10 years, ILC should be used with 5% minoxidil and topical corticosteroid therapy as adjuncts. For those with more than 50% involvement and older than 10 years, topical therapy with diphenylcyclopropenone to elicit cell-mediated sensitization can be used, although brisk allergic contact dermatitis should be anticipated. Topical corticosteroid therapy and ILC are the first choices for localized disease.

G. K. Kim, DO

J. Q. Del Rosso, DO

The clinical features of late onset acne compared with early onset acne in women

Choi CW, Lee DH, Kim HS, et al (Seoul Natl Univ Bundang Hosp, Gyeonggi, Korea)
J Eur Acad Dermatol Venereol 25:454-461, 2011

Background.—Little is known about the clinical characteristics of acne based on the age of onset.

Objectives.—The aim of this study was to investigate the clinical characteristics of patients according to the age of onset of acne and evaluate whether the findings were related to regional differences in the density of *Propionibacterium acnes* or the levels of sebum secretion.

Methods.—A total of 89 women were recruited. The acne lesions were assessed by counting the lesions using standard digital photographs. Digital fluorescent photography for the evaluation of the density of *P. acnes* were taken and quantitative measurements of facial sebum secretion were performed.

Results.—In women with acne, the age of onset was negatively correlated with the number of comedones and the proportion of comedones. By comparing the number of comedones and the proportion of comedones, onset of acne after 21 years of age was defined as late onset acne. In the patients with late onset acne, the number of comedones, the total number of acne lesions and the proportions of comedones were significantly less than in the patients with early onset acne. However, there were no significant differences in the fluorescence density of *P. acnes* or the level of sebum secretion between the two groups.

Conclusions.—The results of this study, using objective evaluation tools, suggest that late onset acne has different clinical characteristics. Other possible factors might explain the clinical differences in late onset acne.

▶ Postadolescent acne vulgaris (AV) has been increasing in the past few years, and little is known about the clinical characteristics of AV based on the age of onset. This is an observational study from Korea of 89 female patients with a clinical diagnosis of AV present over a duration that did not exceed 5 years from onset. The mean age of enrolled patients was 23 years, and the mean age of onset was 21.3 years. This was a study to determine the pattern of change of the clinical characteristics of acne based on the age of onset, with late-onset AV defined as starting after 21 years of age. The age of onset showed a negative correlation with both the number of and the proportion of comedones in the specific facial regions and the entire face (r = −0.418, P = .000; r = −0.293, P = 0.000). However, the lesions in the U-zone (cheeks, perioral region, chin) and the inflammatory lesions showed no correlation with the age of onset. To determine the age of onset and to examine the clinical changes, patients were divided into 4 groups (< 16, 16-20, 21-25, and > 25 years old). In the late-onset group, the comedones and total acne lesions were located more commonly in the U-zone compared with the early-onset group (P = 0.006 and 0.01, respectively). However, inflammatory lesions did not show any regional preference. The density of *Propionibacterium acnes* was assessed by image analyses of fluorescent photography. Sebum secretion levels and the density of *P acnes* were not statistically significant between the 2 groups. Limitations of this study were that the patients were not screened for endocrine abnormalities and baseline androgen levels were not determined. Current and past treatment for patients included in this study were not reported. These findings may help clinicians to direct treatment options for teenagers compared with postadolescent patients with AV according to characteristic lesions. However, the clinical presentation of the individual patient and other associated patient-specific factors will ultimately dictate overall management and selection of therapy.

G. K. Kim, DO

J. Q. Del Rosso, DO

Low-cumulative dose isotretinoin treatment in mild-to-moderate acne: efficacy in achieving stable remission

Borghi A, Mantovani L, Minghetti S, et al (Univ of Ferrara, Italy)
J Eur Acad Dermatol Venereol 25:1094-1098, 2011

Background.—Aimed at the reduction of post-treatment relapse of severe acne, the cumulative dose of oral isotretinoin should be ≥120 mg/kg. However, data on the appropriate oral isotretinoin treatment regimen in mild and moderate acne are lacking.

Objective.—The purpose of this study was to determine the efficacy of an isotretinoin-sparing protocol in inducing permanent remission of mild and moderate acne.

Methods.—In this open, prospective, non-comparative study, 150 patients affected with mild-to-moderate acne were treated with isotretinoin until complete recovery and for a further month of treatment, independent of the total cumulative dose reached. Patients then underwent a 1-year maintenance therapy with adapalene 0.1% cream. Patients were followed up for a further year, without any treatment.

Results.—A total of 139 patients completed the study. Overall, patients received a mean of 80.92 mg/kg cumulative dose of isotretinoin. In the 2-year follow-up, relapse only appeared in 13 patients (9.35%).

Conclusion.—Comparing our findings with published data, this isotretinoin-sparing regimen was shown to be effective in inducing stable remission and preventing acne relapses in patients with mild-to-moderate acne. Low-cumulative dose regimens may potentially lead to a lower incidence of side-effects and to lower costs than higher doses.

▶ Oral isotretinoin therapy is a remarkably effective treatment for severe acne, but it has numerous side effects that are often dose dependent. The authors observed that oral isotretinoin is being increasingly prescribed to patients with less-severe acne vulgaris (AV) in patients who have not responded to conventional therapies. They have also noted that patients achieve remission with cumulative isotretinoin doses of less than 120 to 150 mg/kg. This was an open-label, prospective, noncomparative study of 150 patients with mild-to-moderate AV treated with lower cumulative doses of oral isotretinoin until complete recovery was achieved. Investigators in this study also evaluated the incidence of relapse of AV after a single course of oral isotretinoin followed by maintenance therapy with a topical retinoid. Patients were started on oral isotretinoin less than 0.2 mg/kg/d to reduce the potential for flares. Liver function tests and lipid profiles were evaluated for all patients before treatment and at 6 weeks after the beginning of treatment. Pregnancy tests were carried out before treatment in female patients of child-bearing potential, and oral contraception was started before treatment. The mean cumulative dose received by the patients was 80.92 mg/kg. In the 2-year follow-up, relapses appeared in 13 (9.35%) patients. The rate of relapse in patients that reached a cumulative dose greater than 120 mg/kg showed no statistical significance compared with low cumulative doses ($P = .58$). The authors concluded that lower daily and cumulative doses of oral isotretinoin reduced the risk and severity of side effects and increased patient compliance. A limitation to this study was the lack of age-, sex-, and AV severity—matched controls. To add, patients' previous treatment regimens for AV were not discussed; therefore, it was unknown if these patients truly failed all conventional therapies. The authors also did not mention a washout period before starting oral isotretinoin, and some improvement may have been from previous AV, although this is not likely. The authors concluded that use of low-cumulative-dose courses of oral isotretinoin in mild to moderate AV may have its advantages. Starting oral isotretinoin for a patient with mild to moderate AV may not be practical in the minds of some dermatologists due to medicolegal concerns, which is understandable. However, it may be justified in cases that are truly refractory to other conventional options that optimize the likelihood of success, provided a risk-versus-benefit discussion is completed and informed consent obtained.

G. K. Kim, DO

J. Q. Del Rosso, DO

Iron deficiency and diffuse nonscarring scalp alopecia in women: More pieces to the puzzle

St Pierre SA, Vercellotti GM, Donovan JC, et al (Univ of Minnesota Med School, Minneapolis; Univ of Toronto, Ontario, Canada)
J Am Acad Dermatol 63:1070-1076, 2010

The relationship between nonscarring scalp alopecia in women and iron deficiency continues to be a subject of debate. We review the literature regarding the relationship between iron deficiency and nonscarring scalp alopecia and describe iron-dependent genes in the hair follicle bulge region that may be affected by iron deficiency. We conclude with a description of our approach to the diagnosis and treatment of nonscarring alopecia in women with low iron stores. Limitations include published studies with small numbers of patients, different study designs, and absence of randomized, controlled treatment protocols. Additional research regarding the potential role of iron during the normal hair cycle is needed, as is a well-designed clinical trial evaluating the effect of iron supplementation in iron-deficient women with nonscarring alopecia.

▶ Iron deficiency is a relatively common clinical scenario in certain subgroups of patients with underlying disorders related to chronic use of certain medications (ie, salicylates, nonsteroidal antiinflammatory agents) and in many other normal individuals without other pre-existing diseases. Iron can affect epithelial cell growth, maturation, and division and has been linked to nonscarring alopecia. Although iron deficiency has been linked to nonscarring alopecia, it is still a continued debate as to its role. However, research models using mice models have shown that there may be genes affected by iron stores. This article reviews the literature examining iron deficiency anemia and nonscarring alopecia with an approach to the diagnosis and treatment of this condition. In this study, researchers found in a PubMed search that the genes CDC2, NDRG1, ALAD, and RRM2 are up-regulated in the bulge region that regulates iron. The authors speculate that iron deficiency may alter the hair cycle, and these genes may directly impact hair growth. They also suggest a thorough history, physical, and laboratory workup, including complete blood cell count, iron studies with serum iron total iron-binding capacity, iron saturation, ferritin, thyroid function studies, dehydroepiandrosterone sulfate, free testosterone, and a scalp biopsy. The most sensitive and specific test for iron deficiency was found to be ferritin. The most common cause of iron deficiency anemia is from gastrointestinal or genitourinary sources, but malabsorption caused by celiac disease, gastric bypass, or dietary lack is also a consideration. If iron deficiency is found, iron replacement with 60 mg of elemental iron 2 to 3 times a day is indicated for 6 months, and ferritin levels should be maintained above 50 µg/L. Reversal of iron deficiency may be noted as early as 1 to 3 months depending on how severe the iron deficiency was at baseline before starting oral iron supplementation. Parenteral therapy should be considered if continued iron deficiency is observed after noncompliance or malabsorption are excluded. This study suggests that abnormalities in iron metabolism have been linked to hair loss. However, randomized, placebo-controlled trials are needed to further determine the role of iron supplementation in reversal of hair loss in female patients with nonscarring alopecia who are found to be iron deficient. This study was a comprehensive review of literature and provided a guideline for clinicians to follow if nonscarring alopecia from iron deficiency is suspected in a female patient.

G. K. Kim, DO

J. Q. Del Rosso, DO

Staphylococcus epidermidis: A possible role in the pustules of rosacea
Whitfeld M, Gunasingam N, Leow LJ, et al (St Vincent's Hosp, Sydney, Australia; Monash Med Centre, Melbourne, Australia; et al)
J Am Acad Dermatol 64:49-52, 2011

Background.—Rosacea is a common skin and ocular disease. Cutaneous rosacea is characterized by facial flushing, telangiectasia, papules, and pustules. It is generally regarded as inflammatory in nature. We believed that the role of bacteria as a contributory factor in pustular and ocular rosacea needed to be revisited.

Objectives.—We sought to ascertain whether there is an increase in the bacteria isolated from the (1) pustules of rosacea; and (2) eyelid margins of persons with cutaneous pustular rosacea.

Methods.—Bacterial swabs were taken and cultured from an incised rosacea pustule, the ipsilateral cheek skin, and the eyelid margin of 15 patients with pustular rosacea. Swabs were also taken from the cheek skin and ipsilateral eyelid margin of 15 matched control subjects.

Results.—A pure growth of *Staphylococcus epidermidis* was isolated from a pustule of 9 of 15 patients with pustular rosacea, and no pure growth of *S epidermidis* was isolated from their ipsilateral cheek skin. This was a highly statistically significant increase ($P = .0003$). A pure growth of *S epidermidis* was isolated from the eyelid margins of 4 of 15 patients with pustular rosacea, and no pure growth was isolated from the eyelids of age- and sex-matched control subjects. This was a statistically significant increase ($P = .05$).

Limitations.—This study focuses on the microbial basis of rosacea.

Conclusion.—Our findings suggest *S epidermidis* may play a role in pustular and ocular rosacea.

▶ Rosacea is classified into erythematotelangiectatic (ETR), papulopustular (PPR), phymatous (PhR), and ocular (OcR) subtypes. Although rosacea patients are commonly seen in the outpatient setting and the clinical subtypes are well described, the exact pathogenesis remains unknown. The current study found the pure growth of *Staphylococcus epidermidis* in 9 of 15 patients with rosacea pustules but no growth in ipsilateral surrounding cheek skin. *S epidermidis* was also isolated in 4 of 15 eyelid margins of rosacea patients, whereas no pure growth was found on age- and sex-matched control subjects. Because

S epidermidis is usually a commensal organism, researchers hypothesize that the increase in temperature of skin in rosacea patients may contribute to the pathogenic nature of this bacteria. Antibiotic sensitivities showed that all *S epidermidis* isolates were sensitive to cefoxitin, cephalexin, gentamicin, and vancomycin, and 89% were sensitive to erythromycin and tetracycline. The limitation of this study is that a number of different abnormalities in rosacea pathogenesis are described in the literature, and this report is limited to microbial factors. These results are potentially interesting but not confirmatory regarding the role of this organism in the pathogenesis of rosacea.

S. Bellew, DO

J. Q. Del Rosso, DO

Immediate Reduction in Sweat Secretion With Electric Current Application in Primary Palmar Hyperhidrosis
Shams K, Kavanagh GM (Monklands Hosp, Airdrie, Scotland; Royal Infirmary of Edinburgh, Scotland)
Arch Dermatol 147:241-242, 2011

Background.—Tap water iontophoresis has been widely used for decades to evaluate treatments for hyperhidrosis and determine their mechanism of action. In this method, the patient's hands are soaked in shallow pans filled with tap water or tap water plus drugs such as anticholinergic agents. A novel approach using dry current alone to study primary palmar hyperhidrosis was described.

Methods.—The six patients with hyperhidrosis had no clinically significant comorbid conditions and were not taking medications currently. Baseline sweating was evaluated using the Minor starch-iodine test, in which the patients' palms were subjected to an iodine solution and then starch powder, which causes the hyperhidrotic areas to stain dark blue. Digital photographs were obtained 2 minutes after the starch was applied, then the patients' hands were washed and dried to permit further analysis. Patients self-rated their baseline sweating using a 100-point visual analog scale (VAS), with 0 indicating no sweating and 100 extreme sweating. Next a 4-mA current was applied to the patients' wrists using conductive pads and the Minor starch-iodine test was repeated 1 minute later. Photographs were taken with the current still on, then the current was discontinued and additional photographs were taken 2 minutes later. Patients again rated their level of sweating.

Results.—There was a rapid, substantial reduction in sweating during the period the current was applied. Sweating then returned to baseline levels rapidly after the current was switched off. The mean VAS was 66.2 before the current was applied and 19.2 during current application.

Conclusions.—Dry current application revealed that sweating in primary palmar hyperhidrosis is most likely mediated through an electrochemical focus. Although the exact mechanism is not understood, the rapid temporary interference with ion pumps and/or the innervation of eccrine sweat glands may at least partially explain how iontophoresis functions in patients with hyperhidrosis. The use of the tap water iontophoresis machines may not be necessary, since the tap water may just act as a conductor for current. Less bulky methods for iontophoresis and fewer resources may be required to effectively analyze hyperhidrosis.

▶ Palmar hyperhidrosis is a condition that can be an embarrassing nuisance to patients and difficult to treat. Many patients afflicted with this condition often have exacerbation with stress, heat, and other medical conditions. This is a study examining dry ionotropic current and its effect on anhidrosis. The authors observed the anhidrotic effects of dry iontophoresis in 6 patients with primary palmar hyperhidrosis with no other underlying medical conditions. Baseline sweating and self-rating using a 100-point visual analog scale were assessed. The results revealed that after application, there was a decrease in mean sweating compared with baseline ($P < .001$). Limitations to this study include that there were no controls and the duration of anhidrosis after treatment was not discussed. Also, the authors did not explore whether the effects lasted during exacerbating circumstances. Although ionotropic current helped decrease sweating in this study, additional randomized controlled studies with larger cohorts of patients are needed.

G. K. Kim, DO
J. Q. Del Rosso, DO

Iron deficiency in female pattern hair loss, chronic telogen effluvium, and control groups
Olsen EA, Reed KB, Cacchio PB, et al (Duke Univ Med Ctr, Durham, NC; Dermatology Specialists of Spokane, WA)
J Am Acad Dermatol 63:991-999, 2010

Background.—The literature suggests that iron deficiency (ID) may play a role in female pattern hair loss (FPHL) or in chronic telogen effluvium (CTE).

Objective.—We sought to determine if ID is more common in women with FPHL and/or CTE than in control subjects without hair loss.

Methods.—This was a controlled study of 381 Caucasian women aged 18 years or older with FPHL or CTE seen in the Duke University Hair Disorders Clinic, Durham, NC, and 76 Caucasian women aged 18 years or older from the university environs who had no history or physical findings of hair loss (control subjects). All participants had to have at least a serum ferritin and hemoglobin reading and history of menopausal status.

Results.—When ferritin less than or equal to 15 μg/L was used as the definition, ID occurred in 12.4%, 12.1%, and 29.8% of premenopausal women with FPHL (n = 170), CTE (n = 58), and control subjects (n = 47), respectively, and in 1.7%, 10.5%, and 6.9% of postmenopausal women with FPHL (n = 115), CTE (n = 38), and control subjects (n = 29), respectively. When ferritin less than or equal to 40 μg/L was used as the definition, ID occurred in 58.8%, 63.8%, and 72.3% of premenopausal women with FPHL, CTE, and control subjects, respectively, and in 26.1%, 36.8%, and 20.7% of postmenopausal women with FPHL, CTE, and control subjects, respectively. There was no statistically significant increase in the incidence of ID in premenopausal or postmenopausal women with FPHL or CTE versus control subjects.

Limitations.—The effect of correction of ID on hair loss is unknown.

Conclusion.—ID is common in women but not increased in patients with FPHL or CTE compared with control subjects.

▶ Iron deficiency (ID) has been suggested as a cause of hair loss, especially in females. This study sought to investigate whether ID was more common in women with female pattern hair loss (FPHL) or chronic telogen effluvium (CTE) compared with control subjects. This controlled study included 381 Caucasian women with FPHL or CTE and 76 Caucasian women with no history of hair loss. All participants were older than 18 years and underwent laboratory examinations including iron studies and scalp biopsies. In this study, the authors did not observe a higher prevalence of ID in premenopausal compared with postmenopausal women, regardless of which study group they were in (FPHL vs CTE vs control groups). However, the mean serum ferritin levels of all the premenopausal groups (CTE, FPHL, control) were much lower compared with the postmenopausal groups in this study ($P < .005$), likely related to iron loss associated with menstruation. This study did not show any difference in the prevalence of ID between women with or without hair loss. One weakness of this study was that all patients were Caucasian, and iron deficiency may vary between races. Also, the exact definition of ID (or its severity levels) is problematic, and a selected subpopulation of patients may not be symptomatic. Ultimately, iron supplementation may be beneficial in reducing hair loss in some patients; however, well-documented evidence is lacking. In the future, well-designed, properly powered, placebo-controlled studies are needed, including assessment of variables including age, menstrual status, and ethnicity.

G. K. Kim, DO

J. Q. Del Rosso, DO

Neurogenic Rosacea: A Distinct Clinical Subtype Requiring a Modified Approach to Treatment
Scharschmidt TC, Yost JM, Truong SV, et al (Univ of California, San Francisco; Univ of Michigan, Ann Arbor; Los Angeles Med Ctr, CA; et al)
Arch Dermatol 147:123-126, 2011

Background.—Rosacea occurs in four distinct clinical subtypes and three additional variants. The conditions of 14 patients with rosacea and prominent neurologic symptoms may represent another distinct subtype that requires a different approach to management.

Methods.—The patients had the classic features of rosacea combined with distinct neurologic symptoms and were identified during routine medical appointments. Each offered information about their medical history, disease symptoms, triggers, and treatment responses during clinic visits and telephone interviews.

Results.—Twelve patients were women and 12 were white. Mean age at disease onset was 38 years, with the most prominent symptoms being burning or stinging pain, erythema, and flushing, sometimes along with facial edema, telangiectasias, pruritus, and papules. Symptoms were triggered most often by heat, sunlight, hot showers, stress, exercise, and alcohol consumption. Other triggers were using makeup, eating spicy foods, touching skin, drinking hot beverages, cold weather, and humidity. Seventy-one percent of patients obtained relief by cooling through the use of fans or cold compresses or ice applied to the face or held in the mouth. Forty-three percent had neurologic and 50% had neuropsychiatric conditions. These included complex regional pain syndrome, essential tremor, depression, and obsessive-compulsive disorder. Headaches, Raynaud phenomenon, and rheumatologic disorders such as lupus, rheumatoid arthritis, fibromyalgia, mixed connective tissue disease, and psoriatic arthritis were also common.

Treatments that had provided limited relief included topical metronidazole, topical steroids, and oral antibiotics, usually tetracyclines. Neurologically focused treatments, such as gabapentin, duloxetine, pregabalin, tricyclic antidepressants, and memantine, provided relief to most patients. Occasionally patients benefited from topically formulated neuroleptic agents such as doxepin, glycopyrrolate, amitriptyline, capsaicin, and ketamine. Subsets of patients reported relief from hydroxychloroquine and vasoactive agents.

Conclusions.—Neuronal dysregulation may contribute to the pathogenesis of rosacea, which is not fully understood at this time. The relative importance of each contributing influence has yet to be determined. The patients described may represent a previously unknown subset of patients suffering neurogenic rosacea. A diagnostic and treatment algorithm will guide clinicians in managing patients with suspected neurogenic rosacea. Those with prominent vasomotor symptoms may benefit from vasoactive medications and laser- or light-based therapies. Patients with inflammatory features may respond to traditional topical therapies if their conditions are mild, but may require systemic antibiotics or antimalarial agents if unresponsive to these initial agents. Patients with dysesthesia out of proportion to their flushing or inflammation may be the most difficult to treat. Neuroleptic agents, tricyclic antidepressants, and pain-modifying antidepressants may be the most effective agents for these patients, with N-methyl-D-aspartic acid receptor antagonists, systemic antibiotics, and other topically formulated medications added for some cases. Laser- and light-based interventions should be used with caution because of the heightened sensitivity to heat and light.

▶ This article describes 14 patients with rosacea and neurogenic symptoms such as burning, stinging, pain, flushing, facial edema, and pruritus. A notably high percentage of these patients had either neurologic (43%) or neuropsychiatric

(50%) symptoms. The authors propose that an additional subtype of rosacea should be recognized as neurogenic rosacea. Patients in this subtype can have features of the other known subtypes of rosacea, and a treatment approach is suggested. A key message from this article is the categorization of the types of neurogenic symptoms and treatment recommendations for each. These recommendations do not vary from approaches currently being taken for patients with symptomatic rosacea.

D. Thiboutot, MD

Hair care practices and their association with scalp and hair disorders in African American girls

Rucker Wright D, Gathers R, Kapke A, et al (Johns Hopkins Univ, Baltimore, MD; Henry Ford Health System, Detroit, MI)
J Am Acad Dermatol 64:253-262, 2011

Background.—Few studies have extensively examined the prevalence of hair care practices and their association with scalp and hair conditions in African American girls.

Objectives.—We sought to determine the prevalence of hair care practices and their association with traction alopecia, seborrheic dermatitis (SD), and tinea capitis (TC).

Methods.—A questionnaire was administered to caregivers of African American girls aged 1 to 15 years. Multivariate analyses were performed to determine the association of hair care practices with reported disorders.

Results.—A total of 201 surveys were completed from dermatology (n = 98) and nondermatology (n = 103) clinics. Mean patient age was 9.8 ± 4.4 years. Essentially all respondents reported use of hair oils/grease (99%). Ponytails, braids, and cornrows were worn by 81%, 67%, and 49% of girls, respectively, within the past 12 months. In all, 61% reported hair washing every 2 weeks; 80% used hot combs; and 42% used chemical relaxers. Cornrows were significantly related to traction alopecia among respondents from nondermatology clinics only: adjusted odds ratio = 5.79 (95% CI 1.35-24.8, $P = .018$). Hair extensions and infrequent hair oil use were significantly related to SD: adjusted odds ratio = 2.37 (95% CI 1.03-5.47, $P = .04$) and 3.69 (95% CI 1.07-12.7, $P = .039$), respectively. No significant associations were observed for TC.

Limitations.—Small sample size and disorders reported by caregivers were limitations.

Conclusions.—Certain hair care practices were strongly associated with development of traction alopecia and SD. No association was found between hair washing frequency and SD or TC, or between hair grease use and TC. These results can be used to inform practitioners, advise parents, and adapt treatment regimens to accommodate cultural preferences.

▶ Scalp and hair disorders are among the most common dermatologic diagnoses in African American (AA) girls. This study investigated the prevalence and association of 11 diverse hair care practices and certain scalp and hair conditions in AA girls in a large health care system in metropolitan Detroit, MI, USA.

This cross-sectional study involved a 51-question survey concerning hair care practices and history of physician-diagnosed hair and scalp conditions in AA girls between ages 1 and 15 years. The authors found an association between cornrows and traction alopecia and hair extensions and infrequent oil use with seborrheic dermatitis. However, washing hair every 1 to 2 weeks was not a risk factor for seborrheic dermatitis or tinea capitis. In addition, no significant associations were reported between hairstyles and tinea capitis.

The benefit of the cross-sectional study design is the ability to gather data concerning the frequency of wearing particular hairstyles, using chemical hair treatments, washing hair, and the occurrence of hair or scalp disease among young AA girls in the Detroit area. However, the study design that was implemented included several limitations to the interpretation of the data.

First, a case-control experimental design would offer a control population, so the analysis may have better demonstrated a causal relationship between certain hair practices in AA girls (risk) and scalp and hair changes (disease). In addition, the cross-sectional design leads to a significant amount of collected data that could not be used in the statistical analysis.

Second, relying on nondermatologic health care providers to diagnose dermatologic conditions may lead to decreased accuracy, inconsistency in the data collected, or both.

Third, as the authors described, self-administered surveys may result in misinterpretation of the questions, recall bias, and inaccurate information.

Overall, this article offers valuable information about the frequency of certain hair care practices in AA girls in Detroit and is a starting point for the study of the causal relationship between hair care practices and hair disease. Further studies of different designs will likely shed more light on this topic.

J. Levin, DO

J. Del Rosso, DO

Effectiveness of conventional, low-dose and intermittent oral isotretinoin in the treatment of acne: a randomized, controlled comparative study

Lee JW, Yoo KH, Park KY, et al (Chung-Ang Univ Hosp, Dongjak-Gu, Seoul, Korea)
Br J Dermatol 164:1369-1375, 2011

Background.—The efficacy of conventional isotretinoin treatment ($0 \cdot 5$– $1 \cdot 0$ mg kg^{-1} daily for 16–32 weeks, reaching a cumulative dose of 120 mg kg^{-1}) for acne has been well established. To date, there are many reports regarding the efficacy of low-dose and intermittent isotretinoin treatment in patients with acne. Data comparing these three therapeutic regimens simultaneously, however, are unavailable.

Objectives.—To evaluate the clinical efficacy and tolerability of low-dose and intermittent isotretinoin regimens and to compare them directly with conventional isotretinoin treatment.

Methods.—In this study, 60 patients with moderate acne were enrolled and randomized to receive either isotretinoin at $0\cdot5$–$0\cdot7$ mg kg^{-1} daily (group A), isotretinoin at $0\cdot25$–$0\cdot4$ mg kg^{-1} daily (group B) or isotretinoin at $0\cdot5$–$0\cdot7$ mg kg^{-1} daily for 1 week out of every 4 weeks (group C). The total period of drug administration was 6 weeks in group C, and 24 weeks in groups A and B. Evaluations included global acne grading system (GAGS) scores, lesion counts (inflammatory and noninflammatory), patient satisfaction and side-effects. A 1-year follow-up evaluation after the end of treatment was also performed.

Results.—Differences in GAGS scores were statistically significant between groups A and C ($P < 0\cdot001$) and groups B and C ($P = 0\cdot044$). There was no significant difference between groups A and B. For the number of inflammatory lesions, there were statistically significant differences between groups B and C ($P = 0\cdot048$) and groups C and A ($P = 0\cdot005$). There was no significant difference between groups A and B. For the number of noninflammatory lesions, there were statistically significant differences between groups B and C ($P = 0\cdot046$) and groups C and A ($P = 0\cdot006$). There was no significant difference between groups A and B. These results suggest that the conventional and low-dose regimens have similar efficacy. Intermittent treatment had less effect than either conventional or low-dose treatments. Patient satisfaction was highest in group B ($3\cdot76$), followed by group C ($3\cdot31$), then A ($3\cdot06$), with statistically significant differences between groups A and B ($P = 0\cdot003$) and groups B and C ($P = 0\cdot019$) but no significant difference between groups A and C. This result suggests that the low-dose regimen is superior to other regimens (conventional or intermittent) in terms of patient satisfaction. Side-effects were more frequent with conventional treatment compared with low-dose and intermittent treatments. One year after the end of treatment, two of 16 patients relapsed in group A, three of 17 patients relapsed in group B, and nine of 16 patients relapsed in group C.

Conclusions.—Our study suggests that, when considering tolerability, efficacy and patient satisfaction, low-dose treatment is most suitable for patients with moderate acne.

▶ Oral isotretinoin was first introduced for difficult, treatment-resistant nodulocystic acne vulgaris (AV). However, because of several dose-dependent side effects, there has been a move toward low-dose therapy and intermittent regimens. Use of oral isotretinoin today is not just limited to severe nodulocystic acne but has become more popular for moderate inflammatory AV that is treatment resistant. This is a randomized, prospective, controlled, open study evaluating 3 different doses with 60 Korean patients on oral isotretinoin in 1 of 3 dosing regimens: 0.5 to 1.0 mg/kg daily (group A), 0.25 to 0.4 mg/kg daily (group B), or 0.5 to 0.7 mg/kg daily for 1 week every 4 weeks (group C). At the end of the 24-week study, acne severity based on a global acne grading system, patient satisfaction, and side effects were evaluated. There was no difference between group A and B for inflammatory and noninflammatory lesions ($P = .738$). However, there was a statistically significant difference between groups B and C (*P* = .044) and groups C and A (*P* < .001). The most common side effect was dry, chapped lips (94% in group A, 65% in group B, and 44% in group C). Dry skin was noted in 31% in group A and 6% in group B, and epistaxis was reported in 19% only in group A. There was also only 1 case of elevation of serum levels of hepatic enzymes reported (group A). Regarding relapse rates, group A and B had no statistical differences noted between them (*P* = .478). However, there was a statistical difference in relapse rates between groups A and C (*P* = .002) and groups B and C (*P* = .0015). A limitation to this study was that it was performed in only patients with moderate-severity AV. Also, larger studies with a more diverse group of patients are suggested. Although a high cumulative dose is an important factor in reducing relapse rates, lower doses for moderate-severity AV that is poorly responsive to other therapies may decrease side effects while still achieving therapeutic results that are satisfying to patients.

G. K. Kim, DO

J. Q. Del Rosso, DO

'Follicular Swiss cheese' pattern—another histopathologic clue to alopecia areata
Müller CSL, Shabrawi-Caelen LE (Univ Hosp, Homburg/Saar, Germany; Univ Graz, Austria)
J Cutan Pathol 38:185-189, 2011

Yellow dots are the most useful dermoscopic criterion in the clinical diagnosis of alopecia areata and correspond histopathologically with dilated follicular infundibula. They are found in about 95% of alopecia areata cases and help to differentiate alopecia areata from trichotillomania, telogen effluvium and from scarring alopecias. Histopathology of alopecia areata differs with disease activity and dermatopathologist, therefore, heavily depends on other diagnostic features. Objective of the study was to determine the frequency of dilated follicular infundibula, peribulbar lymphocytic infiltrate, inflammatory infiltrates of lymphocytes and eosinophils within fibrous streamers and a shift to catagen/telogen follicles in alopecia areata. Histopathologic features of 56 specimens of 33 patients were correlated with clinical findings and alopecia areata subtype. Results: 57% of all biopsies showed dilated follicular infundibula, regardless of horizontal or vertical sectioning of the slides. Dilated follicular infundibula showed a maximum occurrence of 66% in the recovery stage of alopecia areata and were seen in 33% of alopecia areata incognita. In conclusion, dilated follicular infundibula, reminiscent of a Swiss cheese in horizontally sectioned slides, is an exceedingly useful criterion in the histopathologic diagnosis of alopecia areata and are of great help in the daily routine to recognize alopecia areata (Fig 2).

▶ Diagnosis of hair disorders by histologic examination can prove vexing for the dermatopathologist. As alopecia may be an evolving condition, criteria

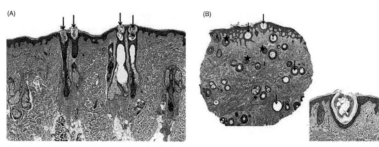

FIGURE 2.—A) Vertical section: Hematoxylin and eosin stained slide, ×100. Note four dilated follicular infundibula filled with orthokeratin. In two follicles, the dilatation extends into the isthmic area. No hair shafts are found. B) Horizontal section: Hematoxylin and eosin stained slide, ×100. Multiple dilated hair follicles, with dilatation ranging from 0.2–0.3 mm, are apparent. Compare the dilated hair follicles (arrows) with those of normal distention (stars). Inset: A vertical section of the same patient shows a distended follicular infundibulum filled with compact orthokeratin and bacteria. (Reprinted from Müller CSL, Shabrawi-Caelen LE. 'Follicular Swiss cheese' pattern – another histopathologic clue to alopecia areata. *J Cutan Pathol.* 2011;38: 185-189, with permission from John Wiley and Sons www.interscience.wiley.com.)

may shift with the stage of disease, and the situation is confounded by insufficient clinical information and suboptimal biopsies.

In videodermoscopy of the scalp, yellow dots composed of dilated follicular infundibula containing sebum, hyperkeratotic debris, and bacteria are seen in 95% of cases of alopecia areata (AA), irrespective of clinical subtype.[1]

The authors of this study sought to examine the use of dilated follicular infundibula, the histologic correlative of yellow dots relative to other histological findings, in the diagnosis of AA. Studying 56 biopsies (25 vertical and 31 horizontal) of various patterns of AA occurring in 33 patients, 57% of cases manifested dilated follicular infundibula. The appearance of multiple dilated follicular infundibula was likened to Swiss cheese in horizontal sections (Fig 2).

Interestingly, other widely discussed histologic findings, such as a peribulbar lymphocytes, lymphocytes and eosinophils in fibrous streamers, and a shift toward catagen/telogen growth phase were studied. A shift in catagen/telogen ratios was observed in 68% of cases overall, whereas a peribulbar lymphocytic infiltrate was seen in just 38% of cases (being a classic and dense swarm of bees in just 7%), and eosinophils within fibrous streamers was identified in just 4% of cases.

In fact, in the difficult distinction of recovery phase AA versus AA incognita (diffuse AA) versus androgenic alopecia, the combination of dilated follicular infundibula and increased catagen/telogen follicles was of particular use in diagnosis of AA.

Lastly, while there is continued debate as to the use of classic vertical versus horizontal sections in the diagnosis of all alopecias, and in this study, horizontal sections more often demonstrated peribulbar infiltrates than did vertical sections (45% vs 28%, respectively), dilated follicular infundibula were reliably found by both methods.

Recognition that AA is an evolving condition, with a variety of histologic clues, and release from the dogmatic and misguided requirement of a peribulbar swarm of bees of lymphocytes, will assist dermatopathologists in rendering an accurate diagnosis in this condition and will improve patient care.

W. A. High, MD, JD, MEng

Reference

1. Tosti A, Whiting D, Iorizzo M, et al. The role of scalp dermoscopy in the diagnosis of alopecia areata incognita. *J Am Acad Dermatol.* 2008;59:64-67.

The efficacy of adapalene-benzoyl peroxide combination increases with number of acne lesions

Feldman SR, Tan J, Poulin Y, et al (Wake Forest Univ, Winston-Salem, NC; Univ of Western Ontario, Windsor, Canada; Centre de Recherche Dermatologique du Quebec Metropolitain, Canada; et al)
J Am Acad Dermatol 64:1085-1091, 2011

Background.—There is no direct correlation between acne severity and lesion numbers and patients with moderate acne may present with varying lesion counts. The fixed-dose adapalene 0.1%-benzoyl peroxide (BPO) 2.5% combination gel is an efficacious and safe acne treatment.

Objective.—We sought to evaluate whether the benefit of adapalene-BPO relative to vehicle varies with baseline lesion counts.

Methods.—Data were pooled from 3 randomized, double-blind, controlled studies, which compared efficacy in 4 treatment groups (adapalene-BPO, adapalene, BPO, and the gel vehicle). Three lesion count subgroups (Low, Mid, and High) were defined based on the number of total, inflammatory, or noninflammatory lesion at baseline. Efficacy of each treatment and benefit of each treatment relative to vehicle were evaluated on the entire population and in all lesion count subgroups. Safety was assessed by local tolerability score and adverse events.

Results.—Adapalene-BPO provided significant benefit relative to vehicle and monotherapies on the entire population and in all lesion count subgroups ($P < .05$). At study end point, the benefit of adapalene-BPO relative to vehicle was greatest in the High subgroup, suggesting that patients with the highest baseline lesion counts contributed the most to the treatment benefit observed in the entire population. This effect was only observed with adapalene-BPO and not with monotherapies. Higher baseline lesion counts did not lead to more related adverse event or worse tolerability score for adapalene-BPO.

Limitation.—These results were generated from clinical trials. Results in clinical practice could differ.

Conclusion.—The relative benefit of adapalene-BPO increases with higher lesion counts at baseline.

▶ Adapalene 0.1%-benzoyl peroxide 2.5% gel (Adap-BP) has been used for most forms of acne vulgaris (AV) except in severe cases. This is a randomized, double-blind, controlled study examining the benefits of an Adap-BP combination with baseline lesion counts. The 4 treatment groups were Adap-BP, Adap, BP, and gel vehicle. Lesion counts were based on the number of total, inflammatory, or noninflammatory (comedonal) lesions at baseline. Specified washout periods were required for patients using topical and systemic treatments, and those with severe acne were excluded from the study. Authors found that Adap-BP exhibited increased benefit with higher baseline lesion counts. Adap-BP was significantly more efficacious than Adap alone, BP alone, and gel vehicle, regardless of the number of lesions at baseline ($P < .05$). The higher the lesion counts (total, inflammatory, and noninflammatory), the greater benefit relative to the vehicle. Also, the progressively greater efficacy with increasing total and noninflammatory lesion counts was observed in both Adap and Adap-BP arms but not with BP, suggesting that the comedolytic effect of Adap may be the main contributing factor. On the other hand, patients with greater acne severity in a clinical study may be more motivated to adhere to treatment, which was not measured. Adap-BP was also shown to be well tolerated and light stable, which may have been another reason patients found this combination to be user-friendly, therefore encouraging compliance. Cost is also a considerable factor to patient compliance, a potential weakness not discussed in this article. In conclusion, Adap-BP gel is a good option for patients with AV, including those with a high number of AV lesions, both inflammatory and comedonal.

G. K. Kim, DO
J. Q. Del Rosso, DO

Investigation of optimal aminolaevulinic acid concentration applied in topical aminolaevulinic acid—photodynamic therapy for treatment of moderate to severe acne: a pilot study in Chinese subjects
Yin R, Hao F, Deng J, et al (Third Military Med Univ, Chongqing, China)
Br J Dermatol 163:1064-1071, 2010

Background.—Aminolaevulinic acid—photodynamic therapy (ALA-PDT) is a novel and effective treatment in acne. However, little is known about the effect of different concentrations of ALA in the treatment of acne in Chinese patients with Fitzpatrick skin type III and IV.

Objectives.—To investigate the efficacy and safety of ALA-PDT in the treatment of moderate to severe acne in Chinese patients and to identify the suitable concentration of topical ALA.

Methods.—One hundred and eighty patients with moderate to severe facial acne were recruited and randomly divided into four groups. Each group was treated with a different concentration (5%, 10%, 15% and 20%) of ALA to the facial lesions on the right side and placebo agent on the left side as control. Each patient was treated once every 10 days for four sessions. The numbers of inflammatory and noninflammatory acne lesions were counted at baseline and at weeks 2, 4, 12 and 24 after the last treatment. Adverse effects were recorded at each follow-up visit.

Results.—After 24 weeks, each side treated by ALA-PDT showed clinical improvement compared with the control side treated by red light alone

$(P < 0 \cdot 01)$. Statistically, significantly more patients treated with 20% ALA than with 15% or 10% ALA achieved complete clearance. Regarding side-effects, a trend towards more serious erythema and pigmentation was observed with increasing ALA concentration.

Conclusions.—Increasing the concentration of ALA seems to be beneficial for improving the results. Considering effectiveness and safety, ALA-PDT using 10% or 15% ALA is suggested to the ideal treatment for moderate to severe acne in Chinese patients with Fitzpatrick skin type III and IV.

▶ Finally, a large controlled study on phototherapy as monotherapy of acne! The authors found a dose-dependent improvement in severe acne vulgaris (AV) treated with aminolevulinic acid (ALA) and red light. Side effects were not intolerable. Most previous studies of ALA photodynamic therapy (PDT) used blue light, which doesn't penetrate deep enough in skin to reach the sebaceous gland. There are many targets for phototherapy of AV. Light could directly lower *Propionibacterium* acnes counts, modulate inflammation, alter follicular plugging, or destroy the sebaceous gland. It isn't known which one(s) were active in this study; in fact, it could be all of them. The light alone also appeared to have some activity, reaching a nearly 2-grade improvement at times. These are encouraging findings. Although the ALA-PDT I have done seems too hard to tolerate for my patients, I can foresee the development of a less-uncomfortable phototherapy in the near future.

G. Webster, MD, PhD

Alopecia areata as another immune-mediated disease developed in patients treated with tumour necrosis factor-α blocker agents: Report of five cases and review of the literature

Ferran M, Calvet J, Almirall M, et al (Hosp Del Mar, Barcelona, Spain)
J Eur Acad Dermatol Venereol 25:479-484, 2011

Background.—Tumour necrosis factor antagonists (anti-TNF-α) have demonstrated the efficacy in different chronic immune inflammatory disorders. Within the spectrum of adverse events, autoimmune diseases have been observed, including cases of alopecia areata (AA).

Objectives.—The objective of the study is to characterize AA developed during anti-TNF-α therapy.

Methods.—We present five new cases and review all the cases reported in the literature (eleven).

Results.—One third of the cases had a positive (personal or family) history of AA. Most of them presented with rapid extensive AA, usually involving the ophiasis area. Prognosis was usually poor, with slight response to treatments. In the cases where anti-TNF-α therapy was maintained, the course did not seem to change.

Conclusions.—Although rare, AA developed during anti-TNF-α therapy might be more frequent than suggested by reports of isolated cases.

Personal and family history of autoimmune disease might alert clinicians to their possible development or relapse once the anti-TNF-α therapy is started.

▶ Tumor necrosis factor (TNF) antagonists are generally regarded as treatment for inflammatory diseases, not as their cause. However, with the increasing use of this class of drugs, an increasing array of new adverse events are being reported. The authors report the occurrence of alopecia areata (AA) during anti-TNF therapy and review the literature. The authors' case series consisted of 3 women and 2 men, all with rheumatic diseases other than systemic lupus erythematosus, being treated with etanercept (n = 3) or adalimumab (n = 2). One of the individuals had a family history of AA, and another had a personal history of mild AA in early childhood. Three of the patients developed AA between 3 and 5 months after anti-TNF therapy was introduced, coinciding with discontinuation of disease-modifying antirheumatic drugs. Clinically, all of the women developed an ophiasis pattern, whereas the men presented with patchy AA. Anti-TNF therapy was withdrawn in 2 patients, 1 of whom had evolved to AA universalis. However, the evolution of the clinical picture was not modified by maintenance or withdrawal of the anti-TNF agents.

The authors reviewed 11 cases of AA associated with anti-TNF therapy in the literature. There were no differences between genders. History of AA was present in 3 cases, while family history was either negative or not available. The anti-TNF agent associated with AA was more frequently a monoclonal antibody (4 cases of infliximab, 5 adalimumab, and 2 etanercept). The time for AA to develop once the anti-TNF agent had been initiated was between a few weeks and 3.5 years. Prognosis was generally poor, with only slight response to treatments and even worsening of the AA. Although the anti-TNF therapy was discontinued in 5 cases, only 2 cases showed improvement with complete regrowth (1 after treatment with cyclosporine), 2 other cases progressed into AA totalis or universalis, and evolution was not reported in 1 case.

This review of the literature gives us insight into a possible concerning adverse effect of TNF therapy. Obtaining appropriate patient history regarding personal and family occurrence of autoimmune disease and appropriate counseling are warranted.

J. M. Weinberg, MD

A Randomized Trial to Evaluate the Efficacy of Online Follow-up Visits in the Management of Acne

Watson AJ, Bergman H, Williams CM, et al (Ctr for Connected Health, Boston, MA; Massachusetts General Hosp, Boston; Harvard Med School, Boston, MA)
Arch Dermatol 146:406-411, 2010

Objective.—To evaluate whether delivering acne follow-up care via an asynchronous, remote online visit (evisit) platform produces equivalent clinical outcomes to office care.

Design.—A prospective, randomized controlled study.

Setting.—Two teaching hospitals in Boston between September 2005 and May 2007.

Participants.—A total of 151 patients with mild to moderate facial acne.

Interventions.—Subjects were asked to carry out 4 follow-up visits using either an e-visit platform or conventional office care. At 6-week intervals, subjects in the evisit group were prompted to send images of their skin and an update, via a secure Web site, to their dermatologist. Dermatologists responded with advice and electronic prescriptions.

Main Outcome Measures.—The primary outcome measure was change in total inflammatory lesion count between the first and last visit. The major secondary outcomes were subject and dermatologist satisfaction with care and length of time to complete visits.

Results.—The mean age of subjects was 28 years; most were female (78%), white (65%), and college educated (69%). One hundred twenty-one of the initial 151 subjects completed the study. The decrease in total inflammatory lesion count was similar in the e-visit and office visit groups (6.67 and 9.39, respectively) ($P = .49$). Both subjects and dermatologists reported comparable satisfaction with care regardless of visit type ($P = .06$ and $P = .16$, respectively). Compared with office visits, e-visits were time saving for subjects and time neutral for dermatologists (4 minutes, 8 seconds vs 4 minutes, 42 seconds) ($P = .57$).

Conclusion.—Delivering follow-up care to acne patients via an e-visit platform produced clinical outcomes equivalent to those of conventional office visits.

Trial Registration.—clinicaltrials.gov Identifier: NCT00417456.

▶ The authors show that acne patients treated by telemedicine visits did as well as those given traditional office visits. I have my doubts about how generally applicable this might be, but it is nonetheless an interesting idea that could be profitably applied. Teens are typically in school during office hours, making visits problematic for some. Moreover, teens, at least those encountered in my practice, are not the most punctual of patients and can cause scheduling problems. After-hours televisits would seem to be an acceptable solution in some cases.

G. Webster, MD, PhD

Migrating Hair: A Case Confused with Cutaneous Larva Migrans
Kim JY, Silverman RA (Ajou Univ School of Medicine, Yongtong-gu, Suwon-si, South Korea; Georgetown Univ Hosp, Falls Church, VA)
Pediatr Dermatol 27:628-630, 2010

Pili migrans is an unusual skin condition in which a hair shaft migrates under the surface of the skin and mimics the parasitic infection, cutaneous larva migrans. If the migrating hair is located on the sole of the foot, it represents a foreign body from an exogenous source. We present a 3-year-old boy with bilateral pili migrans on the soles of his feet, acquired after running around in his socks while at his mother's beauty salon. This case highlights a distinctive presentation of a foreign body penetration of the skin that can easily be confused for and should be differentiated from the parasitic disease, cutaneous larva migrans.

▶ Imbedded hair, pili cuniculati, cutaneous pili migrans, and creeping hair have all been used to describe hair shafts that migrate under the surface of skin, often mimicking cutaneous larva migrans, a parasitic infection. This phenomenon should be considered in the differential diagnosis for serpiginous eruptions. Differential diagnosis for cutaneous larva migrans may include scabies, erythema chronicum migrans, tinea corporis, and cutaneous myiasis. According to the authors, 21 reported cases, including internal source of ingrown hair and external or foreign body sources of hair that penetrate the skin from the outside, have been documented. Some important differences between cutaneous pili migrans and the parasitic infection are that cutaneous larva migrans can move in various directions, leaving a tortuous path, and it tends to be very pruritic. Pili migrans generally moves in a linear fashion and may be asymptomatic or more often painful rather than pruritic. A thorough history would also assist in the diagnosis. Asian hair tends to have the largest cross-sectional area, and this may account for the larger number of cases found in East Asia.

S. Bellew, DO
J. Q. Del Rosso, DO

7 Photobiology

Indoor Tanning — Science, Behavior, and Policy

Fisher DE, James WD (Massachusetts General Hosp and Harvard Med School, Boston; Univ of Pennsylvania School of Medicine, Philadelphia)
N Engl J Med 363:901-903, 2010

Background.—About 10% of the US population use tanning beds each year, including minors. The Food and Drug Administration (FDA) is reviewing the safety of tanning beds and will soon decide whether and how to reclassify tanning lamps and minors' access to them. Concern is related to the increased incidence of melanoma and its accompanying mortality. Melanoma has increased more rapidly than any other cancer, with a 2.7% increase in new melanoma diagnoses in girls and women age 15 to 39 years that may at least partially result from the wider use of tanning beds. The incidences of thicker cutaneous melanomas and regional and distant tumors have also increased. The 9.2% increased annual rate of the latter may indicate a coming surge in advanced melanomas in young women, which has a high risk of death. Possible links between indoor tanning and melanoma and nonmelanoma cutaneous cancers were assessed.

Research.—The International Agency for Research on Cancer (IARC) finds that persons who first used indoor tanning before age 35 years have a relative risk of melanoma of 1.75. A Minnesota study found the adjusted odds ratio was 1.74, with the risk of melanoma increasing as the number of years of tanning and hours of tanning sessions increased.

Exposure to ultraviolet (UV) radiation has also been linked to nonmelanoma skin cancers. The IARC study found that a history of any indoor tanning had a relative risk of 2.25 for squamous cell carcinoma. Most lesions can be treated successfully at an early stage, but metastatic lesions occur in a small minority of cases and are seldom curable. The high incidence of squamous cell carcinoma makes it accountable for 25% to 35% of all skin cancer-n-related deaths.

Mechanisms.—Tanning and cancer share the common molecular intermediate of DNA damage, which activates melanin synthesis. Both p53 and proopiomelanocortin are involved in processing and secreting melanocyte-stimulating hormone (MSH), which activates pigment production in epidermal melanocytes. The tanning industry holds that indoor tanners avoid sunburn better than outdoor tanners. UVA wavelengths are used rather than UVB wavelengths, but both damage DNA and induce discrete mutations. Also, UV radiation can be carcinogenic without causing sunburn. Repeated UV irradiation, and the use of indoor tanning beds specifically,

193

can also induce significant systemic and behavioral consequences. This includes mood changes, pain, and physical dependency. Frequent tanners detected differences between UV-radiating and sham devices, suggesting a reinforcing stimulus. Administering an opiate-receptor blocker to frequent tanners induced withdrawal-like symptoms, again suggesting an addiction. Such sun-seeking behavior may be related to the UV radiation role in cutaneous vitamin D production. Although this may have had a survival advantage in some settings, it can no longer serve as a justification for tanning with vitamin D supplements readily available.

Conclusions.—Several countries have tightened restrictions on indoor tanning. Currently the FDA classifies tanning beds as medical devices in the same class as tongue depressors and adhesive bandages. Skin cancer screening is not currently recommended because its benefit has not been validated in large prospective randomized trials. New drugs to treat metastatic melanoma are working their way through clinical trials to satisfy the FDA's strict safety and efficacy criteria, which are not being applied to indoor tanning devices. Regulating this industry may offer a profound opportunity to prevent skin cancer.

▶ This is a very useful article in alerting dermatologists to the reasons some patients continue to tan despite the knowledge that sunlight can cause skin cancer. Tanning can be addictive for many patients. The illustration in the article is to the point in explaining the mechanism of ultraviolet light—induced damage regardless of the source—outdoor or indoor. Pointing out how indoor tanning is not a safe and sure way to obtain Vitamin D helps dermatologists talk about this issue with patients who might have been misled by the indoor tanning industry. The discussion about legislative changes pertinent to indoor tanning is also useful.

K. Nguyen, MD

Clinical evidence of benefits of a dietary supplement containing probiotic and carotenoids on ultraviolet-induced skin damage
Bouilly-Gauthier D, Jeannes C, Maubert Y, et al (Laboratoires Innéov, Quai Aulagnier, Asnières sur Seine CEDEX, France; Clinique Appliquée à la Dermatologie, Nice, France; et al)
Br J Dermatol 163:536-543, 2010

Background.—*Lactobacillus johnsonii* (La1) has been reported to protect skin immune system homeostasis following ultraviolet (UV) exposure.

Objectives.—To assess the effects of a dietary supplement (DS) combining La1 and nutritional doses of carotenoids on early UV-induced skin damage.

Methods.—Three clinical trials (CT1, CT2, CT3) were performed using different UV sources: nonextreme UV with a high UVA irradiance (UV-DL, CT1), extreme simulated solar radiation (UV-SSR, CT2) and natural sunlight (CT3). All three clinical trials were carried out in healthy women over 18 years of age with skin type II—IV. In CT1, early markers of UV-induced skin damage were assessed using histology and immunohistochemistry. In CT2, the minimal erythemal dose (MED) was determined by clinical evaluation and by chromametry. Chromametry was also used to evaluate skin colour. Dermatologists' and subjects' assessments were compiled in CT3.

Results.—A 10-week DS intake prevented the UV-DL-induced decrease in Langerhans cell density and the increase in factor XIIIa+ type I dermal dendrocytes while it reduced dermal inflammatory cells. Clinical and instrumental MED rose by 20% and 19%, respectively, and skin colour was intensified, as shown by the increase in the $\triangle E^*$ parameter. The efficacy of DS was confirmed by dermatologists and subjects under real conditions of use.

Conclusions.—Nutritional supplementation combining a specific probiotic (La1) and nutritional doses of carotenoids reduced early UV-induced skin damage caused by simulated or natural sun exposure in a large panel of subjects ($n = 139$). This latter result might suggest that DS intake could have a beneficial influence on the long-term effects of UV exposure and more specifically on skin photoaging.

▶ Every so often we come across articles involving clinical trials that are not only compelling but actually make perfect sense. This article is definitely one of them. Dermatologists assess photo-damaged skin for multiple potential problems every day, but we sometimes forget that photo-damaged skin is immunosuppressed skin. Think of what we use phototherapy for in the office, a few minutes of ultraviolet B or A with psoralens. These phototherapy approaches induce a beneficial immunosuppressive effect on lymphocytes, dendritic cells, and mast cells to modify inflammatory processes. So if 3 to 5 minutes is used to control dermatitis, mycosis fungoides, and psoriasis, think of the long list of what 20- to 30-plus years of unsupervised photo exposure does to localized immunity in the skin. This list includes decreased dendritic cell functions for antigen recognition and processing with decreased immune responsiveness, which leads to poor wound healing, lack of tumor surveillance, and increased risk of secondary infections. These hidden defects are what lies beneath the visible signs of photoaging and dermatoheliosis.

The inclusion of antioxidants and other agents that combat reactive oxygen species has increased exponentially in commercial products, as well as in topical and systemic over-the-counter and prescription medications. The potential application of their benefits are discussed in this article based on their activity in photo-damaged skin, before and after the 6-week treatment period. This approach, if proven to produce positive outcomes, can expand significantly if we continue to note a therapeutic impact on the immune mechanisms involved. Table 1 provides a thorough summary of the effect of the probiotics and carotenoids on important cell populations. Evaluation of the impact of these cell lines should be applied to the clinical findings of photodamage because they are directly related to pathogenesis.

An important clinical caveat to interpreting data like these is to make sure that patients do not mistakenly think that there is a sense of complete photoprotection.

TABLE 1.—Effect of Suberythemal Doses of Ultraviolet Daylight (UV-DL) on Skin Immune Cells, Inflammatory Infiltrate and Pigmentation (Clinical Trial 1)

	Before DS Intake		After DS Intake	
	Nonexposed Skin (n = 16)	UV-DL-Exposed Skin (n = 16)	Nonexposed Skin (n = 16)	UV-DL-Exposed Skin (n = 16)
Langerhans cells (protein S100)	623 ± 299	416 ± 148[a]	613 ± 270	545 ± 215[bc]
Dermal dendrocytes (factor XIIIa+)	4245 ± 2038	4915 ± 2144	4215 ± 1996	4118 ± 1982[c]
Dermal inflammatory cells (CD45+)	4.4 ± 2.6	8.4 ± 4.0[a]	4.1 ± 2.2	5.9 ± 3.3[ab]
Active melanocytes (tyrosinase)	296 ± 115	331 ± 83[a]	321 ± 109	363 ± 154[a]
Melanin content (Fontana−Masson)	2809 ± 1166	3801 ± 1355[a]	2795 ± 1133	3296 ± 1197[abc]

DS, dietary supplement. Results are shown as mean ± SD. The square of the cell count mm^{-1} length of *stratum corneum* represents the density of cells mm^{-2} of skin surface. Dermal dendrocyte count was expressed as the number mm^{-2} of factor XIIIa+ cells in the perivascular compartment of the upper dermis. CD45+ cell count was expressed mm^{-2} of skin surface area. Antityrosinase cells were counted in the basal layer of the epidermis. Melanin content was evaluated using digital image analysis after Fontana−Masson staining.
[a]Exposed *vs.* nonexposed area, $P < 0.05$ (Student's *t*-test).
[b]exposed areas before *vs.* after supplementation, $P < 0.05$ (Student's *t*-test).
[c]comparison of exposed *vs.* unexposed areas before *vs.* after supplementation, $P < 0.05$ (Wilcoxon test).

Use of antioxidants, probiotics, or carotenoids does not provide "diplomatic immunity" from using other prevention methods, such as sunblock and avoidance of prime daytime sun exposure. The potential use of a supplement in this case should be as a modifier of disease pathogenesis, not as a photo protectant.

N. Bhatia, MD

Are sunscreens luxury products?

Mahé E, Beauchet A, de Maleissye M-F, et al (Univ of Versailles-Saint Quentin en Yvelines)
J Am Acad Dermatol 65:e73-e79, 2011

Background.—The incidence of skin cancers is rapidly increasing in Western countries. One of the main sun-protection measures advocated is application of sunscreen. Some studies report a failure to comply with sunscreen application guidance. One explanation is their cost.

Objective.—To evaluate the true cost of sunscreen in two situations: a 4-member family spending 1 week at the beach and a transplant patient respecting all the sun protection recommendations.

Methods.—We performed an analysis of prices of sunscreens sold via Internet drugstores in Europe and North America. Standard sunscreen application recommendations were followed. We tested the recommended amount of sunscreen to be applied (ie, 2 mg/cm²).

Results.—Six hundred seven sunscreens from 17 drugstores in 7 countries were evaluated. Median price of sunscreen was $1.7 US per 10 grams. The price decreased with the size of the bottle. The median price for a family varied from $178.2 per week to $238.4 per week. The price decreased by 33% if the family wore UV-protective T-shirts and by 41% if large-volume bottles were used. The median price for a transplant patient varied from $245.3 per year to $292.3 per year.

Limitations.—Anti-UVA activity and topical properties were not evaluated. We tested the recommended amount (2 mg/cm^2) rather than the amount actually used (1 mg/cm^2).

Conclusion.—Under acute sun exposure conditions (a week at the beach), the cost of sun protection appears acceptable if sun protective clothing is worn and large-format bottles and low-cost sunscreens are used. Conversely, in a sun-sensitive population requiring year-round protection, the annual budget is relatively high and patients may require financial assistance to be compliant with sun protection guidelines.

▶ Proper and consistent application of sunscreen or sunblock is one of the many measures advocated by practitioners to help patients reduce exposure to ultraviolet (UV) light and its ensuing harmful effects. Patients, however, do not always comply with this recommendation, and as noted in the article, cost is one major explanation. As a result, Mahe et al sought to evaluate the cost of sunscreen use under 2 scenarios. One scenario was the cost of sunscreen use for a family of 4 during a 1-week beach holiday. The other was for a transplant patient who used sunscreen regularly based on current sun protection guidelines. The purpose of the article was to point out that sunscreen, although important, may pose a financial burden on patients needing year-round protection. Although the details of the article and its methodology are beyond the scope of this commentary, several findings are worth mentioning. The cost of sunscreen was found to be affordable for a family of 4 on 1-week beach vacation; cost varied from $178.2 to $238.4 dollars per week (although the definition of affordable is certainly arguable depending on the family). More importantly, the article found that this amount decreased substantially when UV-protective T-shirts were worn and when low-cost, larger bottles of sunscreen are purchased. In regard to patients—such as renal transplant patients—who are sun sensitive and require year-round use, the cost of daily sunscreen use may be affordable, but it was found that annually, the cost may be burdensome. The conclusion was that these patients may need financial assistance to enhance sunscreen compliance. There were several limitations listed in the study. Additionally, no practical recommendations were provided for how patients were to obtain potentially needed assistance; it was only mentioned that they may need it. Ultimately, the findings of the study were not necessarily surprising. The article did, however, provide practical dispensable advice, such as the importance of using other modalities or approaches, not just sunscreen, for sun protection (such as UV-protective T-shirts) and advising patients to use lower-cost and larger bottles of sunscreen. Overall, the article offers a starting point for much needed discussion and provides important data on the cost of sunscreens that may serve to promote advocacy of patient assistance, especially for children.

B. D. Michaels, DO

J. Q. Del Rosso, DO

An overview analysis of the time people spend outdoors

Diffey BL (Univ of Newcastle, Newcastle upon Tyne, UK)
Br J Dermatol 164:848-854, 2011

Background.—An important factor in determining our exposure to sunlight, and the consequent impact on skin health and vitamin D status, is the time we spend outdoors.

Objectives.—To determine estimates of the typical times per day spent outdoors during weekdays, weekends and holidays during a summer season.

Methods.—A number of published studies giving data on the time per day spent outdoors by people were reviewed and a meta-analysis performed. From these data summary estimates of the average time per day outdoors were extracted.

Results.—Time spent per day outdoors during weekdays and weekends is positively skewed, with a normal distribution of times outdoors during holidays. The *median* times per day outdoors during weekdays and weekends gave pooled estimates of 1·04 and 1·64 h, respectively. Corresponding values for the pooled estimates of mean times outdoors during these two periods were 1·43 and 2·38 h. The mean time per day outdoors during holiday exposure is 5—6 h.

Conclusions.—Summer-long distribution of times spent outdoors on a daily basis exhibits a highly skewed nature that highlights the difference between our adventitious and recreational exposure. Over the course of a summer season, when people are outside, they spend on average of 1—2 h per day outdoors.

▶ Spending time outdoors can have a great impact on skin health. The authors sought to estimate the time of day spent outdoors during the weekdays, weekends, and holidays during a summer season. Inspection of these data indicated that the median time per day outdoors is significantly less than the mean time for weekday and weekend exposure. It was found to be approximately equal for holiday exposure. In a cohort of studies, the time spent outdoors during the weekday and weekend was positively skewed, but there was a normal distribution of times per day outdoors during holidays. The median time per day outdoors during the weekdays and weekends gave pooled estimates of 1.04 and 1.64 hours, respectively. The values for the pooled estimates of mean time outdoors during these 2 periods were 1.43 and 2.38 hours. The mean time per day outdoors during holiday exposure was 5 to 6 hours. Some weaknesses to this meta-analysis are the heterogeneity between the datasets. Because this is a pooled estimate from many different studies, the data should be viewed with caution because of the heterogeneity of each study. Some of these heterogeneities include differences in geographical location, duration, time period during the day, and months of the year the study took place. Also, there may be differences in age, gender, and physical activity level of each individual included in the studies. The conclusion of this article was that during the summer season, people spent on average 1 to 2 hours per day outdoors, which is sufficient for vitamin D synthesis.

G. K. Kim, DO

J. Q. Del Rosso, DO

Adverse effects of ultraviolet radiation from the use of indoor tanning equipment: Time to ban the tan
Lim HW, James WD, Rigel DS, et al (Henry Ford Hosp, Detroita, MI; Univ of Pennsylvania, Philadelphia; New York Univ; et al)
J Am Acad Dermatol 64:e51-e60, 2011

The incidence of melanoma skin cancer is increasing rapidly, particularly among young women in the United States. Numerous studies have documented an association between the use of indoor tanning devices and an increased risk of skin cancer, especially in young women. Studies have shown that ultraviolet exposure, even in the absence of erythema or burn, results in DNA damage. Countries and regulatory bodies worldwide have recognized the health risks associated with indoor tanning. In the United States, 32 states have passed legislation to regulate the indoor tanning industry, but there is an urgent need to restrict the use of indoor tanning devices at the federal level. The Food and Drug Administration is currently reviewing the classification of these devices. For all of these reasons, the Food and Drug Administration should prohibit the use of tanning devices by minors and reclassify tanning devices to at least class II to protect the public from the preventable cancers and other adverse effects caused by ultraviolet radiation from indoor tanning.

▶ This article provides an excellent review of the mechanism of ultraviolet (UV) radiation damage and the latest research into its deleterious effects on the skin. It should be read by all providers who counsel patients on skin care and sun protection, both as a review and to supplement their knowledge on the wealth of evidence that UV light is a proven carcinogen. When the World Health Organization classified tanning beds as a carcinogen in 2009, this provided a lot of ammunition for states to draft and enforce legislation that severely limited their use. The American Academy of Dermatology and other medical groups have used the data presented in this article to help persuade the General and Plastic Surgery Devices Panel to make specific recommendations to the Food and Drug Administration regarding more strict limitations for and reclassification of tanning beds in the hope of developing federal regulations on their use.

The most useful recommendation was that tanning beds be upgraded to a class II device, the same classification as our medical-grade UV light-therapy boxes. This higher classification means that certain controls can be required, such as mandatory performance standards, postmarket surveillance, and patient registries. This would at least ensure that we could better track usage and outcomes for future decisions on regulations and epidemiologic studies. Another recommendation was to develop age restrictions, based on data that shows higher associations with skin cancers when tanning beds are used earlier in life. Many states and countries already have such restrictions in place.

Other suggestions included having different guidelines for different patient skin types and those with family history of skin cancer. I would be surprised to see this particular recommendation become law, because the act of creating legislation based on an individual's genetic makeup would most certainly run afoul of equal rights laws. Indeed, the outcome of these recommendations may be quite timely because the new health care laws are soon to come into effect. If every person will be required to hold a health insurance plan, and more individuals choose to join a government run plan, just how much influence will lawmakers have over the rights of individuals to participate in unhealthy activity?

J. M. Suchniak, MD

Prevalence and Characteristics of Indoor Tanning Use Among Men and Women in the United States

Choi K, Lazovich D, Southwell B, et al (Univ of Minnesota, Minneapolis; et al)
Arch Dermatol 146:1356-1361, 2010

Objectives.—To describe the prevalence and characteristics related to indoor tanning use among adults in the United States in the past year.

Design.—Cross-sectional study.

Setting.—Health Information National Trends Study, 2005.

Participants.—The study included 2869 participants who were white and aged 18 to 64 years; a random subset of 821 participants were also asked questions about skin cancer prevention knowledge and attitudes.

Main Outcome Measures.—The study assessed the prevalence of self-reported use of indoor tanning in the past 12 months and its associations with demographic and lifestyle factors, knowledge, and attitudes.

Results.—Overall, 18.1% of women and 6.3% of men reported tanning indoors in the past 12 months. Women who were older, were less educated, had lower income, and used sunscreen regularly were less likely to report the behavior, while women residing in the Midwest and the South and who used spray tanning products were more likely to report the behavior. Men who were less likely to report the behavior were older and obese but more likely to report the behavior if they lived in metropolitan areas and used spray tanning products. In an open-response format, only 13.3% of women and 4.2% of men suggested that avoidance of tanning bed use could reduce their risks of skin cancer. Greater skin cancer knowledge and higher perceived risk of skin cancer were inversely associated with the behavior in women.

Conclusions.—Prevalence and some characteristics associated with indoor tanning use, such as sunscreen use, differed between women and men in the United States. Most adults did not volunteer avoidance of tanning bed use to prevent skin cancer. Clinician-patient communication on risks of indoor tanning may be helpful to reduce indoor tanning use.

▶ The study confirmed some common accepted notions about indoor tanning, such as that women use indoor tanning more than men, this behavior tapers off as people get older, and that indoor tanning is more prevalent in the Midwest and South. Yet the overwhelming message revealed in this article is that a certain segment of the population still does not understand that indoor tanning can lead to skin cancer. The data show that many respondents are well aware that using hats, sunscreens, and avoiding the sun can help stave off skin cancer but do not understand that getting skin examinations and avoiding tanning beds are also significant in reducing skin cancer risk. These data probably accurately reflect the efforts put in place in the years preceding 2005, when the data were collected, during which most of the messages sent out by the health care industry were targeted to beachgoers, outdoor enthusiasts, college students, and outdoor workers. Because of the rising rates of skin cancers in the late 1990s and early 2000s, there was a strong push by the dermatology community to increase awareness of the dangers of the sun, and indoor sun tanning may have become more popular as an alternative. However, since the data in this study were collected, recent efforts by the health care industry have focused on carcinogenic risks associated with indoor tanning as well. Between the media coverage of the battle between dermatologists and the indoor tanning industry and the new federal tanning tax regulations, I would guess that the number of individuals that know that indoor tanning can cause skin cancer would be much higher now. A follow up study in the next Health Information National Trends Study would reveal whether such efforts are paying off.

Interestingly, this study showed a strong association between indoor tanning use and concomitant spray tanning behavior, not an inverse relationship as one might think. This idea might underlie the possible thinking by some patients that one can get "some" tan while supplementing the color with the "safe" tan (sunless tanning product). I often have patients try this mental trick with me, but I of course tell them this would be akin to wearing half a nicotine patch to still be able to smoke a few cigarettes a day. The idea that getting in the tanning bed for a base tan or "a little" tan is still a prevalent notion in the minds of many patients. Efforts to convey the idea that no ultraviolet-light-induced tan is safe are still clearly in need of reinforcement.

J. Suchniak, MD

Tomato paste rich in lycopene protects against cutaneous photodamage in humans *in vivo*: a randomized controlled trial
Rizwan M, Rodriguez-Blanco I, Harbottle A, et al (The Univ of Manchester and Salford Royal NHS Foundation Trust, UK; Newcastle Univ, Newcastle upon Tyne, UK)
Br J Dermatol 164:154-162, 2011

Background.—Previous epidemiological, animal and human data report that lycopene has a protective effect against ultraviolet radiation (UVR)-induced erythema.

Objectives.—We examined whether tomato paste—rich in lycopene, a powerful antioxidant—can protect human skin against UVR-induced effects partially mediated by oxidative stress, i.e. erythema, matrix changes and mitochondrial DNA (mtDNA) damage.

Methods.—In a randomized controlled study, 20 healthy women (median age 33 years, range 21–47; phototype I/II) ingested 55 g tomato paste (16 mg lycopene) in olive oil, or olive oil alone, daily for 12 weeks. Pre- and post-supplementation, UVR erythemal sensitivity was assessed visually as the minimal erythema dose (MED) and quantified with a reflectance instrument. Biopsies were taken from unexposed and UVR-exposed (3 × MED 24 h earlier) buttock skin pre- and postsupplementation, and analysed immunohistochemically for procollagen (pC) I, fibrillin-1 and matrix metalloproteinase (MMP)-1, and by quantitative polymerase chain reaction for mtDNA 3895-bp deletion.

Results.—Mean ± SD erythemal D_{30} was significantly higher following tomato paste vs. control (baseline, $26 \cdot 5 \pm 7 \cdot 5$ mJ cm^{-2}; control, $23 \pm 6 \cdot 6$ mJ cm^{-2}; tomato paste, $36 \cdot 6 \pm 14 \cdot 7$ mJ cm^{-2}; $P = 0 \cdot 03$), while the MED was not significantly different between groups (baseline, $35 \cdot 1 \pm 9 \cdot 9$ mJ cm^{-2}; control, $32 \cdot 6 \pm 9 \cdot 6$ mJ cm^{-2}; tomato paste, $42 \cdot 2 \pm 11 \cdot 3$ mJ cm^{-2}). Presupplementation, UVR induced an increase in MMP-1 ($P = 0 \cdot 01$) and a reduction in fibrillin-1 ($P = 0 \cdot 03$). Postsupplementation, UVR-induced MMP-1 was reduced in the tomato paste vs. control group ($P = 0 \cdot 04$), while the UVR-induced reduction in fibrillin-1 was similarly abrogated in both groups, and an increase in pCI deposition was seen following tomato paste ($P = 0 \cdot 05$). mtDNA 3895-bp deletion following 3 × MED UVR was significantly reduced postsupplementation with tomato paste ($P = 0 \cdot 01$).

Conclusions.—Tomato paste containing lycopene provides protection against acute and potentially longer-term aspects of photodamage.

▶ Many people believe that everything you ingest, including food, affects body health and function. This single-blinded randomized controlled trial is a great example of this potential and strongly suggests that ingesting tomato paste can ameliorate some of the effects of ultraviolet radiation (UVR).

The objective of this study, stated simply, was to see if daily ingestion of a mixture of lycopene, β-carotene, and other carotenoids found in tomato paste for 12 weeks could help prevent ultraviolet-induced erythema and photodamage. Patients' photodamage was assessed by measuring a specific mitochondrial DNA mutation, collagen production by assessing procollagen 1 level, and elastic and collagen fiber degradation by assessing fibrillin content and matrix metalloproteinase 1 (MMP-1) activation.

The authors found, after 3 months of oral supplementation, an increase in minimal erythema dose (MED) in the tomato paste group versus the control group (nonstatistically significant trend) and a marked increase in the amount of UVR needed to increase erythema 30 units in the tomato paste group only. In addition, the tomato paste group demonstrated significantly decreased MMP-1 activation and increased procollagen 1 deposition as well as fewer mitochondrial DNA mutations. However, changes in elastic protein degradation or fibrillin levels remained unchanged in both groups. It may be that the small sample size may have played a role in the nonsignificant changes seen in the MED and fibrillin degradation between the groups. Therefore, there may be a role for tomato paste in daily moisturizers or as a daily supplement to prevent photodamage. However, further experimentation is needed.

The authors in this study attribute the results of this experiment to the amount of lycopene in the supplied tomato paste. However, this is difficult to determine without a proper control because tomato paste also contains β-carotenes and other carotenoids, which could be contributing to the results demonstrated. Further experimentation may be needed with a variety of controls.

Although patient compliance may be improved by ingesting a pill versus applying a topical product diffusely, it would be interesting to compare the same parameters tested in this experiment after the topical application of a lycopene-containing moisturizer. It may be that only a few days to weeks of topical application would be needed to reach the required steady state dose of lycopene and/or carotenoids in the skin to replicate these photoprotective effects.

J. Levin, DO

J. Del Rosso, DO

Photo-allergic contact dermatitis caused by isoamyl *p*-methoxycinnamate in an 'organic' sunscreen

Ghazavi MK, Johnston GA (Leicester Royal Infirmary, UK)
Contact Dermatitis 64:110-120, 2011

Background.—Isoamyl *p*-methoxycinnamate is derived from cinnamon acid esters and provides an effective waterproof filter for ultraviolet B (UVB) rays. It rarely causes photo-allergic contact dermatitis (PACD), with only two cases reported in 2715 patients studied for 15 years. However, the risk of developing PACD may be increased by the presence of photodermatoses such as polymorphic light eruption and chronic actinic dermatitis.

Case Report.—Woman, 39, reported a polymorphic urticated and papular eruption on sun-exposed areas (except the hands and face) that had been present for 20 years but had worsened at sites where she applied a new, "organic" sunscreen, even the face. The urticated eruption at these sites settled after several days with scaling. She was diagnosed with polymorphic light eruption and a superimposed allergic contact dermatitis and underwent patch testing and photo-patching testing, with patches removed after 2 days. A commercial sunscreen series was applied in duplicate. One set of the patch test samples were irradiated with UVA light, and all patches were read after 4 days. There was a ± reaction to *Myroxylon pereirae* and a ++ reaction to 4-methylbenzylidene camphor, which is used for UV protection in cosmetics, on both irradiated and nonirradiated specimens. This was consistent with a diagnosis of allergic contact dermatitis. The irradiated site also showed a reaction to isoamyl *p*-methoxycinnamate, consistent with a PACD diagnosis. The patient's sunscreen was found to contain isoamyl *p*-methoxycinnamate.

She changed to a sunscreen that did not contain any of the allergens identified and had no further problems.

Conclusions.—Isoamyl p-methoxycinnamate causes a urticated instead of a dermatitis contact reaction and can cross-react with flavorings and fragrances, including M pereirae, as seen in this case, coca leaves, cinnamic acid, and cinnamal. The histamine-releasing effect of cinnamal can cause nonimmunologic contact urticaria, which could have caused the PACD in this patient.

▶ This is a short case report on photoallergic contact dermatitis to isoamyl p-methoxycinnamate in sunscreen. Overall, this article has low clinical importance because of the rarity of photoallergic contact dermatitis to the allergen. In fact, although sunscreen is the most common cause of photoallergic reactions, this is still infrequent. In addition, oxybenzone is the most common allergen in sunscreen. Unspecific reactions such as burning on initial application, exacerbation of preexisting atopic dermatitis, and nonimmunologic forms of urticaria are more likely occurrences.

This article does, however, inadvertently highlight 3 clinically valuable points. First, it reminds the reader that exacerbations of chronic dermatitic conditions may in fact be due to allergic contact dermatitis and that patch tests in these particular instances are warranted. Second, it demonstrates that guessing the culprit allergen based on the most likely allergen according to frequency studies can actually misguide the patient. Only patch tests pinpoint the exact allergen. Finally, the case demonstrates how multiple photo-induced disease entities can frequently coexist in a single photosensitized individual.

P. Saitta, DO

A randomized, double-blind, negatively controlled pilot study to determine whether the use of emollients or calcipotriol alters the sensitivity of the skin to ultraviolet radiation during phototherapy with narrowband ultraviolet B
Skellett A, Swift L, Tan E, et al (Norfolk and Norwich Univ Hosp NHS Foundation Trust, UK; Univ of East Anglia, Norwich, UK)
Br J Dermatol 164:402-406, 2011

Background.—There is contradictory evidence suggesting that emollients increase, decrease or have no effect on minimal erythema dose (MED) or minimal phototoxic dose values prior to phototherapy. Few studies have looked at the in vivo use of emollients or calcipotriol prior to narrowband ultraviolet (UV) B (NB-UVB) treatment.

Objectives.—To investigate whether emollients or calcipotriol alter MED readings of skin on the back of healthy subjects prior to NB-UVB irradiation.

Methods.—Topical agents were applied to the backs of 20 healthy volunteers for 30 min prior to MED testing. These agents were aqueous cream, 50:50 white soft paraffin and liquid paraffin, Diprobase® (Schering-Plough,

Welwyn Garden City, U.K.), Epaderm® (Medlock, Oldham, U.K.) and calcipotriol ointment and cream. A control MED strip was used with no
topical agent applied prior to testing. MED readings were recoded as
integer steps between 1 and 9 (one is lowest MED dose for skin type;
eight is highest; nine is no response, i.e. a higher MED).

Results.—The median MED was between step 5 and 6 for all treatments
and control. There was no significant difference at the 5% level between
control and each topical agent. The study was powered to detect a median
difference of approximately $0 \cdot 4 - 0 \cdot 6$ steps.

Conclusions.—This has important implications at a practical level when
advising patients not to apply creams prior to treatment with NB-UVB.
Studies where agents are applied immediately prior to phototherapy have
been more likely to show that emollients block transmission of UV radiation.
If they are applied at least 30 min prior to treatment, they have no effect.

▶ The impact of emollients on the erythemogenicity of ultraviolet B (UVB) has
been the subject of several studies in the past, some of which have shown that
emollients increase the minimal erythema dose (MED) and others of which
have shown a reduction in the MED or no effect. Similar conflicting results
have been published about the minimal phototoxic dose following application
of emollients, but there are few data concerning the impact of emollients or calcipotriol on the erythemogenicity of narrowband UVB.

To address the impact of topical emollients or calcipotriol on the erythemogenicity of narrowband UVB, the authors applied topical agents to the backs of 20
volunteers 30 minutes before MED testing. There was no significant difference
in MED readings between skin treated with various emollients or calcipotriol
cream or ointment and untreated skin. There was a trend for higher MED readings
for 1 product, Epaderm, indicating that the latter agent appears to block narrowband UVB.

The results of this study should be interpreted cautiously before applying
them to real-life circumstances. In phototherapy units, patients apply topical
agents immediately before phototherapy, not 30 minutes before. Moreover,
there is little control for the thickness with which topical emollients are applied.
In a previous study, thick application of an emollient cream immediately before
phototherapy was shown to block transmission of UVB and increase the MED.[1]
In addition, these authors did not address the potential impact of narrowband
UVB on the stability or efficacy of the irradiated products. Specifically, vitamin
D analogs such as calcitriol are inactivated by narrowband UVB.[2] Calcipotriol is
stable following broadband UVB irradiation, although it is inactivated by UVA.[3]
Nevertheless, it is useful to know that patients who apply their medications
more than 30 minutes before phototherapy with narrowband UVB do not
block the erythemogenicity of that light.

M. Lebwohl, MD

References

1. Lebwohl M, Martinez J, Weber P, DeLuca R. Effects of topical preparations on the
   erythemogenicity of UVB: implications for psoriasis phototherapy. *J Am Acad
   Dermatol.* 1995;32:469-471.

2. Lebwohl M, Quijije J, Gilliard J, Rollin T, Watts O. Topical calcitriol is degraded by ultraviolet light. *J Invest Dermatol.* 2003;121:594-595.
3. Lebwohl M, Hecker D, Martinez J, Sapadin A, Patel B. Interactions between calcipotriene and ultraviolet light. *J Am Acad Dermatol.* 1997;37:93-95.

8 Collagen Vascular and Related Disorders

A systematic review of drug-induced subacute cutaneous lupus erythematosus

Lowe G, Henderson CL, Grau RH, et al (Univ of Utah School of Medicine, Salt Lake City; Univ of Oklahoma College of Medicine; Private Practice of Dermatology, Oklahoma City)

Br J Dermatol 164:465-472, 2011

The initial appearance of subacute cutaneous lupus erythematosus (SCLE) skin lesions in conjunction with Ro/SS-A autoantibodies occurring as an adverse reaction to hydrochlorothiazide [i.e. drug-induced SCLE (DI-SCLE)] was first reported in 1985. Over the past decade an increasing number of drugs in different classes has been implicated as triggers for DI-SCLE. The management of DI-SCLE can be especially challenging in patients taking multiple medications capable of triggering DI-SCLE. Our objectives were to review the published English language literature on DI-SCLE and use the resulting summary data pool to address questions surrounding drug-induced SCLE and to develop guidelines that might be of value to clinicians in the diagnosis and management of DI-SCLE. A systematic review of the Medline/PubMed-cited literature on DI-SCLE up to August 2009 was performed. Our data collection and analysis strategies were prospectively designed to answer a series of questions related to the clinical, prognostic and pathogenetic significance of DI-SCLE. One hundred and seventeen cases of DI-SCLE were identified and reviewed. White women made up the large majority of cases, and the mean overall age was 58·0 years. Triggering drugs fell into a number of different classes, highlighted by antihypertensives and antifungals. Time intervals ('incubation period') between drug exposure and appearance of DI-SCLE varied greatly and were drug class dependent. Most cases of DI-SCLE spontaneously resolved within weeks of drug withdrawal. Ro/SS-A autoantibodies were present in 80% of the cases in which such data were reported and most remained positive after resolution of SCLE skin disease activity. No significant differences in the clinical, histopathological or immunopathological features between DI-SCLE and idiopathic SCLE were detected. There is now adequate published experience to suggest that DI-SCLE does not differ clinically, histopathologically or immunologically from idiopathic SCLE. It should be recognized as a distinct clinical

TABLE 1.—Drugs Identified as Causative of Drug-Induced Subacute Cutaneous Lupus Erythematosus (SCLE) in This Report

Antihypertensives	40 of 117 reported cases: 34·2%
Calcium channel blockers	
Diltiazem[7,10]	6 cases
Verapamil[7,8]	5 cases
Nifedipine[7,10,30]	3 cases
Nitrendipine[31]	1 case
Diuretics	
Hydrochorothiazide[3,10,22]	10 cases
Hydrochlorothiazide + triamterene[6]	3 cases
Chlorthiazide[5]	2 cases
Beta blockers	
Oxprenolol[32]	4 cases
Acebutolol[33]	1 case
Angiotensin-converting enzyme inhibitors	
Enalapril[10]	2 cases
Lisnopril[10]	1 case
Captopril[34]	1 case
Cilazapril[34]	1 case
Antifungals	30 of 117 reported cases: 25·6%
Terbinafine[12,14–16,35–37]	29 cases
Griseofulvin[13]	1 case
Chemotherapeutics	10 of 117 reported cases: 8·5%
Docetaxel[38]	3 cases
Paclitaxel[24,38]	3 cases
Tamoxifen[39]	2 cases
Capecitabine[40,41]	2 cases
Antihistamines	9 of 117 reported cases: 7·7%
Ranitidine[42]	7 cases
Brompheniramine[42]	1 case
Cinnarizine + thiethylperazine[43]	1 case
Immunomodulators	8 of 117 reported cases: 6·8%
Leflunomide[9,17,25,44]	5 cases
Interferon α and β[10,45]	3 cases
Antiepileptics	3 of 117 reported cases: 2·6%
Carbamazepine[46,47]	2 cases
Phenytoin[48]	1 case
Statins	3 of 117 reported cases: 2·6%
Simvastatin[10,49]	2 cases
Pravastatin[10]	1 case
Biologics	2 of 117 reported cases: 1·7%
Etanercept[50]	1 case
Efalizumab[51]	1 case
Proton pump inhibitors	2 of 117 reported cases: 1·7%
Lansoprazole[52]	2 cases
Nonsteroidal anti-inflammatory drugs	2 of 117 reported cases: 1·7%
Naproxen[53]	1 case
Piroxicam[26]	1 case
Hormone-altering drugs	2 of 117 reported cases: 1·7%
Leuprorelin[19]	1 case
Anastrozole[18]	1 case
Ultraviolet therapy	2 of 117 reported cases: 1·7%
PUVA[54]	1 case
PUVA and UVB[20]	1 case
Others	4 of 117 reported cases: 3·4%
Bupropion[55]	1 case
Tiotropium[56]	1 case
Ticlopidine[57]	1 case
Hay with fertilizer[58]	1 case

The numbers in the table represent citations to references, and the drugs reported to be capable of also producing photosensitivity skin reactions other than SCLE in otherwise healthy individuals are presented in italics. PUVA, psoralen plus ultraviolet (UV) A.

Editor's Note: Please refer to original journal article for full references.

constellation differing clinically and immunologically from the classical form of drug-induced systemic lupus erythematosus (Table 1).

▶ Drug-induced subacute cutaneous lupus erythematosus (SCLE) was first described in 1995. Since that time, numerous anecdotal reports have implicated a wide range of drug classes as triggers of drug-induced SCLE. In this systematic review, Lowe et al evaluated data from all English-language reports of drug-induced SCLE published through August 2009 to attempt to answer a number of clinically relevant questions about this disease and its relationship to idiopathic SCLE. Their conclusions based on the 117 reported cases provide useful information for clinicians that will help enable the diagnosis of drug-induced SCLE and thereby potentially prevent overevaluation and treatment of patients who will likely do well simply by discontinuing the triggering drug. Table 1 summarizes drugs and drug classes reported. Key points are as follows:

- Drug-induced SCLE is morphologically, histopathologically, and immunologically indistinguishable from idiopathic SCLE.
- Most cases were in Caucasian women; mean age was 58 years.
- Antihypertensives and antifungals represent the triggering drug classes most often reported.
- Autoantibody positivity was as follows: Ro/SSA, 81%; La/SSB, 48%; histone, 33%. This tends to persist even after drug cessation and rash resolution.
- Median onset of drug-induced SCLE was 6 weeks after commencement of the offending drug (mean, 27.9 weeks; range, 3 days-11 years); it was longest in cases induced by calcium channel blockers and thiazide diuretics (6 months-several years) and shortest in cases induced by antifungal medications (several weeks).
- Most cases resolved within several weeks (mean, 7.3 weeks; median, 4 weeks) of discontinuation of the implicated drug.
- Many drugs implicated in drug-induced SCLE are known photosensitizers.
- Beyond stopping the triggering drug, treatment is often unnecessary, but treatment with topical steroids or calcineurin inhibitors, prednisone, and hydroxychloroquine has been reported.

This review used only English-language reports and may also be limited by publication bias. Cases triggered by drugs previously reported are less likely to be published than cases in which novel drugs are implicated, thereby making it difficult to assess the true frequency of drug-induced SCLE for a given drug class. It is also possible that there is an underreporting of drug-induced SCLE in cases in which patients fail to improve following drug cessation because it is difficult to prove that the drug was the trigger.

This systematic review is highly recommended for any clinical dermatologist for the practical data regarding recognition and management of drug-induced SCLE.

J. T. Clarke, MD

Photoprotective effects of a broad-spectrum sunscreen in ultraviolet-induced cutaneous lupus erythematosus: A randomized, vehicle-controlled, double-blind study

Kuhn A, Gensch K, Haust M, et al (Univ of Muenster, Germany; Univ of Duesseldorf, Germany; et al)
J Am Acad Dermatol 64:37-48, 2011

Objective.—We sought to assess if the exclusive use of a broad-spectrum sunscreen can prevent skin lesions in patients with different subtypes of cutaneous lupus erythematosus (CLE) induced by ultraviolet (UV) irradiation under standardized conditions.

Methods.—A total of 25 patients with a medical history of photosensitive CLE were included in this monocentric, randomized, vehicle-controlled, double-blind, intraindividual study. The test product and its vehicle were applied 15 minutes before UVA and UVB irradiation of uninvolved skin areas on the upper aspect of the back in a random order, and standardized phototesting was performed daily for 3 consecutive days.

Results.—Characteristic skin lesions were induced by UVA and UVB irradiation in 16 patients with CLE in the untreated area, and 14 patients showed a positive test result in the vehicle-treated area. In contrast, no eruptions compatible with CLE were observed in the sunscreen-treated area in any of the 25 patients. This resulted in significant differences ($P < .001$) between UV-irradiated sunscreen-treated versus vehicle-treated areas, and between UV-irradiated sunscreen-treated versus untreated areas. Furthermore, a significant difference ($P < .05$) was observed concerning the age of disease onset and the patient history of photosensitivity. Patients who were younger than 40 years at onset of CLE reported photosensitivity significantly more often than patients with a higher age of disease onset. None of the patients showed any adverse events from application of the test product or the vehicle.

Limitations.—Data resulting from standardized experimental phototesting might not be transferable to a clinical setting.

Conclusion.—These results indicate clearly that the use of a highly protective broad-spectrum sunscreen can prevent skin lesions in photosensitive patients with different subtypes of CLE.

▶ As physicians, we are often quick to offer prescriptions and provide counseling about drug therapy. Our patients often deem prescription therapy more important than nonprescription treatment. This randomized, vehicle-controlled, double-blind study demonstrates how powerful a preventative nonprescription therapy can be for patients with cutaneous lupus erythematosus (LE). The efficacy of a broad-spectrum SPF 60 sunscreen in preventing UV-induced cutaneous lupus erythematosus (LE) lesions in 25 patients known to have UV-inducible skin lesions was clearly demonstrated. The sunscreen agent tested contained ethylhexyl methoxycinnamate, titanium dioxide, zinc oxide, and methylene bis-benzotriazolyl tetramethylbutylphenol. The sunscreen prevented lesions following UV exposure, including UVA and UVB, in all patients, whereas 18 of

25 patients developed histologically confirmed cutaneous LE lesions in nonprotected (either vehicle treated or untreated) skin. The sunscreen was effective for patients with discoid LE, subacute cutaneous LE, and LE tumidus. The article highlights the importance of photoprotection even for patients who may deny photosensitivity because there may be a latency of up to 3 weeks following UV exposure and the onset of new skin lesions. Five of 7 patients in this study who denied a history of photosensitivity developed photo-induced lesions. The authors did not find significant differences in the UV induction of lesions between subtypes of cutaneous LE nor with regard to wavelength of UV light administered (UVA vs UVB); however, given the limited number of patients included (17 with LE tumidus, 3 with subacute cutaneous LE, and 5 with discoid LE), the study was not adequately powered to detect such differences.

Limitations to the study include the enrollment of some patients who had been treated with antimalarials for up to 6 weeks prior to the start of the study. These drugs have photoprotective properties and a long elimination half-life, and it is therefore possible that there was some residual antimalarial-related photoprotection in some of the patients studied. Patients also presumably had relatively mild disease such that they did not require systemic immunosuppressants and could be without antimalarials for at least 6 weeks before the study. Additionally, experimental UV exposure does not replicate natural sun exposure, and application of sunscreens in an experimental setting rarely approximates routine real-world sunscreen use. Finally, previous studies have demonstrated superiority of certain sunscreens in the prevention of cutaneous LE lesions based on their ingredients; the sunscreen used in this study contains ingredients that although available in Europe are not approved by the US Food and Drug Administration.

The article is highly recommended for its excellent review of photosensitivity in cutaneous LE. It is an important prospective, double-blind, vehicle-controlled study that reminds us how beneficial photoprotection alone can be in the management of cutaneous LE.

J. T. Clarke, MD

Malignancy in Systemic Lupus Erythematosus: A Nationwide Cohort Study in Taiwan

Chen Y-J, Chang Y-T, Wang C-B, et al (Taichung Veterans General Hosp, Taiwan; Natl Yang-Ming Univ, Taipei, Taiwan)
Am J Med 123:1150.e1-1150.e6, 2010

Background.—An increased risk of malignancy in patients with systemic lupus erythematosus has been reported, but rarely in Asian populations. We aimed to investigate the relative risk of cancer and to identify the high-risk group for cancer in patients with lupus.

Methods.—We conducted a retrospective, nationwide cohort study that included 11,763 patients with lupus without a history of malignancies, using the national health insurance database of Taiwan from 1996 to 2007. Standardized incidence ratios (SIRs) of cancers were analyzed.

Results.—A total of 259 cancers were observed in patients with lupus. An elevated risk of cancer among those with systemic lupus erythematosus was noted (SIR 1.76; 95% confidence interval [CI] 1.74-1.79), especially for hematologic malignancies (SIR 4.96; 95% CI 4.79-5.14). Younger patients had a greater risk ratio of cancer than the general population, and the risk ratio decreased with age. The risk ratio of cancer decreased with time, yet remained elevated compared with that of the general population. The risk of non-Hodgkin lymphoma was greatest (SIR 7.27) among hematologic cancers. Among solid tumors, the risk was greatest for cancers of the vagina/vulva (SIR 4.76), nasopharynx (SIR 4.18), and kidney (SIR 3.99). An elevated risk for less common cancers, including those of the brain, oropharynx, and thyroid glands, was also observed.

Conclusion.—Patients with lupus are at increased risk of cancers and should receive age- and gender-appropriate malignancy evaluations, with additional assessment for vulva/vagina, kidney, nasopharynx, and hematologic malignancy. Continued vigilance for development of cancers in follow-up is recommended.

▶ An increased risk of malignancy has been described in patients with many rheumatologic diseases, including systemic lupus erythematosus (SLE). This retrospective cohort study evaluated 11 763 patients diagnosed with SLE in Taiwan. Two hundred fifty-nine malignancies were documented after a diagnosis of SLE (2.2% of SLE patients were diagnosed with cancer), demonstrating an overall increased cancer incidence in this patient population. Malignancies were more common in women, and the risk was greatest within the first few years after diagnosis of SLE. This may in part be due to surveillance/detection bias in this group of patients, who undergo more aggressive health screening. It has been postulated that immunosuppressive drugs used to treat SLE may at least partially explain the apparent increased malignancy risk, although this has not been borne out in all studies attempting to answer this question. The authors discuss other possible explanations for the increased risk and make recommendations for screening based on the types of malignancy most often found among their cohort (lymphomas > leukemias > solid tumors). It should be noted that the cohort includes a relatively genetically homogenous group and that risk factors such as smoking, alcohol use, family history of malignancy, and treatment for SLE were not included in the risk analysis. Nonetheless, a large population base was evaluated, and the article serves as a reminder that patients with SLE appear to be at increased risk of malignancy and should at the very least be counseled to avoid behaviors and activities that further increase this risk, to follow up as recommended, and to report unexplained signs or symptoms that may suggest and underlying malignancy (ie, blood in urine, stool, or sputum; persistent cough, unexplained weight loss, unexplained fatigue, etc).

J. T. Clarke, MD

Aortic aneurysms in systemic lupus erythematosus: a meta-analysis of 35 cases in the literature and two different pathogeneses

Kurata A, Kawakami T, Sato J, et al (Kyorin Univ School of Medicine, Tokyo, Japan; et al)
Cardiovasc Pathol 20:e1-e7, 2011

Background.—Aortic aneurysms including dissection are uncommon complications of systemic lupus erythematosus, but the incidence has been increasing with an improved prognosis for this disease. However, the mechanisms contributing to aneurysm formation in systemic lupus erythematosus have not been fully clarified.

Methods.—A meta-analysis of published cases was conducted to clarify the patient characteristics that may contribute to aneurysm formation in systemic lupus erythematosus. A search of relevant studies published over the past 40 years (1969–2008) was carried out in the publications on aortic aneurysms with systemic lupus erythematosus, and 35 cases were identified. The contributing factors to aneurysm formation as well as the patient prognosis were searched for sex, age, duration of corticosteroid treatment, aneurysm site (thoracic and/or abdominal), mortality, evidence of atherosclerotic involvement, and presence or absence of an operation, rupture, dissection, cystic medial degeneration, vasculitis, and hypertension. Each of these factors was assigned to each point score. Based on the point scores, a statistical analysis of rank correlation was thereafter performed.

Results.—The factors correlating with the presence of thoracic or abdominal lesions differed significantly. The presence of thoracic aneurysms correlated with dissection and cystic medial degeneration, whereas abdominal lesions correlated with the finding of atherosclerosis. Thoracic lesions showed a high rate of death, while abdominal lesions were associated with a relatively favorable prognosis. Abdominal lesions were related to the duration of steroid therapy. The other correlations among the various factors were also evaluated, with the finding of cystic medial degeneration associated with vasculitis.

Conclusion.—Two principal patterns emerged from this analysis. One was the fatal nonatherosclerotic thoracic aneurysm which was associated with cystic medial degeneration and probably due to vasculitis. The other was atherosclerotic abdominal aneurysm which was complicated by long-term steroid treatment and it showed a relatively favorable prognosis.

▶ Cardiovascular disease is now the leading cause of death in patients with systemic lupus erythematosus (SLE). Factors such as chronic corticosteroid use and disease-related inflammatory pathways are involved in the increased risk of cardiovascular disease in patients with SLE. Cardiovascular problems linked to SLE include pericarditis, ischemic heart disease, cerebrovascular disease, and vasculitis. Aortic disease is relatively uncommon in SLE patients, but when it occurs, it does so at a younger age than in the general population. In this study, a meta-analysis of reported cases of aortic aneurysm in SLE patients was used to assess the pathophysiology of aortic disease in this population. The authors conclude that the pathogenesis of thoracic aortic aneurysm is related to vasculitis, which leads to dissection and cystic medial degeneration and is usually fatal. Abdominal aortic aneurysms in those with SLE were linked to atherosclerosis and chronic systemic corticosteroid use; these aneurysms were associated with a more favorable prognosis. Antiphospholipid antibody status was not included in the analysis, and the authors were unable to assess whether the presence of these antibodies was linked to aortic disease. As treatments for SLE continue to reduce disease-specific mortality, new complications related to the disease or the treatments will likely emerge. It is important to be aware of the need for cardiovascular monitoring and risk-factor reduction in this patient population.

J. T. Clarke, MD

Efficacy of tacrolimus 0.1% ointment in cutaneous lupus erythematosus: A multicenter, randomized, double-blind, vehicle-controlled trial
Kuhn A, Gensch K, Haust M, et al (Univ of Muenster, Germany; Univ of Duesseldorf, Germany; et al)
J Am Acad Dermatol 65:54-64, 2011

Background.—Topical calcineurin inhibitors are licensed for the treatment of atopic dermatitis; however, the efficacy of tacrolimus in cutaneous lupus erythematosus (CLE) has only been shown in single case reports.

Objective.—In a multicenter, randomized, double-blind, vehicle-controlled trial, we sought to evaluate the efficacy of tacrolimus 0.1% ointment for skin lesions in CLE.

Methods.—Thirty patients (18 female, 12 male) with different subtypes of CLE were included, and two selected skin lesions in each patient were treated either with tacrolimus 0.1% ointment or vehicle twice daily for 12 weeks. The evaluation included scoring of clinical features, such as erythema, hypertrophy/desquamation, edema, and dysesthesia.

Results.—Significant improvement ($P < .05$) was seen in skin lesions of CLE patients treated with tacrolimus 0.1% ointment after 28 and 56 days, but not after 84 days, compared with skin lesions treated with vehicle. Edema responded most rapidly to tacrolimus 0.1% ointment and the effect was significant ($P < .001$) in comparison to treatment with vehicle after 28 days. Clinical score changes in erythema also showed remarkable improvement ($P < .05$) after 28 days, but not after 56 and 84 days. Moreover, patients with lupus erythematosus tumidus revealed the highest degree of improvement. None of the patients with CLE demonstrated any major side effects.

Limitations.—The study was limited by the small sample size.

Conclusion.—Explorative subgroup analyses revealed that topical application of tacrolimus 0.1% ointment may provide at least temporary benefit, especially in acute, edematous, non-hyperkeratotic lesions of CLE patients, suggesting that calcineurin inhibitors may represent an alternative treatment for the various disease subtypes.

▶ Cutaneous lupus erythematosus (CLE) is a chronic inflammatory autoimmune disorder that is primarily confined to the skin. Older treatment such as antimalarials, methotrexate, and thalidomide are efficacious but can have serious side effects. Calcineurin inhibitors are immunomodulators that downregulate T-cell activity. This is a multicenter, randomized, double-blind, vehicle-controlled trial evaluating the efficacy of tacrolimus 0.1% ointment in CLE. The overall mean change from baseline in the total clinical score with tacrolimus 0.1% ointment compared with vehicle in patients with CLE was found to be significant at day 28 ($P = .0040$). However, on day 56, the total clinical score showed marginally significant improvement with topical tacrolimus compared with vehicle ($P = .0496$). The edema score from baseline between tacrolimus 0.1% ointment and vehicle was found to be significant in CLE patients at all visits ($P = .0311$, $P = .0207$, $P = .0251$). For the erythema score, the overall mean change from baseline of tacrolimus 0.1% ointment compared with vehicle was marginally significant ($P = .0475$) in CLE patients on day 28; however, on day 14, 56, and 84, no significant improvement could be found. The authors concluded that tacrolimus 0.1% ointment may be an alternative treatment for active skin lesions to help reduce edema and erythema associated with CLE lesions; however, sustained benefit with prolonged use over 2 to 3 months was not consistently noted.

G. K. Kim, DO

J. Q. Del Rosso, DO

Expression of antimicrobial peptides in different subtypes of cutaneous lupus erythematosus

Kreuter A, Jaouhar M, Skrygan M, et al (Ruhr-Univ, Bochum, Germany; et al)
J Am Acad Dermatol 65:125-133, 2011

Background.—Antimicrobial peptides (AMPs) are small effector molecules of the innate immune system with well-known antimicrobial activity. Skin infections rarely occur in patients with cutaneous lupus erythematosus (CLE), and AMP expression in CLE has not been previously evaluated.

Objectives.—We aimed to determine the expression of several important AMPs in 3 different subtypes of CLE.

Methods.—Skin lesions were analyzed for the gene and protein expression of human β-defensin (hBD)-1, -2, and -3; RNase-7; the cathelicidin LL-37; and psoriasin (S100A7) using real-time reverse transcriptase polymerase chain reaction and immunohistochemistry.

Results.—Skin biopsy specimens of 96 study participants including 47 patients with CLE (15 patients with discoid lupus erythematosus [LE], 11 patients with subacute CLE, and 21 patients with LE tumidus), 34 patients with psoriasis, and 15 healthy control subjects were evaluated in this study. HBD-2, hBD-3, LL-37, and psoriasin were significantly more highly expressed in CLE as compared with healthy controls, and most AMPs were significantly more highly induced in subacute CLE as compared with discoid LE and LE tumidus. AMP gene expression paralleled well with AMP protein expression in CLE and controls. Subacute CLE and discoid LE showed a similar correlation of AMP gene expression (significant correlations between hBD-1 and RNase-7, hBD-2 and hBD-3, hBD-2 and psoriasin, and hBD-3 and psoriasin).

Limitations.—The relatively small number of samples and the lack of analysis of the lesional bacterial colonization are a limitation.

Conclusions.—Several AMPs are increased in CLE at both gene and protein levels. This could explain the low prevalence of skin infections in CLE. It remains to be elucidated whether AMPs play a pathogenic role in CLE.

▶ Cutaneous lupus erythematosus (CLE) is a chronic autoimmune disorder seen in the dermatology setting. Interestingly, skin infections rarely occur in patients with CLE. Antimicrobial peptides (AMPs) may be the reason for this phenomenon observed in CLE patients. AMPs are small effector molecules of the innate immune system known for their antimicrobial activity. Besides their antimicrobial properties, there is evidence suggesting that AMPs also participate in skin immunity through their activity on keratinocyte production of numerous cytokines and chemokines. In this study, participants consisted of 3 groups: patients with CLE including discoid lupus erythematosus (DLE), subacute cutaneous lupus erythematosus (SCLE), and lupus erythematosus tumidus (LET); patients with psoriasis and healthy control subjects were also included in this study. Skin samples of 96 study participants were evaluated with reverse-transcriptase polymerase chain reaction. This study demonstrated that several AMPs such as human B-defensin-2 (HBD-2), and HBD-3, LL-37, and psoriasin were increased in CLE at both the gene and protein levels. Authors also suggest that AMPs may be pathogenetically involved in CLE, particularly the SCLE and DLE subtypes. However, there were some limitations to this study; the sample size of the immunohistochemical part of the study was relatively low, and other subtypes of lupus were excluded (eg, chilblain lupus). Also, skin lesions of SLE were not included. There was no bacterial testing performed in this study, and subclinical infections in CLE lesions could not be excluded. In conclusion, more studies are needed to evaluate the role of AMPs in CLE patients, and it will be interesting to observe whether CLE patients may indeed be protected from skin infections due to increased AMPs.

G. K. Kim, DO
J. Q. Del Rosso, DO

Current and novel therapeutics in the treatment of systemic lupus erythematosus

Yildirim-Toruner C, Diamond B (Columbia Univ Med Ctr, NY; Feinstein Inst for Med Res, Manhasset, NY)
J Allergy Clin Immunol 127:303-312, 2011

Systemic lupus erythematosus (SLE) is a complex autoimmune disease with significant clinical heterogeneity. Recent advances in our understanding of the genetic, molecular, and cellular bases of autoimmune diseases and especially SLE have led to the application of novel and targeted treatments. Although many treatment modalities are effective in lupus-prone mice, the situation is more complex in human subjects. This article reviews the general approach to the therapy of SLE, focusing on current approved therapies and novel approaches that might be used in the future.

▶ In March 2011, the US Food and Drug Administration approved belimumab (Benlysta) for the treatment of systemic lupus erythematosus (SLE). This is the first drug approved for SLE since 1955. This article is a thorough review of therapies currently used in the treatment of SLE, and even more so, of potential novel therapeutic approaches to SLE treatment based on the current understanding of the complex immune pathways involved in the pathogenesis of the disease. The authors provide succinct descriptions of the lupus-related immuno-pathologic basis for each novel therapeutic agent as well as of the proposed mechanism(s) of action of each drug/biologic. Results to date of murine, human open-label, and controlled trials of each agent are described. The authors include data on agents being studied for other autoimmune diseases that may have benefit in SLE, but which have not yet been evaluated in SLE.

This review highlights the complexity of treating a disease with immunologic and clinical features as heterogeneous as SLE. Unfortunately, few of the early trials of the multitude of novel agents discussed focus on cutaneous disease as a primary endpoint; therefore, it is impossible to say which of the agents may be useful for dermatologists treating recalcitrant cutaneous LE. The authors acknowledge the need for dividing patients with SLE into subsets depending on disease manifestations, genetic factors, immunologic parameters, and disease severity. This will allow us to obtain the most useful data with well-designed trials in which appropriate measures of disease activity are used to assess outcome.

This article is recommended for the dermatologist seeking a succinct, yet thorough, review of novel immunologic therapies, many of which are currently in clinical trials, for SLE.

J. T. Clarke, MD

A New Presentation of Neonatal Lupus: 5 Cases of Isolated Mild Endocardial Fibroelastosis Associated with Maternal Anti-SSA/Ro and Anti-SSB/La Antibodies

Guettrot-Imbert G, Cohen L, Fermont L, et al (Centre Hospitalier Universitaire Pitié-Salpêtrière, France; Université Paris V, France; Centre Hospitalier Universitaire Necker-Enfants Malades, France; et al)
J Rheumatol 38:378-386, 2011

Objective.—Maternal anti-SSA/Ro or anti-SSB/La antibodies are associated with neonatal lupus erythematosus syndrome (NLES), especially congenital heart block (CHB), which may be associated with severe endocardial fibroelastosis (EFE) and dilated cardiomyopathy (DCM). A few reports have described severe EFE without CHB associated with anti-SSA/Ro antibodies, with a poor prognosis. EFE has also been observed in biopsies of DCM that had been considered idiopathic. These points, considered in association with 5 unusual cases of mild EFE, led us to consider the relationship between underrecognized cases of isolated autoantibody-associated EFE and DCM that had been considered idiopathic.

Methods.—We analyzed 5 cases of EFE diagnosed *in utero* (n = 4) or after birth (n = 1). In 3 cases, maternal antibody status was discovered because of the EFE diagnosis.

Results.—Endomyocardial hyperechogenicity predominated in the left atrium (n = 3) and mitral annulus (n = 3). No left-heart dysfunction was observed. Two mothers were treated with betamethasone. One mother chose to have a therapeutic abortion, and EFE was confirmed at autopsy. Electrocardiograms at birth (n = 4) did not show CHB. Other manifestations of NLES were present in all cases. One child had right ventricular hypoplasia and underwent a partial cavopulmonary anastomosis. At last followup (4–7 yrs), the other 3 children had normal heart function, and echocardiography showed a normal heart (n = 2) or mild persistent EFE (n = 1).

Conclusion.—Middle-term prognosis of isolated autoantibody-associated EFE may be better than previously reported, although the longterm prognosis remains unknown. We hypothesize that a fetal insult can lead to DCM.

▶ This case series describes 5 pregnancies in which routine second trimester ultrasounds revealed fetal cardiac abnormalities consistent with endocardial fibroelastosis. In all 5 cases, the mothers were found to have or were already known to have SSA/Ro autoantibodies. All infants had cutaneous features of neonatal lupus erythematosus (LE). None of the infants developed heart block; their echocardiographic changes persisted during the antepartum period and resolved after birth, and over 4 to 17 years of follow-up, none developed cardiac disease. Endocardial fibrosis coupled with complete heart block or ventricular dysfunction has been previously associated with Ro antibodies. These cases are unusual in that the endocardial fibrosis was mild, limited to the fetal and early neonatal period, and resolved without later cardiac sequelae in all cases. The authors advise that all mothers in whom fetal ultrasonography demonstrates endocardial fibrosis be evaluated for the presence of circulating anti-Ro/SSA and anti-La/SSB antibodies and suggest that the finding of endocardial fibrosis in the mitral and aortic annuli is specific to neonatal LE. The article describes the array of cardiac abnormalities—not just heart block—that have been reported in the neonatal LE syndrome. Dermatologists are likely to encounter women with SSA/Ro autoantibodies because these have been linked to cutaneous LE in addition to systemic LE, Sjogren syndrome, and other rheumatologic diseases. These patients should be counseled about the risk of neonatal LE and during pregnancy should be monitored closely by experienced subspecialists for evidence of fetal cardiac anomalies that include not only heart block but other abnormalities as well.

J. T. Clarke, MD

Retiform Purpura and Digital Gangrene Secondary to Antiphospholipid Syndrome Successfully Treated With Sildenafil

Gonzalez ME, Kahn P, Price HN, et al (New York Univ School of Medicine)
Arch Dermatol 147:164-167, 2011

Background.—Antiphospholipid antibody syndrome (APS) is an acquired systemic autoimmune disorder manifest by vascular thrombosis and/or pregnancy complications in the presence of antiphospholipid antibodies. The diagnostic criteria for APS include laboratory abnormalities found on two or more occasions at least 12 weeks apart. APS is now recognized as causing recurrent thrombosis in pediatric patients. About half of all patients, pediatric and adult, have an underlying connective tissue disease. Deep venous thrombosis of the lower extremities is the most common clinical presentation. A patient having systemic lupus erythematosus (SLE) and Raynaud phenomenon was reported.

Case Report.—African-American woman, 16, had had SLE for 2 years and Raynaud phenomenon but now exhibited persistently painful and dusky toes after wearing a new pair of boots 2 weeks previously and had more frequent Raynaud episodes. Her nifedipine dose was increased from 30 to 60 mg/d to manage the Raynaud episodes. She continued to take 5 mg/d of prednisone, 1500 mg twice daily of mycophenolate mofetil, 400 mg/d of hydroxychloroquine, and 75 mg twice daily of indomethacin. Her pain worsened, and she developed progressive necrosis of her toes, eventually entering the hospital for evaluation and treatment of impending digital gangrene. Physical examination revealed retiform purpura on the left first and second toes, hemorrhagic bulla on the distal left first toe, and a necrotic ulcer in place of the left second toenail. The left medial sole, left third through fourth toes, and right first through fourth toes evidenced milder purpura with dusky reticulated erythema. Dorsalis pedis pulses were diminished, especially in the right foot. Arterial Doppler studies showed complete absence of blood flow in all the left foot digits and the second through fourth right foot digits.

Biopsy from the peripheral purpuric area on the left first toe showed thrombi in the lumens of small and medium blood vessels throughout the mid and deep reticular dermis, along with partial eccrine gland and overlying epidermal necrosis. Laboratory results included elevated anticardiolipin immunoglobulin M (IgM) antibody levels (which were also elevated 10 months previously) and lupus anticoagulant. The patient was diagnosed with thrombotic vasculopathy secondary to APS. She received enoxaparin, intravenous methylprednisolone, and topical nitroglycerin paste; her dose of nifedipine was doubled. Even with three pairs of socks to keep her toes warm, the pain and necrosis progressed.

On her third day in the hospital nifedipine therapy was discontinued and treatment with 20 mg of sildenafil three times a day commenced. The patient experienced rapid pain relief and a marked increase in dorsalis pedis pulses and fading of the reticular erythema in 24 to 48 hours. Gangrene stabilized, and the patient lost just the tips of her left first and second toes. Sildenafil treatment was continued for 14 months.

Conclusions.—It was believed that sildenafil's vasodilatory and antiplatelet effects helped improve the patient's distal blood flow. Sildenafil is currently approved for use only for erectile dysfunction and pulmonary hypertension. Evidence indicates this selective phosphodiesterase-5 (PDE5) inhibitor also increase capillary blood flow to the fingers and healing digital ulcers in Raynaud's phenomenon and improve digital ischemia. Studies should determine the potential roles of sildenafil and other PDE5 inhibitors in managing cutaneous and extracutaneous vascular thrombosis related to APS.

▶ Sildenafil is a prostaglandin inhibitor that exerts its effects on smooth muscle and also has some antiplatelet activity. The patient described here was on an anticoagulant and a calcium channel blocker but continued to worsen until nifedipine was replaced with sildenafil at which time her symptoms resolved in 2 days. The pathogenesis of antiphospholipid syndrome is not understood, and most attempts at treatment focus on the reduction of inflammation and the dissolution of the fibrin clots in the vessels. However, some theorize that the antibodies in this disease may promote clotting by binding to and activating platelets. Both nifedipine and sildenafil work by separate mechanisms to relax smooth muscle by decreasing the amount of intracellular calcium, yet sildenafil also inhibits platelet activation that is initiated by thrombin. This may account for its superior effect in this patient. However, it would not be surprising to see no benefit from sildenafil in another patient, as pathogenic mechanisms may differ from patient to patient. Furthermore, this patient was also taking 150 mg of indomethacin per day as well as hydroxychloroquine and mycophenolate mofetil, and it is possible that these medicines also played a role in her improvement. Still, this information is encouraging in that we can consider using another medicine in this difficult-to-treat disease. Further research into the use of sildenafil in these patients would be welcome. However, because of their rarity, we are more likely going to depend on case reports or small case series for information on treatment.

J. M. Suchniak, MD

Amyopathic Dermatomyositis
Khambatta S, Wittich CM (Mayo Clinic, Rochester, MN)
Mayo Clin Proc 85:e82, 2010

Background.—Dermatomyositis affects the skin and muscles and may be caused by complement deposits in the blood vessels. This idiopathic microangiopathic disease causes symmetric proximal muscle weakness in most patients. Skin findings typical of the disorder and muscle injury form the basis for the diagnosis. A case was described.

> *Case Report.*—Man, 48, demonstrated rash, cough, shortness of breath, and arthritis. For more than 6 months he had experienced fatigue, fevers, and weight loss. Physical examination revealed increased respiratory rate, hypoxia, and audible fine crackles in both lung bases. Although there was no muscle weakness, multiple joints demonstrated arthritic symptoms. A heliotrope rash, Gottron sign, "mechanic's hands," and the V-sign, all characteristic of dermatomyositis, were present.

Conclusions.—The patient demonstrated a dermatomyositis variant known as amyopathic dermatomyositis, which is not associated with muscle involvement. He also had interstitial lung disease, which has been seen with the amyopathic variant and with classic dermatomyositis.

▶ Amyopathic dermatomyositis is a disorder that manifests with the typical skin signs of dermatomyositis, but without muscle involvement. Given the absence of muscle injury associated with the disease, a stronger suspicion is likely needed, and if typical skin findings are present, this subtype of dermatomyositis must be considered. This diagnosis is also important to consider given the potential for interstitial lung disease and possible malignancy that has been associated with dermatomyositis. Khambatta and Wittich report a case of a 48-year-old man with amyopathic dermatomyositis and provide a concise review of some of the typical skin changes as well as clinical photographs of these skin findings, including the heliotrope rash, Gottron sign, "mechanic's hands," and the V-sign. Given that this variant of dermatomyositis accounts for a smaller percentage of dermatomyositis cases, this review provides a succinct reminder of a variant that can be encountered, and easily misdiagnosed, in clinical practice.

B. D. Michaels, DO

J. Q. Del Rosso, DO

Mycophenolate mofetil treatment in children and adolescents with lupus

Kazyra I, Pilkington C, Marks SD, et al (Belarus State Med Univ, Minsk; Great Ormond Street Hosp for Children, London, UK)

Arch Dis Child 95:1059-1061, 2010

Safety and efficacy data are presented on the use of mycophenolate mofetil (MMF) in 26 children and adolescents with lupus. Data include therapy before and 12 months after starting MMF. 18 of 26 patients had biopsy-proved lupus nephritis. Group 1 were commenced on MMF induction and/or maintenance therapy (n=14), group 2 converted from azathioprine because of inadequate disease control (n=12). 73% of all (10 (71%) group 1 and 10 (83%) group 2) patients experienced a significant improvement in British Isles Lupus Assessment Group score (from median 9.0 to 3.0). Children with hypocomplementaemia increased their C3 significantly in both groups (0.53–1.15 for group 1 and 0.63–1.2 g/l for group 2, p=0.001), and C4 level only in group 1 (0.08–0.17, p=0.01). Renal function and albuminuria improved in those with active nephritis (p≤0.01). Significant improvements were seen in both groups in haemoglobin, erythrocyte sedimentation rate and lymphocyte counts. Prednisolone dose was weaned in both groups, p<0.05. Side-effects were seen in four patients, but none was judged to be severe enough to discontinue treatment. MMF treatment in this cohort of children with lupus seemed to be safe, well tolerated and effective.

▶ Childhood-onset systemic lupus erythematosus (SLE) is often more aggressive than the adult form of the disease. This retrospective study evaluated 26 children and adolescents with SLE treated with mycophenolate mofetil either after not responding to azathioprine therapy or as part of planned induction or maintenance therapy for lupus nephritis. The study is important because mycophenolate mofetil in combination with corticosteroids was recently found to be as effective as cyclophosphamide and corticosteroids (previously the standard of care) for induction and maintenance therapy in adults with lupus nephritis and safer than azathioprine for maintenance therapy. Similar results were observed in this study of pediatric SLE patients, and improvements were also noted in hematologic parameters, corticosteroid doses, and erythrocyte sedimentation rates. Children tolerated mycophenolate mofetil therapy well, with no severe adverse effects, and dosing ranges (20–25 mg/kg/d) were similar to those used in adults. The authors did not comment on cutaneous lupus erythematosus manifestations in this group of patients; however, there are reports of successful therapy with mycophenolate mofetil for adults with recalcitrant cutaneous lupus erythematosus.

J. T. Clarke, MD

Clinical Correlations With Dermatomyositis-Specific Autoantibodies in Adult Japanese Patients With Dermatomyositis: A Multicenter Cross-sectional Study

Hamaguchi Y, Kuwana M, Hoshino K, et al (Kanazawa Univ Graduate School of Med Science, Japan; Keio Univ School of Medicine, Tokyo, Japan; et al)
Arch Dermatol 147:391-398, 2011

Objective.—To clarify the association of clinical and prognostic features with dermatomyositis (DM)-specific autoantibodies (Abs) in adult Japanese patients with DM.

Design.—Retrospective study.

Setting.—Kanazawa University Graduate School of Medical Science Department of Dermatology and collaborating medical centers.

Patients.—A total of 376 consecutive adult Japanese patients with DM who visited our hospital or collaborating medical centers between 2003 and 2008.

Main Outcome Measures.—Clinical and laboratory characteristics of adult Japanese patients with DM and DM-specific Abs that include Abs against Mi-2, 155/140, and CADM-140.

Results.—In patients with DM, anti—Mi-2, anti-155/140, and anti—CADM-140 were detected in 9 (2%), 25 (7%), and 43 (11%), respectively. These DM-specific Abs were mutually exclusive and were detected in none of 34 patients with polymyositis, 326 with systemic sclerosis, and 97 with systemic lupus erythematosus. Anti—Mi-2 was associated with classical DM without interstitial lung disease or malignancy, whereas anti—155/140 was associated with malignancy. Patients with anti—CADM-140 frequently had clinically amyopathic DM and rapidly progressive interstitial lung disease. Cumulative survival rates were more favorable in patients with anti—Mi-2 compared with those with anti—155/140 or anti—CADM-140 ($P<.01$ for both comparisons). Nearly all deaths occurred within 1 year after diagnosis in patients with anti—CADM-140.

Conclusion.—Dermatomyositis-specific Abs define clinically distinct subsets and are useful for predicting clinical outcomes in patients with DM.

▶ Polymyositis (PM) and dermatomyositis (DM) are inflammatory disorders characterized by myositis and, in the case of DM, cutaneous eruptions. Autoimmunity is considered to play a critical role in both diseases with the presence of autoantibodies (Abs) being a prominent feature. This is a retrospective study examining the association of clinical and prognostic features of DM-specific autoantibodies in Japanese adults with DM. Researchers focused on anti—Mi-2, anti-155/140, and anti—CADM-140 and attempted to investigate a correlation between these 3 antibodies with clinical features and prognosis. Serum samples were obtained from 376 adult Japanese patients with DM in Kanazawa University, Japan. Researchers found that interstitial lung disease (ILD) was observed most frequently in patients with anti—CADM-140 Abs, and the incidence of malignancy was highest in patients with anti-155/140 Abs ($P < .001$). Serum KL-6 levels were associated with activity and severity of ILD. Patients with anti—CDM-140 had the lowest prevalence of DM but the highest prevalence of clinically amyopathic DM (*P* < .001 and *P* < .001, respectively). Malignancy was found most frequently in patients with anti-155/140 (*P* < .001). Associated malignancies were observed in 17 of 25 patients with anti-155/140 Abs, with 3 of them having double malignancies. The highest incidences of malignancies were lung, breast, and colon cancer. The prognosis of patients with anti—Mi-2 were favorable with no malignancies found in these patients and with only one showing mild ILD. A limitation to this study was that DM-specific Abs were limited to only Japanese adults within a certain geographic region, and there may have been a center-based bias. Also, other connective tissue diseases were not included in this study to examine the significance of these Abs in other cohorts of patients. To add, not all Abs were included in this study. In summary, this article revealed that classifying patients with DM according to Abs may help guide the physician to focus on particular manifestations with high-risk complications and may guide in prognosis.

G. K. Kim, DO

J. Q. Del Rosso, DO

Drug-induced subacute cutaneous lupus erythematosus: evidence for differences from its idiopathic counterpart
Marzano AV, Lazzari R, Polloni I, et al (Ospedale Maggiore Policlinico, Milan, Italy; et al)
Br J Dermatol 165:335-341, 2011

Background.—Drug-induced subacute cutaneous lupus erythematosus (DI-SCLE) is a lupus variant with predominant skin involvement temporally related to drug exposure and resolving after drug discontinuation. It usually presents with annular polycyclic or papulosquamous eruptions on sun-exposed skin and shows serum anti-Ro/SSA antibodies.

Objectives.—To address the question whether DI-SCLE differs significantly from idiopathic SCLE by virtue of clinical features.

Methods.—Ninety patients with SCLE seen in our departments from 2001 to 2010 were reviewed. Eleven of them diagnosed as having DI-SCLE were evaluated for type of skin lesions, systemic involvement, clinical course, and histopathological, direct immunofluorescence and laboratory findings. The cutaneous features were compared with those of the 79 patients with idiopathic SCLE.

Results.—The cutaneous picture was widespread in 82% of patients with DI-SCLE and in 6% of those with idiopathic SCLE [odds ratio (OR) 66·6, 95% confidence interval (CI) 11·2−394·9; *P* = 0·0001]. Bullous and erythema multiforme (EM)-like lesions were present in 45% of patients with DI-SCLE and in 1% of those with idiopathic SCLE (OR 65·0, 95% CI 6·5−649·6; *P* = 0·0001). Vasculitic lesions were observed in 45% of patients with DI-SCLE and in 3% of those with idiopathic SCLE (OR 32·1, 95% CI 5·1−201·7; *P* = 0·0001). Malar rash occurred in 45% of patients with DI-SCLE and in 6% of those with idiopathic

SCLE (OR 12·3, 95% CI 2·8—54·9; $P = 0·001$). Visceral manifestations were excluded in all patients with DI-SCLE. Anti-Ro/SSA antibodies were found in all but one patient with DI-SCLE and disappeared after resolution in 73% of cases.

Conclusions.—DI-SCLE differs from idiopathic SCLE by virtue of distinctive cutaneous features, particularly the widespread presentation and the frequent occurrence of malar rash and bullous, EM-like and vasculitic manifestations.

▶ Drug-induced subacute cutaneous lupus erythematosus (DI-SCLE) is a drug-associated cutaneous disorder that usually resolves with withdrawal of the inciting agent. However, the clinical presentation of idiopathic subacute lupus erythematosus (SCLE) is similar to that of DI-SCLE with annular polycyclic or papulosquamous lesions. This is a study evaluating the clinical, cutaneous, histopathological, and laboratory differences between DI-SCLE as opposed to idiopathic SCLE. In this study, 11 patients with DI-SCLE were compared with 79 patients with idiopathic SCLE. The authors found that DI-SCLE often differed significantly from idiopathic SCLE by virtue of cutaneous features. In DI-SCLE, the cutaneous features were more widespread, often with involvement of the lower extremities as opposed to idiopathic SCLE. Also, DI-SCLE presented more frequently as bullous lesions and had erythema multiforme (EM)-like features compared with idiopathic SCLE ($P = .0001$). Small vessel cutaneous vasculitis, purpura, and necrotic ulcerative lesions were more frequent with DI-SCLE ($P = .001$). Patients with idiopathic SCLE had more extensive systemic involvement, such as arthralgias, xerophthalmia, and nephropathy, although nephropathy is felt to be relatively uncommon in SCLE. Also, in none of the patients did DI-SCLE evolve into idiopathic SCLE after a mean follow-up of 4 years. The authors concluded that patients with DI-SCLE can present with different cutaneous lesion patterns compared with those with idiopathic SCLE, including bullae, EM-like lesions, and vasculitic manifestations. The number of subjects with DI-SCLE in this analysis was small. Further data are needed to substantiate the conclusions drawn by the authors, although the article does increase the index of suspicion regarding presentations that may vary from "the textbook picture" of SCLE.

G. K. Kim, DO
J. Q. Del Rosso, DO

Antibodies and the Brain: Lessons from Lupus
Diamond B (The Feinstein Inst for Med Res, Manhasset, NY)
J Immunol 185:2637-2640, 2010

Background.—Lupus is a disease characterized by autoantibodies that initiate the inflammatory cascades. All patients with lupus have antinuclear antibodies (Abs) and many have anti-DNA Abs, which are essentially diagnostic of the disease. Anti-DNA Abs titers correlate with renal disease and induce systemic inflammation through a toll-like receptor

(TLR) pathway. Research into the induction and pathogenicity of anti-DNA Abs in systemic lupus erythematosus (SLE) revealed that anti-DNA Abs can be elicited by microbial antigen (Ag), and somatic mutation can lead to the acquisition of DNA binding. Receptor editing in post-germinal center B cells serves as a tolerance mechanism after somatic hypermutation. Renal pathogenicity of anti-DNA Abs may reflect cross-reactivity with renal Ags.

Links to Cognition and Mood.—N-methyl-D-aspartate receptor (NMDAR) is a membrane receptor found in brain neurons. Activation of NMDAR is critical in learning and memory, but prolonged stimulation can cause high calcium influx, leading to apoptotic death of the neuron. As SLE patients live longer, some late disease sequelae are becoming apparent, including frequent, debilitating cognitive impairment and mood disorder. The neurotoxic potential of human lupus Abs cross-reactive with DNA and peptide was evaluated in mice. Neuronal death resulted when Abs were isolated on a peptide affinity column and injected into a mouse hippocampus. Mice pretreated with an NMDAR antagonist were protected from the effects of the Ab. Cerebrospinal fluid (CSF) drawn from a patient with neuropsychiatric SLE (NPSLE) and containing anti-DNA, anti-peptide Abs also mediated neuronal death when injected into mouse hippocampus. Thus anti-DNA, anti-NMDAR cross-reactive Abs are found in serum, CSF, and brain tissue in lupus patients and are neurotoxic in mice. CSF anti-DNA, anti-peptide Ab, and central nervous system (CNS) disease symptoms are significantly related.

The integrity of the blood-brain barrier may be breached by the effects of infection and stress. Mice display cognitive impairment if human lupus Abs gain access to hippocampal neurons. The regional exposure to Ab determines what behavioral deficit develops. Observations in mice are consistent with the clinical features seen in NPSLE. Cognitive impairments and mood disturbances occur independent of disease flares, often with no apparent CNS inflammation. Both an unfavorable serology and a breach in the blood-brain barrier's integrity are needed for CNS damage. The insult to the blood-brain barrier may not be a lupus flare. The neuronal loss observed is noninflammatory. In addition, the concentration of R4A Ab needed to alter synaptic potentials is one tenth the concentration needed to induce neuronal death, explaining why some altered brain functions are transient and some fixed.

Fetal Brain Effects.—Anti-DNA, anti-NMDAR Ab can be toxic to adult brain tissue if it crosses the blood-brain barrier. The fetal brain is constantly exposed to maternal Ab. Studies of the children of mothers with SLE show an increased frequency of learning disabilities. Fetuses of mice immunized to produce high titers of anti-NMDAR Ab have displayed a thin cortical plate, whereas those without this immunization have normal cortical plate. Mice exposed to high titers of anti-NMDAR in utero show delays in acquiring the negative geotaxis reflex. As adults these mice also showed impaired novel object recognition, topologic recognition, and fear extinction. Based on these findings, maternal lupus Ab can damage the fetal brain.

Conclusions.—Ab can produce cognitive and behavioral disturbances in SLE and cause more than one CNS lupus manifestation. The type of manifestation depends on the brain region exposed to the Ab, which depends on the insult to the barrier's integrity. Neurotoxic Abs may mediate brain dysfunction more than previously suspected. B cells do not diversify until after the blood-brain barrier forms. High titers of Ab cross-reactive with brain Ag may cause brain damage if it penetrates brain parenchyma through an insult to the blood-brain barrier. Even in nonautoimmune individuals, behavioral and cognitive impairment may be mediated by the Ab. Some women may have high titers of brain-reactive Ab during pregnancy, and the Ab may alter fetal brain development. Future studies should seek to determine the possible therapeutic applications of the interaction between the immune system and the brain in SLE.

▶ This article does not need a synopsis; it needs complete paragraph-by-paragraph digestion to fully appreciate the findings and to understand the investigators' analysis. One of the first statements of the article, "In the 1980s we knew that essentially all patients with lupus exhibited anti-nuclear antibodies," summarizes the extent that most clinicians understand the pathogenesis of lupus. However, the explanation of an antigen, or antigenic stimulation of that process, was not that simple at the time, which is why the findings explained here are significant. "Autoimmunity," as we define it, still has an antigen as a target, just as any immune process does. Therefore, having a clearer working knowledge of what those antigens are for lupus might pave the way to newer approaches for attempting to block that interaction. The discussion of the anti-N-methyl-D-aspartate receptor antibody and the impact on benefits of neurological components of lupus is particularly fascinating, especially with the potential for controlling the disease during childhood, pregnancy, and other conditions in which the sequelae of autoimmunity might be higher.

N. Bhatia, MD

Biologic Therapy for Systemic Sclerosis: A Systematic Review

Phumethum V, Jamal S, Johnson SR (Prapokklao Hosp, Chantaburi, Thailand; Mount Sinai Hosp, NY; St. Michael's Hosp, Toronto, Ontario, Canada)
J Rheumatol 38:289-296, 2011

Objective.—Biologic agents are increasingly used in the rheumatic diseases. Their role in patients with systemic sclerosis (SSc) is uncertain. Our aim was to evaluate the effectiveness and safety of biologic agents in SSc. We review the evidence for the use of biologic agents to improve inflammatory arthritis, disability, and skin score, and we review adverse effects with biologic agents in patients with SSc.

Methods.—A systematic literature review was performed to identify studies evaluating the use of biologic agents in SSc. Medline, Embase, CINAHL, and Cochrane Database of Systematic Reviews were searched.

A standardized abstraction form was used to extract biologic agent, study design, sample size, treatment effect, and adverse effects.

Results.—A total of 23 studies from 1413 citations were evaluated. Three studies evaluated infliximab, 3 evaluated etanercept, 3 evaluated antithymocyte globulin, 3 evaluated imatinib, 6 evaluated rituximab, and 1 study each evaluated interferon-γ (IFN-γ), IFN-α, relaxin, delipidated, deglycolipidated *Mycobacterium vaccae*, human anti-transforming growth factor ß1 antibody, and oral type I collagen. Studies of etanercept and infliximab suggest improvements in inflammatory arthritis and Health Assessment Questionnaire Disability Index (HAQ-DI). None of the other biologic agents demonstrated reproducible, statistically significant improvements in joint count, HAQ-DI, or skin score.

Conclusion.—Anti-tumor necrosis factor-α agents may improve inflammatory arthritis and disability in SSc. The effect on skin score is uncertain. Adequately powered trials are needed to evaluate efficacy, and longitudinal studies are needed to evaluate longterm safety of these agents in SSc.

▶ Tumor necrosis factor (TNF) is a key cytokine in the development of autoimmune diseases such as rheumatoid arthritis, but there are few data concerning the role that TNF plays in systemic sclerosis. A potential role for anti-TNF agents in the treatment of systemic sclerosis is suggested by mouse models of pulmonary fibrosis in which TNF inhibitors prevent fibrosis and reduce the accumulation of extracellular matrix. Inflammatory arthritis has been reported in 10% to 25% of patients with systemic sclerosis, and TNF blockers have been very effective against inflammatory autoimmune arthritis such as rheumatoid arthritis or psoriatic arthritis. Conversely, TNF inhibitors are associated with the development of autoantibodies and autoimmune diseases such as drug-induced lupus erythematosus. There is a case report of fibrosing alveolitis in a patient with systemic sclerosis who was treated with adalimumab. Moreover, TNF itself suppresses collagen production and stimulates the release of matrix metalloproteinases, which should prevent the development of fibrosis.

To address the potential role of TNF antagonists in the treatment of systemic sclerosis, medical database searches were conducted to look for trials of various biologics for systemic sclerosis. Twenty-three studies were found on therapies including antithymocyte globulin, imatinib mesylate, various interferons, recombinant human relaxin, *Mycobacterium vaccae*, recombinant human anti−transforming growth factor-β1, type I collagen, rituximab, infliximab, and etanercept. In one of the etanercept studies, 15/18 patients (83%) experienced resolution of joint symptoms, and there was a Rodnan skin score reduction from 6.63 to 3.94, but 1 patient had a reduction in pulmonary function.

Many of the studies reviewed were observational studies that showed modest improvements in skin severity scores and in health assessment questionnaires, but the reports were not uniform. This review emphasizes the need for larger prospective controlled trials before we use unproven therapies for this very difficult disease. The review does point out the expected beneficial effects of TNF blockers on inflammatory arthritis in patients with systemic sclerosis.

M. Lebwohl, MD

9 Blistering Disorders

The role of therapeutic plasma exchange in pemphigus vulgaris

Sagi L, Baum S, Gendelman V, et al (Tel Aviv Univ, Israel; Magen David Adom
Natl Blood Services, Ramat Gan, Israel)
J Eur Acad Dermatol Venereol 25:82-86, 2011

Background.—The treatment of pemphigus, an autoimmune bullous disease, is based on the combination of corticosteroids and adjuvant therapies, such as immunosuppressive drugs, anti-inflammatory drugs and immunomodulatory procedures, such as intravenous immunoglobulin and therapeutic plasma exchange (TPE).

Objective.—This study aims to assess our experience with TPE as a steroid-sparing modality in moderate and severe intractable pemphigus patients.

Methods.—A retrospective evaluation for all intractable pemphigus patients treated by TPE in a university-affiliated tertiary referral medical centre between the years 1998 and 2008. Treatment protocol included three TPE treatments weekly for 1−3 months, combined with monthly pulse therapy of dexamethasone and/or cyclophosphamide. Maintenance therapy was based on once/bi weekly TPE treatments or monthly intravenous immunoglobulin.

Results.—Seven patients were included in the study, four with severe pemphigus vulgaris and three with moderate disease. Six of the seven patients responded to TPE: Four patients (57%) achieved complete remission and two patients (28%) achieved partial remission on minimal therapy. Mild adverse effects related to TPE were observed in two patients and included dizziness and mild headache.

Conclusion.—TPE is a well-tolerated effective steroid-sparing agent in recalcitrant pemphigus patients.

▶ In my opinion, therapeutic plasma exchange is an important option for the emergency treatment of pemphigus. This review article shows it can work rather safely (given risks vs benefits) as emergency therapy or as chronic therapy. I have treated 3 patients with this plasma exchange, and all had an obvious and rapid response. I exchanged 2000 to 4000 mL of plasma 3 times a week for 2 weeks. All patients had extensive, active, treatment-resistant pemphigus vulgaris prior to this treatment. All these pemphigus patients were aggressively immunosuppressed to minimize the rebound effect discussed in this article. There are drawbacks. The large volume of plasma exchanged usually required placement of a central venous access line. Besides pemphigus antibodies, plasma exchange also (1) removes clotting factors causing increased bleeding from erosions; (2) removes protective antibodies, potentially increasing susceptibility to sepsis; (3) removes fluid volume, requiring careful monitoring of replacement volumes of albumin or plasma and other fluids; (4) removes immunosuppressive and other drugs from the bloodstream; (5) treatments are expensive; and (6) patients suffer discomfort as they lie on their pemphigus erosions for long periods during treatments.[1]

M. V. Dahl, MD

Reference

1. Swanson DL, Dahl MV. Pemphigus vulgaris and plasma exchange: clinical and serologic studies. *J Am Acad Dermatol.* 1981;4:325-328.

Approach to the patient with autoimmune mucocutaneous blistering diseases

Sami N (Univ of Alabama, Birmingham)
Dermatol Ther 24:173-186, 2011

Autoimmune mucocutaneous blistering diseases (AMBD) are a rare group of dermatoses that can be potentially fatal. There are many subtypes and their clinical presentation can vary from being localized to general involvement. It is crucial that a diagnosis be made as early as possible and appropriate treatments are implemented. This article will discuss the diagnosis and available treatments of the major AMBDs. There are very few case-controlled studies regarding the treatments of these diseases. Most of the treatments used for these diseases are based on anecdotal reports. Hence, a synopsis of the conventional treatments and some brief recommendations will also be discussed. A brief discussion regarding "rescue" therapies that have been used for those patients with more recalcitrant cases of AMBD will also be presented.

▶ This is a nice review of autoimmune blistering diseases, including clinical, histological, and immunopathological features as well as an overview of treatment. Most of the practical information is well known to most dermatologists, but the article can serve as a meaty refresher for them and a basic reference for others. Because autoimmune bullous diseases are well known to dermatologists but not commonly encountered in general ambulatory practice, this reference may assist in expediting review of the material if such a case is suspected in clinical practice.

M. V. Dahl, MD

Pemphigus and Osteoporosis: A Case-Control Study

Wohl Y, Dreiher J, Cohen AD (Tel-Aviv Univ, Israel; Ben-Gurion Univ, Be'er-Sheva, Israel)
Arch Dermatol 146:1126-1131, 2010

Objective.—To investigate the association between pemphigus and osteoporosis.

Design.—Case-control study.

Setting.—A large health care provider organization in Israel.

Participants.—Patients with pemphigus older than 20 years (hereinafter, pemphigus patients) were compared with a sample of age- and sex-matched controls.

Interventions.—Data retrieval from a large community-based medical database regarding health-related lifestyles, comorbidities, use of medications, bone mineral density scans, and drugs for osteoporosis.

Main Outcome Measures.—The prevalence of osteoporosis in patients and controls, use of bone mineral density scans, and drugs for osteoporosis.

Results.—The study included 255 pemphigus patients and 509 controls older than 20 years. Osteoporosis was diagnosed among 40.4% of pemphigus patients compared with 6.5% of controls ($P < .001$; odds ratio [OR], 9.77; 95% confidence interval [CI], 6.34-15.10). After controlling for confounders, including age, sex, and duration of glucocorticosteroid therapy and proton pump inhibitor therapy, the associations with osteoporosis persisted (OR, 4.27; 95% CI, 2.44-7.47; $P < .001$). Similar results were obtained when using cumulative glucocorticosteroid dose. Only 73 pemphigus patients with osteoporosis (70.9%) had undergone a bone mineral density test within the past 10 years. While most pemphigus patients with osteoporosis purchased medications for osteoporosis, including calcium (95.1% of patients), cholecalciferol (89.3%), bisphosphonates (90.3%), or raloxiphene (8.8%), the duration of therapy was short.

Conclusions.—We found an association between pemphigus and osteoporosis, which persisted after controlling for glucocorticosteroid use. Monitoring and treatment of osteoporosis in pemphigus patients was suboptimal in this study.

▶ Glucocorticosteroids remain the mainstay of therapy for patients with pemphigus. Thus, it seems obvious to infer that the incidence of osteoporosis would be higher in pemphigus patients because of prolonged corticosteroid therapy. In this large case-controlled study, the authors examined the prevalence of osteoporosis in pemphigus patients and then controlled for confounders, including duration of glucocorticosteroid therapy. As expected, the prevalence of osteoporosis in pemphigus patients was several times greater than in controls. Interestingly, the association of osteoporosis and pemphigus persisted even when controlling for confounders, suggesting a risk for osteoporosis unrelated to glucocorticosteroid use. The authors suggest that the correlation is due to similarities in the inflammatory pathways of both diseases. This finding strongly suggests that osteoporosis screening and prevention should be considered in all patients with pemphigus, not just limited to those on glucocorticosteroid therapy.

S. M. Purcell, DO

Use of intravenous immunoglobulin therapy during pregnancy in patients with pemphigus vulgaris

Ahmed AR, Gürcan HM (Ctr for Blistering Diseases, Boston, MA)
J Eur Acad Dermatol Venereol 25:1073-1079, 2011

Background.—Pemphigus vulgaris (PV) is a potentially fatal autoimmune disease characterized by the presence of *in vivo* deposition of antibodies against cell surface antigens desmoglein 1 and desmoglein 3 in the epidermis.

Objectives.—To report the treatment outcomes in pregnant PV patients treated with intravenous immunoglobulin (IVIg) therapy.

Methods.—Eight patients with active disease during pregnancy were treated. Patients were treated with a dose of 2 g/kg/cycle. Seven patients were treated for 2 months on post-partum basis. Main Outcome Measures were as follows: (i) pregnancy outcome; (ii) presence of neonatal pemphigus; (iii) post-partum flare; (iv) effect of IVIg on present and future pregnancies; (v) immediate and long-term side-effects in the mother and child.

Results.—Patients ages ranged from 20 to 43 years (mean 29.6). All patients had severe and widespread disease involving the skin and multiple mucous membranes. Patients one to seven responded to IVIg therapy and did not have a post-partum flare. Patient eight could not tolerate IVIg because of intense headaches and significant post-partum flare. None of the neonates had pemphigus. Three patients who completed the IVIg protocol had normal second pregnancies. One patient who did not complete the protocol had a miscarriage during the second pregnancy. Since last observation, none of the patients have had a recurrence of the disease or another pregnancy.

Conclusions.—The data suggests that IVIg can be useful and safe in treating pregnant patients with PV. No long-term adverse effects of IVIg in the mother or in the child were observed based on a long-term follow-up.

▶ Pemphigus vulgaris (PV) typically affects middle-aged adults, therefore often affecting women of child-bearing age. Systemic therapy is usually required, which puts the developing fetus at risk of complications from treatment of the mother. Apparently, 3 infusions of intravenous immunoglobulin (IVIg) once weekly in cycles spaced 3 to 4 weeks apart provides a remission for the mother and a normal outcome for the fetus. In this study, 8 women with PV received IVIg during pregnancy, and all of them completed normal delivery of healthy babies. None of the babies had neonatal pemphigus. Four of the women became pregnant again, and all of these again delivered healthy babies. Remissions were complete, although 1 woman redeveloped PV in a subsequent pregnancy. Seven of the 8 patients developed headaches during treatment. In 1 patient, the headaches were intractable and infusions were stopped. No other major side effects were observed. It makes sense that IVIg might be safe to the fetus; it is more like a blood transfusion than like a potent pharmacologic agent. Nevertheless, there are other considerations,[1] and practitioners considering this therapy should read both this and the article by Dahl[1] thoroughly to ensure consideration of multiple factors.

M. V. Dahl, MD

Reference

1. Dahl MV, Bridges AG. Intravenous immune globulin: fighting antibodies with antibodies. *J Am Acad Dermatol.* 2001;45:775-783.

Therapeutic ladder for pemphigus vulgaris: Emphasis on achieving complete remission
Strowd LC, Taylor SL, Jorizzo JL, et al (Wake Forest Univ School of Medicine, Winston-Salem, NC)
J Am Acad Dermatol 64:490-494, 2011

Background.—Pemphigus vulgaris (PV) is a blistering autoimmune bullous disease that is usually fatal without proper treatment. There are no clear treatment guidelines for PV at this time.

Purpose.—We suggest a standard treatment regimen for patients with PV based on the success of our treatment.

Methods.—A retrospective chart review of 18 patients with PV was conducted to assess response to a similar approach using mycophenolate mofetil (MMF) and prednisone. Diagnosis was confirmed through routine histology, direct immunofluorescence, and indirect immunofluorescence, and patients were followed up for a total average of 35.2 months.

Results.—We achieved complete disease control in 89% of patients using our treatment algorithm. Fourteen of 18 patients achieved complete disease control on therapy with prednisone and MMF. Three of the 4 patients who did not achieve control on MMF and prednisone went on to receive rituximab therapy, and two of those patients achieved disease control on rituximab. The average length of time from initiating therapy to 75% clearance of lesions was 4.5 months. Three of 18 patients were able to discontinue therapy after an average of 3 years and have remained in complete remission for more than 1 year.

Limitations.—This was a retrospective chart review with a small patient sample size.

Conclusions.—The combination therapy of MMF and prednisone is an effective treatment regimen to achieve rapid and complete control of PV. For those patients who fail treatment with MMF and prednisone, rituximab is an efficacious alternative therapy.

▶ Pemphigus vulgaris (PV) is an autoimmune blistering disease that characteristically involves the oral mucosa, scalp, midface, sternum, groin, and pressure points.[1] Patients may present with flaccid blisters or large denuded areas of skin that spread radially with limited stress or pressure on the skin surface. Diagnosis is made by histologic examination with suprabasalar intraepithelial acantholysis, intraepidermal IgG/C3 deposition on direct immunofluorescence, and circulating antibodies detected on indirect immunofluorescence. The authors illustrate a treatment algorithm for management of PV patients. (1) Begin with mycophenolate mofetil (MMF), 1 g twice a day, and prednisone, 1 mg/kg daily; (2) increase MMF dose by 0.5 mg every month (maximum 3 g daily), continue prednisone; and (3) slowly taper if complete control; if not, consider alternate therapies (intravenous immunoglobulin G or rituximab). MMF is generally well tolerated with the most common adverse events being gastrointestinal side effects. This article retrospectively reviewed the charts of 18 patients with PV and found 78% of patients were able to achieve control utilizing the first step of the treatment ladder. Limitations mentioned by authors are those inherent to a retrospective study and small sample size.

S. Bellew, DO

J. Q. Del Rosso, DO

Reference

1. Elder DE, Elenitsas R, Johnson BL. *Lever's Histopathology of the skin.* Lippincott Williams & Wilkins; 2005:254-257.

Clinical efficacy of different doses of rituximab in the treatment of pemphigus: a retrospective study of 27 patients

Kim JH, Kim YH, Kim MR, et al (Yonsei Univ College of Medicine, Seoul, Korea; Univ of Pittsburgh, PA)

Br J Dermatol 165:646-651, 2011

Background.—The treatment of pemphigus is still challenging and some patients with pemphigus are unresponsive to conventional immunosuppressive treatments. Rituximab, a chimeric monoclonal anti-CD20 antibody, binds to the CD20 antigen on the surface of B cells and has been reported to be effective for the treatment of recalcitrant pemphigus.

Objective.—To compare the efficacy of different doses of rituximab in patients with pemphigus who were unresponsive to conventional therapies.

Methods.—Twenty-seven patients with pemphigus who received different doses of rituximab (375 mg m^{-2} per infusion weekly) were analysed retrospectively. We divided the patients into two groups: group 1 ($n = 12$) received two infusions of rituximab and group 2 ($n = 15$) received three or more infusions of rituximab at 1-week intervals. The number of infusions was determined by the choice of each patient. The endpoints of the study were time to disease control, partial remission (PR) and complete remission (CR).

Results.—There was no significant difference in time to achieve PR between the two groups (147 vs. 135 days, $P = 0 \cdot 65$). However, group 2 demonstrated better outcomes than group 1 in time to CR (443 vs. 149 days, $P = 0 \cdot 06$) and relapse rate (0% vs. 67%, $P < 0 \cdot 01$).

Conclusions.—We conclude that three or more infusions of rituximab are more effective than two infusions for the treatment of pemphigus.

▶ This study confirms the responsiveness of pemphigus, a disease that is often difficult to control, to administration of rituximab. Therapies aimed at stopping blister formation often fail, unless other treatments are used to stop or slow the synthesis of pathogenic antibodies. Rituximab depletes the antibody-producing cells, which are a major pathogenic source of the disorder. As circulating antibodies are metabolized, blister formation ceases, and long durable remissions are possible, as evidenced by the data presented in this article. Apparently, 3 infusions spaced 1 week apart are usually sufficient. Remissions take time. A mean of about 5 months after the treatment course was needed to obtain complete remission. Rituximab is expensive and potent, but benefits of treatments often seem to outweigh risks, especially in severely affected patients.

M. V. Dahl, MD

10 Genodermatoses

Cardiac magnetic resonance imaging illustrating Anderson—Fabry disease progression

Imbriaco M, Messalli G, Avitabile G, et al (Univ "Federico II", Napoli, Italy)

Br J Radiol 83:e249-e251, 2010

Anderson—Fabry disease is an X-linked lysosomal storage disorder resulting from a deficiency of the enzyme α-galactosidase A (α-Gal A) and subsequent cellular storage of the enzyme's substrate globotriaosylceramide (Gb3) and related glycosphingolipids. We report a case of Anderson—Fabry disease with cardiac involvement evaluated with cardiovascular MRI. Disease progression was observed despite enzyme replacement therapy.

▶ Anderson-Fabry disease is an X-linked recessive lysosomal storage disorder that is caused by a deficiency of lysosomal enzyme, resulting in severe renal, cerebrovascular, and cardiac disease. Cardiac involvement is common and appears to be the most common cause of death in these patients. The accumulation of glycosphingolipid in the cardiac tissue can lead to left ventricular hypertrophy, arrhythmias, coronary artery disease, and heart failure. This is a case report of a 44-year-old man with Anderson-Fabry disease with cardiac involvement evaluated with cardiovascular MRI to evaluate disease progression. Enzyme replacement therapy (ERT) has been shown to reduce microvascular deposits of globotriaosylceramide in the kidneys, skin, and heart and significantly helps with regression in cardiac hypertrophy. In this case report, there was disease progression despite ERT due to extensive fibrosis in the myocardium. Imaging studies revealed a predilection for the posterolateral wall of the left ventricle in this patient. This case report represents a point of no return when there is progression of cardiac dysfunction despite rescue therapy with ERT. However, more studies are needed and early detection is essential to help reduce morbidity in these individuals. ERT therapy may be less effective in patients of advanced age and in the presence of extensive areas of myocardial fibrosis, which may be an argument for early initiation of ERT in patients with Anderson-Fabry disease.

G. K. Kim, DO

J. Q. Del Rosso, DO

Inherited syndromes

Reyes MA, Eisen DB (Univ of California, San Diego; Univ of California Davis Med Ctr, Sacramento)
Dermatol Ther 23:606-642, 2010

Many inherited skin conditions are associated with underlying malignancies. The astute clinician will be able to recognize many of these cutaneous findings. The identification of these genetic syndromes with cutaneous findings, or genodermatoses, may allow early recognition of internal malignancies and the extension of these patients' life expectancy. Several of these syndromes have established screening and treatment protocols, which should be utilized in the care of affected patients. This article succinctly reviews the dermatologic, clinical, and laboratory findings associated with genodermatoses that have associated internal malignancies. Appropriate treatment and screening recommendations are explored.

▶ This meta-analysis may have more clinically relevant information regarding the screening and treatment of patients with genodermatoses than some of the major textbooks published to date.

The authors provide a high-yield and thorough analysis of genodermatoses that are associated with internal malignancy. Although the authors' stated objective was to help dermatologists identify and diagnose genodermatoses associated with internal malignancy, this review does much more. In addition to being an excellent reference for the diagnosis of genodermatoses, this article provides the epidemiology of the cutaneous and internal manifestations, the prognostic factors, and the appropriate screening, management, and treatment of each genodermatoses in both text and easy reference table format. The thorough epidemiology and prognostic factors reported in this review is important information that can be relayed to the patient as to what can be expected in the years to come.

The detailed review of the required screening and management of each of the reviewed genodermatoses will allow dermatologists to direct physicians of other specialties in the appropriate management of these cases. Therefore, these guidelines may help ensure an early diagnosis of malignancy and an increased survival for many patients. This article is one of the most useful clinically relevant reviews that has been published to date and is highly recommended reading for both dermatology residents and practicing physicians.

J. Levin, DO

J. Q. Del Rosso, DO

Fabry disease in children: correlation between ocular manifestations, genotype and systemic clinical severity
Allen LE, Cosgrave EM, Kersey JP, et al (Cambridge Univ Hosps, UK)
Br J Ophthalmol 94:1602-1605, 2010

Background/Aims.—Fabry disease is an X linked lysosomal disorder associated with severe multiorgan failure and premature death. This study aims to determine the prevalence of ophthalmic manifestations in children with the condition and investigate the correlation with genotype and systemic disease severity.

Methods.—The records of 26 children from 18 pedigrees with Fabry disease undergoing regular ophthalmic and systemic examination were reviewed. All pedigrees underwent *GLA* gene sequencing to determine genotype. Correlations between ocular and systemic phenotype and genotype were investigated.

Results.—Corneal verticillata occurred in 50% of the children in this study (95% CI, 29% to 79%). Children with ophthalmic manifestations were more likely to have loss-of-function *GLA* mutations (p=0.003). Retinal vascular tortuosity was seen in seven children (27%), all of whom had systemic symptoms suggestive of autonomic neuropathy, such as diarrhoea and syncope. These symptoms seemed less prevalent in children without retinal vascular changes, although this did not reach statistical significance (p=0.134).

Conclusion.—Ophthalmic manifestations of Fabry disease are common even in young children with loss-of-function *GLA* gene mutations. Although the limited sample size possibly prevented statistical significance, systemic symptoms of autonomic neuropathy often coexist with retinal vascular changes and may share the same pathogenesis.

▶ Fabry disease is an inherited disorder of lysosomal storage. The interpatient variability of the presentation makes diagnosis difficult in some cases. In addition, eye examinations in this population of patients can be useful, especially if performed early. Ophthalmologic findings are due to deposition of glycosphingolipids that result in corneal verticillata, which is not on its own diagnostic but is highly suggestive of Fabry disease and can be predictive of more severe systemic involvement. This unique ocular finding is significant to the clinician because cornea verticillata can precede systemic presentation. This is a cohort study of 26 children and adolescents undergoing ophthalmologic examinations with symptoms of Fabry disease. Of all the children studied, none had severe corneal manifestations, and 7 had moderate changes. All 7 children with retinal vascular tortuosity had neurological and gastrointestinal symptoms. Five children had cardiac symptoms and auditory symptoms. Ophthalmic manifestations were found in 76% of patients predicted to have no enzyme function. Although the loss-of-function *GLA* mutation correlated with ophthalmologic findings ($P = .003$), the prevalence of cardiac and renal systemic symptoms were higher in genotypes with residual enzymatic activity. Also, the absence of eye signs does not correlate with milder disease, and it could indicate a missense mutation. One limitation to this study was that although ophthalmologic examinations are necessary in this population, corneal verticillata is a highly subjective finding. Larger studies need to be performed to determine if this finding correlates with systemic disease. This study demonstrates that ocular symptoms of Fabry disease may help early recognition of the disease, and those with a strong suspicion should have regular ophthalmologic examinations to ensure early initiation of a treatable disease and its manifestations, affecting several major organs.

G. K. Kim, DO

J. Q. Del Rosso, DO

Adnexal tumours of the skin as markers of cancer-prone syndromes

Kanitakis J (Ed. Herriot Hosp [Pav. R], Lyon, France)
J Eur Acad Dermatol Venereol 24:379-387, 2010

Adnexal tumours of the skin are benign, rarely malignant, primary skin tumours that originate from, or differentiate towards, hair follicles, sebaceous and sweat glands. Although they are usually encountered as single, sporadic tumours, they may occasionally be multiple, hereditary; in that case, they may herald complex genetic syndromes that comprise visceral cancers. Dermatologists should be aware of these adnexal skin tumours, the diagnosis of which may contribute to an early detection of a cancer-prone syndrome with a potentially lethal outcome. The main tumours falling into this category and their associated syndromes are reviewed here.

▶ Adnexal tumors of the skin can represent a group of benign and rarely malignant primary skin neoplasms with a potentially lethal outcome. This is a review of adnexal tumors of the skin and their association with cancer-prone syndromes. Trichilemmomas are benign tumors of the hair follicle that can be associated with Cowden syndrome (multiple hamartoma syndrome). These lesions can begin around the age of 20 years before extracutaneous manifestations such as breast carcinoma or thyroid cancer. Sebaceous tumors are papular, nodular, or cystic-appearing tumors that appear on the face and are a hallmark of Muir-Torre syndrome. They can also appear before or concomitantly with internal malignancies such as colorectal carcinomas and urogenital cancers in 30% to 40% of cases, or in patients with sebaceous carcinoma of the eyelid, which can present as a focal lesion or diffuse simulating chronic blepharitis or conjunctivitis, and can be associated with Muir-Torre syndrome. Cutaneous cysts of the hair follicle are usually benign lesions appearing on the scalp, but multiple lesions in unusual sites (such as limbs) can be a hallmark of Gardner syndrome. These patients can develop multiple adenomatous polyps of the colon and rectum (50%-65% of cases) that invariably undergo malignant transformation as early as 40 years of age. Trichodiscomas and fibrofolliculomas are flesh-colored whitish papules on the face and neck. Multiple lesions may likely be indicative of Birt-Hogg-Dube syndrome, an autosomal dominant disease presenting around the third decade of life and can be associated with renal cell carcinomas and spontaneous recurring pneumothorax, which can be bilateral, thyroid gland carcinoma, and bilateral bullous emphysema. The author concluded that the dermatologist plays a vital role in detecting patients with these potentially lethal syndromes and recommends careful clinicopathologic assessment if these adnexal tumors are observed, especially if multiple or at unusual sites.

G. K. Kim, DO
J. Q. Del Rosso, DO

11 Drug Actions, Reactions, and Interactions

A comparative analysis of cetirizine, gabapentin and their combination in the relief of post-burn pruritus
Ahuja RB, Gupta R, Gupta G, et al (Lok Nayak Hosp and associated Maulana Azad Med College, New Delhi, India)
Burns 37:203-207, 2011

Post-burn pruritis is a very distressing symptom having a reported incidence between 80 and 100%. The mainstay of management of post-burn itch has been with antihistaminics and emollients but the treatment is ineffective in a very large percentage of patients. With the recognition of a distinct itch specific neuronal pathway, which has a complex interaction with pain pathway, a fresh approach to itch management has surfaced with the use of gabapentin. Gabapentin is an antiepileptic drug which has been successfully used to manage neuropathic pain, and is reporting to be successful in management of all forms of itch. With a paucity of randomized trials evaluating the role of gabapentin in post-burn itch management the current study was undertaken to individually evaluate gabapentin, cetirizine and their combination in relieving itch. Twenty patients were randomly recruited in each of the three groups and administered the respective drug(s) in doses determined by initial VAS (visual analog scale) scores. There was no significant difference in all the three groups with respect to mean age, sex distribution, mean percentage of TBSA burn and mean VAS score on day 0. VAS scores were evaluated over next 28 days (days 3, 7, 14, 21 and 28), and no emollients were prescribed for the study period. The initial mean VAS score reduced 95% in gabapentin group compared to 52% for the cetirizine group, which was highly significant ($p < 0.01$). There was a 94% reduction in mean VAS score in the combination group which was comparable to the relief observed with gabapentin alone ($p > 0.05$). Even the onset of action with gabapentin was significantly faster than the cetirizine group as evident from the mean VAS scores on day 3, which decreased 74% in gabapentin group compared to 32% in cetirizine group ($p < 0.01$). Whereas all patients receiving gabapentin (either as monotherapy or in combination with cetirizine) reached an itch free status

(VAS score 0−1) by day 28 only 3/20 patients reached this level with cetirizine alone. It is quite evident from this study that gabapentin is significantly better than cetirizine as monotherapy in relieving post-burn itch and it also has a faster action. The hypothetical combination of a centrally acting drug with a peripherally acting agent did not result in any better control of post-burn itch than monotherapy with gabapentin. No side effects were reported with gabapentin administration but all patients receiving cetirizine reported sedation. There is now a need to relook at the antipruritic protocols in burn management.

▶ This is a nice introductory study to explore new treatments for postburn pruritus, which is unfortunately very common in wounds that are extensive enough to take several weeks or more to heal. Although the itching eventually subsides in most patients as the scar matures, patients are plagued with often intractable itching until then. Many of us still tend to reach for antihistamines for the control of pruritus, in part because of the lack of any better options and our relative inexperience in general dermatologic practice, unless we work with burns regularly.

This article provides some very convincing evidence that the antiepileptic drug, oral gabapentin, provides much better itch relief than does cetirizine. Obviously the study was limited by the sample size and the omission of a placebo group. However, it opens the door to explore gabapentin and perhaps some related antiepileptics as better options for intractable postburn pruritus. The study also helps to confirm what most of us already know—H_1 antihistamines perform poorly to alleviate itching in patients with postburn scars, not to mention some other forms of itching, such as in many patients with atopic dermatitis.

One note of caution is that there are many patients who do not tolerate even lower dosages of gabapentin when they take it for postherpetic neuralgia, as not only somnolence but irritability, dizziness, fatigue, and ataxia are frequent complaints leading to drug cessation. The dosing schedule the authors chose was based on avoiding these side effects by giving 300 mg once daily for non-severe itching and titrating up from there. Although this report revealed virtually no such side effects at these lower dosages, one should still be cautious when considering using gabapentin for itching and should screen patients carefully. Before the use of gabapentin for this form of pruritus becomes commonplace, further large-scale trials are needed to gather firm data regarding efficacy and dosing. Calling this a comparative analysis with such a small study group and without a placebo arm is an overstatement. In addition, gabapentin has been popularized for many off-label uses, many of which may be valid and clinically relevant.

For postburn pruritus, more studies are needed to more thoroughly assess the role of gabapentin.

J. M. Suchniak, MD
J. Q. Del Rosso, DO

Fixed drug eruption caused by etoricoxib – 2 cases confirmed by patch testing
Andrade P, Gonçalo M (Coimbra Univ Hosp, Portugal)
Contact Dermatitis 64:110-120, 2011

Background.—Most fixed drug eruptions (FDEs) are caused by nonsteroidal anti-inflammatory drugs (NSAIDs). Two cases of FDEs caused by etoricoxib, a widely used selective cyclo-oxygenase (COX) isoenzyme 2 inhibitor that is rarely associated with FDEs, were reported.

Case Reports.—Case 1: Woman, 69, had multiple sharp round, 1- to 4-cm erythematous pruriginous patches on her face, upper limbs, and trunk. All had occurred simultaneously within 24 hours of taking 60 mg of oral etoricoxib to manage a febrile episode. The patient had taken etoricoxib 3 years previously without any cutaneous reaction.

Case 2: Woman, 63, had used several NSAIDs to manage osteoarthritic pain. She had lesions on her face and upper and lower limbs after taking NSAIDs, one of which was etoricoxib. This was the second eruption within a month. The first had spontaneously regressed with hyperpigmentation.

Both patients experienced regression of the inflammatory lesions after the suspected drugs were discontinued and mild topical steroids were applied. Both patients had multiple hyperpigmented residual lesions as well. Six weeks after resolution, patch tests with various agents provoked a positive reaction to etoricoxib only on lesional skin 1 and 2 days after exposure. Patients had no reaction to celecoxib or other NSAIDs. Neither patient had a reaction on normal skin. No FDE flares developed after etoricoxib was discontinued.

Conclusions.—Etoricoxib combines high anti-inflammatory activity with a low incidence of side effects, with cutaneous adverse events being quite rare. Despite the pharmacologic similarity of etoricoxib and celecoxib, no cross-reactivity was found.

▶ Fixed-drug eruption (FDE) can be caused by a variety of ingested drugs and other substances, with tetracyclines and nonsteroidal anti-inflammatory drugs (NSAIDs) among the most common. This is a report of FDE to a new COX2 inhibitor, etoricoxib. This drug is not available in the United States. Importantly, the authors state that the drug is a sulfonamide, which may make skin reactions more likely and suggest cross-reaction with other NSAIDs is unlikely.

Interestingly, patch testing induced positivity to etoricoxib on skin previously involved with FDE (sites identified by residual pigmentation) but not on clinically uninvolved normal skin in both cases.

J. F. Fowler, MD

A Prospective Self-Controlled Phase II Study of Imiquimod 5% Cream in the Treatment of Infantile Hemangioma

Jiang CH, Hu XJ, Ma G, et al (Shanghai Jiaotong Univ, China)
Pediatr Dermatol 28:259-266, 2011

Imiquimod has been reported to be efficacious in the topical treatment of uncomplicated infantile hemangiomas (IH). However, due to the natural tendency of IH to involute spontaneously, prior uncontrolled efficacy and safety studies have been called into question. We conducted a prospective self-controlled phase II study of imiquimod initially applied to uncomplicated, proliferative superficial or mixed IHs treating half of each IH once every other night for 16 weeks, leaving the other half untreated. After 16 weeks, an independent dermatologist evaluated the color, area, and volume of each half of the hemangioma. Of the 44 patients treated, the total effective rate was 80% ($n = 35$), with an overall resolution rated as excellent or good rate in 39% of lesions ($n = 17/44$). The relapse rate was 2% ($n = 1$). Side effects were noted in 61% ($n = 27$) including erythema or/and edema ($n = 16\%$, 7), local itching ($n = 7\%$, 3), peeling ($n = 7\%$, 3), erosion ($n = 5\%$, 2), crusting ($n = 55\%$, 24), ulceration ($n = 9\%$, 4), and scarring ($n = 5\%$, 2). Some patients had two or more side effects. Most were judged to be mild to moderate and did not result in treatment being interrupted. Crusting or ulceration was noted to cause post-treatment skin reactions, such as texture change, whereas cases without crusting involuted to almost normal skin. No local infection or systemic reaction was observed. The difference in effective rate and side effect incidence between superficial and mixed IH was not statistically significant. Imiquimod 5% cream can be an effective and safe treatment option for superficial mixed IH in which the superficial component predominates. The recurrence rate is low, but local reactions including crusting can develop and result in post-treatment skin changes.

▶ It was encouraging to see a study that involved this age group and approached the treatment of hemangiomas as both vascular and inflammatory processes. The details of the study are not as important in this article as the discussion, which is an impressive overview of the science of how topical immunomodulators can impact vascular tumors. Although the authors state the caveat that many hemangiomas can spontaneously regress, the findings that a larger vascular tumor has the potential to shrink are significant to both patient and parents, who are often adversely affected by its presence. In addition, children in the age group studied are, by label, not to be considered candidates for imiquimod therapy. What is often forgotten is that patients with tumors requiring intervention such as beta-blockers, corticosteroids, or laser therapy may not be of the age or health status to respond to treatment. The authors specifically point out how similar secondary endpoints of improvement, such as size and color, from therapy with timolol gel were not significantly different from those treated with imiquimod, yet the potential for systemic side effects based on mechanism of action in that age group could be significant and dangerous. In addition, many tumors are small enough to respond to topical therapies, thus sparing the adverse consequences of other treatments.

The homogenous Chinese population chosen for this pediatric study is not an obstacle to interpreting the data, nor is the age group or the overall tumor size, leaving the clinician to process and therefore position the impact of topical therapy individually. However, it was refreshing to read the scientific summary of the impact of imiquimod and interferons on angiogenesis and vascular mediators. The overview of the recruitment of proapoptotic cytokines also summarizes the basis for therapy.

An important observation was that the tumors that best responded to therapy were associated with significant inflammatory reactions, including erythema, crusting, and even symptoms that were dose-limiting. These are significant observations considering how interferon-alfa affects a tumor, but it is also somewhat contradictory to the concept of the findings by the Angiogenesis Foundation[1] and its pivotal publication on the individualized maximal tolerated dose. This study investigated a dose-response protocol in which imiquimod was applied to lesions at gradually escalating doses until the first signs of redness and irritation appear. The study findings suggest that everyone has a threshold of erythema that can be obtained but is still independent of the response, given that the subclinical activity of therapy can still provide resolution of individual targets. These findings are in direct contrast to the authors' finding that response rates correlated with measurable reactions.

Many clinicians ask why imiquimod would work on hemangiomas. After reviewing the article, it is more important to take into account the impact of interferon-alfa, apoptosis, and matrix metalloproteinases, specifically MMP-1 and -9, on the pathogenesis of the vascular tumors. The summary of the science behind the need for application of a topical therapy for a condition that is often self-limiting is important to understanding the utility of the therapy.

N. Bhatia, MD

Reference

1. Li VW, Li WW, Talcott KE, Zhai AW. Imiquimod as an antiangiogenic agent. *J Drugs Dermatol.* 2005;4:708-717.

Exacerbation of Seborrheic Dermatitis by Topical Fluorouracil

Brodell EE, Smith E, Brodell RT (Univ of Richmond, VA; Northeastern Ohio Universities College of Medicine and Pharmacy, Rootstown)
Arch Dermatol 147:245-246, 2011

Background.—When patients were treated with systemic fluorouracil for solid internal malignant neoplasms, it was discovered that fluorouracil effectively destroys clinical and subclinical actinic keratoses (AKs) by targeting rapidly proliferating cells but sparing normal skin. Topical fluorouracil was then shown to clear AKs and minimize internal adverse effects related to the systemic formulation. The topical form can also produce an intense inflammatory response in areas of seborrheic dermatitis.

A small, nonrandomized, open-label study focused on determining whether this inflammatory response could be confirmed prospectively.

Methods.—Twenty patients with five or more facial AKs were given topical 5% fluorouracil twice a day for 2 weeks. The visible or palpable AKs were counted at baseline, and the presence or absence of seborrheic dermatitis was confirmed, along with a determination of its degree as mild or marked. After 2 weeks the presence of erythema, pruritus, and pain or burning was noted at the AK sites to indicate the clinical response to topical fluorouracil. Any inflammatory response in the distribution of seborrheic distribution was also noted. After the fluorouracil was discontinued, a topical water-based emulsion was applied twice a day to the treated areas, with the degree of inflammation in areas of AK and seborrheic dermatitis documented.

Results.—Inflammation developed at the AK sites in all patients. Most of the AKs demonstrated excellent resolution. One patient had mild seborrheic dermatitis, and 11 had marked cases. Eight patients had no seborrheic dermatitis.

An inflammatory response at the seborrheic sites developed in 92% of the patients after the 2 weeks of topical fluorouracil. Patients without seborrheic dermatitis did not develop the inflammation. The severity of the reaction varied considerably. The inflammation resolved in all patients 2 weeks after discontinuing the fluorouracil, leaving just mild postinflammatory erythema.

Conclusions.—The epidermis in AKs and in areas of active seborrheic dermatitis proliferates rapidly, with the keratinocytes serving as prime targets for topical fluorouracil, which inhibits DNA synthesis by inhibiting thymidylate synthetase. Patients with active seborrheic dermatitis who are treated with topical fluorouracil can develop inflammation of the skin of the nasomesial, retroauricular, eyebrow, and glabellar areas similar to what is produced in seborrheic dermatitis. Thus topical fluorouracil given to treat AKs exacerbates preexisting seborrheic dermatitis in its area of distribution. Possibly pretreatment of seborrheic dermatitis with topical fungal azole drugs will minimize the inflammation. Patients given fluorouracil should be warned to expect the inflammation in areas of seborrheic dermatitis as well as in clinical and subclinical AKs.

▶ Seborrheic dermatitis is classified as a neutrophilic dermatosis that can be aggressive in patients who are immunocompromised (eg, acquired immunodeficiency syndrome patients). The explanation of the mechanism of how seborrheic dermatitis flares in this patient group directs us to understanding the reactions in these patients. Topical 5-fluorouracil is considered an antimetabolite, and its efficacy is best seen on epithelial tissue that is considered to have rapid turnover, such as in the gastrointestinal tract and the skin. As the authors describe, its use in the treatment of actinic keratosis is directed at modification of the keratinization defect to impact both clinical and subclinical lesions in the spectrum of photodamaged skin. However, unlike immune response modifiers, the inflammation seen in the affected areas is a consequence of the keratinocyte destruction and not the primary purpose of the active ingredient. The authors also remind us of the mechanisms of irritant versus allergic contact dermatitis induced by topical 5-fluorouracil and that the inflammation created is a secondary phenomenon unlike the mechanisms of immune response modifiers. It is also needs to be understood that photodamaged skin is immunosuppressed skin.[1,2] From there it can be interpreted how the signs of another cellular-mediated process such as seborrheic dermatitis can be exacerbated, since other procellular cytokines as well as neutrophils are recruited into the inflamed areas.

This observation leads us to the 1 missing piece of the study: the patients were all diagnosed with seborrheic dermatitis based on clinical findings without histologic confirmation. As the authors point out, the observed inflammation that develops in the seborrheic distribution goes against an irritant or contact dermatitis-like presentation, but histology before and after treatment to confirm baseline seborrheic dermatitis and the diagnosed flare would be essential for the conclusion. The pitfall there is that the biopsy itself induces an inflammatory response and scarring, which might alter the diagnosis as well, so we rely on the expertise of the clinicians to make the diagnosis and not confuse the inflammation as iatrogenic or as a consequence of baseline dermatoheliosis. The findings and conclusions are solid but therefore pose the issue to us that if we are not screening and even pretreating for seborrheic dermatitis before prescribing this class of therapy, we might be at risk for exacerbation of baseline symptoms that could therefore limit compliance. In any case, recognition of this potential consequence of topical 5-fluorouracil will be useful for management.

N. Bhatia, MD

References

1. Moyal D, Fourtanier A. Acute and chronic effects of UV on skin. In: Rigel DS, Weiss RA, Lim HW, Dover JS, eds. *Photoaging*. New York, NY: Marcel Dekker; 2004:15-30.
2. Schwarz A, Schwarz T. Molecular determinants of UV-induced immunosuppression. *Exp Dermatol*. 2002;11:9-12.

Topical calcitriol restores the impairment of epidermal permeability and antimicrobial barriers induced by corticosteroids
Hong SP, Oh Y, Jung M, et al (Konyang Univ Hosp, Daejeon, Korea; Yonsei Univ Wonju College of Medicine, Korea; et al)
Br J Dermatol 162:1251-1260, 2010

Background.—The active form of vitamin D_3, calcitriol, is widely used for the treatment of psoriasis, with or without topical corticosteroids. Topical corticosteroids are known to disrupt permeability and antimicrobial barriers, even with short-term use. Yet, the effect of topical calcitriol on epidermal permeability and antimicrobial barriers disrupted by topical corticosteroids has not been determined.

Objectives.—To examine the effect of calcitriol on epidermal permeability and antimicrobial barrier function that has been impaired by corticosteroids, as well as to elucidate the mechanism of improvement.

Material and Methods.—Topical calcitriol or the control vehicle was applied to each flank of hairless mice 20 min after treatment with topical clobetasol propionate and repeated every 12 h for 3·5 days. Barrier function assessment, Nile red staining, electron microscopy, immunohistochemistry, Western blotting, and real-time reverse transcriptase—polymerase chain reaction studies were performed 24 h after the last application.

Results.—Epidermis co-treated with topical calcitriol showed an improvement of stratum corneum integrity and barrier recovery, more intense fluorescence staining with Nile red, and an increase in lamellar body (LB) maturation and density, as well as upregulation of major epidermal lipid synthesis-related enzymes (3-hydroxy-3-methylglutaryl-CoA, serine-palmitoyl transferase and fatty acid synthase), mouse beta-defensin 3, cathelin-related antimicrobial peptide and vitamin D receptor.

Conclusions.—We found that topical calcitriol restored both the epidermal permeability and antimicrobial barrier that had been impaired by corticosteroids. This restoration was mediated by both an activation of the cutaneous vitamin D pathway and an increase of epidermal lipids and antimicrobial peptides, promoted by the formation of the LB and the activity of epidermal lipid synthesis-related enzymes.

▶ One of the prime teaching points here is that corticosteroid atrophy involves the epidermis as much as the dermis. Negative keratinocyte differentiation in skin treated with topical corticosteroids, for even a few days, is an important consequence in chronic diseases such as atopic dermatitis and psoriasis in which barrier functions and reduction of transepidermal water loss are essential. The incorporation of calcitriol topically to reverse the consequence in a locally immunosuppressed environment created by corticosteroids can have significant benefit when normal host antimicrobial functions are compromised.

There is a thorough discussion of what cathelicidins are and also of the role of calcitriol in the homeostasis of barrier functions. The clinician must take into account how vitamin D analogs affect these processes because the public interest in vitamin D is increasing out of proportion to the dermatologists' education about it. We also need to take a step back from our routines for treating with topical corticosteroids and understand where adjunctive agents such as calcitriol, retinoids, keratolytics, and similar treatments have potential benefits and can also minimize long-term adverse consequences.

N. Bhatia, MD

Allergic contact dermatitis caused by glycyrrhetinic acid and castor oil
Sasseville D, Desjardins M, Almutawa F (McGill Univ Health Centre, Montréal, Quebec, Canada)
Contact Dermatitis 64:168-169, 2011

Background.—The oil extracted from the seeds of the castor oil plant is used in many lipsticks as a humectant and pigment stabilizer. Rare cases of allergic contact dermatitis to its main fatty acid, ricinoleic acid, and its derivatives have been reported. Glycyrrhetinic acid is derived from the hydrolysis of glycyrrhizic acid, a principal component of licorice root. It has a steroid-like chemical structure and possesses anti-inflammatory, antibacterial, antiviral, and antifungal activities. It is used in the treatment of atopic dermatitis to provide anti-inflammatory and antipururitic effects. A woman who demonstrated allergies to both these agents was reported.

> *Case Report.*—Woman, 19, had a history of eczematous lesions developing where she had contact with costume jewelry and adhesive dressings. She suffered repeated episodes of contact dermatitis on the lips, axillae, and face over the course of 3 years. She believed two lip balms, a deodorant, and a post-sun moisturizing cream caused the problem. Patch testing was initially done using the North American Contact Dermatitis Group baseline series, the antimicrobials/vehicles/cosmetics series, and the four suspected cosmetics. Her positive reactions to colophonium and nickel sulfate were seen as representing past relevance. Each of the four cosmetics produced strong reactions. After determining the ingredients of the cosmetics from their manufacturers, patch testing was repeated, yielding positive reactions to *Ricinus communis* (castor oil plant) seed oil and glycyrrhetinic acid.

Conclusions.—The patient's reactions to *R communis* and glycyrrhetinic acid were concomitant reactions, since the chemical structures of the two molecules are completely different. Her weaker reaction to the higher concentration of glycyrrhetinic acid probably resulted from its anti-inflammatory effect. The recent increase in the use of glycyrrhetinic acid in cosmetics and therapeutic adjunctive products will likely produce more cases of allergic contact dermatitis in the future.

▶ Allergic contact dermatitis (ACD) is an important disease that in 2006 was reported to affect 14.5 million Americans each year. The adverse impact of ACD can be significant in terms of patient morbidity, loss of income due to time off from work, absence from school, and health care-related financial costs for visits to health care providers, patch testing, and other laboratory tests and medications. Once patch testing is performed and the allergen has been identified, recommendations related to avoidance of direct skin contact with allergan-containing triggers is vital to prevent relapse or progression of ACD to a chronic inflammatory or hyperkeratotis dermatosis.

However, in patients with ACD it is often difficult to identify the specific cause. This case report describes a woman who developed ACD from 4 different products in her cosmetic regimen. These 4 products were made by 4 different companies. With the aid of patch testing with all of the ingredients from all 4 cosmetic products, 2 individual ingredients induced a positive patch test reaction. The 2 ingredients were castor oil and glycyrrhetinic acid.

Castor oil is extracted from the seeds of *Ricinus communis*. It is used in most lipsticks as a humectant and pigment stabilizer.

Glycyrrhetinic acid is one of the main components of licorice root and possesses anti-inflammatory properties secondary to its suggested ability to slow the catabolism of cortisol in skin based on basic science research. Glycyrrhetinic acid has been used in "barrier repair" and moisturization products designed to mitigate inflammation associated with atopic dermatitis or irritation associated with some topical medications.

ACD to these 2 chemically unrelated ingredients is relatively uncommon but certainly does occur. However, this case report is a good reminder that any ingredient can potentially trigger ACD despite its widespread use in industry or its anti-inflammatory benefits.

Remember, even topical corticosteroids can occasionally induce ACD depending on their structural class and cross-reactivity.

J. Levin, DO
J. Q. Del Rosso, DO

Allergic contact dermatitis caused by tetrahydroxypropyl ethylenediamine in cosmetic products
Goossens A, Baret I, Swevers A (Univ Hosps Leuven, Belgium)
Contact Dermatitis 64:161-164, 2011

Background.—From 2004 to 2010, five patients developed contact allergic reactions to tetrahydroxypropyl ethylenediamine (INCI), which is used in cosmetics.

> *Case Reports.*—Case 1: Woman, 35, had eczema of 8 months' duration beginning on the back of her hands and spreading to the forearms, legs, and abdomen. Patch testing with the European baseline and rubber series plus her cosmetics yielded positive reactions to nickel sulfate, palladium chloride, and her hand cream, specifically the component INCI. Eczematous lesions on the hands and wrists tied directly to the hand cream applications, but the widespread eczema on the forearms and abdomen was seen as spread from the initial areas. She discontinued hand cream use and symptoms cleared.
>
> Case 2: Woman, 59, had recurrent eyelid dermatitis of 9 months' duration that extended to the face and V of the neck 2 weeks before coming for treatment. She ascribed this to the use of anti-aging creams. Patch testing with an extended European baseline series, cosmetic series, and her cosmetics showed a positive reaction to methylisothiazolinone, found in her shampoo, hair and body cleanser, and the anti-aging creams. INCI was the only ingredient to which she reacted positively on a subsequent test. With avoidance of the allergens, her eczema cleared.
>
> Case 3: Man, 24, had hand dermatitis of 2 months' duration first seen on his right ring finger, then on the backs of both hands and

wrists. Eczema developed on his eyelids 3 days before he saw the dermatologist. The patient was a laboratory technician and noted improvement in his condition during holidays, but deterioration when he returned to work. Patch testing with the European base-line series, rubber series, and ingredients of products to which he was exposed showed positive results to lanolin, benzalkonium chloride, cocamide diethanolamine (DEA), and two cosmetic products that contained lanolin and INCI. The relevance of the DEA was undetermined, but avoidance of the products involved led to complete resolution of symptoms.

Case 4: Woman, 47, had eczema of 2 months' duration mainly on the backs of her hands and fingers. A strong corticosteroid cream and a hydrating cream cleared the condition, but it recurred quickly after they were discontinued. Previous patch tests showed contact allergy to p-phenylenediamine, nickel sulfate, *Myroxylon pereirae*, fragrance mixes I and II in the European baseline series, and nitrile rubber and polyvinylchloride (PVC) gloves she wore at work. Additional patch testing revealed positive reactions to methyldibromo glutaronitrile and INCI. The patient admitted using a hand cream containing INCI and was diagnosed with irritant and allergic contact dermatitis to certain cleansing products.

Case 5: Woman, 49, had recurrent facial eczema of 2 months' duration that was especially pronounced in the mouth and eye area. Previous tests revealed a type I allergy to latex proteins and contact allergy to potassium dichromate, cobalt chloride, nickel sulfate, colophonium, lanolin, *M pereirae*, and fragrance mix I. Repeat patch testing showed positive reactions to colophonium, fragrance mixes I and II, and several components of her own perfumes, perfumes of her husband and sons, and INCI, which was used as a control substance. It was decided the atopic eczema was aggravated by direct and airborne contact with the perfumes, but the relevance of the positive reaction to INCI was puzzling. She may have had contact with products containing it, since she had used several moisturizers in the past.

Conclusions.—INCI is a chelating agent used in cosmetics such as anti-aging products, sunscreens, sunless tanning products, hand creams, moisturizers, deodorants and antiperspirants, shaving preparations, hairsprays, and lubricants and/or spermicides. It is similar to tetrahydroxyethyl ethylenediamine, which is also widely used as a chelating and buffering agent. Four patients had multiple sensitivities, but none reacted to either ethylenediamine dihydrochloride or disodium edetate (EDTA).

▶ This article is a case series describing 5 patients with sensitive skin reactions to tetrahydroxypropyl ethylenediamine (THPED). THPED is a chelating agent used in a wide variety of cosmetic products. Prior to this article, there was only 1 previously published case report of contact allergy to THPED.

In this case series, all of the patients except for 1 tested positive to multiple ingredients including THPED. Therefore, the question becomes, is the positive test result a false-positive secondary to angry back syndrome? Or have the authors of this article stumbled on a new potential allergen? The fact that each patient had a negative action to several ingredients in addition to positive reactions to several ingredients suggests that these patients are less likely to be in the hyperreactive state of angry back syndrome.

Interestingly, patients in all 5 cases had no reaction to chemically similar ingredients, such as ethylenediamine, disodium edetate, or ethylene dihydrochloride, suggesting that the allergic component of THPED may be a unique chemical component not found in these other chemically similar ingredients.

However, in addition to this case series bringing about awareness to a new potential allergen, THPED, it serves as a reminder that allergic reactions can be induced from commonly used ingredients in the cosmetic industry and that any ingredient can induce an allergic reaction.

J. Levin, DO

J. Q. Del Rosso, DO

Chemotherapy-related bilateral dermatitis associated with eccrine squamous syringometaplasia: Reappraisal of epidemiological, clinical, and pathological features

Martorell-Calatayud A, Sanmartín O, Botella-Estrada R, et al (Instituto Valenciano de Oncologia, Valenciaa, Spain; et al)
J Am Acad Dermatol 64:1092-1103, 2011

Background.—A characteristic cutaneous eruption related to the use of cytostatic chemotherapeutic drugs has been described in the literature. This condition appears to be characterized by an erythematous eruption, primarily affecting the intertriginous areas bilaterally, together with eccrine squamous syringometaplasia as the main histologic feature.

Objective.—We sought to establish the epidemiologic, clinical, and histologic characteristics of this poorly defined chemotherapy drug-related eruption.

Methods.—Retrospective data were collected from 21 consecutive patients with this clinical and histopathologic pattern who attended an oncology center between January 1999 and September 2009. Two skin biopsy specimens were obtained from all patients, with the first being taken within 24 hours of onset, and the second 72 to 96 hours after onset.

Results.—The patients analyzed were predominantly female (72%), with a mean age of 52 years (range 10-69 years). The lesions presented clinically as bilateral erythematous plaques affecting both axillae (95%), groin (88%), and side aspects of the neck (48%). The main histologic feature in all cases was eccrine squamous syringometaplasia, characterized by the transformation of the eccrine cuboidal epithelium into two or more layers of squamous cells with intercellular bridges. The onset of the eruption appeared within 30 days (range 2-30 days) after the initiation of the cytostatic agent infusion. The lesions resolved with desquamation and postinflammatory hyperpigmentation. The same cutaneous pattern recurred in up to 50% of patients in whom the oncologist reintroduced the cytostatic treatment.

Limitations.—Small sample size was a limitation.

Conclusions.—We suggest the term "chemotherapy-related bilateral dermatitis associated with eccrine squamous syringometaplasia" to describe this distinctive entity, which is primarily associated with pegylated liposomal doxorubicin infusions and chemotherapeutic regimens used in autologous bone-marrow transplantation.

▶ Chemotherapy-related bilateral dermatitis associated with eccrine squamous syringometaplasia (ESS) has been described in literature after the initiation of chemotherapeutic agents. The aim of this study was to describe a poorly defined entity with clinical and histologic features of a series of patients undergoing cytostatic therapy who developed bilateral intertriginous lesions associated with chemotherapeutic drug administration. Twenty-one patients presented with intertriginous dermatitis shortly after treatment with a chemotherapeutic agent. Clinical findings included pruritus or burning in 14 patients (66%), whereas 7 patients reported no symptoms (34%). The axilla was the most common site (20 patients [95%]) with the groin also being a common site of involvement. In all 21 patients, the onset of the eruption appeared within 30 days after the initiation of chemotherapy. Also, the eruptions were most often observed with pegylated liposomal doxorubicin and cytostatic treatments administered in autologous hematopoietic cell transplantation. However, the pathophysiology was not discussed in this article. There were no abnormal laboratory values observed. Biopsies showed transformation of the eccrine cuboidal epithelium into 2 or more layers of squamous cells with intraductal keratinization. Eruption onset in chemotherapy-related bilateral ESS ranges between 2 and 30 days after chemotherapy infusion. Lesions resolved on an average of 15 days with postinflammatory hyperpigmentation in some cases. The authors stated that a combination of topical and oral corticosteroids were effective for treatment and also suggest that a dose reduction of the chemotherapy agent would aid in treatment-resistant cases. Limitations to this study were the small sample size and single center bias. This article defines a chemotherapy-related cutaneous eruption that is characterized by bilateral, intertriginous, erythematous plaques histologically defined by ESS with chemotherapy-related epidermal changes.

G. K. Kim, DO

J. Q. Del Rosso, DO

Simvastatin-induced myoglobinuric acute kidney injury following ciclosporin treatment for alopecia universalis

Teutonico A, Libutti P, Lomonte C, et al (Miulli General Hosp, Acquaviva delle Fonti, Italy)
NDT Plus 3:273-275, 2010

Alopecia areata can affect the entire scalp (alopecia totalis) or cause loss of all body hair (alopecia universalis). Ciclosporin (CsA) has been suggested for its treatment, with controversial results. Concomitant use of statins and CsA may increase the risk of rhabdomyolysis due to drug-drug interactions.

Here we report the case of a 45-year-old woman treated with CsA for alopecia universalis, who presented a severe myoglobinuric acute kidney injury following the concomitant use of simvastatin. Upon admission to our unit, she was oligo-anuric. Her serum creatinine level was 13.8 mg/dl. CsA and simvastatin therapy were stopped, and haemodialysis treatment was started (eight daily dialysis sessions) until sufficient kidney function was regained. After 1 month, her serum creatinine level was 3.5 mg/dl; after 2 months and onwards (follow-up of 4 months), her serum creatinine level was 1.4 mg/dl and creatinine clearance was 43.2 ml/min.

In conclusion, physicians should be aware of the potential risks of the combined use of CsA and statins. Patients should be advised to report any muscle symptoms when they are on statins and CsA. The laboratory follow-up should include the monitoring of serum creatinine and muscle enzyme levels, blood CsA levels and liver function tests.

▶ Alopecia areata (AA) is a common condition that is usually localized to 1 or more small discoid foci on the scalp which usually reverses spontaneously over time or responds favorably to intralesional corticosteroid injection. In some cases, AA may progress rapidly to involve the entire scalp (alopecia totalis) or entire body (alopecia universalis). This is a case report of a 45-year-old women treated with cyclosporin (CsA) for alopecia universalis, who presented with severe myoglobinuric acute kidney injury with concomitant use of simvastatin. This woman was treated previously with injections of efalizumab without any clinical benefit. She was also started on CsA 150 mg twice daily and azathioprine 50 mg initially. The patient was on CsA for 1 year preceding treatment with simvastatin (20 mg/d). On admission to the hospital, a diagnosis of oligo-anuric myoglobinuric acute kidney injury was made (her serum creatinine of 13.8 mg/dL), which was attributed to concomitant use of simvastatin and CsA. Both drugs were withdrawn, and the patient was started on hemodialysis. After 2 months and beyond, serum creatinine reduced markedly; however, a final diagnosis of chronic kidney disease was made consequent to an episode of severe oligo-anuric myoglobinuric acute kidney injury. Nephrotoxicity is a therapeutic limitation to the use of CsA. The risk of statin-induced rhabdomyolysis is significantly increased when many of these agents are used concomitantly with such drugs as CsA, macrolide antibiotics, and azole antifungal agents (ie, ketoconazole, itraconazole). Both simvastatin and CsA are metabolized by the same hepatic enzyme system (cytochrome 3A4 [CYP 3A4]), as are many other statins, such as atorvastatin and lovastatin. Although this was a case report, there are other reports of this type of interaction with statins due to enzyme inhibition of CYP 3A4 by other drugs. Physicians should be aware of drug interactions such as this, which have established clinical relevance. In some cases, package inserts include important interactions with some statins as contraindications or warnings. Serum creatinine, muscle enzyme levels, blood CsA levels, and liver function tests should be monitored in patients that are on CsA.

G. K. Kim, DO

J. Q. Del Rosso, DO

Stevens—Johnson syndrome and toxic epidermal necrolysis: a review of treatment options
Worswick S, Cotliar J (David Geffen School of Medicine at UCLA; Northwestern Univ Feinberg School of Medicine, Chicago, IL)
Dermatol Ther 24:207-218, 2011

Stevens—Johnson syndrome (SJS) and toxic epidermal necrolysis (TEN) are severe cutaneous reactions that are medication-induced in most instances. While the clinical manifestations of SJS and TEN are well-defined, the optimal treatment for these disorders is not. Case reports have shown benefit with the use of a variety of agents including tumor necrosis factor-alpha inhibitors and cyclophosphamide, whereas thalidomide was associated with an increased mortality. Plasmapheresis and cyclosporine have also demonstrated efficacy anecdotally, albeit with an even smaller number of cases in the literature. Most of the reporting has focused on the use of systemic corticosteroids and intravenous immunoglobulin (IVIG) for these severe reactions. The majority of studies analyzing the use of IVIG in the treatment of SJS/TEN show a benefit, though more recent series cast doubt upon this conclusion. The results of these studies are summarized in this present review study.

▶ Stevens-Johnson syndrome (SJS) and toxic epidermal necrolysis (TEN) are associated with significant morbidity and mortality with treatment options that have been controversial. Patients with SJS have less than 10% of the body surface area (BSA) affected, while TEN is defined as greater than 30% BSA. This article reviews the treatment options of SJS/TEN. In treating SJS/TEN, the most important factor is the identification and withdrawal of the inciting agent, which may be more difficult to determine in elderly patients on multiple drug regimens. Systemic corticosteroids (CS) have been commonly used even though there is a lack of well-controlled evidence proving their efficacy in the treatment of SJS/TEN. Some authors have identified what they believe to be an increased morbidity or mortality when systemic CS are used to treat TEN. Some case reports have been published suggesting a benefit from the tumor necrosis factor (TNF)-alpha inhibitor, etanercept, based on targeting elevated TNF-α levels. Case reports have suggested that adding cyclophosphamide or cyclosporin to CS improves outcomes. According to retrospective studies, plasmapheresis may be an option for patients experiencing deterioration on systemic CS. There are also other studies investigating the role of intravenous immunoglobulin G (IVIG) for the treatment of SJS/TEN, but there is still great controversy on its use. Some studies have suggested that it does not improve outcome and does not affect re-epithelization, and others have found that it decreases the mean time to arrest disease progression. Because the pathophysiology pathways and genetic predisposition of SJS/TEN have not been completely elucidated, there may be different treatments for different stages of the disease or based on how early in the course of the disease treatment is initiated. What also adds to the confusion is that there is wide variability on the dosage and times when therapy is initiated, which confounds standardization of the results of these studies. Because SJS and TEN are rare diseases, these results may be difficult to obtain. Also, there needs to be more multicentered, prospective trials and head-to-head studies evaluating the efficacy of IVIG compared with systemic CS, cyclosporin, and TNF-alpha inhibitors, which is difficult to achieve because of the relative rarity of these disorders and inability to control many variables that can affect outcomes.

G. K. Kim, DO

J. Q. Del Rosso, DO

Toxic Epidermal Necrolysis with Prominent Facial Pustules: A Case with Reactivation of Human Herpesvirus 7
Honma M, Tobisawa S, Iinuma S, et al (Asahikawa Med College, Japan)
Dermatology 221:306-308, 2010

A 37-year-old Japanese man presented with confluent erythemas and progressive erosive lesions on almost the entire body including the oral mucosa and genitalia. This was accompanied with prominent facial pustules. Although a lymphocyte stimulation test was positive only for acetaminophen, he took other agents including carbamazepine for his depression. He was diagnosed as having toxic epidermal necrolysis with prominent facial pustules and treated by methylprednisolone pulse therapy, which resulted in a good response. During the course, human herpesvirus 7 (HHV-7) DNA was detected in his peripheral blood. The HHV-7 reactivation might be related to facial pustulosis, which is occasionally observed in drug-induced hypersensitivity syndrome/drug rash with eosinophilia and systemic symptoms.

▶ Toxic epidermal necrolysis (TEN) is a mucocutaneous disease characterized by tenderness and erythema of skin and mucosa followed by progressive necrosis and sloughing. Usually the underlying cause is drug-induced from the use of antibacterial (ie, sulfonamides), anticonvulsant, analgesic, or allopurinol drugs. The histology of biopsied specimen reveals epidermal separation at the dermal-epidermal junction with overlying epidermal necrosis. Because it is sometimes difficult to distinguish early Stevens-Johnson syndrome (SJS)/TEN from other drug reactions, elevated serum granulysin levels on rapid immunochromato-graphic testing was reported to be useful in diagnosis of SJS/TEN.[1] Drug rash with eosinophilia and systemic symptoms (DRESS), also referred to as drug-induced hypersensitivity syndrome (DIHS), is characterized by fever, an exanthem-like erythematous eruption, facial edema, internal organ involvement (often with elevation of hepatic enzymes), and sometimes human herpes virus-7 (HHV-7) reactivation. Cutaneous involvement can range from faint generalized exanthematous eruption to SJS/TEN. Anticonvulsants (ie, phenytoin, valproic acid, carbamazepine), allopurinol, nonsteroidal anti-inflammatories, and antibi-otics (sulfonamides, dapsone, minocycline) have been associated with DRESS.[2] The current report illustrates a case of a patient with TEN that was possibly induced by acetaminophen (with a positive drug-induced lymphocyte stimulation test) or carbamazepine, which was given simultaneously, with reactivation of HHV-7. The authors hypothesize that because this patient had facial pustulosis, which is an occasional finding in DRESS, that facial pustules may be a sign of HHV-6/7 reac-tivation. Additional case reports need to be rationally evaluated and more studies completed to substantiate these findings, as well as to develop better means of objectively differentiating the drugs that cause specific eruptions in individual cases.

S. Bellew, DO

J. Q. Del Rosso, DO

References

1. Fujita Y, Yoshioka N, Abe R, et al. Rapid immunochromatographic test for serum granulysin is useful for the prediction of Stevens-Johnson syndrome and toxic epidermal necrolysis. *J Am Acad Dermatol.* 2011;65:65-68.
2. Wolf R, Matz H, Marcos B, Orion E. Drug rash with eosinophilia and systemic symp-toms vs toxic epidermal necrolysis: the dilemma of classification. *Clin Dermatol.* 2005;23:311-314.

Irritation and allergy patch test analysis of topical treatments commonly used in wound care: Evaluation on normal and compromised skin

Trookman NS, Rizer RL, Weber T (Colorado Springs Dermatology Clinic PC; Thomas J. Stephens & Associates, Colorado Springs; Beiersdorf Inc, Wilton, CT)

J Am Acad Dermatol 64:S16-S22, 2011

Background.—Topical agents indicated for the treatment of superficial wounds have the potential to cause irritation or allergic contact dermatitis, particularly when applied to an impaired skin barrier.

Objective.—We sought to compare the irritancy potential of 5 topical wound care products commonly used in dermatologic practice on normal and compromised skin.

Methods.—Agents tested included Aquaphor Healing Ointment (AHO) (Beiersdorf Inc, Wilton, CT); bacitracin; Biafine Topical Emulsion (BTE) (OrthoNeutrogena, Los Angeles, CA); Neosporin (Poly/Bac/Neo) (Johnson & Johnson, New Brunswick, NJ); and Polysporin (Poly/Bac) (Johnson &

Johnson). Study 1 assessed cumulative irritation using a modified human repeat insult patch test on normal back skin with an induction phase (test materials applied under occlusive patch 9 times at 48- to 72-hour intervals) and a challenge phase (test materials applied to original and naïve sites for 48 hours, 12-24 days postinduction). Irritation was graded for erythema and type IV allergy skin responses. Study 2 assessed the acute irritation potential of agents on tape-stripped ("wounded") back skin. Test sites were graded for erythema, transepidermal water loss, and skin color (Chroma Meter a*) (Minolta, Osaka, Japan) at 48 and 72 hours poststripping.

Results.—In study 1, cumulative irritation testing in 108 subjects classified AHO, bacitracin, Poly/Bac/Neo, and Poly/Bac as "mild," and BTE as "probably mild." In study 2 at 72 hours, mean clinical grading scores were significantly higher for BTE and Poly/Bac/Neo than AHO. Transepidermal water loss and colorimeter a* values were significantly lower for AHO and bacitracin compared with BTE. No allergic contact dermatitis was seen in either study.

Conclusions.—Patch test studies demonstrated that BTE showed the greatest irritancy potential in both normal and compromised skin whereas AHO showed the least.

▶ The terms allergic and irritant as well as the diagnoses contact dermatitis and irritant dermatitis are confused and mistaken for each other too often. Although it might be trivial to some, many of us truly understand the significance of labeling one's chart with an allergy that limits therapeutic options or of creating an occupational issue based on exposures in which the patient is misdiagnosed with an allergy. In the case of the more popular topical antiinfective agents, as well as a common prescription agent, the label of "allergy" can create unnecessary limitations in wound care, both at home and in the clinic.

The results here were actually well summarized in the discussion: "No evidence of induced allergic contact dermatitis was seen with any of the test products," which was interesting, given the allergens involved. But the key point is that the prevalence of allergy to those products is said in the article to be low, even though awareness is high. The observation that the prescription agent is a stronger irritant than the over-the-counter therapies that contain the known allergens is compelling. The authors state that the presence of parabens and propylene glycol creates part of the irritant potential but that the typical habits of prescribing wound care agents are not affected by the presence of those elements as much as by the warning to patients to look for them on their own by reading content labels when obtaining them over the counter.

So what are the learning points here? That the precise vocabularies of our diagnoses must resonate with those of patients so as to avoid unnecessary limitations; that over-the-counter agents can be more acceptable in a regimen than a prescription product; and that we should carefully scrutinize study data so that we can reinforce definitions for ourselves as well as incorporate other practice options.

N. Bhatia, MD

The risk of infection and malignancy with tumor necrosis factor antagonists in adults with psoriatic disease: A systematic review and meta-analysis of randomized controlled trials

Dommasch ED, Abuabara K, Shin DB, et al (Univ of Pennsylvania, Philadelphia)

J Am Acad Dermatol 64:1035-1050, 2011

Background.—There is a need to better understand the safety of tumor necrosis factor (TNF) inhibitors in patients with psoriatic disease in whom TNF inhibitors are frequently used as monotherapy.

Objective.—We sought to examine the risks of infection and malignancy with the use of TNF antagonists in adult patients with psoriatic disease.

Methods.—We conducted a systematic search for trials of TNF antagonists for adults with plaque psoriasis and psoriatic arthritis. We included randomized, placebo-controlled trials of etanercept, infliximab, adalimumab, golimumab, and certolizumab for the treatment of plaque psoriasis and psoriatic arthritis. Twenty of 820 identified studies with a total of 6810 patients were included. Results were calculated using fixed effects models and reported as pooled odds ratios.

Results.—Odds ratios for overall infection and serious infection over a mean of 17.8 weeks were 1.18 (95% confidence interval [CI] 1.05-1.33) and 0.70 (95% CI 0.40-1.21), respectively. When adjusting for patient-years, the incidence rate ratio for overall infection was 1.01 (95% CI 0.92-1.11). The odds ratio for malignancy was 1.48 (95% CI 0.71-3.09) and 1.26 (95% CI 0.39-4.15) when nonmelanoma skin cancer was excluded.

Limitations.—Short duration of follow-up and rarity of malignancies and serious infections are limitations.

Conclusions.—There is a small increased risk of overall infection with the short-term use of TNF antagonists for psoriasis that may be attributable to differences in follow-up time between treatment and placebo groups. There was no evidence of an increased risk of serious infection and a statistically significant increased risk in cancer was not observed with short-term use of TNF inhibitors.

▶ Tumor necrosis factor α (TNF-α) antagonists are now widely used for psoriatic disease and frequently as monotherapy. Details about the risk of infection and malignancy associated with TNF-α antagonists have been mostly studied in patients with rheumatoid arthritis (RA) or inflammatory bowel disease. As noted by the authors, in the meta-analyses of TNF-α inhibitors in patients with RA, there have been indications of increased risk of infection and malignancy. Consequently, Dommasch et al sought to perform a systemic review and meta-analysis of 20 randomized controlled trials involving 6810 patients to determine the risk of infection and malignancy associated with using TNF-α antagonists in patients with psoriatic disease, including psoriasis (PsO), psoriatic arthritis (PsA), or both. Of the studies reviewed, all patients included in PsA trials were allowed to be on at least 1 concomitant disease-modifying antirheumatic drug, but patients were excluded in the PsO trials if they were on concomitant immunosuppressant therapy. Of the 20 trials, 7 included patients with active PsA (and in 5 of these trials the patients were also required to have active psoriatic skin lesions), and the remaining 13 reviewed trials included patients with moderate to severe PsO.

The results of this large meta-analysis were interesting and of particular importance to dermatologists treating psoriatic disease. The findings of the analysis concluded that there was a small increase in overall infections among patients using short-term TNF-α antagonists for psoriatic disease. However, when this was adjusted for follow-up, there was no statistically significant risk of overall infection. Importantly, there was also no evidence of an increased risk of serious infection. In fact, among the patients who developed infections, the infections were nonserious in 97.6%—the majority having uncomplicated upper respiratory tract infections. In terms of malignancy, there was also no statistically significant increase in the risk of malignancy in psoriatic patients treated with TNF-α inhibitors. However, there were limitations to the study, including the fact the meta-analysis was based on short-term TNF-α antagonist use and not long-term use. This is significant, especially when evaluating potential sequelae such as serious infections and malignancy. The current finding that the risk of malignancy is not a statistically significant risk could potentially change with long-term use, because the authors note that the concern for malignancy "may take years of exposure to accurately define the risk." Moreover, serious infections have been reported previously in patients with TNF-α antagonists, including patients with psoriatic disease, so monitoring by the practitioner to properly screen patients for certain infections (ie, tuberculosis) before starting therapy is suggested. Patients should continue to be monitored for infection during treatment with TNF-α antagonists. Also, the study findings might have been different if the patients were using their TNF-α inhibitor with other immunosuppressive therapy; as the authors note, there is evidence regarding a potential "synergistic effect with the use of anti-TNF agents and other immunosuppressants on the risk of infection and malignancy," although this combination is not consistently utilized in the treatment of psoriasis. Regardless, the results of this meta-analysis are still encouraging and helpful to dermatologists. Overall, this study provides practitioners (and patients) with valuable tangible data that the risk of infection and malignancy associated with short-term use of a TNF-α antagonist may be more favorable than previously thought, at least with regard to use as monotherapy in psoriatic patients.

B. D. Michaels, DO

J. Q. Del Rosso, DO

The cutaneous and systemic manifestations of azathioprine hypersensitivity syndrome
Bidinger JJ, Sky K, Battafarano DF, et al (San Antonio Military Med Ctr, TX)
J Am Acad Dermatol 65:184-191, 2011

Background.—Azathioprine (AZA) hypersensitivity syndrome is a rare side effect that typically occurs early in the initiation of therapy and may include a cutaneous eruption. It is often under-recognized because it mimics infection or disease exacerbation. Until recently, the cutaneous findings associated with AZA hypersensitivity have been reported using nonspecific, descriptive terms without a supportive diagnostic biopsy.

Objective.—To characterize the cutaneous and histologic findings associated with AZA hypersensitivity syndrome.

Methods.—We conducted a retrospective analysis of two cases of AZA hypersensitivity syndrome and describe the cutaneous manifestations and histological findings of each case. A review of the English literature for cases of AZA hypersensitivity or allergic or adverse reactions associated with AZA was performed.

Results.—Sixty-seven cases of AZA hypersensitivity were reviewed; 49% (33/67) had cutaneous manifestations. Of those cases presenting with cutaneous findings, 76% (25/33) had biopsy results or clinical features consistent with a neutrophilic dermatosis, whereas the other 24% (8/33) were reported as a nonspecific cutaneous eruption.

Limitations.—Only case reports in which the skin findings could be classified were reviewed.

Conclusions.—The predominant cutaneous reaction reported in the literature and observed in the present case series is a neutrophilic dermatosis. Hypersensitivity to AZA can manifest along a wide clinical spectrum from local neutrophilic disease to a systemic syndrome. Skin findings may be an important early clue to the diagnosis of AZA hypersensitivity and aid in prompt recognition and treatment of this potentially life-threatening adverse drug effect.

▶ Azathioprine (AZA) is an immunosuppressive agent used as a steroid-sparing option in the treatment of many systemic autoimmune conditions such as inflammatory bowel disease, systemic lupus erythematosus, myasthenia gravis, and others. This is a summary of 2 cases of AZA hypersensitivity syndrome and a review of the literature to better characterize the skin findings. AZA hypersensitivity syndrome is a dose-independent reaction that occurs during the first weeks of therapy. The most common systemic symptoms include fever, malaise, arthralgias, myalgias, nausea, vomiting, diarrhea, and a cutaneous eruption. The most common reported cutaneous manifestations are Sweet's syndrome, erythema nodosum, acute generalized exanthematous pustulosis, leukocytoclastic vasculitis, or nonspecific eruption. The authors found that symptoms and cutaneous findings often improve within 5 days of discontinuing AZA. They suggested that the presence of new skin findings in the absence of infection should alert the clinician to the possibility of AZA hypersensitivity, which can resolve within 2 to 3 days after withdrawal of medication if caught early. Rechallenge is contraindicated because of the potential for a life-threatening shock syndrome. From the review of literature of 75 cases of AZA hypersensitivity, the authors found that 76% had biopsies showing a neutrophilic dermatosis. This was unrelated to the gender, age, or thiopurine methyltransferase (TMPT) levels. Because AZA hypersensitivity has been associated with shock syndrome, clinicians must be aware of cutaneous manifestations that may be a warning that AZA hypersensitivity syndrome is developing, especially in patients who have recently started the drug.

G. K. Kim, DO

J. Q. Del Rosso, DO

Impact of etanercept treatment on ultraviolet B-induced inflammation, cell cycle regulation and DNA damage

Gambichler T, Tigges C, Dith A, et al (Department of Dermatology, Ruhr-University Bochum, Bochum)

Br J Dermatol 164:110-115, 2011

Background.—Current studies indicate that treatment with tumour necrosis factor (TNF)-α blockers plus ultraviolet (UV) B phototherapy results in higher relative Psoriasis Area and Severity Index reduction as compared with TNF-α monotherapy.

Objectives.—This study aimed to investigate the acute impact of etanercept on UVB-induced inflammation, cell cycle regulation and DNA damage.

Methods.—Eleven subjects diagnosed with psoriasis who fulfilled the indication criteria for etanercept treatment were studied. A healthy skin site on the upper back was treated with UVB at 2 minimal erythema doses (MED). After 1, 24 and 72 h punch biopsies were taken from this site. Following the 72 h biopsy etanercept 50 mg was administered subcutaneously. After 48 h, 2 MED was given on healthy skin adjacent to previously treated skin sites. Again, after 1, 24 and 72 h punch biopsies were taken from this site. UVB- as well as UVB plus etanercept-treated skin was assessed by means of colorimetry and immunohistochemical studies for caspase 3, cyclin D_1, interleukin-12, Ki-67, p16, p53, survivin, thymine dimers and TNF-α.

Results.—Erythema formation did not differ significantly between UVB- and UVB plus etanercept-treated sites. Comparisons between UVB- and UVB plus etanercept-treated sites at a given time (1, 24, 72 h) did not result in significant differences in immunoreactivity of the markers investigated, except for cyclin D_1, p53 and survivin. Immunoreactivity of cyclin D_1 and p53 was significantly decreased in UVB plus etanercept-treated sites at 24 h. Survivin expression was significantly higher in UVB plus etanercept-treated skin as compared with UVB monotherapy.

Conclusions.—Our data indicate that combined treatment with broadband UVB and TNF-α blockers might increase the risk of photocarcinogenesis by influencing apoptotic as well as antiapoptotic pathways.

▶ Several studies have looked at the addition of ultraviolet B phototherapy to biologics in the treatment of psoriasis, and many have reported improved response rates. Does biologic therapy impact the effect of ultraviolet B on inflammation and cell cycle regulation or DNA damage? The authors of this study set out to answer that question by exposing healthy skin on the backs of 11 subjects to 2 minimal erythema doses. Punch biopsies were taken from the irradiated skin at 1,

24, and 72 hours. The same patients were then treated with a single 50-mg dose of etanercept, and after 48 hours the same procedure was performed, administering 2 minimal erythema doses of ultraviolet B to the healthy skin of the upper back and repeating biopsies at 1, 24, and 72 hours. Immunohistochemical studies were performed for caspase 3, cyclin D1, interleukin-12, Ki-67, p16, p53, survivin, thymine dimers, and tumor necrosis factor (TNF)—alpha.

Degree of erythema measured by colorimetry was not affected by the addition of etanercept. All of the markers studied were also unaffected by etanercept except for cyclin D1, p53, and survivin. At 24 hours, etanercept treatment resulted in significantly lower cyclin D1 and p53. Survivin was increased by etanercept treatment.

The gene p53 is a tumor suppressor gene that is increased in conditions in which there is DNA damage. p53 protein turns off DNA synthesis allowing time for either DNA repair or for apoptosis. Reduction in p53 levels would, therefore, be expected to contribute to photo-carcinogenesis. Similarly, a reduction in cyclin D1, which regulates the cell cycle, might be expected to enhance photocarcinogenesis. Conversely, survivin is an inhibitor of apoptosis and its increase would also be expected to signal an increase in photocarcinogenesis. Based on these data, the authors speculate that TNF-alpha blockers might increase the risk of photocarcinogenesis.

The authors make important points, but their study is very small, and their statement that TNF-alpha blockers might increase the risk of photocarcinogenesis must be viewed as speculative. To prove that point, we will need registries of thousands of patients treated for many years.

M. Lebwohl, MD

Etanercept: An Overview of Dermatologic Adverse Events
Lecluse LLA, Dowlatshahi EA, Limpens CEJM, et al (Univ of Amsterdam, the Netherlands; Dutch Cochrane Centre, Amsterdam, the Netherlands)
Arch Dermatol 147:79-94, 2011

Objectives.—To provide a comprehensive overview of dermatologic adverse events of etanercept described in the literature (including all study types, case reports, and surveys) and to present information on the occurrence, severity, treatment, and course of these adverse events.

Data Sources.—MEDLINE and EMBASE.

Study Selection.—All reports on individual patients who developed a dermatologic adverse event associated with systemic etanercept treatment for any indication in any type of original article were included.

Data Extraction.—All data were independently extracted by 2 reviewers. Disagreements were resolved by consensus. All articles included (except for case reports/case series) were assessed regarding level of evidence.

Data Synthesis.—In 126 included study reports, a total of 72 separate specific dermatologic adverse events of etanercept were mentioned. In 101 case reports/case series, 153 individual patients with approximately 65 different specific diagnoses (eg, not rash) were reported.

Conclusions.—Etanercept is associated with a wide variety of dermatologic adverse events, many of which were described in study reports, but case reports also described numerous exceptional cases. Although the adverse events are usually mild, some reactions are serious and even potentially life threatening. Therefore, all drug-associated cutaneous abnormalities should be carefully evaluated. Diagnostic steps do not deviate from the norm in these patients, but management of the dermatologic adverse events may need special attention.

▶ Etanercept is a recombinant human tumor necrosis factor (TNF)-α blocker that is currently Food and Drug Administration-approved for treatment of psoriasis, psoriatic arthritis, rheumatoid arthritis, juvenile rheumatoid arthritis, and ankylosing spondylitis. This biologic agent is associated with well-known side effects including injection-site reaction, rare serious infections such as tuberculosis, malignancies, drug-induced lupus, cytopenias, multiple sclerosis, and exacerbation and new onset of congestive heart failure.[1] More specifically, the current article is a systematic review of dermatologic adverse events that are associated with etanercept. The more commonly reported cutaneous side effects are psoriasiform dermatoses, nonmelanoma skin cancers, some forms of lupus erythematosus, and other rare malignant neoplasms. The authors theorize that inhibition of TNF by etanercept can induce overexpression of cutaneous interferon-α, which in turn predisposes to psoriasis. For most of the aforementioned side effects, discontinuation of the drug will yield clinical improvement. However, for many patients on biologics, alternative treatments are scarce at that point. Therefore, treatment discontinuation for mild to moderate adverse events may not be warranted, depending on their nature.

S. Bellew, DO

J. Q. Del Rosso, DO

Reference

1. Menter A, Gottlieb A, Feldman S, et al. Guidelines of care for the management of psoriasis and psoriatic arthritis: section 1. Overview of psoriasis and guidelines of care for the treatment of psoriasis with biologics. *J Am Acad Dermatol.* 2008;58: 826-850.

Occurrence of pustular psoriasis after treatment of Crohn disease with infliximab

Pourciau C, Shwayder T (Henry Ford Hosp, Detroit, MI)
Pediatr Dermatol 27:539-540, 2010

We report a case of pustular psoriasis induced by anti-TNF-α therapy in a 12-year-old boy with inflammatory bowel disease. This is a well-documented phenomenon but remains a clinical challenge, especially when presenting in the pediatric setting.

▶ This is a case report of a 12-year-old boy who was treated successfully for Crohn disease with infliximab. Six months after starting therapy he developed a rash on the left foot that progressed to both distal extremities and was refractory to topical antifungal agents and topical corticosteroids (CS). Three months after the start of the rash, pustules were noted. At the time of his visit, the patient had characteristic psoriasiform lesions affecting the left palms, knees, shins, and dorsal surfaces of the feet with pustules on the lateral sole and desquamation on the volar surfaces of the feet. Infliximab was discontinued and topical CS added with little benefit. Methotrexate 20 mg weekly was started for treatment of the patient's Crohn disease, and the rash cleared within 4 months.

The authors review the literature of tumor necrosis factor (TNF)-alpha antagonist-induced psoriasis and mention that in many cases, cutaneous lesions are managed with topical CS without stopping the TNF blocker. While TNF-alpha antagonist—induced psoriasis is thought to be a class effect, some patients do not develop new lesions of psoriasis when switched to another TNF-alpha blocker. In the current case, methotrexate was effective at controlling the disease in a patient who had discontinued infliximab several months earlier.

This case report adds little to the large body of knowledge that is accumulating about TNF-alpha antagonist—induced psoriasis. It does emphasize that the condition can occur in the pediatric age group. We still don't know why drugs that treat psoriasis in some patients appear to cause psoriasis in others.

M. Lebwohl, MD

Ipilimumab: Unleashing the Power of the Immune System Through CTLA-4 Blockade
Boasberg P, Hamid O, O'Day S (The Angeles Clinic and Res Inst, Los Angeles, CA)
Semin Oncol 37:440-449, 2010

Malignant melanoma is rising faster in incidence than any other malignancy. Long-term remission or "cure" is rare and is almost exclusively limited to therapies that stimulate an immune antitumor response. Ipilimumab is a novel targeted human immunostimulatory monoclonal antibody that blocks cytotoxic T-lymphocyte antigen4 (CTLA-4), an immune-inhibitory site expressed on activated T cells. Ipilimumab is well tolerated as an outpatient infusion therapy. Multiple studies have confirmed significant antimelanoma activity. A randomized trial has documented a survival benefit when ipilimumab was compared to a gp-100 vaccine only arm. The unique mechanism of action of ipilimumab makes assessment of response by conventional criteria difficult. Benefit from ipilimumab can occur after what would be considered progression with World Health Oganization (WHO) or Response Evaluation Criteria in Solid Tumors (RECIST) criteria. New immune response criteria have been proposed. Therapeutic responses peak between 12 and 24 weeks, with slow responses continuing up to and beyond 12 months. The major drug- related adverse side effects (10%—15% grade 3 or above) are immune-related and consist most commonly of rash, colitis, hypophysitis, thyroiditis, and hepatitis. Colonic perforation can occur and patients with diarrhea have to be monitored carefully with strict adherence to treatment algorithms. Algorithms for the treatment of other adverse side effects have been developed. The treatment of immune-related side effects with immunosuppressive agents, such as corticosteroids, does not appear to impair antitumor response. With proper monitoring and management of side effects, ipilimumab is an extremely safe drug to administer. The benefits of ipilimumab will most certainly extend to other malignancies in the near future.

▶ There is no doubt that ipilimumab, a targeted human monoclonal antibody and immune response stimulator with high affinity for CTLA-4, has been the most important development of the last decade in the treatment of metastatic melanoma, not only because it can be used in certain cases as a monotherapeutic agent but also because it actually improves the median and long-term survival in these patients. When CTLA-4 on T cells binds to the costimulatory ligand B7 on antigen-presenting cells, there is inhibition of the immune response. Ipilimumab binds to CTLA-4 and prevents this inhibition of the immune response, increasing the proliferation of activated T cells. This article summarizes years of research and the current state of ipilimumab for the treatment of advanced melanoma. Phase I studies showed that durable responses were obtained with multiple dose regimens, and although data from 3 phase II efficacy trials has shown 1-year survival rates up to 62.4%, a more recent meta-analysis of phase II trials obtained a 1-year survival rate around 25%. Immune-related adverse events were dose dependent. A phase III study showed an improvement in median and long-term survival, response rate, disease control, and progression-free survival in the 2 ipilimumab arms compared with gp100 vaccine alone in HLA-A2.01–positive patients. The addition of the vaccine added no benefits to the overall survival. Studies in HLA-A2.01–negative patients have shown similar results, including similar prevalence of immune-related adverse events. Treatment combinations of ipilimumab with dacarbazine (DTIC) and other chemotherapeutic agents have shown increase in efficacy of therapy. Treatment with ipilimumab has also shown promising results in patients with metastatic disease to the central nervous system, which represents a great advance compared to prior treatments. However, results from ongoing studies are still pending. Also in the article, there is a description of the most common adverse events occurring with ipilimumab, including a pruritic rash that affects nearly 50% of the patients treated, diarrhea and/or intestinal bleeding, hepatotoxicity, and endocrine alterations, including hypophysitis/hypopituitism, with low levels of corticotropin and cortisol as the most commonly seen. Of importance, immunosuppressive therapy for several of these immune-related adverse events does not cause interference with the antitumoral effects of ipilimumab. We are expectant of the results of large ongoing phase III studies for further characterization of ipilimumab's effects in the treatment of advanced melanoma.

B. Berman, MD, PhD
S. Amini, MD

Fas-ligand staining in non-drug- and drug-induced maculopapular rashes

Wang ECE, Lee JSS, Tan AWH, et al (Natl Skin Centre, Singapore)
J Cutan Pathol 38:196-201, 2011

Background.—Morphologically and histopathologically, drug- and non-drug-induced maculopapular rashes can be almost indistinguishable. It has been postulated that Fas-ligand (Fas-L) is involved in the pathogenesis of drug rashes but not in the genesis of rashes, such as viral exanthems, that are not induced by medications.

Aim.—This study sought to determine if epidermal Fas-L is a distinguishing feature in the pathology of drug and non-drug maculopapular rashes.

Methods.—Archived skin biopsies of patients with a confirmed diagnosis of drug or non-drug maculopapular rashes ($n = 10$ each) and positive and negative controls were retrieved for immunohistochemical staining for Fas-L. The proportion of Fas-L-positive skin biopsies were compared. The presence of tissue eosinophilia was also evaluated.

Results.—Ten percent of non-drug-induced rashes were Fas-L positive compared to 50% of drug rashes ($p = 0.05$). Twenty percent of non-drug exanthems had moderate tissue eosinophilia, while 60% from drug rashes had moderate to dense tissue eosinophilia ($p = 0.17$).

Conclusion.—There is a trend toward Fas-L being more prevalent in the epidermis of drug maculopapular rashes, although this did not reach statistical significance. This is possibly because of the small sample size.

▶ In this retrospective pilot study, the authors attempted to demonstrate a relationship between the presence of Fas-ligand and drug-induced maculopapular rashes. As the authors stated in the article, the presence of positive Fas-ligand detected in skin biopsies was more prevalent in the group of patients with drug-induced rashes than in the group of patients with non-drug-induced rashes, but there was no significant statistical difference between the 2 groups. Analyzing separately the group of patients with drug-induced rashes, the presence of Fas-ligand in only 50% of the cases is still too low to establish some degree of correlation. However, the concept is interesting and warrants further investigation in a prospective fashion, with a larger sample size, and establishing clear and objective criteria for the classification of both study groups. At this point, it is too early to conclude that this stain can be useful in the clinical setting.

B. Berman, MD, PhD

S. Amini, MD

Penicillin skin testing in the evaluation and management of penicillin allergy

Fox S, Park MA (Mayo Clinic, Rochester, MN)
Ann Allergy Asthma Immunol 106:1-7, 2011

Objective.—To review the role of penicillin skin testing in the evaluation and management of penicillin allergy mediated by IgE.

Data Sources.—PubMed and OVID search of English-language articles regarding penicillin allergy, penicillin allergy testing, and management of penicillin allergy.

Study Selection.—Articles pertinent to the subject matter were selected and reviewed.

Results.—The major determinant (benzylpenicillin polylysine) detects the greatest number of penicillin allergic patients during skin testing, and the minor determinants of penicillin increase the sensitivity of penicillin skin testing. Penicillin skin testing to the major and minor determinants was found to have a negative predictive value of 97% to 99%. The incidence of systemic adverse reaction to penicillin skin testing is less than 1%.

Conclusion.—A detailed history of the prior reaction to penicillin is an integral part of the evaluation, but it is not accurate in predicting a positive penicillin skin test result. A patient with a negative penicillin skin test result to the major and minor determinants is at a low risk of an immediate-type hypersensitivity reaction to penicillin. Patients with a positive skin test result

TABLE 1.—Penicillin Reagents Used During Penicillin Skin Tests and Outcomes of Penicillin Challenge

Source	Positive Penicillin Skin Test Result, No. (%)	Negative Penicillin Skin Test Result, No. (%)	Patients Challenged With Penicillin, No. (%)	Adverse Reactions to Penicillin Challenge, No. (%)
del Real et al[17b]	49/596 (8.2)	527/596 (88.4)	290	5/290 (1.7)
Jost et al[30]	177/921 (19)	744 (81)	NA	NA
Goldberg et al[18]	73/169 (43)	96/169 (57)	94	4/94 (4.3)
Wong et al[14]	16/91 (18)	75/91 (82)	72	2/72 (2.8)
Gadde et al[10]	55/776 (7.1)	700/776 (90)	649	54/649 (8.3)
Cetinkaya and Cag[32d]	15/147 (10.2)	132/147 (89.8)	NA	NA
Sogn et al[26e]	146/825 (18)	656/825 (80)	566	7/566 (1.2)
Mendelson et al[22]	21/240 (9)	219 (91)	219	3/219 (1.4)
Levine et al[19f]	12/90 (13)	77/90 (86)	77	1/77 (1.3)

Abbreviations: MDM1, penicillin G; MDM2, penilloate, penicilloate, and penicillin G; MDM3, penicillin G and penicilloate; MDM4, penicillin G, penicilloate, and benzylpenicilloyl-N-propylamine; NA, not available.

Editor's Note: Please refer to original journal article for full references.

[a]Note that reactions were considered IgE mediated if the reaction occurred within the first 72 hours unless otherwise specified by the author.

[c]Includes history-positive and history-negative patients.

[b]Penicillin skin test result was indeterminate in 20 patients (3.4%). Patients could have been challenged with any β-lactams, but most patients were given penicillins.

[d]Study tested children without a history of penicillin allergy.

[e]Twenty-three patients (3%) had a penicillin skin test result that was uninterruptible.

[f]Penicillin skin test result was uninterruptible in 1 patient.

should undergo desensitization to penicillin or an alternative antibiotic should be considered (Table 1).

▶ As a dermatologist who specializes in patch testing, I am often asked about skin testing for systemic drug allergy. Several European studies have suggested that patch testing for allergy to certain anticonvulsant agents has some reasonable predictive capacity, and cross-reaction between some topical allergens and systemic agents (eg, neomycin and aminoglycosides) can be shown. Nevertheless, overall there are no reliable skin tests that predict systemic drug allergy or hypersensitivity, with the exception of penicillin. This excellent review discusses the usefulness of skin prick and/or intradermal testing in assessing penicillin allergy, with several points worthy of emphasis. First, patient history is a poor predictor of true penicillin allergy. In the history, it is important to differentiate immunoglobulin (Ig) E–type symptoms (early onset, urticaria, anaphylaxis, etc) as opposed to other types of drug reactions (serum sickness, Stevens-Johnson syndrome, etc). Skin testing is able to detect only IgE-mediated reactions. Second, the "major" allergen—benzylpenicillin polylysine—will identify from 65% to 90% of penicillin allergy cases (Table 1). Adding the "minor determinants" and/or amoxicillin will increase positive yield. If tests to both major and minor determinants are negative, the patient has a small chance (< 1%–3%) of suffering an IgE reaction to oral penicillins. Finally, the skin test itself is generally safe. Reported rates of systemic reactions upon testing are in the range of 1% to 2%. Prick testing should always be performed before intradermal testing, because intradermal testing carries a greater risk of systemic reaction. The conclusion is that skin testing can be useful in assessing true penicillin allergy, especially in patients with an apparent reliable history of possible IgE-mediated hypersensitivity.

J. F. Fowler, MD

12 Drug Development and Promotion

Chemoprevention of Chemically Induced Skin Tumorigenesis by Ligand Activation of Peroxisome Proliferator–Activated Receptor-β/δ and Inhibition of Cyclooxygenase 2

Zhu B, Bai R, Kennett MJ, et al (The Pennsylvania State Univ; et al)
Mol Cancer Ther 9:3267-3277, 2010

Ligand activation of peroxisome proliferator-activated receptor-β/δ (PPARβ/δ) and inhibition of cyclooxygenase-2 (COX2) activity by nonsteroidal anti-inflammatory drugs (NSAID) can both attenuate skin tumorigenesis. The present study examined the hypothesis that combining ligand activation of PPARβ/δ with inhibition of COX2 activity will increase the efficacy of chemoprevention of chemically induced skin tumorigenesis over that observed with either approach alone. To test this hypothesis, wild-type and *Pparβ/δ*-null mice were initiated with 7,12-dimethylbenz[*a*]anthracene (DMBA), topically treated with 12-O-tetradecanoylphorbol-13-acetate to promote tumorigenesis, and then immediately treated with topical application of the PPARβ/δ ligand GW0742, dietary administration of the COX2 inhibitor nimesulide, or both GW0742 and nimesulide. Ligand activation of PPARβ/δ with GW0742 caused a PPARβ/δ-dependent delay in the onset of tumor formation. Nimesulide also delayed the onset of tumor formation and caused inhibition of tumor multiplicity (46%) in wild-type mice but not in *Pparβ/δ*-null mice. Combining ligand activation of PPARβ/δ with dietary nimesulide resulted in a further decrease of tumor multiplicity (58%) in wild-type mice but not in *Pparβ/δ*-null mice. Biochemical and molecular analysis of skin and tumor samples show that these effects were due to the modulation of terminal differentiation, attenuation of inflammatory signaling, and induction of apoptosis through both PPARβ/δ-dependent and PPARβ/δ-independent mechanisms. Increased levels and activity of PPARβ/δ by nimesulide were also observed. These studies support the hypothesis that combining ligand activation of PPARβ/δ with inhibition of COX2 activity increases the efficacy of preventing chemically induced skin tumorigenesis as compared with either approach alone.

▶ The role of prostaglandins in tumorigenesis has been known for many years. Cyclooxygenase (COX) and particularly the isoform 2 (COX2) has been detected in elevated quantities in several human cancers, including colon carcinoma,

273

squamous cell carcinoma of the esophagus, and skin cancer, after its induction by several oncogenes. Inhibition of COX2, the rate-limiting enzyme in the synthesis of prostaglandins, has been shown to decrease expression of bcl-2, and interleukin (IL)-6 (which enhances haptoglobin synthesis) and to induce apoptosis. Prostaglandins are also associated with the development of metastasis, IL-6 with cancer cell invasion, and haptoglobin with implantation and angiogenesis. In addition to specific receptors, prostaglandins may also modulate peroxisome proliferator-activated receptors (PPAR). One isoform in particular, PPARβ/δ, has been found in high levels in the nucleus of, and has an important constitutive role in, the epithelium, including intestine and keratinocytes. Prior studies have demonstrated that upon stimulation, PPARβ/δ inhibits epidermal cell proliferation; PPARβ/δ-dependent inhibition of skin tumorigenesis (chemoprevention) is found after topical application of the ligand GW0742; nonsteroidal antiinflammatory drugs (NSAIDs) attenuate carcinogenesis by inhibiting PPARβ/δ expression or activity (or both); and combining COX2 inhibition and ligand activation of PPARβ/δ increase chemoprevention. This interesting murine-controlled study showed that dietary COX2 inhibitor (nimesulide), topical activator of PPARβ/δ (GW0742), and the combination of both, were capable of enhanced chemoprevention, decreased tumor multiplicity, and decreased tumor size distribution in wild-type mice compared with PPARβ/δ-null mice. However, some mechanisms were determined to be PPARβ/δ-independent and still must be elucidated in future studies. PPARβ/δ-dependent mechanisms included enhancement of terminal differentiation correlated with the obtained increased expression of keratin 1 (K1) protein, antiinflammatory activity correlated with the reduction in the expression of TNF-alpha mRNA, the inhibition of IL-6, and the reduction in accumulation of infiltrating PMN. In regard to apoptosis, only nimesulide was able to increase the apoptotic signaling in mouse keratinocytes, probably through PPARβ/δ-independent pathways. This study shows the molecular basis of one of the multiple factors involved in chemoprevention of skin tumorigenesis and shows in part that a multifactorial approach is still necessary to obtain a certain degree of effective chemoprevention. Randomized Phase II studies have shown that the addition of COX2 inhibitors to chemotherapeutic regimens have significantly increased progression-free survival compared with the control group in patients with metastatic melanomas, previously unresponsive to chemotherapy alone; and retrospective studies have shown a short-term (<5 years) protective effect for the development of nonmelanoma skin cancer in NSAID users compared with nonusers. This is a controversial and interesting field that needs further evaluation.

B. Berman, MD, PhD
S. Amini, MD

Efficacy and Safety Evaluation of a Novel Botulinum Toxin Topical Gel for the Treatment of Moderate to Severe Lateral Canthal Lines

Brandt F, O'Connell C, Cazzaniga A, et al (Dermatology Res Inst, Coral Gables, FL; et al)
Dermatol Surg 36:2111-2118, 2010

Background.—Botulinum toxin type A (BoNTA) is commonly injected to treat facial wrinkles. Complications include pain, erythema, bruising, and potential infection. RT001 Botulinum Toxin Type A Topical Gel (RT001) is under development for the treatment of lateral canthal lines (LCLs).

Objective.—To assess the efficacy and safety of RT001 for the treatment of LCLs using a randomized, double-blind, repeat-dose, placebo-controlled study design.

Methods & Materials.—Healthy adult subjects were randomized to receive RT001 (N=19) or placebo (N=17) applied to their lateral canthal areas (LCAs). To evaluate safety of repeat exposure, treatment was administered at baseline and week 4. The primary efficacy measure was improvement in baseline LCL severity using the Investigator's Global Assessment of Lateral Canthal Line at Rest (IGA-LCL) Severity Scale.

Results.—At 8 weeks, 19 (50%) LCAs treated with RT001 showed a 2-point or greater improvement in baseline IGA-LCL severity, versus none (0%) of the placebo-treated subjects ($p<.001$); 36 (94.7%) LCAs treated with RT001 showed a 1-point or more improvement in baseline IGA-LCL severity, versus five (14.7%) placebo-treated LCAs ($p<.001$). There were no treatment-related adverse events.

Conclusion.—RT001 was well tolerated and demonstrated an improvement in LCLs.

▶ This study was extremely well conducted, as it was placebo controlled and randomized. It also thoroughly investigated the adverse event profile, including antibody detection, electrocardiogram, metabolic panels, and careful evaluation of the seventh cranial nerve at all follow-up visits. It is notable that no subjects had weakness or paralysis of unintended muscle groups, suggesting that the topical formulation remains where it is applied. Whether this holds true without occluding the site remains to be seen. What was missing was a longer follow-up period, not only to further assess safety, but to determine how long the clinical effects last.

Should larger studies confirm that the drug is efficacious, it would be a welcome addition to dermatologists to offer an alternative to patients who fear needles or who experience more pain, or to avoid the complication of bruising. However, this botulinum toxin formulation may also be of interest to practitioners who are not regularly using the injectable versions now, as it is simpler to use, noninvasive, and seemingly relatively side-effect free, therefore making it less time consuming and less risky.

If approved, the interesting question will be whether it will perform as well as the current injectable products on the market. If head-to-head comparisons show equivalence, the invasive administration of botulinum toxin may certainly lose much of its appeal. Of course this study only looked at lateral canthal lines, and it remains to be seen if it can perform as well in other areas of the face. In addition, axillary, palmar, or plantar hyperhidrosis would be important disorders to assess with a topical formulation. Perhaps most exciting is that the study proves that the drug is stable in a topical formulation and is capable of inhibiting acetylcholine at the level of the neurons. One can hope that this or other formulations may be developed to treat other conditions such as hyperhidrosis, blepharospasm, or migraine headaches.

J. M. Suchniak, MD

Efficacy and Safety of a Novel Botulinum Toxin Topical Gel
West TB (The West Inst for Skin Laser & Body Contouring, Chevy Chase, MD)
Dermatol Surg 36:2119-2120, 2010

Background.—The injection of botulinum toxin A (BoNTA) is an extremely popular cosmetic procedure, but the ability to deliver a molecule as large and complex as BoNTA through the skin is an even more impressive milestone. Injection has been facilitated by combinations of effective topical anesthetics, pain-minimizing interventions, and a carefully refined injection technique by an experienced practitioner. Currently, injectable BoNTA is a minor procedure with no downtime, relatively little pain and few side effects in most cases. Some patients, however, see the injection as a major barrier to their use of BoNTA treatments. Topical application would eliminate that hurdle but other disadvantages accompany this novel topical gel.

Topical Application Issues.—Topical BoNTA application requires that the patient wait 30 minutes in the physician's office after application. This may be unacceptable to some patients who want to leave immediately. In addition, with the unveiling of topical BoNTA, untrained persons may be able to obtain and use this product in the "wrong" areas and produce serious adverse side effects. If these become common, it may be difficult to explain that the problem was with the inexperienced, untrained person who applied the product rather than with the product itself. The result could negatively influence the use of BoNTA in any form by scaring away potential patients. It could also lead to increased governmental regulation for both forms of BoNTA.

Conclusions.—Topical application of BoNTA would be preferable to injection, especially in treating axillary, palmar, and plantar hyperhidrosis. However, the ease of use and possible ease of obtaining a topical gel is attended by a number of downsides. Efforts are needed to determine how best to avoid potential misuse. A balance must be struck between enthusiasm for new developments and concern over safety with respect to current and potential patients.

▶ This commentary regarding the safety and efficacy of a new botulinum toxin (BoNTA) topical gel reveals some interesting information we all need to keep in the backs of our minds as newer compounds such as this are brought forward into the BoNTA market. Topical BoNTA is making its way through the US Food and Drug Administration process and may be very useful, as the author points out, for those patients who are needle phobic, despite the fact that the morbidity and adverse events (AEs) associated with the proper injection of BoNTA is relatively small. It is pointed out that if such a product is brought to market, its benefits for patients with hyperhidrosis—axillae, palms, and soles—holds great promise. Optimal dosing and frequency trials for these indications are still necessary for proper usage. The concern of the author, and rightly so, is that if such a product is made easily available too soon, it could lead to some using it incorrectly and with risk of potential AEs (including with overuse). If dosing information is inaccurate, it could lead to more concerns associated with BoNTA use overall, which really may not be justified. The author stresses that the manufacturer must focus on how this product should be used correctly and minimize misuse—misuse will be detrimental to overall BoNTA use.

This potential product will be a major breakthrough if studies bear out what is known thus far; needleless delivery of BoNTA is intriguing, and we are all awaiting further clinical studies to see where we end up with this novel idea.

M. H. Gold, MD

New Drugs and New Molecular Entities in Dermatology
Eaglstein WH, Corcoran G (Univ of Miami, FL; Celgene Corp, Summit, NJ)
Arch Dermatol 147:568-572, 2011

Objective.—To identify and analyze the possible reasons that so few drugs with new molecular entities (NMEs) are first developed for "dermatologic diseases," especially diseases treated primarily by dermatologists.

Design.—Systematic review and analysis. IMS Health (the pharmaceutical industry worldwide product database) was searched using the terms *first launch*, *topical*, and *skin/dermatological* for the preceding decade. These terms were used for inclusion but not exclusion so that intravenous and oral agents were also identified if they were for skin or dermatologic use. The US Food and Drug Administration (FDA) New Molecular Entities Drug and New Biologic Approvals Web site for the 10 years from 1999 to 2009 was examined for approval of dermatologic agents. To determine the frequency of drug development for dermatologic drugs compared with other fields, the total number of NMEs by therapeutic category for the 5-year period 2005 to 2009 was assessed.

Results.—Worldwide, the total number of NMEs for diseases treated primarily by dermatologists for almost a decade was 13. Using the FDA Web site, 5 NMEs for diseases treated primarily by dermatologists were approved in 10 years.

Conclusions.—The major factors precluding NME development for dermatologic diseases seem to be (1) the economic potential of dermatologic drugs, (2) the benefit-to-risk relationship, (3) the limited number of surrogate end points and "soft" semiquantitative end points, and (4) the limited or inadequate basic knowledge of the pathophysiologic characteristics of skin diseases.

▶ Skin diseases continue to be the most common among all disease states; however, the total number of approved and available new molecular entity (NME) drugs used for diseases treated primarily by the dermatologist is relatively small. NME drugs are defined by the Food and Drug Administration as those drugs with an active ingredient that has never been marketed in the United States in any form. In essence, it is considered a drug with a new active ingredient or a novel mechanism of action. But why are such NME drugs not produced for dermatology? Eaglstein and Corcoran perform a systematic review and analysis to answer this question, and their findings shed light on this important concern. Based on their findings, there are 4 variables: the economic potential for drug manufacturers of new dermatologic drugs; the perceived poor benefit-to-risk relationship of drugs for nonlethal conditions, such as many dermatologic diseases; the limited number of surrogate end points in dermatologic disease that, if available, may result in a more predictable development path for a new drug; and the knowledge of skin disease necessary to formulate new drugs, which to date is limited in many areas. The suggested variables are supported by interesting facts and analyses that provide a much-needed point for discussion on this topic. For example, drugs for heart disease and other life-threatening diseases simply have higher investment return than dermatologic drugs, with the exception of biologics for psoriasis, many of which were developed for other disorders such as rheumatoid arthritis. In 2009, atorvastatin (Lipitor) sales worldwide reached $12.45 billion; for clopidogrel (Plavix) it was $9.29 billion. By comparison, only 2 topical drugs in 2007 exceeded the $200 million total. Could this trend, however, be changing with the advent of biologic agents? According to the authors, given the recent billion dollar plus revenues for biologics, it may result in a stronger interest in NME development for dermatologic therapies. Nevertheless, to date, only 5 NME drugs have been approved in the last 10 years for diseases treated primarily by the dermatologist. Ultimately, this article provides an important review on the current state of dermatologic therapies and offers significant insight on what should be a priority topic for discussion among leaders in dermatology.

B. D. Michaels, DO
J. Q. Del Rosso, DO

13 Miscellaneous Topics in Clinical Dermatology

12-Month Controlled Study in the United States of the Safety and Efficacy of a Permanent 2.5% Polyacrylamide Hydrogel Soft-Tissue Filler
Narins RS, Coleman WP III, Rohrich R, et al (New York Univ, White Plains; Tulane Univ, New Orleans, LA; Univ of Texas Southwestern Med Ctr, Dallas; et al)
Dermatol Surg 36:1819-1830, 2010

Objective.—To evaluate the safety and efficacy of a 2.5% polyacrylamide hydrogel in the aesthetic enhancement of nasolabial folds.

Methods and Materials.—The safety and efficacy of a polyacrylamide hydrogel were compared with those of nonanimal stabilized hyaluronic acid (NASHA) in 315 subjects in a double-blind, randomized, multicenter, noninferiority trial with a 12-month follow-up. The primary efficacy end point was mean change in Wrinkle Assessment Scale (WAS) scores at 6 months. The primary safety end point was rate of serious adverse events (AEs) through 12 months after treatment.

Results.—Polyacrylamide hydrogel was as effective as NASHA, and effectiveness persisted throughout the 12-month follow-up. Treatment-related AEs occurred with equal incidence; most were mild to moderate, transient, and related to injection procedure. One serious AE (infection) was thought to be related to treatment with polyacrylamide hydrogel; it resolved within 5 days after appropriate treatment.

Conclusion.—This 2.5% polyacrylamide hydrogel offers promise as a long-lasting soft tissue filler. It is well tolerated, as effective as NASHA in correction of nasolabial folds, and persistent. Longer evaluation is required to evaluate longer-term safety and demonstrate duration of effect beyond 12 months (Figs 1-4, Tables 4 and 5).

▶ In this clinical trial, the authors evaluated a permanent 2.5% polyacrylamide hydrogel soft-tissue filler as compared with nonanimal stabilized hyaluronic acid (NASHA), a hyaluronic acid filler, in a side-by-side comparison for nasolabial folds for a duration of 12 months. The permanent 2.5% polyacrylamide hydrogel soft-tissue filler has demonstrated ability[1] that it does not migrate within the tissues after injection because of its large molecular size, high cohesive properties, and vessel ingrowth from surrounding tissues. The hydrogel is homogenous and contains no microparticles or microspheres, and its filling

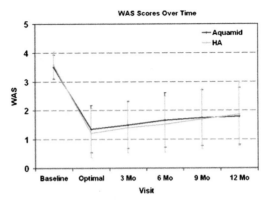

FIGURE 1.—Wrinkle Assessment Scale (WAS) scores over time (mean ± SD) (0 = no wrinkles 5 = very deep wrinkles, redundant fold). Polyacrylamide hydrogel was as effective as nonanimal stabilized hyaluronic acid (HA) in achieving WAS improvement, and the effect persisted throughout the 12 months of post-treatment follow-up. (Reprinted from Narins RS, Coleman WP III, Rohrich R, et al. 12-month controlled study in the United States of the safety and efficacy of a permanent 2.5% polyacrylamide hydrogel soft-tissue filler. *Dermatol Surg.* 2010;36:1819-1830, with permission from John Wiley and Sons, www.interscience.wiley.com.)

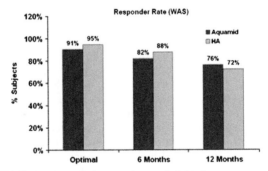

FIGURE 2.—Wrinkle Assessment Scale responder rate. Individual treatment success rates were high for each treatment group throughout the 12 months of post-treatment follow-up. (Reprinted from Narins RS, Coleman WP III, Rohrich R, et al. 12-month controlled study in the United States of the safety and efficacy of a permanent 2.5% polyacrylamide hydrogel soft-tissue filler. *Dermatol Surg.* 2010;36:1819-1830, with permission from John Wiley and Sons, www.interscience.wiley.com.)

effect is immediate, which helps differentiate it from other long-lasting fillers. A total of 315 individuals were enrolled in this clinical trial and followed for 12 months. The Wrinkle Assessment Scale was used as the primary efficacy end point, and at 6 months, the permanent 2.5% polyacrylamide hydrogel soft-tissue filler was found to be noninferior to the NASHA. The efficacy was maintained at the 12-month follow-up. Safety of the permanent 2.5% poly-acrylamide hydrogel soft-tissue filler was evaluated and found to be no different in this evaluation as compared with NASHA. One serious adverse event (AE) infection was found in the permanent 2.5% polyacrylamide hydrogel soft-tissue filler group, deemed related to the treatment, and resolution was noted after 5 days of appropriate therapy. The results show that the permanent 2.5%

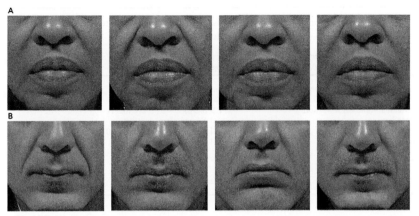

FIGURE 3.—(A) Female subject at baseline prior to treatment, at the optimal treatment visit, and at 6 and 12 months after the optimal treatment visit. (B) Male subject at baseline prior to treatment, at the optimal treatment visit, and at 6 and 12 months after the optimal treatment visit. (Reprinted from Narins RS, Coleman WP III, Rohrich R, et al. 12-month controlled study in the United States of the safety and efficacy of a permanent 2.5% polyacrylamide hydrogel soft-tissue filler. *Dermatol Surg.* 2010;36:1819-1830, with permission from John Wiley and Sons, www.interscience.wiley.com.)

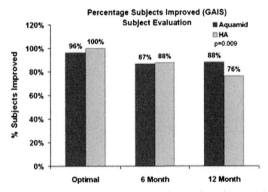

FIGURE 4.—Global Aesthetic Improvement Scale evaluation by subjects. Subject perception of improvement was significantly greater 12 months after treatment for those treated with 2.5% polyacrylamide hydrogel than for those treated with nonanimal stabilized hyaluronic acid (HA) ($p = .009$). (Reprinted from Narins RS, Coleman WP III, Rohrich R, et al. 12-month controlled study in the United States of the safety and efficacy of a permanent 2.5% polyacrylamide hydrogel soft-tissue filler. *Dermatol Surg.* 2010;36:1819-1830, with permission from John Wiley and Sons, www.interscience.wiley.com.)

polyacrylamide hydrogel soft-tissue filler is as effective as NASHA for correction of the nasolabial folds at 12 months. The authors also state that although AEs were not very different with the products except for 1 serious infection, one must be aware that permanent fillers have been associated with biofilm formation and bacterial infections, although the incidence with this filler seems very low.

We are, as a group, afraid of permanent fillers in the United States. We are afraid of the potential AEs that may be associated with them, although studies

TABLE 4.—Improvement in Wrinkle Assessment Scale (WAS) Scores from Baseline to 6 Months

WAS Improvement from Baseline	Polyacrylamide Hydrogel ($n = 210$)	Control ($n = 105$)	Difference (Hydrogel−Control)
Improvement from baseline to 6 months			
N	203	100	
Mean ± standard deviation	1.8 (0.90)	2.1 (0.91)	
Median	1.8	2.0	
Minimum, maximum	−1.0, 4.0	−0.5, 4.0	
Adjusted mean	1.83	2.02	−0.185
95% lower bound			−0.342

Model includes treatment, center, baseline WAS.
WAS is six-level scale: 0 = no wrinkles, 5 = very deep wrinkles, redundant fold.

TABLE 5.—Incidence of All Adverse Events (AEs) Through 12-Month Post-Treatment Follow-Up

AE Type	% Polyacrylamide Hydrogel Subjects ($n = 210$)	Control Subjects ($n = 105$)
Acneform papules	1.0	1.9
Bruising	73.8	76.2
Discoloration	1.4	0.0
Dysesthesia	0.5	0.0
Edema	65.7	79.0
Induration	1.4	0.0
Infection	0.5	0.0
Inflammation	2.4	2.9
Itching	17.6	22.9
Nodule formation	1.4	1.9
Pain	25.7	34.3
Redness	53.3	58.1
Tenderness	44.8	55.2
Tingling	2.4	1.0
Uneven distribution or small subcutaneous lump	0.5	7.6
Other injection site reaction	4.3	5.7
Other adverse event*	28.1	21.0
Subjects with ≥ 1 AEs	88.1	85.7

*The most frequently reported events categorized as "other adverse events" were complaints of pain (back, arm, leg) and the common cold.

such as this clearly show a very small AE rate for biofilm formation, less than 0.5%.[2-4] Perhaps a longer study is needed for safety concerns to be alleviated, but proper injection technique and patient selection are crucial in keeping these AEs at a low rate. Also, clinicians must be made familiar with the signs and symptoms of biofilm formation and bacterial infections and must know which therapies are appropriate when confronted with one of these AEs. However, in the right patient, permanent fillers can have an acceptable place, although at this time, US physicians appear not to welcome these as much as physicians from other countries. Longer-term safety studies after Food and

Drug Administration approval may be the answer to put these fears to rest and give clinicians more comfort when choosing these fillers for their patients.

This was a well-done study showcasing a new permanent dermal filler. These do not have the acceptance of hyaluronic acid fillers in the United States, mainly from fear of biofilm formation, which may or may not be truly accurate based on the results of studies such as this; they occur but rarely. Education, identification, and early treatment are needed if they occur.

M. H. Gold, MD

References

1. de Cássia Novaes W, Berg A. Experiences with a new nonbiodegradable hydrogel (Aquamid): a pilot study. *Aesthetic Plast Surg.* 2003;27:376-380.
2. Zarini E, Supino R, Pratesi G, et al. Biocompatibility and tissue interactions of a new filler material for medical use. *Plast Reconstr Surg.* 2004;114:934-942.
3. von Buelow S, von Heimburg D, Pallua N. Efficacy and safety of polyacrylamide hydrogel for facial soft-tissue augmentation. *Plast Reconstr Surg.* 2005;116:1137-1146.
4. Liu HL, Cheung WY. Complications of polyacrylamide hydrogel (PAAG) injection in facial augmentation. *J Plast Reconstr Aesthet Surg.* 2010;63:e9-e12.

A Double-Blind, Randomized, Placebo-Controlled Health-Outcomes Survey of the Effect of Botulinum Toxin Type A Injections on Quality of Life and Self-Esteem

Dayan SH, Arkins JP, Patel AB, et al (Univ of Illinois at Chicago; DeNova Res, Chicago, IL; Univ of Kentucky, Lexington)
Dermatol Surg 36:2088-2097, 2010

Background.—Although studies show that botulinum toxin type A (BoNTA) can positively influence one's first impression, little research has been conducted to measure the effect that BoNTA has on mental well-being.

Objective.—To determine the effects that BoNTA injections for the treatment of facial wrinkles had on quality of life (QOL) and self-esteem.

Methods and Materials.—One hundred participants received treatment with BoNTA or placebo saline in this double-blind randomized placebo-controlled survey. All participants completed a health outcomes survey consisting of Quality of Life Enjoyment and Satisfaction Questionnaire—Short Form and Heatherton and Polivy State Self-Esteem measurements before injection and 2 weeks and 3 months after injection.

Results.—Statistically significant improvements ($p < .05$) in participants treated with BoNTA were observed in answers to QOL questions regarding physical health, mood, household activities, overall life satisfaction, body satisfaction, self-consciousness, intellect, self-worth, appearance, comprehension, weight satisfaction, attractiveness, and sense of well-being. Increases in overall self-esteem and appearance-, social-, and performance-related self-esteem were observed in participants treated with BoNTA.

Conclusion.—Our findings showed that BoNTA injections result in improvements in QOL and self-esteem. In addition, BoNTA-naïve participants demonstrate greater improvements in QOL and self-esteem than

TABLE 1.—Significant Differences Between OnabotulinumtoxinA and Placebo

	p-Value	
	2 Weeks	3 Months
Body appearance		.05
Satisfaction with weight		.02
Feeling good about one's self	.045	
Physical health	.05	
Household activities	.05	
Overall life satisfaction and contentment		.04

TABLE 2.—Difference within Each Group

	p-Value			
	2 Weeks		3 Months	
	BoNTA	Placebo	BoNTA	Placebo
Body appearance	.01	.025		
Weight			.05	
Less self-consciousness	.03	.03	.01	.01
Perceived self-intellect	.008	.008		
Feeling good about one's self	.002		.002	
Appearance	<.001		<.001	
Confidence in understanding things	.04	.04		.01
Attractiveness			.03	
Total self-esteem	.004		.01	
Social-related self-esteem			.05	
Performance-related self-esteem	.003			
Appearance-related self-esteem	.002		.01	
Mood	.015			
Family relationships	.01			
Overall life satisfaction and contentment	.003		.05	

The results presented represent significant differences from baseline scores for placebo and botulinum toxin type A (BoNTA) groups at 2 weeks or 3 months.

participants previously exposed to BoNTA. Moreover, BoNTA-familiar participants demonstrated sustained improvement in QOL and self-esteem relative to BoNTA-naïve participants, even when injected with placebo (Tables 1-3).

▶ This is an important article that demonstrates scientifically that injections of botulinum toxin type A (BoNTA) can markedly change an individual's quality of life (QOL). In this study, the authors injected 50 people with BoNTA and 50 people with placebo. The patients were followed up at 2 weeks and at 3 months after completion of their injections. The authors performed QOL assessments to determine if the injections had an effect on various parameters of daily life activities and overall well-being. They found that by injecting BoNTA they were able to achieve a statistically significant increase in improvements in physical health, mood, household activities, overall life satisfaction, body satisfaction, self-consciousness, intellect, self-worth, appearance, comprehension, weight satisfaction, attractiveness, and sense of well-being. They also noted that there was

TABLE 3.—Change Score Differences Between OnabotulinumtoxinA and Placebo

	p-Value	
	2 Weeks	3 Months
Feeling good about one's self	.006	.02
Appearance	.04	.02
Attractiveness	.04	
Sense of doing well	.04	
Total self-esteem	.04	
Mood	.01	
Overall life satisfaction and contentment	.01	.04

The results represent significant differences in change in scores between baseline and 2 weeks and to 3 months. The comparison is made between the resulting change in score, or "change score," for the botulinum toxin type A (BoNTA) and placebo groups.

some improvement in some of the placebo participants, especially body appearance at 2 weeks and perception of self-consciousness and confidence over baseline at 2 weeks and 3 months, which was an interesting finding. They also found that those patients who had previous BoNTA injections had higher QOL improvements than BoNTA-naive patients but both more so than placebo. This study provides scientific evidence for what many of us have known for many years: BoNTA injections change lives, making one's QOL better.

M. H. Gold, MD

Comparison of Two Botulinum Toxin Type A Preparations for Treating Crow's Feet: A Split-Face, Double-Blind, Proof-of-Concept Study

Prager W, Wissmüller E, Kollhorst B, et al (Dermatologikum Hamburg, Germany; SClderm GmbH, Hamburg, Germany; et al)
Dermatol Surg 36:2155-2160, 2010

Background.—This is the first double-blind, randomized, proof-of-concept study to compare the clinical effectiveness of botulinum toxin type A (BoNTA) free of complexing proteins with a BoNTA complex (BTXCo) in the treatment of crow's feet.

Patients and Method.—Twelve U of each product were compared in an intra-individual study in 21 participants with a facial wrinkle scale (FWS) score of 2 to 3. Evaluations were done for up to 4 months. Subjects with an improvement of at least 1 point on the FWS were considered responders.

Results.—One month after treatment, the percentage of responders was slightly higher for the BoNTA side (95%) than the BTXCo side (90%). After 4 months, both sides still showed good efficacy, with an 84% response rate and greater than 30% FWS reduction (no statistically significant difference between the products). After 1 month, FWS score at rest was approximately 66% lower for BoNTA, versus 63% lower for BTXCo. After 4 months, FWS reduction was approximately 50%.

Conclusion.—Both botulinum toxin A products displayed high efficacy and good tolerability at a dose ratio of 1:1, with no statistically significant

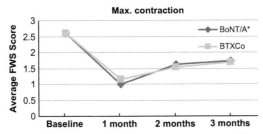

FIGURE 2.—Mean Facial Wrinkle Scale scores at maximum contraction before and after treatment with botulinum toxin type A free of complexing proteins and botulinum toxin type A complex evaluated by a blinded investigator. (Reprinted from Prager W, Wissmüller E, Kollhorst B, et al. Comparison of two botulinum toxin type A preparations for treating crow's feet: a split-face, double-blind, proof-of-concept study. *Dermatol Surg.* 2010;36:2155-2160, with permission from John Wiley and Sons www.interscience. wiley.com.)

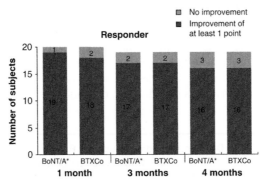

FIGURE 3.—Response rate at maximum contraction after treatment with botulinum toxin type A free of complexing proteins and botulinum toxin type A complex. Responders are defined as participants with an improvement in Facial Wrinkle Scale score of at least 1 point. (Reprinted from Prager W, Wissmüller E, Kollhorst B, et al. Comparison of two botulinum toxin type A preparations for treating crow's feet: a split-face, double-blind, proof-of-concept study. *Dermatol Surg.* 2010;36:2155-2160, with permission from John Wiley and Sons www.interscience.wiley.com.)

differences between them. The high response rates observed after 4 months suggest a good effectiveness beyond this observation period (Figs 2-5).

▶ This is the first clinical trial that compared 2 BoNTA preparations in the treatment of "crow's feet" (laterial periocular lines). One side of the patient was injected with BoNTA, and the other side was treated with a newer BoNTA—one free of complexing proteins usually associated with BoNTA—called BTXCo. BTXCo is free of complexing proteins through a unique purification process; having a high load of foreign protein is thought to be an important risk factor for the formation of neutralizing antibodies, with subsequent loss of therapeutic efficacy. Although this is reported as a theoretical outcome, it is not frequently seen in clinical practice.

Twenty-one patients were entered into this clincial study, and 12 units of each toxin was injected into a crow's feet area in a randomized fashion. Evaluations

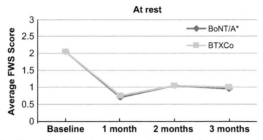

FIGURE 4.—Mean Facial Wrinkle Scale scores at rest before and after treatment with botulinum toxin type A free of complexing proteins and botulinum toxin type A complex evaluated by a blinded investigator. (Reprinted from Prager W, Wissmüller E, Kollhorst B, et al. Comparison of two botulinum toxin type A preparations for treating crow's feet: a split-face, double-blind, proof-of-concept study. *Dermatol Surg.* 2010;36:2155-2160, with permission from John Wiley and Sons www.interscience.wiley.com.)

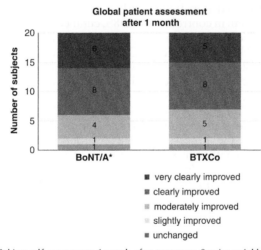

FIGURE 5.—Subject self assessments 1 month after treatment: 9-point wrinkle scale ranging from −4 (very strong worsening of crow's feet) to +4 (very marked improvement of crow's feet). (Reprinted from Prager W, Wissmüller E, Kollhorst B, et al. Comparison of two botulinum toxin type A preparations for treating crow's feet: a split-face, double-blind, proof-of-concept study. *Dermatol Surg.* 2010;36:2155-2160, with permission from John Wiley and Sons www.interscience.wiley.com.)

were made at 1, 3, and 4 months following the injections. At 1 month, the percentage of responders was slightly higher for the BoNTA side (95%) versus BTXCo (90%). After 4 months, both sides showed continued good efficacy, with an 84% response rate and 30% facial wrinkle score reduction (no statistical difference between groups). Both products showed similar efficacy with only 1 adverse effect noted, which was thought to be unrelated to treatment.

This study demonstrates that BTXCo is a useful product for injection into crow's feet and demonstrates efficacy similar to BoNTA.

M. H. Gold, MD

Where does the antigen of cutaneous sarcoidosis come from?

Kurata A, Terado Y, Izumi M, et al (Kyorin Univ School of Medicine, Tokyo, Japan; Tokyo Med Univ, Japan; et al)
J Cutan Pathol 37:211-221, 2010

Background.—The antigen pathway of cutaneous sarcoidosis remains obscure. We have investigated topographic involvement of inflammatory cells and lymphatic vessels.

Methods.—Eleven cutaneous biopsies from eight patients were studied, along with controls from other granulomatous disorders and various skin lesions. Markers for lymphocytes, dendritic cells (DCs), and lymphatic vessel endothelial cells were detected using immunohistochemistry.

Results.—S100$^+$ and CD1a$^+$ immature DCs (Langerhans cells) occurred more frequently within the epidermis, whereas S100$^+$, fascin$^+$, or CD83$^+$ maturing DCs occurred more frequently beneath the epithelium in cutaneous sarcoidosis cases than in controls (e.g. CD83, cutaneous sarcoidosis vs. other granulomatous disorders: $r = 0.557$, $p = 0.011$). Fascin$^+$ and CD83$^+$ mature DCs were often closely attached to CD3$^+$ T-lymphocytes around dermal granulomas. D2-40$^+$ lymphatic vessels were often found surrounding dermal granulomas, especially those located in the deeper dermis, in contrast to fascin$^+$ blood vessels.

Conclusions.—Antigen-capturing by immature DCs seems to take place initially in the epidermis, followed by maturation of DCs. These mature DCs may present the processed antigen to T-lymphocytes that cause dermal granulomas either in the interstitium of the upper dermis, or in or around lymphatic vessels of the lower dermis. Environmental antigen could be verified by skin test.

▶ In this article, investigators performed a topographic study of 9 patients with sarcoidosis with cutaneous involvement (8 with systemic disease, and 1 with disease limited to skin). Using a variety of cases, investigators examined the distribution of antigen-presenting cells and other lymphoid-derived cells, compared with other granulomatous and nongranulomatous conditions.

Similar to a prior investigation,[1-4] the authors found a significantly increased number of CD1a+ immature antigen-presenting cells within the epidermis overlying the epithelioid cell granulomas (ECGs). The investigators also documented a significantly increased number of mature antigen-presenting cells in the "subepidermal" layer of the dermis (essentially the papillary dermis and grenz area), as determined with immunostains for fascin or CD83 (markers of maturation). Lastly, the authors observed increased marking with D2-40 at the periphery of the ECGs, particularly in the deeper granulomas, indicating that compressed and destroyed lymphatics exist at the edge of the granulomas; however, this feature was not unique to sarcoidosis and was observed in other granulomatous conditions.

Synthesizing this information, the authors speculate that the antigen of sarcoidosis, at least in skin disease, may be cutaneously derived, with immature antigen cells of the epidermis first coming in contact with an unknown but environmentally derived stimulus, with subsequent migration and maturation of dendritic cells into the upper dermis. Furthermore, certain populations of T-cells, including CD4+/CD45RO+ cells, may be stimulated during the early activation and migration of dendritic cells.

Admittedly, this study cannot wholly exclude the possibility of hematogenous deposition of mature dendritic cells, unrelated to the overlying immature counterpart, as an alternative explanation for the same "mapped" findings, but the authors note a lack of clear involvement of blood vessels in the distribution of ECGs to mitigate against this alternative mechanism.

Ultimately, the number of cases in this study is small. Although the nationality and ethnicity of the patients is not specified, given the origins of the research work, one might wonder whether this has applicability of sarcoidosis as it is observed in the United States, where blacks and particularly blacks in the southern states are preferentially affected. Still, it may provide titillating and indirect support for limited evidence that cutaneously derived antigens, such as *Propionibacterium* spp, fungi, or other environmental exposures (insecticides, agricultural products, or microbial bioaerosols) may be involved in the disease process.

W. A. High, MD, JD, MEng

References

1. Martin AG, Kleinhenz ME, Elmets CA. Immunohistologic indentification of antigen-presenting cells in cutaneous sarcoidosis. *J Invest Dermatol.* 1986:625-629.
2. Oswald-Richter KA, Drake WP. The etiologic role of infectious antigens in sarcoidosis pathogenesis. *Semin Respir Crit Care Med.* 2010;31:375-379.
3. Terčelj M, Salobir B, Harlander M, Rylander R. Fungal exposure in homes of patients with sarcoidosis—an environmental exposure study. *Environ Health.* 2011;10:8.
4. Ali MM, Atwan AA, Gonzalez ML. Cutaneous sarcoidosis: updates in the pathogenesis. *J Eur Acad Dermatol Venereol.* 2010;24:747-755.

The Effect of Combined Steroid and Calcium Channel Blocker Injection on Human Hypertrophic Scars in Animal Model: A New Strategy for the Treatment of Hypertrophic Scars

Yang J-Y, Huang C-Y (Chang Gung Memorial Hosp and Univ, Taipei, Taiwan; Taipei Med Univ, Taiwan)
Dermatol Surg 36:1942-1949, 2010

Background.—Hypertrophic scars (HScs) are inelastic scars that can cause functional loss and disfigurement. Decorin regulates collagen fibrillogenesis, and its expression is lower in HScs than in normal skin and during wound healing.

Objective.—To evaluate the efficacy of combined verapamil and triamcinolone in treating HScs.

Methods.—Excised human HSc fragments from surgically treated burned patients were divided into three groups: A (normal saline), B (verapamil), and C (verapamil and triamcinolone). The specimens were bilaterally implanted in the back of nude mice, treated using intralesional injections, and observed for 4 weeks. We compared the fibroblast viability and proliferation, decorin staining, and scar weights to evaluate treatment efficacy.

Results.—Viability and proliferation of HSc fibroblasts from groups B and C were significantly lower at all time intervals after transplantation ($p<.001$). Treatment (Groups B and C) stimulated strong decorin staining by 4 weeks. Nonsignificant differences in changes in scar weight were observed between groups.

Conclusions.—We present the first evidence of verapamil-augmented decorin expression spatially correlated with collagen bundles in HScs. Combination therapy can reduce the dosage of each drug but achieve equal or better efficacy than monotherapy, reducing the side effects of a single drug.

▶ Calcium channel blockers, particularly verapamil, have been evaluated in clinical trials several times in the past as monotherapeutic agents or in combination with corticosteroids for the treatment of hypertrophic scars and keloids. It has been shown that the intralesional injection of verapamil reduces extra cellular matrix collagen production and promotes collagenase synthesis. In this study, the authors injected human hypertrophic scars into an animal model to evaluate the effect of verapamil (V) alone or in combination with triamcinolone (TAC) at a cellular level. For example, there was a significant reduction in the number of fibroblasts in the group treated with V + TAC when compared with the control group ($P = .008$), and between the 2 V groups, including V alone, compared with the control group ($P = .01$). Other interesting findings included (1) a strong increase in the expression of decorin (a proteoglycan inhibitor of fibroblast proliferation and migration, usually decreased in hypertrophic scars) to normal levels in V-treated groups compared with the control group, with the increase stronger in the V + TAC group, and (2) a trend showing more scar tissue weight loss in the 2 V-treated groups, which cannot be attributed to the study drugs alone. This study adds more evidence to the existent clinical findings showing that calcium channel blockers may be used as adjuvant therapeutic agents to the standard of care (ie, intralesional corticosteroid injection) to reduce adverse events with the latter or both. At this point, there is no reason (or evidence) to believe that verapamil can be used as a monotherapeutic agent for hypertrophic scars. Further studies are needed testing different dose regimens to determine any real future for calcium channel blockers as part of the armamentarium for the treatment of hypertrophic scars and keloids.

B. Berman, MD, PhD
S. Amini, MD

A comparison of wound healing between a skin protectant ointment and a medical device topical emulsion after laser resurfacing of the perioral area

Sarnoff DS (Cosmetique Dermatology, Laser & Plastic Surgery LLP, NY)
J Am Acad Dermatol 64:S36-S43, 2011

Background.—Currently, there is no standard of care for postlaser resurfacing treatment of the face. Ideally, treatment should speed re-epithelialization and reduce downtime, with minimal irritation.

Objective.—This study compared the wound healing efficacy and safety of Aquaphor Healing Ointment (AHO) (Beiersdorf Inc, Wilton, CT) and Biafine Topical Emulsion (BTE) (OrthoNeutrogena, Los Angeles, CA) treatment after laser resurfacing of the perioral area.

Methods.—In this double-blind, split-face study, 20 subjects with perioral rhytides received fractional carbon dioxide laser resurfacing. AHO and BTE were applied to opposite sides of the face 4 times daily after the resurfacing procedure. Clinical grading of erythema, edema, epithelial confluence, crusting/scabbing, subjective irritation, and general wound appearance were assessed using 5-point scales on days 2, 4, 7, and 14. Subjects ranked the two treatment sites daily as to which side of their face looked better.

Results.—AHO resulted in significantly less erythema (days 2 and 7) and crusting/scabbing (days 2, 4, and 7) and higher epithelial confluence (day 4) than BTE ($P \leq .042$). Subjective irritation assessments demonstrated significantly less stinging, itching, and tightness at day 2 and tightness at day 7 with AHO than with BTE ($P \leq .049$). General wound appearance was graded significantly higher for AHO on days 2 and 7 ($P \leq .049$). Significantly more subjects preferred AHO to BTE ($P \leq .046$).

Limitations.—This was a small study in a homogenous population of white women.

Conclusions.—AHO exhibited superiority to BTE in several wound healing parameters and in overall wound condition.

▶ There are many choices to use on ablative wounds. This study demonstrates that Aquaphor healing ointment performs better than Biafine topical emulsion. The study is well done, and the data appear convincing. The results from this apparent fractional resurfacing are remarkable. The settings, the healing period, and the results would suggest that these patients were receiving a nonfractional treatment.

E. A. Tanghetti, MD

A comparison of postprocedural wound care treatments: Do antibiotic-based ointments improve outcomes?
Draelos ZD, Rizer RL, Trookman NS (Duke Univ School of Medicine, Durhama, NC; Thomas J. Stephens & Associates, CO; Colorado Springs Dermatology Clinic PC)
J Am Acad Dermatol 64:S23-S29, 2011

Background.—Topical antibiotic ointments are commonly used for the postprocedural treatment of superficial wounds created during dermatologic procedures. We propose that antibiotics may not be necessary for healing these wounds, have the potential to cause allergic contact dermatitis, and may contribute to the development of antibiotic resistance.

Objective.—We sought to compare the efficacy and safety of a nonantibiotic, petrolatum-based ointment (Aquaphor Healing Ointment [AHO], Beiersdorf Inc, Wilton, CT) and an antibiotic-based first-aid ointment (Polysporin [Poly/Bac], Johnson & Johnson, New Brunswick, NJ) for the treatment of wounds created by removal of seborrheic keratoses.

Methods.—In this double-blind study, 30 subjects each had two seborrheic keratoses removed from their trunk or abdomen; one wound was treated with AHO and one with Poly/Bac twice daily. Clinical grading of wound healing and subjective irritation was assessed at days 7, 14, and 28 postwounding. Adverse events were recorded.

Results.—Clinical grading assessment showed no differences between wounds treated with AHO versus Poly/Bac for erythema, edema, epithelial confluence, crusting, and scabbing at any time point. Subjective irritation assessment showed wounds treated with Poly/Bac had a significant increase in burning at week 1, whereas no differences were seen between treatments for stinging, itching, tightness, tingling, or pain. One case of allergic contact dermatitis was reported after Poly/Bac treatment.

Limitations.—This was a relatively small study.

Conclusions.—This study demonstrated that the petrolatum-based skin protectant ointment AHO provided equivalent efficacy for wound healing as a combination antibiotic first-aid ointment. Antibiotics may not be necessary to achieve satisfactory wound healing and may cause allergic contact dermatitis.

▶ There are obvious growing concerns among medical professionals, researchers, government agencies, and the public at large regarding antibiotic resistance. This concern is applicable to topical antibiotics used for wound care as well. In addition to resistance issues, topical antibiotics, especially neomycin and bacitracin, are also known to be a cause of allergic contact dermatitis. Given concerns over the common practice of using a topical antibiotic for superficial wound healing, Draelos et al sought to compare the efficacy of a topical antibiotic versus a topical nonantibiotic petrolatum-based ointment for superficial wound healing. Thirty subjects in all were included in the study, with each patient having 2 superficial wound sites evaluated (caused by shave removal of seborrheic keratoses): one wound site was treated with a topical antibiotic and the other with a nonantibiotic petrolatum-based ointment. Although the study size was small and the study included only evaluation of superficial wounds, the results still merit consideration. Based on the study, there was equal efficacy of wound healing between the 2 topical products. In fact, the antibiotic ointment had been shown to cause a significant increase in skin burning in week 1 and also induced 1 case of allergic contact dermatitis. All other symptoms of stinging, itching, pain, tingling, and tightness were otherwise the same with both topical therapies. The value of this study is that as a general rule, there is actually no need for application of a topical antibiotic ointment in superficial wound healing over a nonantibiotic petrolatum-based ointment. If implemented by physicians, the practice of using a nonantibiotic petrolatum-based ointment should help with issues such as sensitization and bacterial resistance, all the while having equal efficacy on superficial wound healing. Overall, this is another important article for review on this subject and, hopefully, for clinical application. In fact, both reviewers have stopped routinely recommending application of a topical antibiotic to wound sites after basic dermatologic surgical procedures, such as skin biopsies (eg, shave, saucerization, punch) and excisions, including at sutured repair sites.

B. D. Michaels, DO

J. Q. Del Rosso, DO

A genome-wide association study to identify genetic determinants of atopy in subjects from the United Kingdom
Wan YI, Strachan DP, Evans DM, et al (Univ Hosp of Nottingham, UK; St Georges' Med School, London, UK; Univ of Bristol, UK; et al)
J Allergy Clin Immunol 127:223-231, 2011

Background.—A genetic component in the development of atopy has been identified. However, numerous heritability models have been proposed with inconsistent replication of susceptibility loci and genes.

Objective.—We sought to use a genome-wide association study approach to examine genetic susceptibility to atopy, which was defined as increased specific IgE levels, positive skin prick test (SPT) responses, or both, within a large discovery cohort and 3 additional white populations.

Methods.—Single nucleotide polymorphisms (SNPs) across the genome were tested for association with increased specific IgE levels (≥ 0.35 kU$_A$/L) in the British 1958 Birth Cohort (1083 cases and 2770 control subjects; Illumina 550K Array) to 1 or more allergens, including house dust mite (Der p 1), mixed grass, or cat fur. Independent replication of identified loci ($P \leq .05$) was assessed in 3 case-control cohorts from the United Kingdom (n = 3225). Combined analyses of data for top signals across cohorts were conducted for atopic phenotypes: increased specific IgE levels (1378 cases and 3151 control subjects) and positive SPT responses (1058 cases and 2167 control subjects).

Results.—A single SNP on chromosome 13q14 met genome-wide significance ($P = 2.15 \times 10^{-9}$), and a further 6 loci ($4.50 \times 10^{-7} \leq P \leq 5.00 \times 10^{-5}$) showed weaker evidence for association with increased specific IgE levels in the British 1958 Birth Cohort. However, no SNPs studied showed consistent association with atopy defined by increased specific IgE levels, positive SPT responses, or both in all study cohorts.

Conclusions.—Seven putative atopy loci were identified using a genome-wide association study approach but showed limited replication across several white populations. This study suggests that large-scale analyses with results from multiple populations will be needed to reliably identify key genetic factors underlying atopy predisposition.

▶ The authors attempted to identify genes associated with predisposition to atopy, using loci identified in a prior longitudinal study started in 1958 in the United Kingdom and obtaining DNA from study subjects who met the definition criteria of atopy (ie, increased specific immunoglobulin (IgE) levels and 1 or more reactions to allergens including house dust mites, mixed grass, and cat fur) during 2002 to 2004. Single nucleotide polymorphisms (SNP) across candidate regions were used to replicate the top signals in 3 independent cohorts from the United Kingdom using atopy as increased specific IgE levels, positive skin prick test, or both. The authors did not obtain replicated evidence for the atopy susceptibility loci found in the original study. Another interesting finding suggested that the genetic influence on specific IgE levels probably resulted from a large number of loci with modest effects. One SNP showed association with atopy across 2 studies; however, it did not show association with IgE levels, indicating that it may play a role in sensitization to allergens. Two SNPs were found to be associated with atopy susceptibility. Additional testing tightening the definition of atopy to specific IgE 3.5 kU/L or greater did not identify SNPs that met genome-wide significance. Questions that remain open include the study of black and Asian populations, which epidemiologically have more visits related to atopic dermatitis than whites (which is the group studied in these cohorts); considering atopic dermatitis as a chronic/recurrent disease instead of a pure immediate hypersensitivity reaction (IgE-dependent) condition; and considering atopic dermatitis as a result (among other factors) of a Th1:Th2 imbalance. Further studies are needed to uncover the role of multiple loci in the etiology, risk, and susceptibility to develop atopic dermatitis.

B. Berman, MD, PhD

S. Amini, MD

Clinical, dermoscopic, and histopathologic features in a case of infantile hemangioma without proliferation
Oiso N, Kimura M, Kawara S, et al (Kinki Univ Faculty of Medicine, Osaka-Sayama, Japan)
Pediatr Dermatol 28:66-68, 2011

Infantile hemangioma precursors or those without a proliferative phase may mimic a port-wine stain. We describe a case of infantile hemangioma precursor, which proved to be Glut-1 positive in biopsy, with the dermoscopic features of red round globular vessels, red comma-like vessels, and red linear vessels. These dermoscopic features should help to distinguish infantile hemangioma precursors or those with an absent or minimal growth phase from a port-wine stain.

▶ Infantile hemangiomas (IH) are the most common vascular tumors in childhood, affecting approximately 1% to 2% of all newborns. IH typically presents within days to weeks after birth and have an initial proliferative phase followed by a stable plateau period with subsequent involution of the tumor. However, IH with minimal or no proliferation have been described and labeled as "plaque-telangiectatic hemangiomas," "abortive hemangiomas," or "minimal-growth hemangiomas."[1-3] These entities may sometimes be confused with port-wine stains (PWS), a relatively common capillary malformation. One distinguishing feature of IH from other vascular tumors and malformations is immunoreactivity for glucose transporter (Glut)-1.

In this brief case report, Oiso et al highlight the use of dermoscopy in evaluating vascular birthmarks. Their patient, a 5-month-old girl with a 5 × 3 cm, asymptomatic, well-demarcated, dark-reddish macule on the right lower leg, was initially thought to have a PWS. Dermoscopic features of the patient were polymorphous: red round globular vessels, red comma-like vessels, and red linear vessels.[4] These findings suggested to the authors that the lesion might not be a PWS. Superficial PWS typically demonstrate red, round globular vessels under dermoscopy; deeper PWS reveal red linear vessels. Histologic evaluation and Glut-1 positivity aided to confirm the diagnosis of IH in this patient.

This is a provocative and interesting finding, although it is difficult to extrapolate ideas from only 1 case. Further investigations are needed to confirm that the finding of red comma-like vessels are more highly suggestive of infantile hemangiomas with minimal or no proliferation than port-wine stains.

T. S. Chen, MD

S. Fallon Friedlander, MD

References

1. Chiller KG, Passaro D, Frieden IJ. Hemangiomas of infancy: clinical characteristics, morphologic subtypes, and their relationship to race, ethnicity, and sex. *Arch Dermatol.* 2002;138:1567-1576.
2. Corella F, Garcia-Navarro X, Ribe A, Alomar A, Baselga E. Abortive or minimal-growth hemangiomas: immunohistochemical evidence that they represent true infantile hemangiomas. *J Am Acad Dermatol.* 2008;58:685-690.
3. Makkar HS, Frieden IJ, Hemangioma Investigator Group. Abortive hemangiomas: a unique morphologic variant of infantile hemangiomas. Oral communication session 4. 16th International Workshop on Vascular Anomalies, ISSVA; June 14—17, 2006; Milan, Italy.
4. Vázquez-López F, Coto-Segura P, Fueyo-Casado A, Pérez-Oliva N. Dermoscopy of port-wine stains. *Arch Dermatol.* 2007;143:962.

An Audit of Behcet's Syndrome Research: A 10-year Survey

Esen F, Schimmel EK, Yazici H, et al (Istanbul Univ, Turkey; Univ of Mississippi Med Ctr, Jackson; NYU Hosp for Joint Diseases)
J Rheumatol 38:99-103, 2011

Objective.—Data suggest that the use of disease control groups and proper use of power calculations were neglected in published reports. We surveyed these and other methodological shortcomings in reports published within the last decade about one specific topic, Behcet's syndrome. We reason that recognizing such methodological shortcomings will lead to better quality clinical and basic science articles.

Methods.—Articles published in the 15 highest impact factor journals on rheumatology, ophthalmology, dermatology, and general medicine between January 1999 and January 2009 were searched for original reports on Behcet's syndrome. Study designs (study types and time element), control groups, demographic data, use of power calculations, and reporting of negative results were specifically tabulated.

Results.—Most studies on Behcet's syndrome were cross-sectional (83%). Prospective longitudinal studies were few (7%). In a considerable proportion of papers (21%), some basic demographic data were missing. Power calculations were rare (3%) even in randomized controlled trials and were not considered at all in clinical hypothesis-testing. Disease control groups were present in slightly over half of clinical and laboratory original research, while just 13% of genetic association studies included disease controls. Only 12% of all reports concerned mainly negative outcomes.

Conclusion.—A considerable number of the published research articles have methodological weaknesses. The generalizability of what we observed in Behcet's syndrome to other research topics needs to be formally studied.

▶ The authors of this study put a spotlight on research methodologies that may serve as a model for future evaluation of evidence-based medicine. Their results are eye-opening in that they expose what most of us have known all along but have either forgotten to question or have just become too jaded because it is so prevalent. First, proper investigational techniques of disease states and statistical evaluations of data are extremely rare. Second, prospective longitudinal studies provide the best epidemiologic data for disease prevalence and outcomes but were rarely detected in the 10-year study period. Third, disease control groups were also found in less than half of the studies but are essential in determining specificity of the data. Perhaps most puzzling is why so many of the studies chose not to rely on using power calculations in interpreting their data.

There may be many reasons for this lack of detail. Time constraints could stifle long-term studies because of researchers being required to accomplish more in a shorter period of time, especially if they also frequently see patients in clinic. Researchers at universities may be under the gun to publish more often, and the ever-present issue of funding may also contribute to the lack of well-conducted studies. In the end, however, the fact remains that the most useful data are those culled from well-designed, prospective, investigational studies with proper controls and conclusions backed by established statistical analyses. This study is helpful in reminding us that while much of our collective knowledge on a subject comes from peer-reviewed journals, we should always remain skeptical and critical.

J. M. Suchniak, MD

Targeted treatment of pruritus: a look into the future
Tey HL, Yosipovitch G (Wake Forest Univ School of Medicine, Winston-Salem, NC)
Br J Dermatol 165:5-17, 2011

Recent advances in pruritus research have elucidated mediators and neuronal pathways involved in itch transmission, and this fast emerging knowledge may possibly be translated into new therapies in the near future. In the skin and peripheral nerves, potential mediator and receptor therapeutic targets include the H4 histamine receptor, protease-activated receptor 2, serine proteases, cathepsin S, peripheral mu- and kappa-opioid receptors, interleukin-31, transient receptor potential vanilloid 1 and 3, fatty acid amide hydrolase, nerve growth factor and its receptor, acetylcholine, and the Mas-related G protein-coupled receptors. In the spinal cord, gastrin-related peptide and its receptor, as well as substance P and its receptor neurokinin receptor-1 serve as potential therapeutic targets. In the brain, reduction of itch perception and modulation of emotions may possibly be achieved through drugs acting on the anterior cingulate cortex. Clinically, management of pruritus should be instituted early and should address the skin pathology, peripheral neuropathy, central sensitization, and the cognito-affective aspects of the disease.

▶ Currently known and newer pathways and mediators of pruritus that can be targeted for the development of new treatments are discussed in this article. Histamine H3 and H4 receptors have recently been linked to inflammation through modulation of dendritic cells and T cells, being potentially useful in atopic dermatitis (AD). Independently or overlapping with histamine are the protease-activated receptor (PAR)-2 and PAR-4 pathways, which have been found to be elevated in AD. In addition to modulation through PAR-2, serine proteases participate in the epidermal barrier function and skin inflammation. Nafamostat and tetracyclines (including doxycycline and minocycline) belong to this group, along with the cysteine protease inhibitor targeting cathepsin S: E-64. Mu-opioid receptor antagonists and kappa-opioid agonists have proved to be of value for the treatment of pruritic conditions. Topical naltrexone 1% cream has also been tested with good results.

Possible new targets include interleukin-31, which is mostly produced in Th2 lymphocytes and is found elevated in AD lesions; transient receptor potential vanilloid (TRPV)-1 and -3, which upon activation by high-potency (8%)

capsaicin or tacrolimus desensitize C-fibers; and activation of cannabinoid receptors, which decreases histamine effects, may reduce the activity of TRPV1 receptors, and suppresses neuronal enzyme fatty acid amide hydrolase. Neurotrophins such as keratinocyte- and mast cell—derived nerve growth factor (NGF) and NGF receptors (tropomyosin-related kinase A [TrkA]), neurotrophin 4, and brain-derived neurotrophic factor have been found to be increased in AD and other pruritic conditions; these have been targeted with monoclonal antibodies to significantly improve pruritus and AD lesions. Acetylcholine release blockage from presynaptic nerve terminals by subcutaneous injection of botulinum toxin has decreased pruritus in some studies during treatment of lichen simplex chronicus and neuropathic itch. Toll-like receptor 7, found in C-fiber sensory neurons mediating nonhistaminergic pathways, gastrin-releasing peptide (GRP) and the GRP receptor, located in the dorsal root ganglia, and dorsal horn of the spinal cord, respectively, have shown promising results in mice. Mas-related G protein coupled receptors are expressed in peripheral neurons and activated by peptides that also promote the expression of GRP in the spinal cord. Substance P, a well-known itch mediator and the central neurokinin receptor-1, has been antagonized with various compounds, obtaining good results and reducing itch from several sources. Lysophosphatidic acid is synthesized by the enzyme autotaxin, the levels of which correlate with pruritus levels in cholestatic patients. Finally, antidepressants including selective serotonin reuptake inhibitors, mirtazapine, serotonin-noradrenalin reuptake inhibitors, and gamma-aminobutyric acid—ergic compounds such as gabapentin and pregabalin inhibited the cingulate cortex in mice, which in humans has been found to be active in AD patients after histamine administration. All these compounds need to be tested for pruritus in randomized clinical trials before any conclusions can be reached and any formal recommendations given. Other treatments in clinical trials, such as omalizumab, an anti-immunoglobulin-E monoclonal antibody, and bepotastine, a second-generation H1 receptor antagonist that also inhibits some inflammatory reactions, were not discussed in this article.

B. Berman, MD, PhD

S. Amini, MD

A Case of Xanthoma Disseminatum with Spontaneous Resolution over 10 Years: Review of the Literature on Long-Term Follow-Up

Park HY, Joe DH, Kang HC, et al (Chonnam Natl Univ Med School, Gwangju, Korea)
Dermatology 222:236-243, 2011

Xanthoma disseminatum (XD) is a rare and potentially progressive non-Langerhans-cell histiocytosis. To date, a few cases of XD with spontaneous complete resolution have been described. The present report describes a 16-year-old girl who presented with yellow to red-brown papules and nodules on her eyelids, cheeks, axillae, back and buttocks. Indirect laryngoscopy showed multiple xanthomatous plaques on the larynx, posterior pharynx, epiglottis, and vocal cords. Additional findings were polyuria, polydipsia, and amenorrhea. Skin biopsy and electron microscopy results confirmed the diagnosis of XD. The patient was treated with fenofibrate, simvastatin, desmopressin, and sex-hormone replacement therapy. Her skin lesions began to slowly fade 6 years after disease onset, eventually resolving spontaneously and completely, but leaving an atrophic scar, frank anetoderma, and persisting diabetes insipidus. This case report together with a review of the English-language literature on the long-term follow-up of XD patients provides additional information on the natural history of this disease.

▶ Xanthoma disseminatum is a rare non-Langerhans cell histiocytosis. It classically presents with the symptom triad of diabetes insipidus, cutaneous xanthomas, and xanthomas of the mucous membranes. As noted in the article, the natural history of the disease is generally benign, but lesions in critical anatomic sites, such as the respiratory and central nervous system, can contribute to an increase in the morbidity and mortality of xanthoma disseminatum. Three clinical patterns exist: a persistent form, a progressive form with systemic involvement, and a self-healing form with spontaneous resolution. Park et al report a case of spontaneous resolution of xanthoma disseminatum over a 10-year period, except for sequelae of atrophic scarring, anetoderma, and persistent diabetes insipidus. Up to now, there have only been a few reports of spontaneous resolution, and overall not much is known about its natural course because of the rarity of the disorder and the paucity of long-term follow-up reports. To this end, this article provides a review of the literature to distill information on the course of the disease as well as providing detailed information about the disease itself. In addition, the article provides a thorough and useful summary, in table form, of the some of the comparative clinical, histologic, and treatment features of xanthoma disseminatum versus other differential diagnoses, including juvenile xanthogranuloma, papular xanthoma, generalized eruptive histiocytosis, progressive nodular histiocytosis, multicentric reticulohistiocytosis, Langerhans cell histiocytosis, and eruptive xanthomas. With regard to the course of the disease, the article reviewed 13 reported cases with long-term follow-up. Of the 13 cases, 8 showed clinical improvement—4 with partial remission and 4 with complete remission. Five of the cases showed progressive or persistent disease. These results led to the conclusion that the prognosis of xanthoma disseminatum is unpredictable but with the possibility of spontaneous regression. Given that spontaneous regression on long-term follow-up was seen in approximately one-third of the cases, continuous monitoring of these patients is emphasized. Important features were also noted in patients with spontaneous complete regression. Namely, although the disease itself had resolved, all of these patients were left with atrophic scars and anetoderma. Furthermore, in the patients that had undergone complete regression, the only systemic involvement reported was diabetes insipidus. Overall, this article provides a detailed review of xanthoma disseminatum and helps yield further information into the long-term course and prognosis of this disorder.

B. D. Michaels, DO
J. Q. Del Rosso, DO

An approach to the patient with retiform purpura

Wysong A, Venkatesan P (Stanford Univ, CA; Duke Univ Med Ctr, Durham, NC)
Dermatol Ther 24:151-172, 2011

Retiform purpura consists of branching purpuric lesions caused by a complete blockage of blood flow in the dermal and subcutaneous vasculature. The differential diagnosis for retiform purpura is broad, including vasculitides of the small and medium vessels as well as microvascular occlusion due to thrombotic, infectious, and embolic phenomena. Determining the etiology of this important dermatologic sign can be a diagnostic challenge; however, an organized approach can improve the speed and accuracy of diagnosis and identify an effective treatment. This review focuses on early recognition, evaluation, and treatment of hospitalized patients with retiform purpura. Specifically, vasculitis, protein C and S deficiencies, heparin necrosis, warfarin necrosis, antiphospholipid antibody syndrome, disseminated intravascular coagulation, cryoglobulinemia, calciphylaxis, and cholesterol embolization syndrome will be discussed in detail. These conditions are commonly seen in consultative dermatology and can have multiorgan involvement, complicated laboratory evaluation, and long-term therapeutic implications.

▶ Hospitalized patients with retiform purpura can present a diagnostic challenge to consulting physicians. There are numerous potential causes for retiform purpura and many may have multiorgan involvement and potentially significant sequelae if not properly diagnosed. To help the clinician with a more focused diagnostic approach when presented with this finding, this article by Wysong et al provides a complete but succinct method of how to deal with a hospitalized patient with retiform purpura, most specifically, those disease states involving microvascular occlusion leading to retiform purpura. The article provides not only comprehensive information on the differential diagnosis, physical examination findings, and workup, but also includes concise tables that have such information as clinical features, biopsy, and laboratory findings. A workup algorithm is also included. Helpful advice is also offered when appropriate, such as the need to perform a skin biopsy on all hospitalized patients with retiform purpura and to ensure it is from a tender area—as that area will most likely demonstrate the histologic changes needed to determine if there is microvascular occlusion. Treatment options for the various causes of retiform purpura are discussed, and a table of the commonly used anticoagulant therapies is provided complete with dosing, monitoring suggestions, and antidotes. Overall, the article is well-organized and comprehensive and serves as a good review and efficient reference for all dermatologists who perform hospital consults.

B. D. Michaels, DO

J. Q. Del Rosso, DO

Approach to the hospitalized patient with targetoid lesions

Hughey LC (Univ of Alabama, Birmingham)
Dermatol Ther 24:196-206, 2011

Approaching the hospitalized patient with skin disease can be daunting. This article focuses on a practical approach to the patient with targetoid lesions. The discussion focuses on differentiating erythema multiforme from Stevens—Johnson syndrome and toxic epidermal necrolysis. In addition, the article offers a concise review of the broader differential diagnosis of targetoid lesions including ecthyma gangrenosum, fixed drug eruption, erythema multiforme-like drug reaction, vasculitis, acute hemorrhagic edema of infancy, erythema chronicum migrans, connective tissue diseases, and blistering diseases.

▶ In this article, the author performs a helpful and thorough review of exactly how to approach a patient with targetoid lesions. Initially, the article reviews the terminology and classification of erythema multiforme (EM), Stevens-Johnson syndrome (SJS), and toxic epidermal necrolysis (TEN) and their distinguishing factors, as well as reviewing different types of targetoid lesions. A brief summation of the differentiating factors between EM and SJS/TEN is provided in tabular form based on lesion morphology, percentage detachment, distribution, and etiology. As important, the author meticulously discusses the potential disease states that can present with targetoid lesions. For each disease state, the author provides important information on how each disease may present (including the presenting form of the targetoid lesion), diagnostic clues and considerations to help the practitioner ascertain each diagnosis, and treatment suggestions. An easy-to-use algorithm is also made available to help practitioners establish a baseline differential diagnosis of the potential cause of the presenting targetoid lesion. In general, the article offers a valuable review for any dermatologist needing a quick, but thorough source when assessing a hospitalized (or nonhospitalized) patient with targetoid lesions.

B. D. Michaels, DO

J. Q. Del Rosso, DO

The Modified Patient and Observer Scar Assessment Scale: A Novel Approach to Defining Pathologic and Nonpathologic Scarring

Fearmonti RM, Bond JE, Erdmann D, et al (Duke Univ Med Ctr, Durham, NC; Univ of Pennsylvania School of Medicine, Philadelphia)
Plast Reconstr Surg 127:242-247, 2011

Background.—Scarring is a highly prevalent and multifactorial process, yet no studies to date have attempted to distinguish pathologic from nonpathologic scarring.

Methods.—This article defines and proposes methods of classifying pathologic scarring as it pertains to clinical presentation.

Results.—The authors propose a new scar scale that incorporates pain and functional impairment.

Conclusions.—The modified Patient and Observer Scar Assessment Scale is the first of its kind to factor in the functional deficits pain and pruritus of scarring into measurements of associated morbidity. This scale has great potential in evaluating patient response to treatment and analyzing clinical outcomes.

▶ Scarring can have significant impact on patient quality of life, not only from a cosmetic perspective but also from a functional perspective. The question is not will there be a scar—it is how will the final scar look, and will it affect the patient from a functional standpoint. It is important to distinguish pathologic from nonpathologic scarring to determine the prevalence, for research and understanding the different biological mechanisms involved, and for improving prevention and treatment. What sets the scale described in this article apart from other existing scar scales is that it incorporates quality of life and the impact of pain, pruritus, and functional impairment. Better understanding of scars will stimulate more research and development of new treatments. This scale will help to define and bring attention to pathologic scarring in future research studies.

R. I. Ceilley, MD

B. A. Kopitzki, DO

Bimatoprost Ophthalmic Solution 0.03% for Eyebrow Growth
Elias MJ, Weiss J, Weiss E (Nova Southeastern Univ/Broward General Med Ctr, Davie, FL; Univ of Miami, FL)
Dermatol Surg 37:1057-1059, 2011

Background.—Bimatoprost ophthalmic solution 0.03% is an established treatment for ocular hypertension that has the side effect of stimulating eyelash hypertrichosis. The beneficial applications of such an effect led to the medication being offered as a cosmetic agent. Bimatoprost is the only prescription agent given Food and Drug Administration (FDA) approval for use to treat inadequate eyelashes. Two cases of bimatoprost successfully stimulating fuller eyebrow growth were reported.

Case Reports.—Case 1: Hispanic man, 52, was dissatisfied with the thinning of his eyebrows that began 6 months previously in association with dieting. Physical examination revealed mild thinning of crescentic hair along the superior edge of the orbit, with neither scarring nor a characteristic geometric pattern of hair loss. No newly growing short hairs with tapered ends or broken shafts were noted on dermatoscopic evaluation of the eyebrows. The patient's complete blood count, complete metabolic profile, thyroid studies, and hormone levels were within normal limits; no biopsy was performed because the patient refused the procedure. The tentative diagnosis was benign generalized diffuse thinning of the eyebrow hair, and the patient expressed a desire for topical therapy to improve the eyebrows' appearance. Bimatoprost ophthalmic solution 0.03% was applied to both eyebrows with the same applicator used for eyelashes each night for 16 weeks. The patient had markedly improved eyebrow growth and was quite satisfied. He experienced no side effects and estimated he used one 2.5-mL container per month.

Case 2: Hispanic woman, 46, was concerned about the diffuse thinning of her eyebrows, which had been occurring for 8 years. Her complete blood count, complete metabolic profile, thyroid studies, and hormone levels were within normal limits; no biopsy was done because the patient feared it would worsen her appearance. Bimatoprost ophthalmic solution 0.03% was used on both eyebrows for 12 weeks. Her eyebrows were thicker, longer, and darker after treatment. She experienced no side effects and was very satisfied with the outcome. She has continued the bimatoprost treatment and uses about one 2.5-mL container each month.

Conclusions.—Bimatoprost is a prostamide $F_{2\alpha}$ analog whose chemical structure resembles that of prostaglandin $F_{2\alpha}$ analogs. Prostaglandin receptors are found in the dermal papilla and the outer root sheath of the hair follicle. Apparently they play a role in the development and regrowth of hair follicles in mice. Animal studies show that bimatoprost alters the eyelash hair cycle by increasing the proportion of hair follicles in the anagen phase and lengthening the time spent in this phase. The exact mechanism by which it works is unclear, but multiple clinical trials have found it to be both safe and effective. The patients experienced greater total drug exposure because the eyebrow has a larger surface area than the upper lid margin, but neither patient developed adverse reactions.

▶ Bimatoprost ophthalmic solution 0.03% has been used for treatment of ocular hypertension (glaucoma). More recently, this agent has been rebranded for the cosmetic purpose of promoting increased growth and greater density of eyelashes. This is a case report of 2 patients successfully treated with bimatoprost to achieve a more full appearance of eyebrows. Although the exact mechanism of action of bimatoprost is unclear, animal studies have found that treatment with bimatoprost results in changes to the eyelash hair cycle by increasing and prolonging the duration of the anagen phase. The first patient in this study was a 52-year-old Hispanic man with thinning eyebrows possibly related to a new diet and no other associated medical causes. After 16 weeks of nightly application of bimatoprost ophthalmic solution 0.03% to both eyebrows, the patient had markedly improved appearance and thickness of the eyebrows. The second individual was a 46-year-old Hispanic woman with diffuse thinning of her eyebrows for 8 years. She was placed on nightly application of bimatoprost ophthalmic solution 0.03% and returned with noticeable results. Importantly, biopsies were not performed on either patient (mostly because of the delicate eyebrow location), and no laboratory examinations were performed in an attempt to assess any underlying causes of decreased eyebrow density or hair loss. Also, because there were no controls provided in this study, spontaneous resolution could not be ruled out in either case; however, this seems unlikely, especially in the latter case of 8 years duration. More studies are needed to determine the overall safety and efficacy, especially in lighter-pigmented individuals who have more of a risk of hyperpigmentation. Neither patient experienced adverse reactions. The authors determined that bimatoprost can be used safely on the eyebrows; however, with an N = 2 study size, this conclusion is premature as a definitive statement. Overall, in patients who are very bothered by thin eyebrows without a known underlying cause (ie, hypothyroidism, aggressive plucking), this approach seems reasonable, provided the patient is adequately informed and consents to treatment after a benefit-versus-risk discussion is completed.

G. K. Kim, DO

J. Q. Del Rosso, DO

Early White Discoloration of Infantile Hemangioma: A Sign of Impending Ulceration

Maguiness SM, Hoffman WY, McCalmont TH, et al (Children's Hosp Boston, MA; Univ of California, San Francisco)
Arch Dermatol 146:1235-1239, 2010

Objective.—To evaluate the relationship between early white discoloration of infantile hemangioma (IH) and ulceration.

Design.—Retrospective cohort study.

Setting.—Tertiary referral center.

Patients.—A case series of 11 infants with early white discoloration of IH are described. An additional 55 infants with IH, aged 3 months, were evaluated retrospectively from a photograph archive to further explore the relationship between early white discoloration and presence or development of ulceration.

Main Outcome Measures.—Patient demographics and hemangioma size, location, and subtype are documented. Sensitivity and specificity of white discoloration in relationship to ulceration are estimated.

Results.—Ten of the 11 infants in the case series were girls (90%); all IHs were of segmental or indeterminate subtype. Average age at first ulceration was 2.6 months, with average age at healing 5.2 months. No intervention halted progression of ulceration. Of the 55 additional 3-month-old infants, 14 had white discoloration and 12 of these 14 had or developed ulceration (86%). When the hemangioma was either white or slightly white, sensitivity for predicting ulceration was 1.00 (95% confidence interval [CI], 0.78-1.00), with a specificity of 0.68 (95% CI, 0.51-0.81). In contrast, in infants with either slightly white or no white discoloration, the sensitivity for not developing ulceration was 0.80 (95% CI, 0.52-0.96), with a specificity of 0.95 (95% CI, 0.83-0.99), suggesting that a lack of substantial white discoloration early in infancy indicates low risk of ulceration.

Conclusion.—Early white discoloration of infantile hemangioma is highly suggestive of impending ulceration.

▶ Infantile hemangiomas (IH) are the most common benign vascular tumors of infancy. Complications include ulceration, infection, airway obstruction, and visual impedance, with ulceration being the most common and occurring in 15% of cases. Risk factors for ulceration include hemangiomas that are segmental, large, exhibit combined superficial and deep involvement, and/or are located in the anogenital region, on the lip, or on the chest. Once ulceration occurs, hemangiomas can be painful, are more likely to scar, and may require several medical interventions for treatment.

In this study, the authors report on an early white discoloration of hemangiomas and its association with the development of ulceration. A case series of 11 infants with early white discoloration resulted in all patients developing ulceration. Furthermore, a retrospective evaluation of 55 patients demonstrated that white or slightly white discoloration had a sensitivity of 100% for predicting ulceration. In contrast, patients with slightly white or no white discoloration had a sensitivity of 80% for not developing ulceration. Histopathologic sections from 2 excised white hemangiomas showed areas of superficial dermal fibrosis correlating with clinically white areas. The areas of early fibrosis are likely to exhibit decreased vascularity, making those sites more susceptible to ulceration from even slight trauma.

This case series is small, and patients were not randomly selected to be followed over time. White discoloration does occur without subsequent ulceration, and a large, truly prospective study would be required to substantiate the sensitivity and specificity of this putative association. Dermoscopic examination of areas of white discoloration would also be interesting.

This observation is significant because the finding can be observed easily by visual inspection. These results suggest that the presence of early white discoloration mandates careful follow-up. In addition, it may prove to be an important indication for early interventions, such as a topical or oral beta-blocker (ie, propranolol, timolol) to avoid development of ulcers or to facilitate quicker healing.

S. Fallon Friedlander, MD

J. Q. Del Rosso, DO

Chronic pruritus — pathogenesis, clinical aspects and treatment
Metz M, Ständer S (Charité-Universitätsmedizin Berlin, Germany; Univ Hosp of Münster, Germany)
J Eur Acad Dermatol Venereol 24:1249-1260, 2010

Chronic pruritus is a major symptom in numerous dermatological and systemic diseases. Similar to chronic pain, chronic pruritus can have a dramatic impact on the quality of life and can worsen the general condition of the patient considerably. The pathogenesis of itch is diverse and involves a complex network of cutaneous and neuronal cells. In recent years, more and more itch-specific mediators and receptors, such as interleukin-31,

gastrin-releasing peptide receptor or histamine H4 receptor have been identified and the concept of itch-specific neurons has been further characterized.
Understanding of the basic principles is important for development of
target-specific treatment of patients with chronic pruritus. In this review,
we summarize the current knowledge about the pathophysiological principles of itch and provide an overview about current and future treatment
options.

▶ Pruritus can be a symptom of many dermatologic dermatoses. Similar to urticaria, if the pruritus persists for more than 6 weeks, it is defined as chronic. The
epidemiological data on chronic pruritus are scarce, but investigations have
identified chronic itch better in the general population as related to specific
diseases. Keratinocytes can be activated to produce and release inflammatory
and pruritogenic substances by various innate mechanisms, toll-like receptors
(TLR), ultraviolet (UV) light, or thermoreceptors. Mast cells can release histamine
and cause induction or modulation of itch. Pruritus is mediated by free nerve
endings of nonmyelinated nerve fibers that are located at the dermoepidermal
junction and within the epidermis. Pruritus-specific nonmyelinated C nerve fibers
exist that respond only to histamine. G protein-coupled receptors that mediate
chloroquine-induced pruritus have been identified in sensory neurons. Therapy
for pruritus is directed at eliminating triggers for itch, such as overheated rooms,
insulating clothing, and warm beds. In addition, wool should be avoided. Other
exogenous factors can also intensify the perception of itch, such as hot spices,
alcohol, hot beverages, and medications (ie, beta-blockers and allopurinol).
H1-antihistamines are a popular treatment option in chronic pruritus because
they are affordable and have been proven to help, although drowsiness can be
problematic. Anticonvulsants such as gabapentin have often demonstrated potent
analgesic effects and have been approved for neuropathic pain. Other medications
such as naltrexone have also been used as an opioid receptor antagonist but are
helpful in some cases of pruritus. Also, antidepressants such as selective serotonin
reuptake inhibitors have been documented to help with chronic pruritus. UVA and
UVB have also been used in the past to help with chronic pruritus. Future treatment of pruritus includes H4 receptor antagonists, K-opioid receptor agonists,
and neurokinin 1-receptor antagonists. In conclusion, this is a thorough review
of chronic pruritus, its pathophysiology, and treatment, with options to consider
in refractory cases.

G. K. Kim, DO
J. Q. Del Rosso, DO

Association of Hearing Loss With PHACE Syndrome
Duffy KJ, Runge-Samuelson C, Bayer ML, et al (Med College of Wisconsin,
Milwaukee; et al)
Arch Dermatol 146:1391-1396, 2010

Background.—PHACE syndrome describes a spectrum of anomalies
associated with large facial infantile hemangiomas and characterized by

posterior fossa malformations, hemangiomas, arterial anomalies, coarctation of the aorta and cardiac defects, and eye abnormalities. With improved recognition and imaging practices of infants with PHACE syndrome, additional associations have been identified. To our knowledge, the potential association of ipsilateral hearing loss and PHACE syndrome has not been previously emphasized.

Observations.—We describe 6 patients, 4 with definite and 2 with probable PHACE syndrome, according to the new diagnostic criteria, and associated auditory deficiencies. One patient had isolated conductive hearing loss; 2 patients had isolated sensorineural hearing loss; 1 patient had mixed hearing loss (both conductive and sensorineural components); and 1 patient had hearing loss that was inconclusive at the time. Also, 1 patient had conductive loss and auditory neuropathy and auditory dyssynchrony. Four of the 6 patients had magnetic resonance imaging features of lesions consistent with intracranial hemangiomas involving auditory structures. All 6 patients had facial hemangiomas in a nearly identical distribution ipsilateral to the ear with the hearing loss, with involvement of the proposed facial segments S1 and S3, the affected ear, the periauricular region, and the midoccipital area of the scalp.

Conclusions.—There is an underrecognized risk of hearing loss in patients with PHACE syndrome, although the exact nature of such deficiencies can vary. Patients with PHACE syndrome who have cutaneous hemangiomas involving the ear should be evaluated for intracranial hemangiomas and monitored for hearing loss. Early detection and therapy of intracranial hemangiomas may slow or stop tumor growth, resultant hearing loss, and structural damage.

▶ PHACE syndrome is characterized by the association of a facial infantile hemangioma greater than 5 cm with posterior fossa defects, arterial anomalies, cardiac anomalies, coarctation of the aorta, eye abnormalities, supraumbilical raphe, and sternal clefts. The standard workup for this syndrome is magnetic resonance imaging/angiography of the head and neck, echocardiogram, cardiac exam, ophthalmologic examination, and 4-extremity blood pressure reading.

This article suggests that hearing evaluation should be part of the workup of a patient with confirmed or suspected PHACE syndrome because both conductive and sensorineural hearing impairment can be associated with this disorder. Importantly, patients with PHACE syndrome who pass their newborn screening may later develop hearing abnormalities given the natural course of growth of infantile hemangiomas during early infancy. Therefore, the authors recommend repeat hearing evaluations at 6 to 9 months and 12 to 18 months of age. Given the noninvasive nature of audiologic evaluation and the plausibility of infantile hemangiomas affecting hearing, baseline and repeat hearing evaluations seem appropriate in the management of a patient with PHACE syndrome.

M. G. Osofsky, MD

S. Fallon Friedlander, MD

Becker Nevus With an Underlying Desmoid Tumor: A Case Report and Review Including Mayo Clinic's Experience

Sciallis GF, Sciallis AP (Mayo Clinic, Rochester, MN)
Arch Dermatol 146:1408-1412, 2010

Background.—Becker nevus is a nevoid melanosis, referred to as Becker nevus syndrome when it is associated with other anomalies. Our objectives were to report the occurrence of a Becker nevus with an underlying desmoid soft-tissue tumor; to review Mayo Clinic's experience with Becker nevi, concentrating on Becker nevi associated with bone, vascular, neural, and other soft-tissue abnormalities; to inform physicians of the Becker nevus syndrome; and finally to alert clinicians to evaluate a Becker nevus with its associations in mind.

Observations.—A 46-year-old woman had a Becker nevus with an underlying desmoid-type fibromatosis (desmoid tumor) presenting clinically as a "painful dimple" within the nevus. Review of medical records for 1997 through 2006 at Mayo Clinic, Rochester, Minnesota, yielded 52 patients with Becker nevi, 12 of whom had an associated bone, vascular, neural, congenital, or other soft-tissue abnormality, ranging from liposarcoma to an accessory areola.

Conclusions.—We add to the literature a unique case of desmoid-type fibromatosis immediately beneath a Becker melanosis, which presented as a painful dimple. We hope to raise awareness that a Becker nevus may be associated with other abnormalities, including an infiltrative soft-tissue tumor. We also emphasize the importance of follow-up, including inspection of not only the surface but also the deep tissues underlying the Becker nevus.

▶ The authors of this retrospective case review of 52 patients with Becker nevi at Mayo Clinic found 23% with confirmed associated anomalies. Investigators propose definitions of disorders associated with a Becker nevus as follows: (1) Becker melanosis—pigmentary macular changes; (2) Becker nevus—macular pigmentation and associated contiguous adnexal changes involving follicular components, smooth muscle hamartomas, desmoid tumors, dermal and subcutaneous alterations, and epidermal tumors; (3) Becker nevus syndrome—in addition to the foregoing 2 categories (ie, Becker melanosis and Becker nevus), associated abnormalities including ipsilateral hypoplasia of the breast, hypoplasia of underlying muscle, lipoatrophy, and underlying skeletal anomalies. Histologically, Becker nevus displays hyperplasia, hyperpigmentation of basal keratinocytes, elongation of rete ridges, and increased hair follicles and/or smooth muscle unassociated with surrounding adnexa. Although Becker nevi are not generally associated with malignancy, patients nevertheless should be monitored and evaluated periodically for underlying changes. This is illustrated by the case report in which a 46-year-old woman with Becker nevus was found to have an underlying desmoid tumor.

S. Bellew, DO
J. Q. Del Rosso, DO

Vitamin D-effective solar UV radiation, dietary vitamin D and breast cancer risk

Edvardsen K, Veierød MB, Brustad M, et al (Univ of Tromsø, Norway; Univ of Oslo, Blindern, Norway; et al)
Int J Cancer 128:1425-1433, 2011

Vitamin D is well known for its important role in calcium and phosphor homeostasis. Recent research suggests that vitamin D also prevent some type of cancers. We studied solar vitamin D effective UV radiation (VD dose), dietary vitamin D, sun-seeking holidays, use of solarium, frequency of sunburn and breast cancer risk in a large population-based cohort study. A total of 41,811 women from the prospective Norwegian Women and Cancer Study, aged 40–70 years at baseline, were followed from 1997/1998 to 2007. Dietary vitamin D intake was calculated at baseline. Information on historical VD dose was used as a proxy for cutaneously obtained vitamin D status. Cox proportional hazards model was used. We adjusted for age, height, BMI, baseline menopausal status, use of hormone replacement therapy, use of oral contraception, alcohol, mother's history of breast cancer, mammography and parity. During 8.5 years of follow-up, 948 new cases of breast cancer were registered using data from the Norwegian Cancer Registry. We found no significant associations between VD dose, or vitamin D intake, or sun-seeking holidays, or use of solarium, or frequency of sunburn, and breast cancer risk. Relative risks (95% confidence intervals) for highest versus lowest category were 1.17 (0.95–1.44), 0.95 (0.75–1.21), 1.07 (0.87–1.32), 0.93 (0.76–1.14) and 1.10 (0.89–1.36), respectively. Our results do not support an association between vitamin D status, and breast cancer risk.

▶ Vitamin D homeostasis, whether achieved by dietary intake or solar radiation, may have a positive effect on cancer survival. Previous studies have supported an increase in vitamin D levels with a reduction in breast cancer. This large population-based cohort study of 41 811 women followed over a 10-year period failed to support an association between vitamin D status and breast cancer reduction.

J. L. Smith, MD

Botulinum Toxin Type A vs Type B for Axillary Hyperhidrosis in a Case Series of Patients Observed for 6 Months

Frasson E, Brigo F, Acler M, et al (Cittadella Hosp, Padua, Italy; Univ of Verona, Italy)
Arch Dermatol 147:122-123, 2011

Background.—Botulinum toxin type B (BT-B) is being more widely used for axillary hyperhidrosis, but the effective dose remains to be determined. A comparison of BT-B and botulinum toxin type A (BT-A) was conducted to judge their antihyperhidrotic effects when delivered via intra-axillary injection.

Methods.—Ten patients (age 23 to 54 years) with idiopathic focal axillary hyperhidrosis since childhood participated in a bilateral paired, single-blinded, randomized study. Their conditions had not responded to other nonsurgical treatments. Each patient received BT-A unilaterally and BT-B contralaterally. All underwent a pretreatment examination and objective quantification of sweat production at rest. The quinizarin sweat test was used to define the hyperhidrotic area. Gravimetric measures were used to evaluate sweat production over 5 minutes. Assessments were done before treatment as well as 1 and 2 weeks and 1, 3, and 6 months after BT injection. Each patient received 20 injections in each axilla. The 20 U of BT-A were diluted with 1 mL of 0.9% sterile physiologic saline solution without preservative; the 2500 U of BT-B were diluted with 0.5 mL of the same saline solution. Toxin was injected in amounts of 0.025 mL for BT-B and 0.050 mL for BT-A intradermally using a 20-gauge needle. Patients also completed questionnaires to document subjective responses such as the beginning and duration of benefit and satisfaction with treatment.

Results.—Axillary sweat production was reduced in all patients until the 6-month assessment. Sweat weight and area diminished significantly more on the BT-B side than on the BT-A side. Treatment satisfaction scores were also significantly higher for the BT-B than for the BT-A treatments until the third month. Treatment responses were noted earlier with the BT-B injections than the BT-A injections, with the mean time to initial effect being 3.0 days (range 1 to 7 days) for BT-B and 14.3 days (range 7 to 20 days) for BT-A. Subjective benefits also lasted longer with the BT-B than the BT-A (17.3 versus 12.9 weeks, respectively). The intradermally injected BT-A and BT-B were both well tolerated, although some patients reported mild pain, particularly with BT-B. None of the patients developed hematomas at the injection site or systemic adverse effects.

Conclusions.—BT-B was more effective in managing axillary hyperhidrosis than BT-A, reducing sweat production and area size. Both the objective and the subjective results favor the use of BT-B for treating bilateral axillary hyperhidrosis, making it both safe and effective. Future research should focus on how BT-A and BT-B affect the autonomic and motor nervous systems and the duration of effects on these systems.

▶ Axillary hyperhidrosis is a common debilitating disorder of excess sweating that can adversely affect patients' daily activities. Current treatment options include topical antiperspirants (both over-the-counter or prescription strengths), botulinum toxin, oral medications (anitcholinergics, beta blockers, clonidine), local surgery to remove sweat glands, or endoscopic thoracic sympathectomy. Botulinum toxin blocks signals at the neuromuscular junction of sweat glands via inhibition of acetylcholine. Botulinum A subtype (BT-A) and B subtype (BT-B) are commercially available. The study is a bilateral paired, single-blinded, randomized study of 10 patients with axillary hyperhidrosis. Investigators found that both toxins provided improvement of symptoms, while BT-B was found to provide earlier development of anhidrotic areas. BT-B use produced higher patient satisfaction scores and had a longer-lasting effect than BT-A. Contraindications for botulinum toxin include pregnancy, neuromuscular diseases, and blood clotting disorders.[1] Limitations of the study include small sample size and the fact that it was a single-blinded study. As the authors suggest, a future double-blind study detailing results using BT-A and BT-B in a larger number of patients, evaluation of their effects on autonomic and motor nervous systems, and comparison of the relative duration of their effects may be warranted.

S. Bellew, DO

Reference

1. Vorkamp T, Foo FJ, Khan S, Schmitto JD, Wilson P. Hyperhidrosis: evolving concepts and a comprehensive review. *Surgeon.* 2010;8:287-292.

Effect of Aqueous Cream BP on human stratum corneum *in vivo*
Tsang M, Guy RH (Univ of Bath, UK)
Br J Dermatol 163:954-958, 2010

Background.—Aqueous Cream BP is widely prescribed to patients with eczema to relieve skin dryness. The formulation contains sodium lauryl sulphate (SLS), a chemical that is a known skin irritant and a commonly used excipient in personal care and household products. The chronic effects of Aqueous Cream BP application on skin barrier function have not been determined.

Objectives.—To characterize and assess skin barrier function of healthy skin after application of Aqueous Cream BP and to study the physical effects of the formulation on the stratum corneum (SC).

Methods.—The left and right volar forearms of six human volunteers were each separated into treated and control sides. The treated sides of each forearm were subjected to twice daily applications of Aqueous Cream BP for 4 weeks at the end of which concomitant tape stripping and transepidermal water loss (TEWL) measurements were made. The untreated sides of the forearms were not exposed to any products containing SLS during the study period.

Results.—Changes in SC thickness, baseline TEWL and rate of increase in TEWL during tape stripping were observed in skin treated with Aqueous Cream BP. The mean decrease in SC thickness was $1 \cdot 1 \, \mu m$ (12%) ($P = 0 \cdot 0015$) and the mean increase in baseline TEWL was $2 \cdot 5 \, g \, m^{-2} h^{-1}$ (20%) ($P < 0 \cdot 0001$). Reduced SC thickness and an increase in baseline TEWL, as well as a faster rate of increase in TEWL during tape stripping, were observed in 16 out of 27 treated skin sites.

Conclusions.—The application of Aqueous Cream BP, containing ~1% SLS, reduced the SC thickness of healthy skin and increased its permeability to water loss. These observations call into question the continued use of this emollient on the already compromised barrier of eczematous skin.

▶ Despite the many potential disadvantages of using surfactants in cleansers and surfactant emulsifiers in moisturizers, they are necessary evils. Without surfactants we would not be able to cleanse the skin of dirt and oils or combine the hydrophilic and hydrophobic components of a moisturizer into one cosmetically elegant formulation. Sodium lauryl sulfate (SLS) is an example of an anionic surfactant that is well known for its irritation potential. Anionic surfactants have the most potential to interact with skin lipids and proteins and, therefore, are viewed as having the most negative effects on the epidermal permeability barrier. Despite the potential of anionic surfactants to induce stratum corneum (SC) disruption, dehydration, and irritation, they are often used in mild moisturizers as emulsifiers because of their organoleptic qualities.

The premise of this study and its conclusion revolve around the many reports of skin irritation secondary to SLS in atopic dermatitis (AD) patients as well as a previous study conducted with children. In this study, 56% of children reported a stinging sensation after using the Aqueous Cream BP product, which contains 1% SLS, and this cream elicited a higher level of discomfort compared with the other creams tested.

The objective of this study was to determine the effect of an Aqueous Cream BP containing SLS on the SC permeability barrier function of patients with AD. The Aqueous Cream BP used in this experiment is an emollient cream containing 1% SLS as a surfactant emulsifier. The authors found that areas that used the Aqueous Cream BP had an increase in transepidermal water loss (TEWL) from baseline and decreased SC thickness compared with the control, which the authors contribute to the SLS in the formula.

There are several limitations to the study design of this article. First, SC barrier function and the level of disruption of the proteins and lipids are assumed here based on the elevation of TEWL measurements. It has been discussed in other recent articles[1] that TEWL measurements may not be the most reliable marker of SC barrier function and that other methods may be more reliable to determine specific details related to barrier function impairment.

Secondly, the authors assume that the SLS is the sole reason for the barrier disruption seen. To confirm this conclusion, there needs to be a control formula without SLS. The explanation of what was used as the control seemed somewhat lacking in this report.

If what is concluded in this study is true, then the question becomes, "what about those formulas that use SLS in lower concentrations?" Many authors today claim that the irritation potential of some anionic emulsifiers can be diminished by partially neutralizing them with other cationic ingredients or adding other nonionic emulsifiers to keep their concentration low in the formula. However, another perspective is that all surfactant and surfactant emulsifiers affect the SC permeability barrier. This is supported by the evidence of relative changes in the SC barrier function and in proteins and lipids of the SC, with anionic, nonionic, and cationic surfactants. It may be that surfactants and surfactant emulsifiers are necessary evils, and minimizing damage in patients with sensitive skin may require a low concentration in the formula. However, this too needs further experimentation.

Overall, I compliment the authors for looking into a subject that has been overlooked by many, that is, that emulsifiers are surfactants that have the same if not more potential to damage the SC permeability barrier.

J. Levin, DO

J. Q. Del Rosso, DO

Reference

1. Levin J, Miller R. A Guide to the ingredients and potential benefits of over-the-counter cleansers and moisturizers for rosacea patients. *J Clin Aesthet Dermatol.* 2011;4:31-49.

Depth profiling of stratum corneum biophysical and molecular properties
Mohammed D, Matts PJ, Hadgraft J, et al (School of Pharmacy, London, UK; London Innovation Centre, Egham, UK)
Br J Dermatol 164:957-965, 2011

Background.—The barrier function of the skin may be characterized by a number of biophysical and molecular methods. Variation in the barrier properties as a function of depth has not been explored in detail.

Objectives.—To characterize changes in corneocyte surface area, corneocyte maturity, selected protease activities and transepidermal water loss (TEWL) in the ventral forearm with increasing depth.

Methods.—The left mid-ventral forearm of 22 healthy volunteers was selected as the study site. After tape stripping, corneocyte maturity and surface area were assessed. The protease activity of the desquamatory kallikrein proteases, KLK5 and KLK7, and inflammatory tryptase was measured using a fluorogenic probe assay. Protein content and TEWL were also recorded.

Results.—Corneocyte maturity and surface area decreased with increasing number of tape strippings, i.e. depth into the skin. More mature corneocytes were typically larger than less mature corneocytes. The protease activities of both the desquamatory and inflammatory enzymes together with the protein content were highest in the outer layers of the stratum corneum and decreased with depth. As expected, TEWL increased as more stratum corneum layers were removed. There were no statistical differences between men and women or caucasian and black subjects for all of the parameters studied.

Conclusions.—The techniques used in this study provide rapid noninvasive measures of the spatial distribution of corneocyte maturity and surface area as well as protease activity and protein content within different levels of the stratum corneum layers. The methods used will allow mechanistic insight into the effects of formulation excipients and active ingredients on epidermal turnover and skin barrier function.

▶ The objectives of this experiment are to characterize specific stratum corneum (SC) protease activity, transepidermal water loss (TEWL), and corneocyte surface area and maturity as a function of SC depth on the left midventral forearm using minimally invasive tape stripping analysis. The authors found that proteases, especially kallikrein 5, are increased near the top layers of the SC. These proteases are increased at the top layers and are likely to allow for activation of antimicrobial peptides (ie, cathelicidin) and to facilitate desquamation. Corneocyte maturity and surface area were also found to be greatest in the top layers of the SC. This is consistent with what is known about the progression of keratinocyte differentiation upward from the stratum basale layer to the stratum corneum. TEWL, a crude measure of SC permeability barrier function, was the lowest at the top layers of the SC. Because the SC is thought to be the major rate-limiting step in reducing skin permeation by exogenous agents, it makes sense that the highest level of "barrier function" is at the top layers of the skin (upper SC). The authors postulate that the increased barrier function at the uppermost layers of the SC is secondary to the greater amount of cross-linking of the cornified envelope in these layers, although an intact intercellular lipid membrane is a major contributing factor in regulating TEWL. The major results found in this experiment are consistent with SC basic science already known, validating the techniques used in this experiment.

In addition to the stated objectives and corresponding results in the abstract of this article, this experiment compared the above investigated parameters in men versus women and in white versus nonwhite skin. The only significant differences found in these comparisons were increased protein content in the outer layers of the SC in women versus men and white versus nonwhite skin. The specific protein or proteins that are increased is unknown, and the significance of the increased protein content is also undetermined.

Only after understanding normal skin SC mechanisms and functionality can we begin to understand the alterations seen in skin disease. Now that the authors have characterized these important properties of the SC of healthy skin with minimally invasive techniques, we can begin to characterize the properties of the SC as they relate to aberrations associated with specific skin diseases. Such disease-specific characterizations allow for a better understanding of the pathogenesis of the disease and the role of specific SC changes if any are present. Whether the SC changes contribute to the pathogenesis of a given disorder, or are "sideline bystanders," requires further study. Nevertheless, the data allow for development of novel approaches to disease management that targets specific abnormalities.

Overall, this experiment was well designed despite the small number of subjects involved. However, it remains to be seen how revolutionary the results of this experiment are given what is known today about the basic science of the SC.[1]

J. Q. Del Rosso, DO

J. Levin, DO

Reference

1. Del Rosso JQ, Levin J. The clinical relevance of maintaining the functional integrity of the stratum corneum in both healthy and disease-affected skin. *J Clin Aesthet Dermatol.* 2011;4:22-42.

Superantigens in dermatology

Maclas ES, Pereira FA, Rietkerk W, et al (New York Med College)
J Am Acad Dermatol 64:455-472, 2011

Superantigens (SAgs) are virulent polypeptides that are produced by a variety of infectious organisms. They are capable of causing nonspecific T cell activation by circumventing normal antigen processing in the human host. The genetic makeup of the host plays a role in conferring susceptibility or protection against SAgs. They are linked to a variety of conditions, ranging from toxic shock syndrome to recurrent toxin-mediated perineal erythema. The early recognition of signs and symptoms of SAg-mediated illnesses is important to ensure prompt medical treatment.

▶ Superantigens (SAgs) are virulent polypeptides that are produced by infectious agents. This is a review of literature discussing the pathophysiology of SAgs and the diseases they cause. Diseases such as staphylococcal toxic shock syndrome (TSS) and Kawasaki disease (KD) are both SAg-mediated illnesses. TSS is a progressive, systemic illness associated with staphylococcal infection involving specific organism strains. Streptococcal TSS is usually associated with severe necrotizing soft tissue infection. KD is a purely clinical diagnosis based on documenting certain criteria, and up to 25% of patients can be affected with coronary artery aneurysms. The treatment of KD consists of a single dose of intravenous immunoglobulin and long-term aspirin therapy. Kawasaki-like syndrome has also been identified from exposure to SAgs and may be seen in adults with advanced human immunodeficiency virus disease. It is characterized by a rash, mucositis, edema of hands and feet, conjunctivitis, and arthralgia. Other diseases such as plaque/guttate psoriasis, cutaneous T-cell lymphoma (CTCL), and atopic dermatitis (AD) appear elicited or exacerbated by SAgs in some cases. Patients with CTCL are susceptible to *Staphylococcus aureus* infection, which may lead to both neoplastic and reactive T cells. In psoriasis, researchers have found that the presence of staphylococcal SAgs has been linked with more severe disease. In atopic dermatitis, the same SAgs have been known to exacerbate the disease. The reduction of bacterial load by antibiotics or phototherapy causes clinical improvement. Staphylococcal scalded skin syndrome (SSSS) is caused by infection with exfoliative toxin-producing *S aureus*. Other typical features of SAg-mediated illness such as acral edema, strawberry tongue, and mucositis are often present and resolve rapidly following antibiotic therapy. The link between SAgs and other diseases has also been identified, and further research is needed to elucidate its role in various skin conditions.

G. K. Kim, DO

J. Q. Del Rosso, DO

Adverse effects of propranolol when used in the treatment of hemangiomas: A case series of 28 infants

de Graaf M, Breur JMPJ, Raphaël MF, et al (Univ Med Ctr Utrecht, The Netherlands)

J Am Acad Dermatol 65:320-327, 2011

Background.—Infantile hemangioma (IH) is a frequently encountered tumor with a potentially complicated course. Recently, propranolol was discovered to be an effective treatment option.

Objective.—To describe the effects and side effects of propranolol treatment in 28 children with (complicated) IH.

Methods.—A protocol for treatment of IH with propranolol was designed and implemented. Propranolol was administered to 28 children (21 girls and 7 boys, mean age at onset of treatment: 8.8 months).

Results.—All 28 patients had a good response. In two patients, systemic corticosteroid therapy was tapered successfully after propranolol was initiated. Propranolol was also an effective treatment for hemangiomas in 4 patients older than 1 year of age. Side effects that needed intervention and/or close monitoring were not dose dependent and included symptomatic hypoglycemia (n = 2; 1 patient also taking prednisone), hypotension (n = 16, of which 1 is symptomatic), and bronchial hyperreactivity (n = 3). Restless sleep (n = 8), constipation (n = 3) and cold extremities (n = 3) were observed.

Limitations.—Clinical studies are necessary to evaluate the incidence of side effects of propranolol treatment of IH.

Conclusions.—Propranolol appears to be an effective treatment option for IH even in the nonproliferative phase and after the first year of life. Potentially harmful adverse effects include hypoglycemia, bronchospasm, and hypotension.

▶ Infantile hemangiomas (IH) are vascular tumors that often gradually involute with time. In some cases, IH can become complicated and life threatening. Propanolol is a nonselective β-blocker shown to be effective for treatment of IH. This is a study of 28 children with complicated IH. Patients were started on 1 mg/kg/d in 2 or 3 divided daily doses and increased up to 4 mg/kg/d in some patients. Before initiation of medication, all patients received an electrocardiogram and serial photographs of the IH. The mean age of the infants was 6 months. After 1 week of treatment, lesions improved, with change in depth of color and considerable softening to palpation both observed. One patient was on propranolol and oral prednisone and could not be tapered off of the prednisone early because of rebound growth of the IH after attempts to decrease the prednisone. Potential side effects of propranolol include symptomatic hypoglycemia, especially at doses over 4 mg/kg. In this study, 11% of patients (3 of 28) had to discontinue propanolol because of bronchospasm. The authors suggest that propanolol may be safer than systemic corticosteroids. Limitations of this study were the small sample size and absence of a control; however, the latter is difficult to allow for in cases of IH that are complicated. However, with no control, it was difficult to determine if these lesions may have spontaneously resolved without treatment. Propanolol has many side effects that may be detrimental to a growing infant, and risks versus benefits should be carefully weighed before starting this medication.

G. K. Kim, DO

J. Q. Del Rosso, DO

Timolol Maleate 0.5% or 0.1% Gel-Forming Solution for Infantile Hemangiomas: A Retrospective, Multicenter, Cohort Study
Chakkittakandiyil A, Phillips R, Frieden IJ, et al (Hosp for Sick Children, Toronto, Canada; Royal Children's Hosp, Victoria, Australia; Univ of California at San Francisco; et al)
Pediatr Dermatol 29:1-4, 2011

Therapeutic options for superficial infantile hemangiomas (IH) are limited. Recently, timolol maleate gel, a topical nonselective beta-blocker, has been reported as a potentially effective treatment for superficial IH. This study is an extension of a previously published pilot study designed to further investigate the efficacy and safety and to identify predictors of good response of topical 0.5% or 0.1% timolol maleate gel-forming solution. This was a retrospective cohort study including patients enrolled from five centers. Patientswere included if theywere treated with timololmaleate 0.1% or 0.5% gel-forming solution and had photographic documentation of the IH and at least one follow-up visit. Patients with concomitant active treatment using other IH treatments were excluded. The primary endpoint was change in the appearance of IH as evaluated using a visual analog scale (VAS). Data from 73 subjects were available for final analysis. Timolol maleate gel-forming solution 0.5% was used in 85% (62/73) of patients, the remainder being treated with 0.1%. The median age at treatment initiation was 4.27 months (interquartile range [IQR] 2.63–7.21 mos), and patients were treated for a mean of 3.4 ± 2.7 months. All patients except one improved, with a mean improvement of $45 \pm 29.5\%$. Predictors of better response were superficial type of hemangioma ($p = 0.01$), 0.5% timolol concentration ($p = 0.01$), and duration of use longer than 3 months ($p = 0.04$). Sleeping disturbance was noted in one patient. This study further demonstrates the efficacy and tolerability of topical timolol maleate and gradual improvement with longer treatment in patients with superficial IH.

▶ Any dermatologist who sees patients with infantile hemangiomas (IHs) will find this report useful. While the use of systemic propranolol has changed forever how we manage complicated infantile hemangiomas (IHs), most of the IHs that we see are not complicated and do not warrant systemic treatment. Nonetheless, parents want them gone. Infantile hemangiomas most often occur in highly visible areas on the head and neck, and parents are forced to endure the inevitable comments of family members and strangers alike. Luckily, a readily available topical version of a nonselective β-blocker exists in the form of timolol maleate ophthalmic gel-forming solution.

This study retrospectively looks at the effects of topical timolol maleate gel-forming solution (0.05% or 0.1%) twice daily without occlusion on 79 infants with IH. While the mean age of onset of IH was 3 weeks (± 3 weeks), the median age at which treatment was started was 4.3 months. Note that there was a wide age range at which treatment was started. Most lesions were located on the head and neck (85%) and were solitary (70%). No significant side effects were noted. Sleep disturbance was noted in 1 patient. Improvement was noted in all but 1 patient over an average treatment time of 3.4 months. The best responses were seen with superficial hemangiomas and those treated for longer durations.

In terms of safety, there have been cases of systemic absorption with the ophthalmic use of timolol solution with typical β-blocker side effects reported: wheezing, bradycardia, and respiratory depression. Timolol gel-forming solution has less insignificant bioavailabilty in adults than the standard solution. Nonetheless, topical β-blocker therapy should be used with caution, especially around the eye where absorption is greater.

Because this study was not prospective or controlled, there was significant variability as to when the medication was started. Ideally, for the greatest response, timolol maleate 0.5% gel-forming solution applied twice daily should be started at the earliest signs of IH and continued throughout the typical growth period of the hemangioma, 3 to 6 months. Consider use of timolol gel-forming solution in the treatment of any hemangioma that could benefit from earlier regression.

A. Zaenglein, MD

Aesthetic Dermatology for Aging Ethnic Skin
Davis EC, Callender VD (Callender Skin and Laser Ctr, Glenn Dale, MD)
Dermatol Surg 37:901-917, 2011

Background.—Dark-skinned patients manifest the signs of skin aging differently than their fair-skinned counterparts in that the former exhibit more intrinsic facial aging, whereas the later shows more photodamage. Nevertheless, common cosmetic procedures can be used in skin of color to treat the signs of aging.

Objective.—To provide updated clinical information on the use of cosmetic procedures for skin aging in darker phototypes for the safe treatment of this population.

Methods.—A Medline literature search was performed for publications on the safety and efficacy of botulinum toxin, dermal fillers, chemical peels, laser and light-based devices, and microdermabrasion for the treatment of skin aging specifically in ethnic populations.

Results.—Similarly to light-skinned patients, botulinum toxin and dermal fillers provide fast, effective results in skin of color, with fewer complications than with traditional surgery and no downtime. More-invasive procedures, such as chemical peeling, laser resurfacing, and microdermabrasion, can also be effective, but it is important to exercise caution and remain within certain parameters given the greater risk of dyschromias in this population.

Conclusion.—With the proper knowledge of how to treat aging skin of color, these patients can experience the benefits of cosmetic procedures while minimizing the risks.

▶ There are clear differences in the appearance, biochemistry, and inflammatory response when comparing various ethnic skin types. Therefore, it seems reasonable to assume that ethnic skin may have varied responses to cosmetic procedures and therapies.

It was the objective of this article to discern and compare the patterns of aging in white skin versus skin of color in addition to gathering and reporting clinical evidence regarding the safety and efficacy of botulinum toxin injections, lasers, fillers, and chemical peels in skin of color.

This is a thorough meta-analysis detailing most considerations and concerns when evaluating and conducting the above-mentioned cosmetic procedures in patients with skin of color. This article may serve as a comprehensive guide for both physicians who already treat various ethnic skin types and those who may primarily see patients with white skin.

Some of the salient differences between white skin and skin of color mentioned in this article include the patterns of intrinsic and extrinsic aging, effectiveness and duration of certain botulinum toxins, and the increased potential for postinflammatory hyperpigmentation in skin of color.

When comparing skin types, whether it is female versus male skin or different ethnic backgrounds, it is becoming more apparent that there are differences beyond our appearance when comparing skin types. More studies may be needed to clearly understand these differences in skin disease, skin aging, as well as response to medications and cosmetic procedures.

J. Levin, DO

J. Q. Del Rosso, DO

Development of a Photographic Scale for Consistency and Guidance in Dermatologic Assessment of Forearm Sun Damage

McKenzie NE, Saboda K, Duckett LD, et al (Univ of Arizona, Tucson)
Arch Dermatol 147:31-36, 2011

Objectives.—To develop a photographic sun damage assessment scale for forearm skin and test its feasibility and utility for consistent classification of sun damage.

Design.—For a blinded comparison, 96 standardized 8 × 10 digital photographs of participants' forearms were taken. Photographs were graded by an expert dermatologist using an existing 9-category dermatologic assessment scoring scale until all categories contained photographs representative of each of 4 clinical signs. Triplicate photographs were provided in identical image sets to 5 community dermatologists for blinded rating using the dermatologic assessment scoring scale.

Setting.—Academic skin cancer prevention clinic with high-level experience in assessment of sun-damaged skin.

Participants.—Volunteer sample including participants from screenings, chemoprevention, and/or biomarker studies.

Main Outcome Measures.—Reproducibility and agreement of grading among dermatologists by Spearman correlation coefficient to assess the correlation of scores given for the same photograph, κ statistics for ordinal data, and variability of scoring among dermatologists, using analysis of variance models with evaluating physician and photographs as main effects and interaction effect variables to account for the difference in scoring among dermatologists.

Results.—Correlations (73% to >90%) between dermatologists were all statistically significant $(P < .001)$. Scores showed good to substantial agreement but were significantly different $(P < .001)$ for each of 4 clinical signs and the difference varied significantly $(P < .001)$ among photographs.

Conclusions.—With good to substantial agreement, we found the development of a photographic forearm sun damage assessment scale highly feasible. In view of significantly different rating scores, a photographic reference for assessment of sun damage is also necessary (Table 1).

▶ Standard communication and consistent assessments are 2 things that enable doctors to understand each other and offer somewhat interchangeable and reliable care from one doctor to the next. The objective of this article is to present and evaluate an objective grading method of forearm sun damage via photographic evaluation for consistency in dermatologic assessment. Using the authors proposed scale shown in Table 1, the study found good to excellent agreement among 6 dermatologists at a high level of statistical significance. Nevertheless, there were differences in how the physicians rated the photographs.

Objective grading methods are used throughout medicine. A classic example is the New York Heart Association classification of the stages of heart failure. Having an objective grading method promotes consistent communication between physicians, allows the development of standardized treatment dependant on the stage of the disease, and assists in reasonable determination of the prognosis based on the stage of disease. Using a similar grading for forearm sun

TABLE 1.—Distribution of Reference Standard Initial Grading by Category and Clinical Sign

Category	Level	Fine Wrinkling	Coarse Wrinkling	No. Abnormal Pigmentation	Global Assessment
None	0	2	9	5	6
Low	1	12	5	12	10
	2	7	11	7	8
	3	11	8	10	9
Moderate	4	6	5	4	5
	5	10	14	13	14
	6	21	10	19	17
Severe	7	15	19	13	15
	8	9	7	10	6
	9	3	8	3	6

damage may similarly allow the development of a standardized treatment regimen and an accurate risk assessment for skin cancer development based on the stage of the disease within the classification.

There are several limitations to the scale proposed. First, the scale was created using 1 physician's assessment as the reference standard instead of using objective measurements or physician consensus. As mentioned in the article, physicians can be biased based on the population of patients who come to their office. Therefore, a physician that deals mostly with the elderly would likely evaluate "average" sun damage as being more mild in severity than other physicians who see younger patients with less sun damage.

Second, the dermatologists used the proposed scale without any training or seeing a photographic reference standard for the different categories and their severity levels. Perhaps with proper training and reference standards, there may be less variation among dermatologists. Third, there is an impaired ability via photography to evaluate the topographic features, such as hyperkeratotic changes, including those that are more palpable than visible.

Despite the limitations, this is an important study, and it may provide the impetus for a more standardized way of assessing sun damage of the forearm.

J. Levin, DO

J. Q. Del Rosso, DO

Gender aspects in skin diseases
Chen W, Mempel M, Traidl-Hofmann C, et al (Technische Universität München, Germany)
J Eur Acad Dermatol Venereol 24:1378-1385, 2010

Gender differences in medicine have been recognized in anatomy, physiology, as well as in epidemiology and manifestations of various diseases. With respect to skin disorders, males are generally more commonly afflicted with infectious diseases while women are more susceptible to psychosomatic problems, pigmentary disorders, certain hair diseases, and particularly autoimmune as well as allergic diseases. Significantly, more female sex-associated dermatoses can be identified than the male sex-associated dermatoses. Dermatoses in the genital area differ between men and women. Gender differences also exist in the occurrence and prognosis of certain skin malignancies. The mechanisms underlying gender differences in skin diseases remain largely unknown. Differences in the skin structure and physiology, effect of sex hormones, ethnic background, sociocultural behaviour and environmental factors may interact to exert the influences. A better understanding of gender differences in human health and diseases will allow the development of novel concepts for prevention, diagnosis and therapy of skin diseases (Table 1).

▶ This study is meta-analysis concerning the differences in skin structure and function and skin disease in men versus women.

Although the title Gender Aspects in Skin Disease implies that this article only discusses gender differences with regard to cutaneous disorders, this article

TABLE 1.—Skin Diseases with Significant Female Predominance (Except Female Genital or Pregnancy Diseases)

High (Female/Male Ratio ≥9)	Moderate (Female/Male Ratio 5–8)	Low (Female/Male Ratio 2–4)
Autoerythrocyte sensitization syndrome	Lichen sclerosus et atrophicus	Rhematoid arthritis
Disseminated discoid lupus erythematosus	Chronic venous insufficiency/varicose vein/ulcus cruris venosum	Scleroderma
Lupus erythematosus (adult)	Morton interdigital neuroma	Antiphospholipid antibody syndrome
Sjögren syndrome	Verrucae planae juveniles	Temporal giant cell arteritis
Type III hereditary angioedema	Multiple eccrine hidrocystomas	Chronic immune thrombocytopenic purpura
Frontal fibrosing alopecia (Kossard)	Loose anagen hair syndrome	Chronic urticaria
Graham–Little syndrome		Cutaneous adverse drug reaction (including Stevens–Johnson-syndrome/toxic epidermal necrolysis)
Central centrifugal cicatricial alopecia		Erythromelalgia
Chronic telogen effluvium		Lichen planopilaris
Trichotillomania		Polymorphous light eruption
Fox–Fordyce disease		Actinic prurigo
Rosacea fulminans		Prurigo pigmentosa
Acne excoriée		Granuloma annulare
Lichen nuchae		Necrobiosis lipoidica
Perioral dermatitis		Sarcoidosis
Melasma		Erythema nodosum
Hori nevus		Partial lipodystrophy
Dercum's disease		Ota nevus
Angioma serpiginosum		Adult tinea capitis
Hidradenoma papilliferum		Trichilemmal cyst/proliferating trichilemmal cyst
Erosive adenomatosis of nipple		Pilomatricoma
Multiple dermatofibroma		Cylindroma
Mammary Paget's disease		Eruptive syringoma
		Subungual glomus tumour
		Angiokeratoma of Mibelli
		Subcutaneous panniculitis-like T-cell lymphoma
		Primary cutaneous large B-cell lymphoma, leg type
		Lentigo maligna

appropriately discusses more than disease alone. In addition to succinct reporting of which skin diseases are more common in men compared with women and vice versa in Table 1, this article also explores the differences between men and women with regard to skin structure, function, genetics, immune function and responses, and sociocultural backgrounds. Most of the differences in men versus women can be explained by hormonal differences; however, some differences need further discovery.

Only with examining the basic science and function of skin on a molecular level can we begin to understand the differences in men versus women in skin disease. This article offers a great starting point to a subject that, upon further discovery, may be more complex than just a simple initiator (hormones) and promoter (environment). However, with what information is known today concerning the differences in skin in men versus women, the most central explanation we have is clearly related to hormonal influences.

J. Levin, DO

J. Q. Del Rosso, DO

Prevalence of benign cutaneous disease among Oxford renal transplant recipients

Lally A, Casabonne D, Imko-Walczuk B, et al (Oxford Radcliffe Hosps, UK; Univ of Oxford, UK; et al)

J Eur Acad Dermatol Venereol 25:462-470, 2011

Background.—The burden of malignant and benign cutaneous disease among renal transplant recipients (RTR) is substantial. Little attention is given to non-malignant skin problems in the literature despite their potential impact on quality of life or on aesthetics — which may contribute to poor compliance with immunosuppressive medications post-transplantation.

Objectives.—The aim of this study was to examine prevalence of benign cutaneous disease in a group of RTRs and identify risk factors for individual cutaneous conditions.

Methods.—All cutaneous findings were recorded in a single full body skin examination of 308 RTRs. Data on medical, transplant and medication history were obtained from questionnaire and medical records. Odds ratios were calculated to look at associations between benign cutaneous diseases and various potential risk factors after controlling for gender, age, time since transplantation and skin type.

Results.—Cutaneous infections such as viral warts (38%), fungal infection (18%) and folliculitis (27%) were common and usually chronic. A range of pilosebaceous unit disorders were observed with hypertrichosis being strongly associated with ciclosporin ($P < 0.0001$). Other iatrogenic cutaneous effects included gingival hyperplasia (27%) and purpura (41%). We identified seborrhoeic warts and skin tags in 55% and 33% respectively. Inflammatory dermatoses were rare (< 2%) apart from seborrhoeic dermatitis (9.5%).

Discussion.—In this first comprehensive study on prevalence of benign cutaneous diseases in a UK transplant population, a wide range of skin disorders was identified. It is therefore important that RTRs have access to dermatology services post-transplantation for appropriate management of benign cutaneous conditions as well as early detection of cutaneous malignancy and education regarding risks of sun exposure.

▶ Much has been studied and written about the increased incidence of skin cancers in renal transplant recipients and other immunosuppressed patients. This is the first comprehensive evaluation of nonmalignant cutaneous disorders that occur in renal transplant recipients in the United Kingdom. The study population had a mean age of 52 years and a longer time after transplantation than previous studies that often evaluated a younger population. A high prevalence of benign cutaneous disease was revealed, most of which were iatrogenic or infectious and many of which were listed in the abstract. Some of these were related to specific immunosuppressive agents, and some were related to the duration of immunosuppression.

The significance of this article is that it demonstrates the prevalence of cutaneous conditions in this patient population, which, although nonmalignant, can be very distressing. Some of these conditions, such as hypertrichosis, acne, or warts, can be frustrating and can affect the quality of life enough to potentially influence adherence to immunosuppressive regimens. Recognizing and managing these nonmalignant cutaneous conditions is important for primary care physicians and transplant teams to address, and access to dermatologic care should be made readily available for this patient population.

E. M. Billingsley, MD

Diagnosis and treatment of the neutrophilic dermatoses (pyoderma gangrenosum, Sweet's syndrome)
Dabade TS, Davis MDP (Mayo Clinic, Rochester, MN)
Dermatol Ther 24:273-284, 2011

Neutrophilic dermatoses include a spectrum of disorders with similar histologic appearance and pathologic processes. Clinically, however, they have different physical manifestations and associations. This group includes two diseases for which dermatologists are commonly consulted in the hospital, namely pyoderma gangrenosum and acute febrile neutrophilic dermatosis, or Sweet's syndrome. Evaluation is challenging, and many therapeutic approaches have been described for both. The previously reported diagnostic criteria, physical descriptions, differential diagnosis, workup, and treatment options are reviewed. A practical approach to pyoderma gangrenosum and Sweet's syndrome for the provider is described.

▶ Pyoderma gangrenosum (PG) and Sweet syndrome are often reasons for hospital consultation, and the evaluation can be difficult and challenging for clinicians. To this end, Dabade and Davis present a well-written and comprehensive review of these 2 disease states. Careful attention is paid to all aspects of the diseases, including a review of the description of the lesions, the differential diagnoses that must be considered, the workup, and the treatment options. As noted in the article, a wide differential exists when presented with ulcerations on a patient, including PG. As the authors consider PG a diagnosis of exclusion, the proper workup is crucial. The review provides the relevant diagnostic criteria for the 4 forms of PG and a thorough approach to a patient with PG ulcerations, complete with tables. An approach for patients with recalcitrant PG ulcerations is also provided along with a thorough list of potential treatments. No less attention is provided to Sweet syndrome, and a similar review with tables is provided on diagnostic criteria, workup considerations, and treatment options. Additionally, each treatment option for Sweet syndrome includes a reference citation that is representative of the highest level of evidence published. Ultimately, this article is a nice one-stop reference source for the clinician when presented with either PG or Sweet syndrome.

B. D. Michaels, DO
J. Q. Del Rosso, DO

Conceptual Approach to the Management of Infantile Hemangiomas
Fay A, Nguyen J, Waner M (Harvard Med School, Boston, MA; West Virginia Univ School of Medicine, Morgantown; St Luke's/Roosevelt Hosp Ctr, NY)
J Pediatr 157:881-888, 2010

Background.—The best outcomes of hemangioma treatment are achieved using a multidisciplinary approach. Treatment goals include preservation of life and sight, but also consider outward appearance, psychosocial health, and family dynamics. The decision to treat depends largely on the location and size of lesions, patient age, systemic involvement, and family desire. A case-specific interventional strategy relies on the subtype, stage, and depth of the lesion as well as other factors. A rationale for treatment selection and review of emerging therapies for infantile hemangioma were offered.

Treatment Planning.—The diagnosis of infantile hemangioma is often obvious but ultrasound scans, magnetic resonance imaging, angiography, or biopsy may be needed. A diagnosis of hemangioma relies on clinical presentation and a positive histochemical response to glucose transporter protein type 1. Factors driving the decision to intervene include anatomic location and size of the lesion and patient age. Subtype, stage, and depth of the lesion dictate how to intervene. Hemangiomas can be focal or segmental; the two types behave differently and vary in treatment response. Focal lesions are more easily resected; segmental ones are more destructive, are more likely to ulcerate and signal systemic involvement, and more often need a systemic approach. Hemangiomas progress through proliferative, dormant, and involutional stages, which respond to varying treatment protocols. Lesions are found in the skin (cutaneous), under the skin (subcutaneous), or both (compound).

Treatment Options.—Systemic corticosteroids were the mainstay of treatment for segmental, orbital, airway, and other large hemangiomas but adverse effects include behavior disturbances, Cushingoid appearance, growth delay, and hypertension. Young age, high doses, and prolonged treatment are associated with a greater frequency of adverse effects. Intralesional corticosteroids reduce the refractive error in children with periocular focal hemangiomas or medium-size subglottic hemangiomas, but risk blindness and other complications. Topical corticosteroids are a low-risk, low-reward option for superficial hemangiomas when laser treatment is unavailable. Imiquimod produces modest clinical results but can cause severe erythema and crusting. Interferon (INF) α-2a should not be used for infantile hemangiomas. Vincristine is used as a second-line therapy for corticosteroid-resistant life- or sight-threatening hemangiomas but can cause gastrointestinal upset, fever, headache, and neuropathies.

Beta-blocking agents offer promise for treating segmental, orbital, and life-threatening hemangiomas, but their usefulness for focal lesions is unsupported. Propranolol has replaced corticosteroids as the first-line treatment for segmental, orbital, airway, and other large, aggressive hemangiomas, but no standard protocol is being used.

The pulse dye laser (PDL) is effective for superficial hemangiomas and can be combined with local corticosteroid injections or surgical excision for compound lesions. Complications include minor blisters, ulceration, crusting, textural change, scarring, and changes in pigmentation. Fractional photothermolysis generates a microgrid pattern of independent thermal columns in the dermis that stimulate collagen remodeling and allow rapid epithelial recovery. It is especially useful for late treatment of involuted hemangiomas. The carbon dioxide laser is useful for airway hemangiomas but can cause post-laser subglottic stenosis.

Surgical approaches have changed considerably, as have the indications for this approach. Previously only life- or sight-threatening cases and end-stage reconstruction merited surgical intervention, but the rapid, definitive effect of surgery allows one to avoid missing early psychological milestones. Delaying surgery can miss the tissue-expanding effect of proliferating subcutaneous hemangiomas. Advances in anesthesia, surgical technologies, and surgical techniques have improved surgical success. Drawbacks include a significant risk of hemorrhage that requires intensive hemostatic maneuvers. The enhanced hemostasis now available has allowed safe dissection in previously inaccessible regions. Surgeons can also combine their surgeries with later laser treatments. Airway and periocular hemangiomas along with refractory lesions are managed primarily using surgical excision. Eyelid and orbit surgery is designed to avoid amblyopia, astigmatism, strabismus, blepharoptosis, and permanent facial deformity. Early excision of lip hemangiomas can promote suckling and improve outcomes.

Conclusions.—The diversity of hemangioma presentations requires individualization of evaluation and treatment planning. No single modality or subspecialist can treat all hemangiomas, but ophthalmologists, otolaryngologists, dermatologists, and radiologists can contribute by identifying morbidities and initiating preventive measures.

▶ In some cases, infantile hemangiomas (IHs) can have not only threatening physical consequences but also sequelae related to the psychosocial well being of the patient. In the last several years, effective treatments for infantile hemangiomas continue to be a topic of interest, and treatment modalities have expanded. Even with these advances, no one single treatment option is effective for all types of IHs, thus, proper evaluation of each patient and development of a treatment plan is important. To this end, Fay et al provide insightful considerations when approaching the treatment of IHs and, although not a study, the article is constructive to physicians in many respects. The article addresses important planning suggestions regarding when and how to intervene in the treatment of infantile hemangiomas. In addition, the authors also provide a thorough review of the current medical treatment options, including their effectiveness and adverse effects. Interventional treatment alternatives covered include the available pharmacologic therapies to laser treatment to considerations for surgical management. Overall, the article is a thorough and thoughtful source of review on this topic and, ultimately, is a beneficial review for any practitioner who evaluates IHs.

B. D. Michaels, DO

J. Q. Del Rosso, DO

Use of complementary and alternative medicine among adults with skin disease: Updated results from a national survey

Fuhrmann T, Smith N, Tausk F (Univ of Rochester Med Ctr, NY)

J Am Acad Dermatol 63:1000-1005, 2010

Background.—In the United States, complementary and alternative medicine (CAM) is used for a variety of diseases, including those of the skin. An estimate of the prevalence of CAM use among adults with skin disease using the alternative health supplement of the 2002 National Health Interview Survey (NHIS) has been published.

Objective.—We sought to analyze the 2007 NHIS data to update the prevalence of CAM use among adults with skin disease in the United States.

Methods.—We conducted a cross-sectional survey using the 2007 alternative health supplement of the NHIS.

Results.—Among those reporting skin problems in the past year, 84.5% (95% confidence interval 76.9-92.0) used CAM. Only 1.1% of this group (95% confidence interval 0.7-1.6) used CAM specifically for skin disease. Adjusting for race, sex, income, education level, and region, those reporting skin problems were more likely to use CAM than those who did not report skin problems (adjusted odds ratio 2.5, $P \leq .002$, 95% confidence interval 1.4-4.4). Vitamin/mineral and herbal supplements were the most common CAM modalities used among those with skin disease in general, and among those who used CAM specifically for skin problems.

Limitations.—As this is not a dermatology-focused database, the definition of skin disease is limited. It was not possible to comment on trends between the 2002 and 2007 data because the 2007 survey was significantly changed.

Conclusion.—CAM use among adults with skin problems in the United States continues to be common. Addition of a specific dermatology supplement to a future NHIS survey would allow for population-based estimates not only of CAM use but of associations with other comorbid conditions among adults with skin disease in the United States.

▶ As expected, complementary and alternative medicine (CAM) is used commonly in the United States, including for skin diseases. In the past, data have been compiled on CAM use in the National Health Interview Survey (NHIS). In 2007, however, new information on CAM use was made available in the NHIS. Fuhrmann et al sought to analyze and update this surveyed information as it relates to skin disease. Although the percentage of patients that used CAM specifically for skin disease was found to be only 1.1% in the group, CAM use among patients who have had skin disease within the previous year of the survey was found to be as high as 84.5%. This represents a definitive increase in CAM use from the prior 2002 survey period. In addition, the most common type of CAM options used were herbal and vitamin/mineral supplements. Overall, although the study meets its objective, the results in this survey are not surprising. However, the article does provide an important reminder to dermatologists that patients do in fact use other non-physician-prescribed medicinal modalities such as herbal and mineral supplements—and at an increasing rate. The article also provides a nice table of some of the more common herbal supplements used by patients among those reporting skin problems. Ultimately, dermatologists need to keep in mind the increasing use of CAM treatments by patients when managing their skin diseases, and to that end, this article is a beneficial review.

B. D. Michaels, DO

J. Q. Del Rosso, DO

Skin Conditions That Bring Patients to Emergency Departments
Baibergenova A, Shear NH (Univ of Toronto, Ontario, Canada)
Arch Dermatol 147:118-120, 2011

Background.—Dermatologic conditions requiring medical treatment are found in an estimated 19% to 27% of the population, yet only about 7% of all outpatient clinic visits involve dermatologic complaints. This may reflect the usually benign nature of most skin conditions, which often have a low acute mortality. The epidemiology of emergency department (ED) visits for skin conditions was investigated.

Methods.—The National Ambulatory Care Records System, kept by the Canadian Institute for Health Information, provided the data that were analyzed. The records of patients who visited EDs in Ontario between

April 1, 2002 and March 31, 2007 and had a principal diagnosis of diseases of the skin and subcutaneous tissues were reviewed. The diagnoses were made by ED physicians in most cases, and there was no way to discern if the patient was seen by a consulting dermatologist.

Results.—Skin complaints accounted for 3.3% of all the ED visits, with the annual average of skin-related visits being 173,395. Male and female patients were represented fairly equally. The mean age of the patients was 39.4 years, but infants and patients over age 80 years were particularly over-represented. Seventy-five percent were assigned non-urgent or semi-urgent status, with just 2% qualifying as emergencies. Discharge home was the final disposition in 94% of cases; 4% required hospital admission. Over half of the visits involved skin and subcutaneous tissue infections. Other disorders noted were dermatitis, urticaria, and skin appendage disorders, with bullous disorders accounting for only 0.06% of the visits. The most common infectious diagnosis was cellulitis, found in 30.4% of patients but 71.4% of those requiring hospital admission. The ED visits showed a seasonal variation, with the highest numbers found in July and August and the lowest in February.

Conclusions.—Patients seldom seek emergency care for dermatologic diseases. The seasonal variations noted probably reflect the heat, humidity, outdoor activities, and insect bites common in the summer peak and the lack of these in the winter lull. A significant percentage of patients were diagnosed with cellulitis. Other studies have indicated that about 20% of cases diagnosed in the ED as cellulitis were revised to other diagnoses after being seen by specialists in dermatology and infectious diseases. The conditions that mimic cellulitis and may complicate its diagnosis should be identified to determine if the diagnosis is skewed by the attending physician's specialty.

▶ Overall, there is a lack of both data and studies on the epidemiology of skin conditions that present to the emergency room (ER). Baibergenova and Shear performed a retrospective review of a large Canadian medical administrative database to help provide further insight on this topic. Not surprisingly, more than half of ER visits relating to skin conditions were for infections, with cellulitis being the most commonly diagnosed infectious etiology. Cellulitis was also responsible for greater than two-thirds of skin-related hospital admissions. Presenting conditions did, however, vary based on age, with infections the most common presenting condition among adults and dermatitis and urticaria more common among infants and preschool-age children, respectively. Seasonal variation in ER visits was also noted. The summer months of July and August had the largest peak for skin conditions presenting in the ER, which was hypothesized to be possibly related to causative triggers such as heat/humidity, increased outdoor activities, and insect bites. The limitation in the study is that although it was a large study, it was based solely on information from Canadian ER visits. Also, as was noted by the authors, the diagnoses were made by ER physicians with no way of verifying if the diagnoses were also verified by a consulting dermatologist, leaving the possibility of overdiagnosis of skin conditions such as cellulitis. Despite this limitation, the study does provide further relevant information on dermatologic conditions presenting in the ER and provides a framework for potential further studies in this area.

B. D. Michaels, DO

J. Q. Del Rosso, DO

Dermatoscopy use by US dermatologists: A cross-sectional survey

Engasser HC, Warshaw EM (Minneapolis Dept of Veterans Affairs Med Ctr, MN; Univ of Minnesota Dept of Dermatology; Chanhassen)
J Am Acad Dermatol 63:412-419, 2010

Background.—Although dermatoscopy is widely used in Europe and Australia, little is known about dermatoscopy use by US dermatologists.

Objective.—We sought to estimate the prevalence of dermatoscopy use by US dermatologists and examine associations with practice characteristics.

Methods.—We conducted a cross-sectional survey of all US fellows of the American Academy of Dermatology.

Results.—Of 8501 eligible recipients, 3238 (38.1%) surveys were completed and returned. Of respondents, 48% used dermatoscopy (n = 1555). Dermatoscopy use was associated with the following characteristics: age younger than 50 years ($P < .0001$), female sex ($P = .0001$), practice location in the Northeast ($P < .0001$), involvement in resident teaching ($P < .0001$), and dermatoscopy training ($P < .0001$). The main reasons for not using dermatoscopy included: lack of training (39.7%), lack of interest (32.5%), time required for dermatoscopic examination (27.6%), and belief dermatoscopy would not affect clinical decisions (15.2%).

Limitations.—Low response rate and potential response bias were limitations.

Conclusions.—Approximately half of respondents used dermatoscopy in their practice. Not surprisingly, dermatoscopy users were more likely to be younger, involved in resident teaching, or have training in dermatoscopy.

▶ Dermatoscopy is a noninvasive technique to visualize morphologic features that are not visible to the naked eye, serving to assist primarily in the diagnosis of pigmented lesions and some nonpigmented skin disorders. Dermatoscopes are modified magnifying devices permitting the visualization of pigmented structures and vessels in the epidermis and superficial dermis.[1] The current cross-sectional survey of US dermatologists found approximately half of the responders use dermatoscopy (1555/3238), and these physicians were more associated with younger age, teaching institutions, previous dermatoscopy course participation, and owning at least 1 dermatoscopy book. The main reasons for not using dermatoscopy include lack of training, lack of interest, length of time required, and the belief that its use would not change their clinical decisions. As stated by the authors, limitations of this study include low response rate of 38%, response bias, and predefined choices that may limit analysis options. Dermatoscopy is a useful adjuvant in the clinicians armamentarium and its use is increasing. Over time, its use is expected to increase among dermatologists.

S. Bellew, DO

J. Q. Del Rosso, DO

Reference

1. Zalaudek I, Kreusch J, Giacomel J, et al. How to diagnose nonpigmented skin tumors: a review of vascular structures seen with dermoscopy: part I. melanocytic skin tumors. *J Am Acad Dermatol.* 2010;63:361-374.

Lichen Planus Occurring after Influenza Vaccination: Report of Three Cases and Review of the Literature

Sato NA, Kano Y, Shiohara T (Kyorin Univ School of Medicine, Tokyo, Japan)
Dermatology 221:296-299, 2010

Although influenza vaccine is thought to be effective and safe, it occasionally causes systemic reactions such as toxic epidermal necrolysis, bullous pemphigoid, lichen planus (LP), etc. The period of increased risk of developing these events was different depending on the immune responses induced by the vaccination. We report 3 cases of LP which appeared after an influenza vaccination. Our cases indicate that the period of increased risk of developing vaccine-related LP was concentrated within 2 weeks after vaccination, and that the vaccine alone represents a triggering factor necessary for immune alteration sufficient for the development of LP. Because these adverse events tend to develop over a predictable time course, the time of onset may give an important clue to the diagnosis of vaccine-related diseases. We suggest that a history of recent vaccination should be sought in all patients presenting with linear LP.

▶ An adverse effect may be vaccine-induced if a clear time period between the event and the vaccination can be established. The influenza vaccine has been associated with a number of skin diseases, such as toxic epidermal necrolysis, Sweet's disease, erythema nodosum, Gianotti-Crosti syndrome, vasculitis, bullous pemphigoid, pemphigus, and lichen planus (LP). Although most cases of vaccine-induced LP have been associated with the hepatitis B vaccine, the current case report illustrates 3 patients who developed linear LP 2 weeks after influenza vaccine injection. Because the risk of developing LP is approximately within 2 weeks of vaccination, clinicians should routinely ask about recent history of vaccine administration in all patients with linear LP.

S. Bellew, DO

J. Q. Del Rosso, DO

Nevus simplex: A reconsideration of nomenclature, sites of involvement, and disease associations

Juern AM, Glick ZR, Drolet BA, et al (Med College of Wisconsin, Milwaukee; George Washington Univ Med School, DC; et al)
J Am Acad Dermatol 63:805-814, 2010

Background.—Nevus simplex (NS) is a common birthmark on the forehead, glabella, upper eyelids, and nape. More widespread involvement can be confused with port-wine stains (nevus flammeus) and other vascular birthmarks.

Objectives.—To further categorize the anatomic locations in infants with extensive NS and evaluate for any possible disease associations.

Methods.—We conducted a retrospective review of patients with extensive NS seen at two tertiary care centers.

Results.—Twenty-seven patients with extensive NS were identified. All had at least one typical site of involvement: glabella (77.8%), nape (59.3%), and eyelids (55.6%). Additional sites were the scalp, including the vertex, occiput, parietal (66.7%); nose (66.7%); lip (59.2%); lumbosacral skin (55.6%); and upper and mid back (14.8 %).

Limitations.—Retrospective nature of the study and relatively small sample size.

Conclusions.—We propose the term "nevus simplex complex" for NS with more widespread involvement beyond the typical sites. Consistent use of the term "nevus simplex" will aid in correct diagnosis and appropriate management of these birthmarks.

▶ Nevus simplex (NS) is commonly known as the "salmon patch" and is one of the most common birthmarks noted in the pediatric population. Although the forehead, glabella, and nape are the most common areas, other sites can be affected and frequently confused with port-wine stain (nevus flammeus). NS is differentiated from nevus flammeus in that it resolves spontaneously within 2 years. This is a retrospective study of 27 patients with 9 having a family history of NS. Also, 4 of 27 had a family history of another vascular anomaly with 40% of cases being infantile hemangioma. All patients had at least 1 typical site affected. The most common sites were the glabella (77.8%), nape (59.3%), and eyelids (55.6%). Certain association patterns were noted. All patients with upper cutaneous lip involvement had glabellar stains (n = 8), all patients with lower lip lesions had upper lip involvement (n = 4), and those with NS on the upper back had a lumbosacral NS (n = 3). Sizes ranged from 0.2 to 10 cm. Lesions on the forehead were typically wedge- or V-shaped, and most were ill-defined ovals. There were no underlying abnormalities detected on magnetic resonance imaging, with no cases showing a spinal cord abnormality. The authors suggest that in patients with an NS without other cutaneous abnormalities such as hypertrichosis, a dermal sinus or pit, lipoma, or deviated gluteal cleft, performance of imaging studies provides a low yield. In conclusion, identification of NS is essential for clinicians to avoid diagnostic confusion and help reassure parents of the benign nature of this condition.

G. K. Kim, DO

J. Q. Del Rosso, DO

Procedural dermatology training during dermatology residency: A survey of third-year dermatology residents
Lee EH, Nehal KS, Dusza SW, et al (Memorial Sloan-Kettering Cancer Ctr, NY; Laser and Skin Surgery Ctr of New York)
J Am Acad Dermatol 64:475-483, 2011

Background.—Given the expanding role of multiple surgical procedures in dermatology, resident training in procedural dermatology must be continually assessed to keep pace with changes in the specialty.

Objective.—We sought to assess the third-year resident experience in procedural dermatology during residency training.

Methods.—This survey study was mailed to third-year dermatology residents at 107 Accreditation Council for Graduate Medical Education (ACGME)-approved dermatology residency programs in 2009.

Results.—A total of 240 residents responded (66%), representing 89% of programs surveyed. Residents assume the role of primary surgeon most commonly in excisional surgery (95%) and flap and graft reconstruction (49%) and least often in Mohs micrographic surgery (18%). In laser and cosmetic procedures, the resident role varies greatly. Residents believed they were most prepared in excisional surgery, botulinum toxin, and laser surgery. Residents believed it was sufficient to have only knowledge of less commonly performed procedures such as hair transplantation, tumescent liposuction, and ambulatory phlebectomy. Of responding residents, 55% were very satisfied with their procedural dermatology training during residency.

Limitations.—Individual responses from residents may be biased. Neither residency program nor dermatologic surgery directors were surveyed.

Conclusion.—This survey confirms dermatology residents received broad training in procedural dermatology in 2009, in keeping with ACGME/ Residency Review Committee program guidelines. The results provide feedback to dermatology residency programs and are an invaluable tool for assessing, modifying, and strengthening the current procedural dermatology curriculum.

▶ The aging population, which has an increased incidence of skin cancer, combined with a more appearance-conscious society that encourages greater demand for cosmetic services, has prompted a survey study of the quality and extent of residency training in procedural dermatology. The current study offered participation of 107 Accreditation Council for Graduate Medical Education-approved dermatology residency programs in 2009. Procedural dermatology is a subspecialty of dermatologic surgery that includes cutaneous oncology, reconstructive surgery, and cutaneous cosmetic procedures. Surveys mailed to third-year residents addressed residency program characteristics, didactic education in procedural dermatology, scope of resident training in procedural dermatology, resident expectations, and resident confidence in and overall satisfaction with procedures. Results indicate that didactic training in procedural dermatology continues to include lectures and journal clubs with even greater exposure to cadavers and live demonstrations. Residents are performing more excisional surgeries and botulinum toxin denervations and using injectable fillers. In contrast, residents have much more limited roles in Mohs micrographic surgery (MMS) and nail surgery. As the authors state, a higher volume of MMS cases coupled with active mentoring may be needed to master MMS. The practice of nail surgery on cadavers may improve competence in nail cases.

Limitations of this study include results based on surveys derived solely from residents. Determination of competency was based on self-assessment and not on a comparison of logs or objective evaluation of resident competency. Future studies comparing plastic surgery and ear, nose, and throat residents with dermatology residents may be of interest. Also, results may change slightly with the inclusion of osteopathic dermatology residents, who may have more hands-on surgical-procedural experience during their training.

S. Bellew, DO
J. Q. Del Rosso, DO

Toll-like receptors and skin
Ermertcan AT, Öztürk F, Gündüz K (Celal Bayar Univ, Manisa, Turkey)
J Eur Acad Dermatol Venereol 25:997-1006, 2011

Toll-like receptors are important pattern recognition receptors which have key roles in both innate and adaptive immune responses. They are strongly associated with the pathogenesis of inflammatory and autoimmune diseases. Furthermore, Toll-like receptors have also been implicated in the pathogenesis of several skin diseases such as skin infections, psoriasis, acne vulgaris, lichen planus, Behçet's disease, leprosy, syphilis, Lyme disease, atopic dermatitis and allergic contact dermatitis, mycosis fungoides, non-melanoma skin cancers and melanoma. In this manuscript, the structure and functions of Toll-like receptors in immune responses, their impact on skin diseases and recent advances on therapeutic usage have been reviewed.

▶ Living organisms have immune systems that have a way of discriminating self from nonself. Toll-like receptors (TLRs) are major recognition receptors important as a first line of defense in innate immunity and also contribute to adaptive immunity. This article discusses the structure and function of TLRs, and their role in the pathogenesis of certain dermatologic disorders. TLRs are a group of glycoproteins that function as surface transmembrane receptors located on the cell membrane and allow these cells to recognize specific ligands, usually found in microbes and also some nucleic acids, allowing for immune activation.

TLR signaling utilizes MyD88-dependent pathways that drive inflammatory processes leading to mediator release (ie, cytokines). The most important epidermal cells expressing TLRs include keratinocytes, Langerhans cells, dermal monocytes, mast cells in the dermis, endothelial cells, and skin stromal cells. TLRs have also been implicated in many immune and inflammatory diseases, cancers, and wound healing. Skin diseases related to TLRs include melanoma, psoriasis, lichen planus, acne vulgaris, rosacea, leprosy, atopic dermatitis, non-melanoma skin cancers, systemic lupus erythematosus, ultraviolet injury, bacterial infections, and viral infections. Also, the activation of TLRs has been of pharmacologic interest. Imiquimod was the first TLR agonist approved for use in humans, exhibiting antiviral and antineoplastic properties. Other drugs such as calcineurin inhibitors, nicotinamide, and retinoids (ie, trans-retinoic acid, adapalene, tazarotene) have also been shown to affect TLRs and aid in the treatment of certain dermatoses. More studies are needed to further evaluate the relationship between skin disease and directed TLR-based treatments.

G. K. Kim, DO

J. Q. Del Rosso, DO

Topical nitroglycerin: A promising treatment option for chondrodermatitis nodularis helicis

Flynn V, Chisholm C, Grimwood R (Scott and White Memorial Hosp Clinic and Texas A&M Health Science Ctr College of Medicine, Temple)
J Am Acad Dermatol 65:531-536, 2011

Background.—Chondrodermatitis nodularis helicis (CNH) is a painful nodule that often interferes with sleep and occurs on the helix or antihelix of the ear in older patients. Although several case reports describe a variety of seemingly effective surgical and conservative treatment options, well-studied treatment modalities have varying efficacy rates and can often demonstrate disappointing results.

Objectives.—The purpose of this study was to evaluate the efficacy of 2% topical nitroglycerin for the treatment of CNH.

Methods.—A retrospective chart review was performed in 12 patients given the diagnosis of CNH who received 2% topical nitroglycerin twice daily for therapy. Therapeutic efficacy was determined by identifying improvement in the appearance and symptomatology of the lesion.

Results.—A total of 13 lesions in 12 patients were treated, with 12 (92%) lesions demonstrating improvement with the use of topical nitroglycerin. Eight of 13 (61.5%) CNH lesions developed complete clearance and resolution of symptoms, requiring no further treatment. Four of 13 (30.8%) lesions were found to have only symptomatic improvement, and these patients continued to use the ointment as needed. One of 12 (8.3%) patients found no benefit with the treatment but had also failed multiple other treatments modalities.

Limitations.—Limitations include the small number of patients treated and the retrospective nature of the study.

Conclusions.—Topical nitroglycerin demonstrated efficacy in treating both the symptoms and lesional appearance of CNH in a noninvasive manner, with an overall success rate that is comparable with other published methods.

▶ There are multiple treatment options for chondrodermatitis nodularis helicis (CNH)—and for good reason, because many have varying degrees of efficacy, with a high recurrence rate even with surgical intervention. According to this study by Flynn et al, a promising new treatment may prove to be a beneficial option: topical nitroglycerin. The study involved a retrospective chart review and was admittedly limited in size: only 12 patients (with a total of 13 lesions) were included in the analysis. However, based on their findings, topical nitroglycerin 2% applied twice a day showed a 92% improvement (either clinical or symptomatic improvement) in CNH lesions. Complete clinical clearance was achieved in 61% of patients (8 of 13 lesions) and of those that did not clear, symptomatic improvement was achieved in 30.8% (4 of 13). It should be noted that 2 patients received other concomitant therapy: 1 also had an intralesional corticosteroid injection, and the other used pressure-reducing measures. Adverse effects were also limited to 2 reports, 1 of headache and 1 of headache and dizziness. Both were cleared by either decreasing the amount of nitroglycerin ointment applied or diluting the concentration of the ointment with petroleum jelly. Beyond its potential effectiveness, the benefit of this approach is that it is also noninvasive and cost-effective. The report notes that two 30-g tubes of topical nitroglycerin average approximately $25. Given these benefits, even if clinical clearance is not obtained, the ointment can be used on an as-needed basis for symptomatic control, as noted in the article. In general, the article provides good initial evidence of a potentially promising treatment for CNH and one that may eventually warrant consideration for use when further studies (including comparative studies) can be performed.

B. D. Michaels, DO

J. Q. Del Rosso, DO

Prospective Study of the Frequency of Hepatic Hemangiomas in Infants with Multiple Cutaneous Infantile Hemangiomas

Horii KA, for the Hemangioma Investigator Group (Children's Mercy Hosps and Clinics, Kansas City, MO; et al)
Pediatr Dermatol 28:245-253, 2011

Multiple cutaneous infantile hemangiomas have been associated with hepatic hemangiomas. Screening of infants with five or more cutaneous infantile hemangiomas with abdominal ultrasound is often recommended. The aim of this study was to determine the frequency with which hepatic hemangiomas occur in infants with five or more cutaneous infantile hemangiomas compared to those with one to four cutaneous infantile hemangiomas and to characterize the clinical features of these hepatic hemangiomas. A multicenter prospective study of children with cutaneous infantile hemangiomas was conducted at pediatric dermatology clinics at Hemangioma

Investigator Groups sites in the United States, Canada, and Spain between October 2005 and December 2008. Data were collected, and abdominal ultrasonography was performed on infants younger than 6 months old with five or more cutaneous infantile hemangiomas and those with one to four cutaneous infantile hemangiomas. Twenty-four (16%) of the 151 infants with five or more cutaneous infantile hemangiomas had hepatic hemangiomas identified on abdominal ultrasound, versus none of the infants with fewer than five (p = 0.003). Two of the 24 infants with hepatic hemangiomas received treatment specifically for their hepatic hemangiomas. Infants with five or more cutaneous infantile hemangiomas have a statistically significantly greater frequency of hepatic hemangiomas than those with fewer than 5. These findings support the recommendation of five or more cutaneous infantile hemangiomas as a threshold for screening infants younger than 6 months old for hepatic hemangiomas but also demonstrate that the large majority of these infants with hepatic hemangiomas do not require treatment.

▶ Infantile hemangiomas (IHs) are common in infants; however, the presence of 6 or more cutaneous IHs is less common. The presence of multiple hemangiomas on the skin has been a marker for liver hemangiomas, and a screening abdominal ultrasonography is recommended for infants with 5 or more cutaneous IHs. This is a multicenter prospective study conducted between 2005 and 2008 of infants aged less than 6 months with 6 or more cutaneous IHs compared with those with 1 to 4 IHs. An abdominal ultrasound was performed on these infants to screen for hepatic hemangiomas. If the abdominal ultrasound identified 1 or more hepatic hemangiomas, a complete blood count, thyroid function tests, stool guaiac, chest radiograph, and echocardiogram were performed. No hepatic hemangiomas were found on abdominal ultrasound in the 50 infants with 1 to 4 cutaneous IHs, whereas 24 of 151 (16%) infants with 5 or more cutaneous IH had solitary or multiple IHs ($P = .003$). Comparison of these 2 groups of infants with 5 or more cutaneous IHs with and without hepatic hemangiomas showed no significant differences in gestational age, preterm birth (< 37 weeks), birth weight, race, ethnicity, sex, multiple gestation, in vitro fertilization, chorionic villus sampling, placental anomalies, or preeclampsia. Only 1 infant with a hepatic hemangioma had hepatomegaly on clinical abdominal examination. Of the 24 infants with hepatic hemangiomas, 8 had solitary and 16 had multiple liver lesions; no significant association between number of cutaneous IHs and actual number of hepatic hemangiomas was noted ($P = .39$). This study represented the relationship between cutaneous and hepatic hemangiomas. This prospective study confirms that infants with hepatic hemangiomas requiring treatment for liver disease in this study population was low (8%). Also, hepatic hemangiomas can cause symptomatic liver disease. Other studies have classified liver hemangiomas into groups based on the pattern of involvement within the liver, which may be of interest to study in the future. This study indicates that there is a greater risk for hepatic hemangiomas with more than 5 cutaneous hemangiomas, and therefore an ultrasound is warranted in these infants.

Because ultrasounds are noninvasive and inexpensive, they can assess individuals who are at a risk for developing symptomatic hepatic hemangiomas.

G. K. Kim, DO

J. Q. Del Rosso, DO

Should one offer an unsolicited dermatologic opinion? Ethics for the locker-room dermatologist

Bercovitch L (Brown Univ and Rhode Island Hosp, Providence)
J Am Acad Dermatol 65:134-136, 2011

Background.—Suppose a dermatologist in a locker room recognizes a lesion on the upper back of another person changing clothes after a workout. It appears to be variegated in color, is about 1 to 2 cm in size, and resembles a malignant melanoma. Should the dermatologist offer an unsolicited opinion in these circumstances? What legal, moral, and ethical considerations are involved?

Legal Issues.—As a bystander the dermatologist has no legal responsibility to act, but should she choose to intervene, there is a legal duty to act in a reasonable manner. However, the exact actions and duties that accompany an unsolicited diagnosis are unclear. It is a legal gray area. Offering unsolicited advice does not meet the legal definition of an established doctor-patient relationship, so no liability should be incurred.

Moral and Ethical Concerns.—There is no strict moral obligation to offer an unsolicited opinion, even though doing so would be an act of beneficence. The degree of moral obligation depends on the urgency and seriousness of the problem, the severity of any consequences for inaction, the degree to which it is obvious that something is wrong, whether the condition is treatable, the certainty of the diagnosis, and the presumption that a stranger would want the dermatologist's advice. The dermatologist is not actually an ordinary bystander because of her specialized medical expertise. She may sense a professional duty and obligation to help sick and suffering patients, but must weigh that against her personal moral beliefs regarding respecting others' privacy. In addition, unsolicited medical advice, although it offers benefits for the patient and physician, can also have risks. The casual visual inspection may prompt a false diagnosis, may lead the individual to undergo expensive and possibly unneeded interventions that carry their own morbidity, or may cause the individual to develop anxiety or depression while awaiting a definitive diagnosis. The person may also become upset because of the invasion of her privacy.

Conclusions.—Should the dermatologist decide to intervene in the situation, the best course of action would be to introduce herself as a dermatologist and simply state that something on the individual's back caught her eye. Then she should suggest that the individual might want to contact her physician to have it evaluated. As a guideline, the dermatologist might consider whether she would appreciate such an intervention and weigh it against any privacy or anxiety-producing effect that might occur.

▶ In the visual specialty of dermatology, patients often literally wear their diagnoses on their sleeve. This dermatoethics discussion presents a problem for dermatologists when a potentially life-threatening diagnosis can be made at a glance without the individual soliciting an opinion or even being aware of having been evaluated.

Unsolicited medical advice, like other medical interventions, carries both risks and benefits to the patient and physician. Dr. Bercovitch makes the point that there is no legal duty in this case, as a patient-doctor relationship has not been established. However, as physicians, we are called to more than legal duties and if a life-threatening diagnosis is suspected, there is a moral obligation to at least inform the individual. Even with these good intentions, a physician must act carefully to protect the individual as much as possible and protect themselves as a physician.

For the protection of the individual, he suggests ensuring their privacy for any conversation that might occur, allowing that the suspected diagnosis is not absolute without further evaluation and taking care to avoid self-promotion (appearance of soliciting), particularly for financial gain.

For the self-protection of the physician, he advises that any act of intervention imposes a legal duty to act in a reasonable manner, especially because good-Samaritan statutes and malpractice insurance may not protect from "gross negligence" or "willful or wanton reckless acts" such as creating unnecessary anxiety over a mistaken diagnosis.

This is an issue that dermatologists consider every day. It is an ethical concern and a legal gray area with questionable liability, as unsolicited advice should not meet the legal definition of the doctor-patient relationship, but the term "should" does not provide definitive legal protection. Thus, it imposes the burden of reasonableness, which is expected both ethically and legally.

A. Torres, MD, JD

14 Pigmentary Disorders

Vitiligo linked to stigmatization in British South Asian women: a qualitative study of the experiences of living with vitiligo
Thompson AR, The Appearance Research Collaboration (ARC) (Univ of Sheffield, UK; et al)
Br J Dermatol 163:481-486, 2010

Background.—Vitiligo is a visible condition that is more noticeable in darker-skinned people. Beliefs about illness have been linked to psychosocial adjustment. There is some evidence that such beliefs may be influenced by cultural factors. Surprisingly little is known about beliefs in relation to vitiligo.

Objectives.—The study sought to explore in depth the ways in which British Asian women manage and adjust psychosocially to vitiligo, and the potential role of ethnicity and culture in this process.

Methods.—In-depth semistructured interviews were conducted with seven British women of South Asian decent and analysed using the qualitative method of template analysis.

Results.—Participants described feeling visibly different and all had experienced stigmatization to some extent. Avoidance and concealment were commonplace. Experiences of stigmatization were often perceived to be associated with cultural values related to appearance, status, and myths linked to the cause of the condition.

Conclusions.—The findings of this study present a unique in-depth analysis of British South Asians living with vitiligo and suggest there is a need for further research to explore cultural associations of disfigurement and of adjustment to chronic skin conditions. Furthermore, they suggest that in addition to individual therapeutic interventions there may be a need for community interventions aimed at dispelling myths and raising awareness of sources of support and treatment.

▶ In this small study of 7 British women of South Asian decent, the investigators tried to determine the effect of vitiligo on psychological adjustment using in-depth semistructured interviews analyzed using the qualitative method of template analysis. The authors state that our current understanding of the roles played by ethnicity and culture in psychosocial adjustment to vitiligo is limited by lack of empirical investigation generally and a reliance on quantitative assessment, which often uses measures that lack cultural sensitivity. The reason for their study was to explore ways in which British South Asian women psychosocially adjust to vitiligo and the role of ethnicity and culture. Patients ranged from ages 19 to 52, and all had lesions on visible parts of the body. Several themes surfaced, including status, stigma, and cultural practices. Patients described feelings of rejection and shame by family members and efforts to hide them from society, which caused patients to feel stigmatized. Difficulty with families being able to get the patient "married off" in an arranged marriage was frequently heard. Another theme was loss of ethnic identity, as lighter skin identified the patient with other races and ethnic groups. Many of the participants described feeling disgusted with their disease, had low self-esteem, and were shame-prone. Some stated their intimate relationships were affected because of fear of rejection or of being exposed. Although most patients practiced avoidance and concealment to hide their disease, some coped by confronting others and explaining it. Denial, wishful thinking, minimizing their disease and overcompensating by being extra nice to others were other reported coping mechanisms. Vitiligo was felt to be an ongoing burden because of its chronicity and the inability to predict its course, other than its persistence. One common falsehood in the South Asian community was reported in this article—that vitiligo is caused by eating fish and drinking milk at the same time, which adds feelings of guilt to affected patients. The authors state that findings of this study suggest the need for dermatology staff to assess cultural associations of vitiligo and particularly to consider psychosocial impact in relation to personal relationships, intimacy, perceptions of cause, and social support. Those offering psychosocial support may also need further guidance in conducting culturally sensitive assessments around these areas. Lastly, the results also suggest that there may be a need for community interventions aimed at dispelling myths and raising awareness of sources of support and treatment. The small size of this study affects the generalizability of its findings. Nevertheless, this study directly addresses many important insights regarding the psychological effects of vitiligo in a particular ethnic group and enhances the cultural competence of dermatologists.

A. Pandya, MD

Vitiligo in children and adolescents: association with thyroid dysfunction
Cho SB, Kim JH, Cho S, et al (Yonsei Univ College of Medicine, Seoul, Korea)
J Eur Acad Dermatol Venereol 25:64-67, 2011

Background.—The clinical characteristics of vitiligo in children and adolescents with an emphasis on thyroid dysfunction have only been reported in a few studies.

Objective.—The purpose of this study was to examine the characteristics of children and adolescents with vitiligo and compare the incidence of thyroid dysfunction between them and controls without vitiligo at the same age.

Methods.—A retrospective analysis of 324 Korean children and adolescents with vitiligo was performed. The results of thyroid function screening tests in them ($n = 254$) were compared with controls ($n = 122$).

Results.—Of the total 324 children and adolescents with vitiligo, vitiligo vulgaris was the most common type (42.3%) and the most commonly involved site was the face (54.6%). A total of 15 of 254 (5.9%) patients screened for thyroid function were diagnosed with thyroid disease (four had Hashimoto's thyroiditis; two, Graves' disease; seven, subclinical hypothyroidism; and two, subclinical hyperthyroidism). None of the 50 patients with segmental vitiligo showed any thyroid dysfunction ($P = 0.047$). There was no significant difference in the incidence of thyroid disease between children and adolescents with vitiligo and the control group, in which seven of 122 (5.7%) showed thyroid dysfunction.

Conclusion.—In this study, we demonstrated the characteristics of children and adolescents with vitiligo and also observed no significant difference in the incidence of thyroid disease between children and adolescents with vitiligo and the control group.

▶ In this large study, the authors performed a retrospective review of children with generalized and segmental vitiligo and compared the incidence of thyroid disease in these groups to a control group of dermatology patients with other skin problems. They found no difference in the incidence of thyroid disease between those with generalized vitiligo and control subjects. Interestingly, none of the children with segmental vitiligo had thyroid abnormalities. This study questions the belief that the frequency of autoimmune thyroid disease is higher in children with vitiligo than in normal control subjects. Although there is some evidence of a higher frequency in adults, the data for children are lacking. It also reminds us that segmental vitiligo is different in many ways from generalized vitiligo, likely with a different pathogenesis that has yet to be elucidated. At this time, there isn't good evidence for a need to routinely screen every child with vitiligo for thyroid disease, particularly those with segmental vitiligo.

A. Pandya, MD

A prospective, randomized, split-face, controlled trial of salicylic acid peels in the treatment of melasma in Latin American women

Kodali S, Guevara IL, Carrigan CR, et al (Univ of Texas Southwestern Med Ctr)
J Am Acad Dermatol 63:1030-1035, 2010

Background.—Melasma, a common disorder of hyperpigmentation, is often resistant to therapy. Although salicylic acid peels have been reported to be useful for patients with recalcitrant melasma, controlled trials are lacking.

Objective.—We sought to determine the efficacy of salicylic acid peels when added to hydroquinone in the treatment of melasma.

Methods.—Twenty Latin American women with moderate to severe bilateral melasma were treated with a series of 20% to 30% salicylic acid peels every 2 weeks for a total of 4 peels on one side of the face along with 4% hydroquinone cream to both sides of the face twice daily. The primary efficacy variable was reduction in pigmentation of the peeled side compared with the unpeeled side using narrowband reflectance spectrophotometry.

Results.—Eighteen patients completed the study. Although both sides had significant reduction in pigment intensity, there was no difference between the peeled and unpeeled side with all outcome measures.

Limitations.—Patients were limited to Latin American women and only 4 peels were performed.

Conclusion.—A series of four 20% to 30% salicylic acid peels are not effective in the treatment of melasma when added to twice-daily 4% hydroquinone cream.

▶ Melasma is a common disorder of hyperpigmentation that often involves the cheeks, forehead, and upper cutaneous lip. Although melasma can affect all people, it is more common in Fitzpatrick skin types IV to VI who live in areas of increased ultraviolet radiation. A number of topical and physical treatment modalities are currently available, with all therapies fraught with variability in response. One of the most common depigmenting agents is hydroquinone (HQ). HQ is a hydroxyphenolic compound that inhibits the enzyme tyrosinase, thereby halting the conversion of dihydroxyphenylalanine to melanin. Some studies report a beneficial effect of using superficial peeling agents such as salicylic acid, glycolic acid, or 20% trichloracetic acid for treatment of recalcitrant melasma. Peeling agents have also been reported to be used adjunctively to enhance the penetration of depigmenting agents. This prospective study evaluated 20 Latin American women over a period of 8 weeks and found that the addition of 20% to 30% salicylic acid peels did not result in statistically significant improvement in melasma. Perhaps a larger study involving more patients may yield different results. Overall, 4% HQ and the salicylic acid were both well tolerated.

S. Bellew, DO

J. Q. Del Rosso, DO

Sequential Treatment with Triple Combination Cream and Intense Pulsed Light is More Efficacious than Sequential Treatment with an Inactive (Control) Cream and Intense Pulsed Light in Patients with Moderate to Severe Melasma

Goldman MP, Gold MH, Palm MD, et al (Univ of California at San Diego; Tennessee Clinical Res Ctr, Nashville; et al)
Dermatol Surg 37:224-233, 2011

Background.—Triple combination (TC) cream is a stable combination of fluocinolone acetonide 0.01%, hydroquinone 4%, and tretinoin 0.05% and is currently the only hydroquinone-containing drug approved by the Food and Drug Administration for the treatment of melasma.

Objective.—To evaluate the safety and efficacy of TC cream when used sequentially with intense pulsed light (IPL) treatments in patients with moderate to severe melasma.

Materials & Methods.—This was a 10-week, split-face study in which 56 patients with symmetrical melasma lesions were treated with TC cream on one side of the face and an inactive control cream on the other side of the face. Patients also had two IPL treatments at weeks 2 and 6. (Topical treatment was suspended during IPL treatments ± 1 day.)

Results.—Melasma severity was significantly less with TC cream and IPL than with inactive cream and IPL at weeks 6 ($p=.007$) and 10 ($p=.002$). Improvement in melasma was greater with TC cream and IPL than with inactive cream and IPL according to investigator and patient evaluations at weeks 6 and 10 ($p<.001$ for both time points). Treatment with TC cream and IPL was well tolerated.

Conclusion.—The results of this study suggest that TC cream and IPL treatment is an effective and safe treatment option for patients with melasma.

▶ This 10-week split-face controlled study compared the combination of intense pulsed light (IPL) therapy and triple combination (TC) cream with the combination of IPL and vehicle cream in 56 patients with melasma. The side to receive the TC cream was determined in a random manner. The IPL treatments were given at weeks 2 and 6. Fluence varied from 14 to 18 J/cm^2 so that mild darkening of the pigmented areas occurred without production of an erythematous footprint. The second IPL treatment typically used a fluence 10% higher than the first IPL treatment. The primary outcome measure was an investigator global assessment (IGA) that rated the melasma on a scale of 0 (clear) to 4 (severe). The authors found that the combination of the TC cream and IPL gave better results than IPL + vehicle. At week 6, 41% (n = 23) of patients in the TC cream group and 15% (n = 8) in the vehicle cream group were clear or almost clear. At week 10, 57% (n = 32) of patients in the TC cream group and 23% (n = 13) in the vehicle cream group were clear or almost clear. Thirty percent of both investigators and patients rated the improvement in melasma as excellent at week 10. Irritation was mild to moderate and occurred predominantly on the side receiving TC cream, most likely because of tretinoin.

Although this study suggests that combining IPL and TC cream is effective for melasma, it is possible that the predominant improvement seen in the patients was due to the TC cream alone. Indeed, another arm, in which the TC cream was used without the IPL treatment, may have shown results equivalent to treatment with the cream + laser. Although it has been suggested that IPL is useful for melasma, most studies have enrolled lighter skinned patients with mild to moderate melasma, not the typical dark melasma seen in women from Latin America and South Asia. Indeed, in this study, 93% of the patients were classified as moderate and only 7% as severe.

In general, nonvalidated subjective evaluations, such as IGA, are less accurate than the melasma area and severity index or, even better, narrow-band reflectance spectrophotometry. Had the authors used these outcome measures, which are more objective, reproducible, reliable, and validated, the results would have been easier to interpret. In summary, TC cream appears to be effective in the treatment of melasma. The jury is still out regarding the role of IPL for patients with melasma, especially those with more severe disease.

A. Pandya, MD

A Pilot Study of Intense Pulsed Light in the Treatment of Riehl's Melanosis
Li Y-H, Liu J, Chen JZS, et al (No. 1 Hosp of China Med Univ, Shenyang, China; Sheftel Associates Dermatology, Tucson, AZ; et al)
Dermatol Surg 37:119-122, 2011

Background.—Riehl's melanosis is a pigmented dermatosis manifesting as a brown or bluish reticulate pigmentation on the face and neck. Its cause is unknown, but suspected etiologies include photoallergic reaction to coal tar-n-derived pigments, bromides, or optical whitener; anxiety; sunlight overexposure; and long-term use of photoallergic drugs. The Japanese regard Riehl's melanosis as pigmented contact dermatitis, and researchers in South Africa consider poor nutrition to be a predisposing factor. No effective treatment has been identified, but unsatisfactory attempts with long-term vitamin C administration, topical bleaching agents, and sun protection have been tried. Intense pulsed light (IPL) is successful against melanocytic lesions. The efficacy and safety of IPL to manage Riehl's melanosis was investigated in a split-face design.

Methods.—Five women and a man with Riehl's melanosis (age 27 to 54 years) and Fitzpatrick skin type IV were treated. One side of the face was randomly chosen to receive IPL while the other side was untreated and served as a control. Serial treatment was delivered with cut-off filters of 590, 640, and 695 nm and fluences between 11 and 17 J/cm^2. A triple pulse mode, pulse width 3 to 4 ms, and a delay time of 35 to 40 ms were used. Slight cutaneous erythema was the end point. Patients could not use any bleaching agents, topical steroids, or systemic drugs during the trial. A dermatologist evaluated photographs of the patients to determine global improvement using a 5-point scale (no, slight, moderate, good, and excellent improvement). Biopsy specimens were also collected at baseline and 1 month after the last treatment on bilateral preauricular areas of the face and stained with the Fontana-Masson method. Patients were asked about any adverse effects. Pigmentation and redness were compared between the treated and untreated sides using a skin melanin index (MI) and erythema index (EI) on the forehead, canthus, cheekbone, cheilion, and submaxilla. Trends on each site with time were evaluated using a repeated measurement data assessment.

Results.—After 6 months, one patient had excellent improvement and five had good improvement. After 8 to 10 treatment sessions, the epidermis and dermis of the treated side showed a significantly greater reduction in melanin than on the control side. Mean MI and EI values were diminishing, with the treated side declining more rapidly than the control side. All patients experienced mild to moderate, but tolerable pain. Erythema and slight edema occurred but resolved within a few hours. One patient developed postinflammatory hyperpigmentation (PIH) on the chin after 3 sessions but resolved in 1 month. No patients experienced blistering, scarring, or hypopigmentation, and all were able to resume daily activities immediately after treatment. No relapse occurred over the 6-month follow-up.

Conclusions.—Satisfactory management was achieved with IPL for Riehl's melanosis. Overall the MI and EI results indicate that IPL can accumulatively eliminate the melanin and erythema of Riehl's melanosis in both the epidermis and the dermis. The mean MI/EI value on the control side also demonstrated some decrease in these symptoms. Skin biopsies showed that IPL removed melanosomes from the epidermis and melanin deposition from the dermis. IPL was both safe and effective, with therapeutic efficacy correlating to the number of sessions and anatomical sites.

▶ This study is significant because it presents intense pulsed light as a novel treatment for Riehl melanosis. The authors did their best to capture true improvement by performing a split-face trial and measuring improvement in both subjective and objective manners. Unfortunately, there are many weaknesses in this study. There were a paucity of subjects and no mention of whether topical lightening creams were also applied by the subjects prior to or during the study. Biopsies were done before and after completion of the study, and a "substantial reduction of melanin in both epidermis and dermis with IPL treatment" was noted. There is no mention how the amount of melanin was quantified except to say that the Fontana-Masson stain was used. In these patients, 8 to 10 treatments were performed. This does not translate into an acceptable treatment modality for most patients given the copious treatments and costs associated with them.

E. Graber, MD

Role of apoptosis and melanocytorrhagy: a comparative study of melanocyte adhesion in stable and unstable vitiligo

Kumar R, Parsad D, Kanwar AJ (Postgraduate Inst of Med Education and Res, Chandigarh, India)
Br J Dermatol 164:187-191, 2011

Background.—Apoptosis and melanocytorrhagy have been proposed as mechanisms of melanocyte disappearance although there are few controlled studies.

Objectives.—We undertook this project to study melanocyte morphology and adhesion defects in patients with stable and unstable disease in controls.

Methods.—In this comparative study we included seven patients with stable disease and seven patients with unstable vitiligo. We cultured perilesional skin melanocytes from these patients with stable and unstable vitiligo and studied for morphological changes, adhesion to collagen type IV and caspase 3 expression. Melanocytes were also treated with okadaic acid and annexin V expression was then checked and compared between controls and patients with stable and unstable vitiligo.

Results.—Perilesional skin melanocytes from patients with unstable vitiligo revealed some significant morphological changes. Melanocytes from unstable vitiligo showed significantly low adhesion to collagen type IV compared with control and stable vitiligo melanocytes. Our results showed that caspase 3 and annexin V staining was significantly greater in melanocytes cultured from unstable vitiligo compared with the control.

Conclusions.—In this study we demonstrated that melanocytes in the patients with unstable vitiligo were in their detachment phase, which ultimately leads to apoptosis of these cells, whereas melanocytes cultured from controls and from patients with stable vitiligo were morphologically normal without any adhesion defects. These morphological and adhesion findings support the theory of melanocytorrhagy as the primary defect underlying melanocyte loss in unstable vitiligo.

▶ In this study, the authors studied a small group of patients with stable vitiligo and compared them to a small group with unstable vitiligo. Biopsies were taken from the border of lesions in both sets of patients. The results showed that melanocytes cultured from patients with unstable vitiligo have greater ultrastructural abnormalities than those with stable vitiligo. They also showed a defective growth pattern and decreased ability to adhere to type VII collagen. This supports the hypothesis that melanocytes in vitiligo patients have defective adhesion, which could explain their loss in active lesions. The article supports melanocytorrhagy as the cause of melanocyte loss in patients with unstable vitiligo. The authors suggest that this technique may help clinicians in selecting appropriate patients for grafting, because patients with unstable vitiligo tend to do poorly with such procedures. Because of the expense and effort associated with culturing and testing melanocytes from skin biopsies in these patients, this technique is not practical for day-to-day practice in choosing patients for grafting but serves as an interesting addition in the important search for the cause of vitiligo.

A. Pandya, MD

Vitiligo

Viles J, Monte D, Gawkrodger DJ (Vitiligo Society, London, UK; Univ of Sheffield, UK)
BMJ 341:c3780, 2010

Background.—Vitiligo is a progressive disease that shows periods of activity interspersed with inactivity. Rarely does spontaneous repigmentation occur. A case was reported illustrating many treatments and complications associated with vitiligo.

Case Report.—Man, 40, first developed small white lines around the cuticles of his left hand. He was diagnosed with leukoderma and told it would resolve spontaneously. More patches appeared and he was told this was vitiligo. Six months later he had spots on the right hand, then pigment loss spread rapidly for 12 to 18 months. A dermatologist prescribed "light" use of a steroid cream over the affected areas, which now included a patch on the right side of his mouth and eventually patches all over his hands and body. His general practitioner sent him to a homeopathic hospital for holistic treatment, since no other treatments were currently available; however, these proved unsuccessful. The patient consulted a psychologist because of his stressful job and was advised to try meditation, since stress is believed to contribute to vitiligo. The patches did not become worse for 2 years but there was no repigmentation.

Pigment loss worsened when the patient changed to a more stressful job. He now had two large facial patches along with patches over the rest of his body. He was referred to a research program where he received psoralen and ultraviolet A (PUVA) twice a week. Rapid, noticeable repigmentation resulted. Within 1 month the facial patches had repigmented, although in a shade darker than his normal skin. After 1 year his legs and calves repigmented in a lighter shade than normal. Because the PUVA treatment appeared to be increasing the white patches, he was switched to narrow-band UVB, which noticeably improved repigmentation except on the hands or feet. After completing 250 sessions, that treatment was stopped with no further repigmentation. Where the white patches were the skin is thin, especially on the hands, requiring use of a high number sun protection cream. The patient also uses tacrolimus ointment on affected facial areas. He believes the way other people react to his depigmented skin is the disease's main effect. The psychological impact is especially painful.

Conclusions.—Vitiligo onset is usually in the second or third decade. Its rate of progression is highly variable. Narrow-band UVB is safer and more effective treatment than PUVA. Current recommendations are to limit treatment to 200 for patients with lighter skin color but allow those with darker skin to undergo more. The loss of pigment after phototherapy is not unusual. Vitiligo produces an extreme emotional effect, which this patient experienced. The patient also served as an expert patient and was able to observe the inadequate knowledge about this disease in the curriculum of medical schools and general practitioner courses. Often only 1 or 2 weeks of dermatologic instruction is provided. Vitiligo has several characteristics common to autoimmune diseases. As many as 30% of patients develop autoimmune thyroid disease. A family history of thyroid problems, diabetes, or other endocrine disorders is often found. Patients with vitiligo have circulating autoantibodies and T lymphocytes against melanocyte antigens, with the resultant loss of functioning melanocytes in the depigmented macules of vitiligo. This patient also developed diabetes and rheumatoid arthritis, which have autoimmune components. Further research is needed to better understand the causative mechanisms and genetics of vitiligo in order to better treat it.

▶ For as many articles as we read, or as much research as we might absorb, there is nothing more educational to the physician than the patient's experience with his or her disease. The evolution from the onset to the adaptation, the signs and symptoms, and the acceptance of chronicity are all powerful historical components of specific disease states. Many of us do not adequately take into account the patient's perspectives as we attempt to understand their needs. The patient with vitiligo clings to certain needs and concerns because as the author portrays in this article, he did not do anything to deserve his fate and did not have any choice in exposing his ailment to the outside world. Vitiligo carries the double-edged sword of being strikingly visible and also having several potential systemic associations that can emerge at any time. As stated in the article, "I felt that the visual effect my depigmented skin had on other people was the main effect of the disease. The psychological impact was quite painful, and took some time to overcome..." As we read his experience, it is an important reminder about the extent patients will go to find the help they need. He also made an important discovery in the search for care: other than dermatologists, medical students and resident physicians receive little organized training on skin diseases. This is an important reminder to dermatologists that some level of support and tolerance has to be demonstrated when encountering patients who have been treated by other specialists or have sought alternative therapies. Patients may endure significant expense, frustration, and even despair when their treatments fail or when they come to accept that many diseases do not have adequate therapeutic regimens or cures. The physician contributor states it clearly in his portion of the article: "The reaction of Darryl's doctors in referring him for homoeopathic treatment illustrates the feeling of powerlessness that doctors may experience and the desperation of patients when faced with a disease like vitiligo, for which there is little effective treatment." There are few times in a career when an allopathic physician suggests homeopathic therapies, thus demonstrating that the approach of many of our chronic diseases deserves more than just a prescription pad. Support, compassion, and understanding the patient's experience may often prove to be equally or more therapeutic.

N. Bhatia, MD

A double-blind, randomized, placebo-controlled trial of topical tacrolimus 0·1% vs. clobetasol propionate 0·05% in childhood vitiligo
Ho N, Pope E, Weinstein M, et al (Univ of Toronto, Ontario, Canada)
Br J Dermatol 165:626-632, 2011

Background.—Both clobetasol propionate 0·05% (CP 0·05%) and tacrolimus 0·1% (T 0·1%) ointments have been shown to be efficacious and safe in treating vitiligo in the paediatric population.
Objectives.—To assess efficacy and safety of these two therapies compared with each other and with placebo.

Methods.—In this prospective study, children aged 2—16 years with vitiligo, stratified into 'facial' ($n = 55$) and 'nonfacial' ($n = 45$) groups, were randomized into three arms: CP 0·05% ointment ($n = 30$), T 0·1% ointment ($n = 31$) and placebo ($n = 29$) for 6 months. Successful repigmentation, defined as > 50% improvement, was evaluated by comparing photographs taken at baseline and at 2, 4 and 6 months.

Results.—In the facial group, 58% of the CP 0·05% group responded successfully compared with 58% of the T 0·1% group, and in the nonfacial group, 39% of the CP 0·05% group responded compared with 23% of the T 0·1% group ($P > 0·05$). There was a significant difference in response between the CP 0·05% group vs. placebo ($P < 0·0001$) and the T 0·1% group vs. placebo ($P = 0·0004$). Spontaneous repigmentation was evaluated as 2·4%. No significant clinical adverse events were noted in any group.

Conclusions.—Both CP 0·05% and T 0·1% ointments offer similar benefit in paediatric vitiligo, both facial and nonfacial. The facial lesions responded faster than the nonfacial ones.

▶ This is a well-done study of 100 children, ages 2 to 16 years, that compares the efficacy of clobetasol propionate 0.05% versus tacrolimus 0.1% ointment versus placebo in the treatment of segmental and nonsegmental vitiligo. Participants were further stratified into facial and nonfacial involvement. Participants were treated a total of 6 months. To limit risk of side effects, the clobetasol group received intermittent therapy, 2 months of clobetasol, 2 months petroleum jelly, then 2 more months of clobetasol. The other groups received continuous therapy throughout the 6 months. Efficacy was defined by a > 50% improvement in pigmentation. The results showed that both were effective, with clobetasol edging out tacrolimus in total clearance rates. For the facial group, both treatment groups had a 58% successful response rate. Twenty-two percent of patients treated with clobetasol had a complete response versus 11% in the tacrolimus group. For the nonfacial group, the response rates were lower at 39% for the clobetasol group and 10% for the tacrolimus group. Total repigmentation rates were 13% and 10%, respectively. The repigmentation rate in the placebo group was 2.4%, with only 2 of the 29 patients having a > 50% improvement. Mild side effects, primarily irritation, were reported in about one-third of patients in all groups.

Other interesting findings in the study included the repigmentation patterns. Four patterns of pigmentation, follicular, diffuse, marginal, and mixed, were examined. In the clobetasol group, a diffuse pattern was mostly seen, while a mixed/diffuse pattern was seen in the tacrolimus-treated group. Follicular pigmentation was seen more frequently in the placebo-treated group. Another interesting finding in the study was the frequency of associated autoimmune disorders. It was found that 8 participants had abnormal associated autoimmune findings at baseline (6 with abnormal TSH, 1 with low B1 level, and 1 with thrombocytopenia). None of these patients were symptomatic at the time.

A. Zaenglein, MD

Future research into the treatment of vitiligo: where should our priorities lie? Results of the vitiligo priority setting partnership
Eleftheriadou V, Whitton ME, Gawkrodger DJ, et al (Univ of Nottingham, UK; Vitiligo Society, London, UK; Royal Hallamshire Hosp, Sheffield, UK; et al)
Br J Dermatol 164:530-536, 2011

Background.—Vitiligo is the most frequent depigmentation disorder of the skin and is cosmetically and psychologically devastating. A recently updated Cochrane systematic review 'Interventions for vitiligo' showed that the research evidence for treatment of vitiligo is poor, making it difficult to make firm recommendations for clinical practice.

Objectives.—To stimulate and steer future research in the field of vitiligo treatment, by identifying the 10 most important research areas for patients and clinicians.

Methods.—A vitiligo priority setting partnership was established including patients, healthcare professionals and researchers with an interest in vitiligo. Vitiligo treatment uncertainties were gathered from patients and clinicians, and then prioritized in a transparent process, using a methodology advocated by the James Lind Alliance.

Results.—In total, 660 treatment uncertainties were submitted by 461 participants. These were reduced to a list of the 23 most popular topics through an online/paper voting process. The 23 were then prioritized at a face-to-face workshop in London. The final list of the top 10 treatment uncertainties included interventions such as systemic immunosuppressants, topical treatments, light therapy, melanocyte-stimulating hormone analogues, gene therapy, and the impact of psychological interventions on the quality of life of patients with vitiligo.

Conclusions.—The top 10 research areas for the treatment of vitiligo provide guidance for researchers and funding bodies, to ensure that future research answers questions that are important both to clinicians and to patients.

▶ Because of the small number of well-done trials, it is often difficult to provide treatment recommendations for vitiligo in clinical practice that are based on a large body of strong data. This study surveyed 461 patients with vitiligo as well as clinicians caring for vitiligo patients to prioritize research questions. The results can then be used to guide future research for this disorder. Sixty-six percent of responses (302 of 461) were from patients, 31% (142 of 461) were from health care professionals, and 3% were from other sources. Overall, 660 uncertainties that specifically related to the treatment of vitiligo were gathered during the consultation stage. The uncertainties were organized into groups and then ranked by 230 participants. A final list of 23 uncertainties was prioritized in a face-to-face workshop, resulting in the top 10 treatment uncertainties. These included psychological interventions, immunosuppressive agents, phototherapy, calcineurin inhibitors, gene therapy, hormonal interactions, and camouflage plus psychological intervention for vitiligo.

This study is a useful guide for researchers, pharmaceutical companies, and research-granting agencies in determining which avenues should be pursued in vitiligo research. Combining the opinions of patients and physicians adds needed relevance to questions and challenges surrounding the management of vitiligo that is greatly needed. The importance of psychological intervention that evident from this consensus highlights the mental stress that vitiligo causes to those who are affected.

A. Pandya, MD

15 Practice Management and Managed Care

Mobile teledermatology in the developing world: Implications of a feasibility study on 30 Egyptian patients with common skin diseases
Tran K, Ayad M, Weinberg J, et al (Memorial Sloan-Kettering Cancer Ctr, NY; Al-Azhar Univ, Cairo, Egypt; Univ of Pennsylvania School of Medicine, Philadelphia; et al)
J Am Acad Dermatol 64:302-309, 2011

Background.—The expansion of store-and-forward teledermatology into underserved regions of the world has long been hampered by the requirement for computers with Internet connectivity. To our knowledge, this study is one of the first to demonstrate the feasibility of teledermatology using newer-generation mobile telephones with specialized software and wireless connectivity to overcome this requirement in a developing country.

Objective.—We sought to demonstrate that mobile telephones may be used on the African continent to submit both patient history and clinical photographs wirelessly to remote expert dermatologists, and to assess whether these data are diagnostically reliable.

Methods.—Thirty patients with common skin diseases in Cairo, Egypt, were given a diagnosis by face-to-face consultation. They were then given a diagnosis independently by local senior dermatologists using teleconsultation with a software-enabled mobile telephone containing a 5-megapixel camera. Diagnostic concordance rates between face-to-face and teleconsultation were tabulated.

Results.—Diagnostic agreement between face-to-face consultation and the two local senior dermatologists performing independent evaluation by teleconsultation was achieved in 23 of 30 (77%) and in 22 of 30 (73%) cases, respectively, with a global mean of 75%.

Limitations.—Limited sample size and interobserver variability are limitations.

Conclusion.—Mobile teledermatology is a technically feasible and diagnostically reliable method of amplifying access to dermatologic expertise in poorer regions of the globe where access to computers with Internet connectivity is unreliable or insufficient.

▶ Mobile telephones are now an integral part of daily communications, and the transmission of data and images are getting faster every day. Relevant to

355

dermatology, image resolution is improving with every new model of mobile phones. For a large part of the underserved population, in the United States and abroad, cell phones are the only way people in underdeveloped regions can tap into the technologic advancement of high-speed, instant communication in the modern world, as there is no infrastructure for fast Internet in these regions. The article describes a study to see if fast mobile telephone image and data transmission can be a useful tool to give dermatology diagnostic care to a group of 30 patients in a remote region of Egypt. The study found that there is a high and acceptable concordance (77%) rate between the on-site dermatologist, albeit a junior dermatologist, and the off-site senior dermatologists, who formed their diagnoses based on transmitted cell phone images and typed up relevant history on the same cell phone. History information was taken via a series of multiple choice questions typed up by the junior on-site dermatologist.

The cell phone used in this study is the Samsung U900, which offers adequate 5-megapixel image resolution, but it cannot take panoramic pictures of affected areas. No current cell phone can take panoramic pictures of large body surface areas with good resolution. This capability is important when it comes to locating all lesions, and examining patients completely and thoroughly so as not to miss important clues besides the obvious lesions patients present to us. The limited keyboard on cell phones makes it impractical to type up a complete, relevant history for patients in the freestyle format, and of course, it would be impractical to use current small cell phone keyboards to type up history in a busy clinic with 30 to 50 patients a day. The on-site personnel will still need to perform biopsies in case diagnosis cannot be made by visual inspection alone. The authors pointed out the many limitations of the study and the current technology in incorporating mobile teledermatology, namely, the level of training between the junior and senior dermatologists is different, patients must have lesions on the skin for participation, and there was no histologic confirmation of the diagnosis of equivocal cases. In the United States, any medical record transmission technology must be HIPPA compliant—another limitation of this technology and the involved Clickdoc Web site that stores these data.

This is an intriguing peek at what the future might hold for the accessibility of care issue in dermatology and a potential opportunity to incorporate into a practice. Of course, there are pros and cons. Imagine there is no patient in your office in a typical day. Just you in front of the computer! This working model may become a reality if our goal is to provide service to the vast dermatologically undeserved areas to compensate for the maldistribution of our workforce.

K. Nguyen, MD

Costs and cost-effectiveness analysis of treatment in children with eczema by nurse practitioner vs. dermatologist: results of a randomized, controlled trial and a review of international costs

Schuttelaar MLA, Vermeulen KM, Coenraads PJ, et al (Univ of Groningen, the Netherlands)
Br J Dermatol 165:600-611, 2011

Background.—In a randomized, controlled trial (RCT) on childhood eczema we reported that substituting nurse practitioners (NPs) for dermatologists resulted in similar outcomes of eczema severity and in the quality of life, and higher patient satisfaction.

Objectives.—To determine costs and cost-effectiveness of care provided by NPs vs. dermatologists and to compare our results with those in studies from other countries.

Methods.—We estimated the healthcare costs, family costs and the costs in other sectors alongside the RCT. All the costs were linked to quality of life [Infants' Dermatitis Quality of Life Index (IDQOL), Children's Dermatology Life Quality Index (CDLQI)] and to patient satisfaction (Client Satisfaction Questionnaire-8) to determine the incremental cost-effectiveness ratio (ICER). We also examined all the reported studies on the costs of childhood eczema.

Results.—The mean annual healthcare costs, family costs and costs in other sectors were €658, €302 and €21, respectively, in the NP group and €801, €608 and €0·93, respectively, in the dermatologist group. The ICER in the NP group compared with the dermatologist group indicated €925 and €751 savings per one point less improvement in IDQOL and CDLQI, respectively, and €251 savings per one point more satisfaction in the NP group at 12 months. The mean annual healthcare costs and family costs varied considerably in the six identified studies.

Conclusions.—Substituting NPs for dermatologists is both cost-saving and cost-effective. The treatment of choice is that provided by the NPs as it is similarly effective to treatment provided by a dermatologist with a higher parent satisfaction. International comparisons are difficult because the types of costs determined, the units and unit prices, and eczema severity all differ between studies.

▶ Eczematous dermatitis that emerges in childhood is often a chronic disease process, typically related to atopic diathesis, that can be accompanied by significant expenditure of costs to health care and the patient. In a randomized controlled trial by Schuttelaar et al, the authors sought to compare the cost and cost-effectiveness between nurse practitioners (NPs) versus dermatologists in the treatment of childhood chronic eczema. In this report, 180 patients were randomized to either a dermatologist or an NP for care. Costs (including health care-related, family-related costs, and other costs) were linked to quality of life and patient satisfaction. In essence, the study found that treatment performed by NPs resulted in both cost-savings and cost-effectiveness. Moreover, not only were there similar outcomes in terms of therapeutic and quality of life outcomes, but patient satisfaction was higher in the NP group. The authors concluded that the "treatment of choice is that provided by NPs." Ultimately, there were limitations in the study. For example, the authors note that the study in the NP arm was mainly carried out by 1 NP, and thus patient satisfaction may have been biased by the characteristics of that individual NP and cannot be generalized to care from NPs in general. This study was also performed solely in the Netherlands. Six studies performed in other countries (not the United States) were included for comparison, but international comparisons were admittedly noted to be difficult. Therefore, application and extrapolation of this study to other countries such as the United States may not necessarily correlate. Regardless, the findings of this study are interesting and deserve attention by dermatologists for further consideration, especially in light of the emerging role of physician extenders in dermatology.

B. D. Michaels, DO
J. Q. Del Rosso, DO

Skin Cancer Prevention Educational Resources: Just a Click Away?
Forsea A-M, Kovalyshyn I, Dusza SW, et al (Elias Univ Hosp, Bucharest, Romania; Memorial Sloan-Kettering Cancer Ctr, NY)
Dermatol Surg 36:1962-1967, 2010

Background.—The general public and health professionals are increasingly choosing the Internet to access skin cancer prevention information.

Objectives.—To identify the optimal mechanism for finding skin cancer educational resources through the Internet and to characterize the resources currently available on-line.

Methods.—A survey of experts involved in skin cancer prevention, followed by standardized searches through popular general Internet search engines using a list of 10 terms relevant to skin cancer prevention resources.

Results.—Internet search was the preferred modality for identifying skin cancer educational resources of all survey participants. The five most-trusted Internet sites identified by the survey participants ranked within the top 10 most findable web sites using general search engines. Ninety-six of 1,000 web pages retrieved using general web-search engines provided information regarding specific skin cancer prevention resources. Seven databases were identified that catalogued educational resources from multiple sources. Peer-reviewed analysis of the outcomes associated with the educational resources was available for only four of 489 resources identified (2.7%).

Conclusions.—Information on skin cancer educational resources available on the Internet is abundant but redundant, and direct access to these resources remains difficult. No sites were identified that comprehensively catalogued and characterized the resources available from the leading providers.

▶ "If you can't beat 'em, join 'em" is to me the best phrase to describe how to deal with the Internet as a physician. We have entered the era of overexposure to medicine online, and patients now come to us often having done some homework first. Many would say that patients went from "Doctor, what do I have?" with an open mind to "Doctor, I have this condition!" with a printout in hand and a diagnosis already made. So, it behooves us to be tolerant of the "too little knowledge is dangerous" phenomenon and make patients more involved and, therefore, responsible in their care.

In some ways, physicians are like cornerbacks and safeties on a football team's defense. We don't know the routes that the receivers are going to run and they are a step ahead of us, but we have to respond effectively and expeditiously, and keep up. The same issue applies with the Internet. We cannot keep up with every potential website or source that a patient is going to search so we are usually at least 1 step behind them as far as their mindset after they perform their own research. As the authors point out, there has not been a standardization of information about skin cancer education for patients and they list multiple common resources. The problem is that the Web sites that dermatologists would reflexively seek out for assistance are not often the first ones that appear on a patient's search through an engine such as Google or Yahoo. As a result, the images and information may not be consistent with standards of care or at the very least be informative enough for a patient's education.

Many dermatology practices have links to certain online resources on their own Web site or even go further to provide images of skin cancer as well as important screening tools for a patient. These methods are important and should be encouraged, but, as we see, they are not standardized for the public. As the authors humorously state at the end, online information is changing fast enough that many of the Web sites and information sources listed in their article might be considered obsolete at the time of publication. So, using the football analogy, it is back to the playbook to keep up.

N. Bhatia, MD

DERMATOLOGIC SURGERY AND CUTANEOUS ONCOLOGY

16 Nonmelanoma Skin Cancer

Alopecia of the Scalp After Ineffective Treatment of Bowen's Disease Using Red Light 5-Aminolevulinic Acid Photodynamic Therapy: Two Case Reports
Letada PR, Uebelhoer NS, Masters R, et al (Naval Med Ctr San Diego, CA)
Dermatol Surg 36:1786-1789, 2010

Background.—Skin diseases such as nonmelanoma skin cancer, Bowen's disease (BD), and other inflammatory and immune disorders are managed using 5-aminolevulinic acid photodynamic therapy (ALA-PDT). First, the ALA is applied, usually topically, then, after cellular uptake, the ALA is metabolized into protoporphyrin IX, which is irradiated with wavelengths of light in its excitation spectrum. This produces cytotoxic reactive oxygen species (ROS) that disrupt the adjacent tissue. Two cases of alopecia of the scalp developed after ineffective red-light ALA-PDT for BD. The mechanisms by which this may have developed and clinical implications for the use of ALA-PDT in other terminal hair-bearing areas were noted.

Case Reports.—Case 1: Woman, 79, reported having two 2- to 3-cm crusted, hyperkeratotic plaques located close together on her vertex scalp for 2 years. BD and hypertrophic actinic keratosis were identified from shave biopsy. Red-light ALA-PDT was selected as treatment because of the large area involved and the patients' strong preference to avoid surgery. Her hair was trimmed and curettage performed judiciously, then topical 20% ALA was applied under occlusion. The area was incubated overnight, then irradiated using a 633-nm light-emitting diode continuous-wave red-light source. Treatments were repeated at monthly intervals using 252 and 300 J. A month after the third treatment the bulk of clinical involvement had diminished significantly but a discontinuous, scaly plaque intermixed with patchy alopecia in the treatment area was seen. Residual BD was confirmed on biopsy, prompting Mohs surgery.

Case 2: Woman, 30, had a history of cystic fibrosis, bilateral lung transplantation, and immunosuppressive medication. She had a

6- × 5-cm erythematous, crusted plaque on the vertex scalp that punch biopsy identified as BD with significant follicular extension. Red-light ALA-PDT was chosen because of the extensive scalp involvement and the patient's strong desire to avoid surgery. A single session of ALA-PDT was conducted, using a total dose of 230 J. After 6 weeks the area involved was smaller but discontinuous hyperkeratotic plaques remained. These were identified on biopsy as residual BD. The patient's hair had thinned over the treatment area, and she had a 1-cm peripheral rim of alopecia. Ten weeks after ALA-PDT the central thinning remained but the alopecia rim had nearly resolved. Bitemporal scalp tissue expansion was performed, followed by Mohs surgery with primary closure.

Conclusions.—ALA-PDT used for basal cell cancer and BD has been associated with nonscalp hair loss previously, but these cases of scalp alopecia are the first reported. ALA preferentially accumulates in rapidly proliferating keratinocytes, so the red-light PDT treatment may have damaged follicular germinative cells in the bulb and bulge, causing longer-term hair loss. In Case 2 the alopecia may also have resulted from selective uptake of the ALA by normal pilosebaceous units, disrupting normal follicular germinative structures after PDT. The red light can penetrate as deeply as 5 mm into the skin, which is deeper than the germinative structures of hair follicles. It is also possible that normal and BD-affected follicles were caught up in the localized treatment-related anagen effluvium. Successful treatment of BD with ALA-PDT ranges from 60% to 100%; the failure in the reported cases remains unexplained. Large tumor burden and follicular involvement in deeper structures may have contributed. Based on the alopecia reported and the high likelihood of treatment failure, red-light ALA-PDT is not recommended for patients who have extensive BD in high-density terminal hair-bearing areas. It may, however, be of use in reducing unwanted hair in normal skin. Actinic keratosis and acne are often treated with much lower doses of light and shorter incubation periods. In addition, many institutions employ blue-light ALA-PDT for treating actinic keratosis, which penetrates less deeply than red light. Hair loss may also be related to the inherent qualities of scalp hair. Further study is needed to determine efficacy and to outline treatment parameters for the use of red-light ALA-PDT to reduce hair.

▶ This series of 2 case studies suggests that treating Bowen disease (squamous cell carcinoma in situ) on the scalp can be inadequate when using photodynamic therapy even with deeper penetrating red light. There is also a suggestion that high-dose red light with aminolevulinic acid could potentially lead to alopecia. This could be because of tumor and heating caused by the high-dose therapy. The dose of light of 100 J to 200 J is much higher than recommended for typical treatments. The red light source used in this study could have dosimetric issues because it is not calibrated on a regular basis.

E. A. Tanghetti, MD

A cost analysis of photodynamic therapy with methyl aminolevulinate and imiquimod compared with conventional surgery for the treatment of superficial basal cell carcinoma and Bowen's disease of the lower extremities

Aguilar M, de Troya M, Martin L, et al (Hospital Costa del Sol, Marbella, España)
J Eur Acad Dermatol Venereol 24:1431-1436, 2010

Background.—Superficial basal cell carcinoma (sBCC) and Bowen's disease (BD) are usually slow-growing, low-grade malignancies that mainly affect older persons. Surgery is often the first choice of treatment and the modality with the lowest failure rate. However, non-invasive procedures, such as topical methyl aminolevulinate photodynamic therapy (MAL-PDT) and imiquimod, are increasingly demanded by dermatologists and patients, because of their generally favourable efficacy and adverse effects profile and their excellent cosmetic outcome.

Objective.—To assess the cost of MAL-PDT and of treatment with imiquimod for primary non-melanoma superficial cutaneous carcinomas compared with conventional surgery, thereby calculating the total medical cost, and the direct and indirect costs.

Setting.—We collected data on 67 patients with 86 tumours (32 sBCC, 54 BD). Patients were treated between May 2006 and April 2007 at the Dermatology Department of the Costa del Sol Hospital in Marbella, Spain. The mean cost and mean cost per complete clinical response were calculated for each therapeutic option.

Results.—After 2 years of follow-up, a complete response was observed in 89.5% of the MAL-PDT group, 87.5% of the imiquimod group and 97.5% of the surgery group. The difference in costs when compared with the surgery group was a mean saving per lesion treated of 307 euros for the imiquimod group, and 322 euros for the MAL-PDT group.

Conclusions.—Although surgery proved to be more effective treatment, our results suggest that its average cost is greater than that of non-invasive therapy for the treatment of non-melanoma superficial cutaneous carcinomas on the lower limbs, at least after the first 2 years of follow-up.

▶ This study provides an interesting insight into the costs involved in treating commonly encountered skin cancers such as superficial basal cell carcinoma (sBCC) and Bowen disease (BD) of the lower leg. Although the analysis of both direct and indirect costs in this study are more applicable to an academic institution or large health care clinic setting, it gives dermatologists based in smaller office settings an insight into the cost-efficiency of various therapies for superficial nonmelanoma skin cancer on the lower extremities. It is generally agreed that surgery on the lower extremities in the elderly is prone to more complications and delayed healing. Before we put down our scalpel in favor of methyl aminolevulinate photodynamic therapy MAL-PDT or imiquimod on the basis of this article, there are several additional considerations. The analysis in this article is based on a 2-year follow-up period in which imiquimod and MAL-PDT had clearance rates in the range of 90% and surgery more than 97%.

Based on a recent systematic review of topical imiquimod and 5-fluorouracil, the "gold standard" for evaluating therapeutic efficacy is 5 years, the strength of evidence for imiquimod as monotherapy for sBCC is weak, imiquimod is not approved by the Food and Drug Administration in the United States for treatment of BD, and compliance issues may arise with topical therapy because of the duration of therapy or need for rest periods if associated inflammation is brisk and/or symptomatic.[1,2] Additionally, a recent study noted that in a significant number of cases of biopsy-proven sBCC and BD that were treated with Mohs surgery, invasive carcinomas were present and hence were more likely to recur with nonsurgical modalities.[2]

We are in an era of global economic recession, and close scrutiny of how health care dollars are allocated has become universal. Studies evaluating the cost-efficiency of dermatologic therapies such as this one are likely to appear more frequently in our literature.

G. Martin, MD

References

1. Love WE, Bernhard JD, Bordeaux JS. Topical imiquimod or fluorouracil therapy for basal and squamous cell carcinoma a systematic review. *Arch Dermatol.* 2009;145:1431-1438.
2. Izikson L, Seyler M, Zeitouni NC. Prevalence of underdiagnosed aggressive non-melanoma skin cancers treated with Mohs micrographic surgery: analysis of 513 cases. *Dermatol Surg.* 2010;36:1769-1772.

Complete Clinical Response to Cetuximab in a Patient with Metastatic Cutaneous Squamous Cell Carcinoma
Miller K, Sherman W, Ratner D (Columbia Univ, NY; Columbia Univ Med Ctr, NY)
Dermatol Surg 36:2069-2074, 2010

Background.—There are no established first-line agents to manage metastatic cutaneous squamous cell carcinoma (cSCC), so targeted therapies are being explored. Cetuximab is an epidermal growth factor receptor (EGFR) antibody that has proved effective against EGF-n-expressing solid tumors. High levels of EGFR are expressed by metastatic cSCC, but the efficacy of cetuximab has not yet been evaluated. A patient with in-transit and distant metastases of cSCC was treated with serial infusions of cetuximab.

> *Case Report.*—Man, 79, had a 5.5- × 5.9-cm wound on his back for 6 months before coming for treatment. Initially the lesion was diagnosed as a decubitus ulcer but biopsy proved it was infiltrative SCC. He was diagnosed with stage 2 disease. Wide surgical margins were required to maximize the probability of removing the lesion completely. Mohs micrographic surgery was performed with 2-cm margins around the clinically visible tumor and surrounding erythema. Frozen section revealed no lymphovascular invasion or neurotropism in the tumor. Horizontal frozen section confirmed

the margins were clear. The defect created measured 10.5×8.5 cm and extended to the muscularis level. Primary closure was performed, then adjuvant radiation therapy was planned, but within 2 months the patient developed a 4- $\times$ 4-cm violaceous, firm subcutaneous nodule several centimeters lateral to the resection. An in-transit metastasis was suspected, and punch biopsy revealed infiltrating SCC with no epidermal connection. A right axillary mass was found and confirmed by computed tomography (CT) to be a 3.8-cm necrotic lymph node with atypical epithelial cells suspicious for SCC.

Systemic treatment was recommended, and cetuximab was chosen because of its relative lack of side effects and ease of administration. The patient began a 4-week cycle of cetuximab 400 mg/m^2 on day 1, then 250 mg/m^2 weekly for 3 weeks. Cycles were scheduled to be repeated at 6-month intervals. After one 4-week cycle the subcutaneous nodule showed marked clinical regression, and follow-up CT showed the right axillary necrotic lymph node had shrunk to 1.2 cm. A second cycle of cetuximab infusions 6 months later achieved complete clinical remission with no CT evidence of nodal disease, resolution of the necrotic node, and no evidence of lymphadenopathy. The patient has had a third cycle and no abnormalities remain. The only adverse effect with the cetuximab was a pruritic, papulopustular, acneiform rash with periungual inflammation during the first cycle that persisted through the second cycle. Treatment with cetuximab will continue at 6-month intervals.

Conclusions.—The Food and Drug Administration (FDA) has approved cetuximab for the treatment of head and neck cancer and EGFR-positive colorectal cancer. It has proved effective in combination with current standard treatment for EGFR-expressing tumors. Adding cetuximab to radiotherapy also improves disease control and overall survival for patients with locoregionally advanced SCC of the head and neck. Clinical trials of cetuximab for patients with cSCC with in-transit or metastatic disease are needed.

▶ Metastatic cutaneous squamous cell carcinoma (SCC) remains a difficult entity to treat. There are no accepted first-line treatments that have been validated using prospective, randomized clinical trials. Cisplatin has been used as a first-line agent, but it has a significant side-effect profile. Increasing interest has been shown in using targeted therapies for metastatic SCC. This case report shows a complete clinical response to cetuximab. It is exciting given the favorable side-effect profile compared with some of the more traditional agents used to treat metastatic SCC. Because this adds to other case reports showing success using cetuximab, it lays further groundwork for clinical trials for its use in metastatic SCC.

R. Ceilley, MD
B. Kopitzki, DO

Expression of the Sonic hedgehog pathway in squamous cell carcinoma of the skin and the mucosa of the head and neck

Schneider S, Thurnher D, Kloimstein P, et al (Med Univ of Vienna, Austria)
Head Neck 33:244-250, 2011

Background.—Activation of the hedgehog pathway may contribute to carcinogenesis. This study characterizes the expression pattern in squamous cell carcinoma of the skin and the head and neck.

Methods.—Tissue microarrays were constructed with samples of squamous cell carcinoma of the skin and the head and neck. All tissue samples were immunohistochemically stained for 7 Hedgehog pathway molecules.

Results.—Significant ($p < .0001$) overexpression of all evaluated molecules could be observed in the tumor samples compared with healthy control tissues. Expression of Gli-2 showed significant upregulation and that of Smoothened and Patched significant downregulation in head and neck compared with skin carcinoma. High expression of Sonic hedgehog correlates significantly ($p = .001$) with poor overall survival in patients with head and neck cancer.

Conclusions.—Hedgehog signaling is differentially regulated in squamous cell carcinomas of the skin and the head and neck. Sonic hedgehog expression may serve as a prognostic factor in patients with head and neck cancer.

▶ This well-conducted investigation provides good primary evidence for the existence of Sonic hedgehog pathway proteins in squamous cell carcinomas of the skin and oral mucosa. Since it has been established that this pathway is implicated in basal cell nevus syndrome as well as wild-type basal cell carcinomas (BCCs), and increased amounts of Sonic hedgehog ligand have been demonstrated in numerous other noncutaneous tumors such as medulloblastoma, pancreatic, and prostate tumors, it seems logical that aberrations of this pathway might be found in the tumors of squamous cells that obviously share similar homology to basal cells.

This study appropriately included normal controls, but it is puzzling why only a few normal skin and mucosal biopsies were included. The results would have generated stronger evidence if the normal sample size was equivalent to that of the test subjects. The evidence not discussed is that a few patients did not show any upregulation of hedgehog pathway proteins. This, coupled with the fact that mucosal lesions were more consistently associated with Gli-2 expression, whereas skin lesions were associated more consistently with smoothened and patched expression, speaks to the fact that this pathway may only partially explain the dysregulation involved, or possibly that the aberration may be transient in the evolution of the tumors.

Although this is a good initial study, much larger studies are needed to elucidate which of the many hedgehog pathway proteins are specifically involved, as novel topical and oral treatments that target the Sonic hedgehog pathway are currently being investigated. Thinking forward, it would be extremely useful for these anticipated drugs to have a formal indication for squamous cell carcinomas should this pathway prove to be implicated, so that reimbursement issues would be less of a hindrance.

J. M. Suchniak, MD

Evaluation of Patient-Perceived Satisfaction with Photodynamic Therapy for Bowen Disease

Hu A, Moore C, Yu E, et al (Univ of Western Ontario, London, Ontario)
J Otolaryngol Head Neck Surg 39:688-696, 2010

Objective.—To formally evaluate patient concerns and patient-perceived satisfaction with photodynamic therapy (PDT) using topical application of 5-aminolevulinic acid for Bowen disease (BD).

Design.—Initial focus groups and mailout questionnaire.

Setting.—Tertiary care hospital.

Methods.—A novel 32-item self-reported patient satisfaction questionnaire was mailed out to all patients treated with PDT for BD from January 1, 2000, to March 31, 2008.

Main Outcome Measures.—A written questionnaire addressing side effects experienced, self-perceived effectiveness, and the personal and social consequences of PDT.

Results.—One hundred thirty-two adults were treated with PDT for BD over this time period. Ninety-five patients (47% male, 53% female) completed the questionnaire. A majority (>90%) indicated a very favourable impression of the effectiveness of PDT for BD and that side effects were mild. The most significant side effects were a burning sensation (21%) and crusting or scabbing (14%). Side effects were judged to be predictable. The process of treatment and overall time demands were judged by only 7% of respondents to be problematic. The most substantial limitations with PDT were social limitations secondary to treatment (26%), self-consciousness (28%), and skin appearance in the immediate posttreatment period (30%). Respondent reliability in response to questions was excellent.

Conclusions.—PDT is favourably received by those diagnosed with BD. PDT resulted in a high degree of perceived satisfaction for those patients with BD. Based on these data, PDT is supported as a viable method of treatment for BD.

▶ The use of photodynamic therapy (PDT) for the treatment of Bowen disease (BD) has been found to be efficacious while providing an excellent cosmetic result. In comparison with cryosurgery, surgical excision, curettage and electro-desiccation, 5-fluorouracil topical imiquimod, or topical diclofenac for the treatment of BD, PDT appears to demonstrate superior results when efficacy, safety, and cosmetic outcomes are compared. For many of us who are experienced in using PDT, this approach often is used as initial therapy for the treatment of BD, particularly for larger lesions (> 2 cm) in cosmetically sensitive areas, on the hands, or on the distal lower extremities. Until now, patient-perceived satisfaction has not been systematically evaluated. When we offer our patients with BD the various treatment options, the discussion of side effects and social impact on their lives is often the determining factor in patient acceptance of a particular treatment. This study, the first of its kind to evaluate patient-perceived satisfaction rating a number of treatment related issues, provides clinicians with cogent evidence regarding patient-perceived satisfaction with PDT (> 90% in this study). The results of this study will go a long way in helping those of us performing PDT on BD to educate our patients regarding its use and associated expectations. Additionally the study results should help create an awareness among physicians regarding PDT as a viable treatment option for BD with regard to efficacy, safety, and cosmetic outcome.

G. Martin, MD

Recurrent basal cell carcinoma following ablative laser procedures

Jung D-S, Cho H-H, Ko H-C, et al (Pusan Natl Univ, Busan, Korea)
J Am Acad Dermatol 64:723-729, 2011

Background.—In Korea, many patients diagnosed with basal cell carcinoma (BCC) have a history of laser ablations of undiagnosed lesions.

Objective.—To evaluate the clinical/pathological and surgical features of BCC developing from undiagnosed lesions following laser ablations (not full-face cosmetic ablations) and to compare them with primary BCCs.

Methods.—This study enrolled 359 patients with 373 biopsy-proven BCC lesions. All of the patients were treated by Mohs micrographic surgery (MMS) at the Department of Dermatology, Pusan National University Hospital from 1998 to 2008. BCC was classified by previous treatment history of lesion ablative laser: post-laser BCC vs primary BCC. We conducted a retrospective study through clinical photographs, pathology slides, and MMS sheets.

Results.—Among 373 BCCs, 58 lesions (15.5%) were post-laser BCCs. The post-laser BCC group was younger (59.9 vs 65.4 years, $P = .001$), but had a longer disease interval until pathologic diagnosis (7.18 vs 3.33 years, $P < .0001$) than the primary BCC group. The post-laser BCC group had a greater frequency of the micronodular pattern (22.4% vs 10.8%, $P = .01$), required more stages of excision (2.69 ± 1.63 vs 2.15 ± 1.05, $P < .001$), and had fewer cases with one Mohs stage excision (10.3% vs 27%, $P = .006$) than the primary BCC group.

Limitations.—We could not identify the type of laser used in all 58 cases; instead, we supposed that most of the patients were likely treated with the carbon dioxide laser.

Conclusions.—The results demonstrated that the post-laser BCC group had a longer disease interval to diagnosis, a more aggressive histologic pattern, and required more stages of excision in MMS than the primary BCC group.

▶ This article suggests that the laser surgeon should be absolutely sure that the lesion being treated is benign and not malignant. A pigmented basal cell carcinoma in Asians can mascarade as a benign nevus. Perhaps it would be better to tangentially remove these lesions if treatment is desired with appropriate pathology rather than to destroy the target without histologic analysis. The use of a laser procedure to remove ("ablate") a skin lesion does not excuse the clinician from confirming the diagnosis histologically, which is the standard of care with a few notable exceptions (ie, cryotherapy of actinic ketatoses, veruccae in children, irritated seborrheic keratosis; scissor removal of pinpoint achrochordons). Should a problem arise later, it is difficult to justify that a lesion removed by laser ablation was not evaluated histologically for confirmation of diagnosis.

E. A. Tanghetti, MD

J. Q. Del Rosso, DO

Bowen's Disease Associated with Human Papillomavirus Infection of the Nail Bed

Aguayo R, Soria X, Abal L, et al (Hosp Universitari Arnau de Vilanova, Lleida, Spain)
Dermatol Surg 37:116-118, 2011

Background.—Bowen's disease is often found on areas of the skin that have been exposed to the sun and represents an in situ type of squamous cell carcinoma (SCC). Most lesions appear without any identifiable cause, and they are often diagnosed incorrectly as onychomycosis, vulgar wart, nail dystrophy, paronychia, or pyogenic granuloma. Pathogenesis for finger lesions includes ultraviolet radiation, other types of ionizing radiation, exposure to hydrocarbons, arsenic exposure, and human papillomavirus (HPV) infection. Immunosuppression also plays a role. A case of SCC of the finger was reported.

Case Report.—Woman, 54, had had progressive right thumbnail dystrophy lasting a few months. Asymptomatic hyperkeratotic plaque under the nail had caused onycholysis that extended to the nail folds. The lesion was diagnosed as a viral wart based on two biopsies. The patient had no history of trauma or exposure to arsenic, but her medical history included ischemic heart disease, arterial hypertension, diabetes mellitus, and a hysterectomy performed 13 years previously for a disease the patient could not recall. The finger lesion was completely excised, with histopathologic analysis revealing a papillomatous and highly hyperkeratotic lesion with epithelial architectural disorder, dyskeratotic keratinocytes, and larger atypical cells with large nuclei in the upper epidermal layers. Digital Bowen's disease was diagnosed.

Two years later the patient had a relapse at the same site that was removed. HPV genotyping studies were performed using polymerase chain reaction and nucleic acid hybridization. The results of both were positive for HPV 16. Pathologic archives helped to identify the disease causing the hysterectomy as cervical intraepithelial neoplasia.

Several months later the patient developed a new lesion on the third finger of her left hand that had the same clinical and histopathologic features, indicating digital Bowen's disease. Genotyping found positive results for HPV 16 and 6.

Conclusions.—The predominant HPV type found in periungual Bowen's disease is HPV 16. Lesions are most often found in index (42%) or middle (29%) fingers and the right hand is more often affected than the left. This patient had an in situ cervical SCC removed 13 years previously, and HPV 16 is one of the types classified as having a high oncogenic potential. This history led to the suspicion that there was viral transmission from the genital region to the fingers.

▶ This article presents a case of a middle-aged woman who developed 2 lesions of Bowen disease of the nail unit on 2 different digits. She also had an in situ cervical squamous cell carcinoma diagnosed years earlier. All 3 neoplasms tested positive for human papillomavirus (HPV) 16, suggesting viral transmission through autoinnoculation. The article suggests that when seeing female patients with digital Bowen disease, referral to a gynecologist should be strongly considered to exclude the presence of occult malignancy of the female genitourinary tract, especially the cervix.

E. M. Billingsley, MD

A new American Joint Committee on Cancer staging system for cutaneous squamous cell carcinoma: Creation and rationale for inclusion of tumor (T) characteristics

Farasat S, Yu SS, Neel VA, et al (Johns Hopkins Univ, Baltimore, MD; Univ of California, San Francisco; Massachusetts General Hosp and Harvard Med School, Boston; et al)
J Am Acad Dermatol 64:1051-1059, 2011

Background.—The incidence of cutaneous squamous cell carcinoma (cSCC) is increasing. Although most patients achieve complete remission with surgical treatment, those with advanced disease have a poor prognosis. The American Joint Committee on Cancer (AJCC) is responsible for the staging criteria for all cancers. For the past 20 years, the AJCC cancer staging manual has grouped all nonmelanoma skin cancers, including cSCC, together for the purposes of staging. However, based on new evidence, the AJCC has determined that cSCC should have a separate staging system in the 7th edition AJCC staging manual.

Objective.—We sought to present the rationale for and characteristics of the new AJCC staging system specific to cSCC tumor characteristics (T).

TABLE 2.—Definition of Cutaneous Squamous Cell Carcinoma Tumor (T) Staging System in 7th Edition of American Joint Committee on Cancer

TX	Primary tumor cannot be assessed
T0	No evidence of primary tumor
Tis	Carcinoma in situ
T1	Tumor ≤2 cm in greatest dimension with <2 high-risk features*
T2	Tumor >2 cm in greatest dimension with or without one additional high-risk feature,* *or* any size with ≥2 high-risk features*
T3	Tumor with invasion of maxilla, mandible, orbit, or temporal bone
T4	Tumor with invasion of skeleton (axial or appendicular) or perineural invasion of skull base

*High-risk features include depth (>2-mm thickness; Clark level ≥IV); perineural invasion; location (primary site ear; primary site nonglabrous lip); and differentiation (poorly differentiated or undifferentiated).

Methods.—The Nonmelanoma Skin Cancer Task Force of AJCC reviewed relevant data and reached expert consensus in creating the 7th edition AJCC staging system for cSCC. Emphasis was placed on prospectively accumulated data and multivariate analyses. Concordance with head and neck cancer staging system was also achieved.

Results.—A new AJCC cSCC T classification is presented. The T classification is determined by tumor diameter, invasion into cranial bone, and high-risk features, including anatomic location, tumor thickness and level, differentiation, and perineural invasion.

Limitations.—The data available for analysis are still suboptimal, with limited prospective outcomes trials and few multivariate analyses.

Conclusions.—The new AJCC staging system for cSCC incorporates tumor-specific (T) staging features and will encourage coordinated, consistent collection of data that will be the basis of improved prognostic systems in the future (Table 2).

▶ This article summarizes the work of the Nonmelanoma Skin Cancer Task Force of the American Joint Committee on Cancer (AJCC), who was given the charge of developing improved staging criteria for cutaneous neoplasms for the 7th edition of AJCC staging. In the past, all nonmelanoma skin cancers were grouped together. By basing the current staging criteria on cutaneous squamous cell carcinoma criteria, and separating out Merkel cell carcinoma as a separate system, it will allow collection of prospective data for future evidenced-based staging that is more specific to a given tumor type. Unlike prior staging systems for these cancers, this is based on data-derived, evidence-based medicine. High-risk features are now explicitly included in T staging, such as tumor size, thickness, Clark's level, and presence of perineural invasion, and the system also accounts for anatomic site and degree of histologic differentiation (Table 2). The authors clearly explain the rationale for the new criteria and allow the reader to understand the challenging undertaking of delineating these prognostic variables.

This new staging system, with clear definition of tumor characteristics, will provide the basis for future clinical trials and allow for prognostic studies across multiple centers.

E. M. Billingsley, MD

A randomized comparative study of tolerance and satisfaction in the treatment of actinic keratosis of the face and scalp between 5% imiquimod cream and photodynamic therapy with methyl aminolaevulinate
Serra-Guillen C, Nagore E, Hueso L, et al (Instituto Valenciano de Oncología, Valencia, Spain)
Br J Dermatol 164:429-433, 2011

Background.—Photodynamic therapy (PDT) and imiquimod are two excellent treatments for actinic keratosis but are often not well tolerated by patients.

Objectives.—To ascertain which treatment is better tolerated and which produces greater patient satisfaction. A secondary objective was to determine the factors related to the patient's tolerance to each treatment.

Methods.—Patients with at least five actinic keratosis lesions on the face and scalp were selected. The patients were randomized to receive treatment with PDT with methyl aminolaevulinate or treatment with imiquimod. Tolerance, satisfaction and predisposition to repeat the treatment were evaluated.

Results.—Most patients exhibited good or acceptable tolerance to both PDT and imiquimod treatment. There was a higher percentage of patients treated with PDT (93%) who were very satisfied compared with imiquimod (62%) ($P = 0.004$). Most patients treated with either one of the two options would repeat the same treatment. No significant relationship was found between age, sex, working time exposed to the sun, phototype and hair colour and the tolerance to both treatments.

Conclusions.—Both PDT and imiquimod are treatments that are generally well tolerated. While both treatments provide a high level of satisfaction, PDT appears to be slightly superior in this regard.

▶ The authors are to be commended for this study, which attempted to ascertain whether photodynamic therapy (PDT) with the photosensitizer methyl aminolevulinate, or imiquimod, is better accepted by patients treated for actinic keratoses (AKs) and which factors influence the level of patient tolerance. However, the latter was not accomplished, and the former is a vague conclusion at best. Although the authors noted enrolling only patients with > 5 AKs, there was no further mention of the number of AKs each patient had or how the number of AKs ranged between study participants and therefore no way to assess whether correlations existed between number of AKs, tolerance, and satisfaction. In addition, the PDT group included pretreatment curettage, which meant that there could have been less local reaction. The PDT group also had postcare with cryotherapy, Zimmer device, or fusidic acid cream, thus affecting posttreatment tolerance, which was assessed immediately after treatment. By contrast, the imiquimod group had no pre- or posttreatment care and was assessed at peak or near peak of their inflammatory response at 4 weeks later.

The authors recognized the importance of follow-up, and did so at 1 month, when they evaluated satisfaction and obtained their statistically significant result: 93% (27 of 29) of patients treated with PDT were very satisfied, as opposed to only 62% (18 of 29) of patients treated with imiquimod. Although statistically significant, an analog scale (0—4, dissatisfied; 5—7, moderately satisfied; and 8—10, very satisfied) was used, making reliable assessment difficult. Patients may not have ascertained much difference between a 7 and an 8, but they perhaps would have responded differently had the choices been "dissatisfied," "moderately satisfied," and "very satisfied." This is especially important in light of the finding that 3% of PDT subjects were moderately satisfied compared with 38% of imiquimod subjects, bringing the total of very and moderately satisfied subjects to 96% and 100%, respectively. How many of those moderately satisfied subjects responded with a 7, and how would this have affected the statistically significant finding? Furthermore, satisfaction 1 month after completion of treatment could have been influenced by the visible removal of lesions by curettage in the PDT group, which does not reflect comparison versus PDT alone. Similarly, it would have been helpful to assess the number of cleared lesions and need for repeat therapy. Patients often undergo more than one session of any form of therapy for AKs, including PDT or topical imiquimod, which may certainly affect their perceptions of satisfaction.

Despite delving into epidemiology, what this study was unable to assess were the qualitative traits that cause patients to have disparate treatment preferences. For example, do they have 4 hours to spend in the dermatologist's office, or would they prefer to apply a cream at home 3 times per week? Will they be compliant with application? How well can they tolerate discomfort?

To summarize, this article concluded that patients experienced a marginal degree of greater satisfaction with PDT than imiquimod. To verify and delve deeper into this claim, future studies should incorporate a larger sample size and more women, evaluate the effect of repeat treatments, establish clearance rates, closely evaluate baseline status including AK lesion counts, use 2.5% and 3.75% imiquimod creams for comparison, and attempt to accurately tease out qualitative patient treatment preferences.

A. Torres, MD, JD

Dermoscopy-guided surgery in basal cell carcinoma

Caresana G, Giardini R (Pathology Unit — Istituti Ospitalieri di Cremona, Italy)
J Eur Acad Dermatol Venereol 24:1395-1399, 2010

Background.—In basal cell carcinoma (BCC), excision margins between 3 and 10 mm, according to site, size, borders, previous treatment and histology, can allow for radical excision in at least 95% of cases.

Objective.—The objective was to ascertain whether dermoscopy can detect more accurately the lateral borders in BCCs than clinical examination alone, and allow us to obtain radical excision in more than 95% of cases with only 2-mm excision margins.

Methods.—A prospective study was performed of 200 consecutive BCCs of the head and neck removed with 2-mm dermoscopically detected excision margins. Morpheaform BCC, deeply recurrent BCC, BCC in Gorlin-Goltz syndrome, BCC located in sites not accessible through dermoscopy and superficial multifocal BCC were excluded. All cases of excised BCC were submitted to a uniform method of histological examination of the whole specimen with serial parallel sections at 2-mm intervals.

Results.—In only three cases did surgical excision with 2-mm margins prove to be inadequate; in the remaining 197 cases, the excision margins were tumour-free. The comparison of clinical and dermoscopic extension measurement showed concordance in 131 cases (65.5%). In 69 cases (34.5%), dermoscopic evaluation showed a larger peripheral extension.

Conclusions.—These results indicate that 2-mm dermoscopically detected excision margins can achieve histologically confirmed complete excisions in 98.5% of cases.

▶ The stated objectives of this study on dermoscopy-guided surgery in basal cell carcinoma (BCC) were to ascertain whether dermoscopy can detect the lateral borders of a BCC more accurately than clinical examination alone and to allow us to obtain complete excision in more than 95% of cases with only 2-mm surgical margins. This goal seems to have been met because the rate obtained was 98.5%. However, a couple of aspects of the study design may have skewed the results in this direction. One flaw was that the surgeon who determined the clinical margin then subsequently determined the dermoscopy margin. One can make the case that because the same operator made the clinical and dermoscopic determination, there is less variability in ability to determine margins among operators. However, it also means that any inherent bias by the investigator as to the usefulness of dermoscopy being superior could lead to a more laissez-faire approach to the clinical margin. This is especially evident in the fact that if the dermoscopy margin was uncertain, the margin was extended 2 mm beyond that margin, but it is unclear whether clinical uncertainty was given that same latitude. Also, the significance of these findings are discussed in the context of international guidelines that recommend anywhere from 3- to 10-mm surgical margins to achieve a 95% or better excision rate. These guidelines are not universally accepted internationally (eg, United States). Another interesting point is that complete (radical) excision would be 94.4% tumor-free if less than 1 mm was added to clinical margins (131 + 55 = 186/197) and 97.4% if up to 1-mm margin was added to the clinical margin (181 + 55 + 6 = 192/197), leading me more to question the international guidelines or to consider making the margin 3 mm if it is clinically not 100% clear. Lastly, the degree of experience of the dermoscopist was not clarified to assess the feasibility of this approach.

This tool does not give any indication as to the depth of the tumor. The entire specimen in this study was serially cross-sectioned in a bread-loaf fashion, then pathologic margins were evaluated histologically. It is well established that complete margin control is not attainable with this method. Hence, a significant proportion of residual tumors potentially would be missed, placing the patient at a higher risk of recurrence. It is a study with good concepts; however, it raises the questions discussed here and warrants a longer-term follow-up and en face complete histologic margin control.

A. Torres, MD, JD

Basaloid squamous cell carcinoma of the skin
Boyd AS, Stasko TS, Tang Y-W (Vanderbilt Univ, Nashville, TN)
J Am Acad Dermatol 64:144-151, 2011

Background.—Basaloid squamous cell carcinoma (BSCC), an aggressive tumor of the aerodigestive tract, was described over 20 years ago, and its defining histologic parameters remain largely unchanged. While rare reports have noted cutaneous metastatic deposition, primary tumors have not been previously described.

Objective.—Although most cutaneous malignancies with basaloid features comprise variants of basal cell carcinomas, a subset exhibit histologic attributes suggestive of more aggressive tumors. We evaluated 3 such tumors submitted to our dermatopathology service over a 6-month period.

Methods.—Immunohistochemical stains useful in differentiating the lineage of cutaneous malignancies with basaloid-appearing tumor cells were employed. Human papillomavirus (HPV) detection and typing were performed by using polymerase chain reaction and sequencing.

Results.—The tumor cells expressed high molecular weight cytokeratin (34βE12) and cytokeratin 5/6 but not Ber-EP4 or bcl-2. This pattern of immunohistochemical staining and the histologic attributes of the neoplasms are inconsistent with those expected in better defined cutaneous basaloid malignancies but are characteristic of BSCC. Two of the tumors arose in the inguinal crease of middle-aged men, and two patients were known to be immunosuppressed. HPV genotype 33 was detected in the tumor tissue from both inguinal lesions.

Limitations.—The number of cases available for evaluation is small and any prognostic implications therefore tenuous.

Conclusions.—The differential diagnosis of cutaneous malignancies exhibiting basaloid cells should include BSCC, a tumor with an unusual pattern of immunohistochemical staining and a potentially poor prognosis.

▶ Basaloid squamous cell carcinoma (BSCC) is a rare aggressive tumor of the aerodigestive tract. The most common presenting symptoms are bleeding and hoarseness. By the time the diagnosis is made, the cancer is often at an advanced stage, and distant metastasis is reported to be present in up to 75%. In other words, prognosis is typically poor; however, when BSCC is compared with poorly differentiated squamous cell carcinoma (SCC) of the same location, a recent retrospective study from China has shown no significant difference in prognosis between the 2.[1] Treatment is generally rendered using surgery with postoperative chemotherapy and/or radiation therapy in combination. There has been an association with the human papillomavirus in some cases. Histologically, the tumor can have a basaloid appearance with fibrotic stroma, peripheral palisading, atypical mitosis, and squamous atypia. Immunohistochemical evaluation shows positivity for high molecular weight cytokeratin (34βE12) and cytokeratin 5/6, but is negative for basal cell carcinoma markers Ber-EP4 or bcl-2 further substantiating

BSCC diagnosis. A limitation of this study is the small number of cases studied
($n = 3$) that were submitted to a dermatopathology laboratory.

S. Bellew, DO

J. Q. Del Rosso, DO

Reference

1. Wang LC, Wang L, Kwauk S, et al. Analysis on the clinical features of 22 basaloid
squamous cell carcinoma of the lung. *J Cardiothorac Surg*. 2011;6:10.

Axillary basal cell carcinoma: additional 25 patients and considerations
Betti R, Crosti C, Moneghini L, et al (Univ of Milan, AO San Paolo, Italy;
Università degli Studi di Milano-Fondazione IRCCS Ca' Granda — Ospedale
Maggiore Policlinico, Milano, Italy)
J Eur Acad Dermatol Venereol 25:858-860, 2011

Background.—Axillary basal cell carcinoma represents a rarely described
occurrence in world literature.

Objective.—To report our 14 years' experience of axillary basal cell
carcinomas.

Methods.—A review of Pathology department database is given.

Results.—Twenty-five further patients with axillary basal cell carcinomas
of 7367 basal cell carcinomas diagnosed are reported. These represent
a percentage of 0.33%. The average age of patients was 64.96 years, not
significantly different from the average age of patients with overall basal
cell carcinomas. No patient had had previous radiant or immunosuppressive treatment or axillary sunburn. No patient had basal cell naevus
syndrome. The subtypes involved were superficial and nodular. No patient
of 17 patients followed up had recurrences or metastasis after 5 years of
follow-up.

Conclusion.—Axillary Basal cell carcinomas are rare. No particular predisposing or risk factor is recorded. They do not seem to be significantly
more aggressive than other basal cell carcinomas.

▶ The axilla is a sun-protected body site and a rare location for basal cell
carcinoma (BCC) to develop. This is a review of 25 cases of axillary BCCs
recorded over a 15-year period focusing on the role of sun exposure and subtypes
of BCC found. In this study, axillary BCCs represented less than (0.33%) of all
cases of basal cell carcinoma. There were no predisposing factors identified,
such as a history of sunburn in the area, radiation treatment, or immunodeficiency.
The histological subtypes involved were superficial (16 cases), nodular (7 cases),
fibroepithelioma (1 case), and mixed superficial and nodular (1 case). There were
no cases of infiltrative or morpheaform histologic pattern. Although sun exposure
was a factor that was not identified as a risk, there was no control group. In addition, self-reports of sun exposure may be unreliable. Also, previous history of BCC
and other skin cancers was not known. Information on whether these BCCs were
primary lesions or recurrent lesions would have also been helpful. This study may

indicate that although the axilla is thought to be a sun-protected area, no area on the body is truly protected. Development of BCCs in these unusual areas of the body may be due to the sun's reflective properties, or greater exposure in reality than what is perceived. To add, this study emphasizes the importance of a complete body examination on the part of the dermatologist with skin cancer that may be present in hidden areas.

G. K. Kim, DO

J. Q. Del Rosso, DO

The sap from *Euphorbia peplus* is effective against human nonmelanoma skin cancers

Ramsay JR, Suhrbier A, Aylward JH, et al (Mater Radiation Oncology Centre, Brisbane, Queensland, Australia; Queensland Inst of Med Res, Brisbane, Australia; Peplin Biotech Ltd, Brisbane, Queensland, Australia)
Br J Dermatol 164:633-636, 2011

Background.—The sap from *Euphorbia peplus*, commonly known as petty spurge in the U.K. or radium weed in Australia, has been used as a traditional treatment for a number of cancers.

Objective.—To determine the effectiveness of *E. peplus* sap in a phase I/II clinical study for the topical treatment of basal cell carcinomas (BCC), squamous cell carcinomas (SCC) and intraepidermal carcinomas (IEC).

Methods.—Thirty-six patients, who had refused, failed or were unsuitable for conventional treatment, were enrolled in a phase I/II clinical study. A total of 48 skin cancer lesions were treated topically with 100−300 μL of *E. peplus* sap once daily for 3 days.

Results.—The complete clinical response rates at 1 month were 82% ($n = 28$) for BCC, 94% ($n = 16$) for IEC and 75% ($n = 4$) for SCC. After a mean follow-up of 15 months these rates were 57%, 75% and 50%, respectively. For superficial lesions < 16 mm, the response rates after follow-up were 100% for IEC ($n = 10$) and 78% for BCC ($n = 9$).

Conclusions.—The clinical responses for these relatively unfavourable lesions (43% had failed previous treatments, 35% were situated in the head and neck region and 30% were > 2 cm in diameter), are comparable with existing nonsurgical treatments. An active ingredient of *E. peplus* sap has been identified as ingenol mebutate (PEP005). This clinical study affirms community experience with *E. peplus* sap, and supports further clinical development of PEP005 for the treatment of BCC, SCC and IEC.

▶ Ramsay and colleagues report a pilot study that is the first series of patients with nonmelanoma skin cancer treated with the sap from *Eupohorbia peplus*, which is known as petty spurge or radium weed. Previously there was 1 published case report and multiple anecdotal reports from the community of its effectiveness. Forty-eight tumors in 36 patients were treated with 3 daily applications of the sap directly onto lesions under occlusion. The side effects and the appearance of the cancer sites were then evaluated clinically at 1, 6, and 12 months. A complete response (meaning complete clinical clearance with biopsy-confirmation) was seen in 57% of basal cell carcinomas (BCCs), 75% of intraepithelial carcinomas (IECs), and 50% of squamous cell carcinomas (SCCs). For superficial lesions that were less than 16 mm in diameter, the response rate was 100% for IEC (n = 10) and 78% for BCC (n = 9). Overall, the treatment was well tolerated, with the most severe side effects being pain in lesions that were very large in size.

This is a valuable study that affirms the community experience of *E. peplus* sap for the treatment of BCCs and superficial SCCs. The results of the study are impressive given the high number of difficult lesions included in the study (lesions on the head and neck, large tumors, and those that had failed previous treatments). The high clearance rate for small superficial lesions suggests a future role of this treatment for superficial BCC and SCC in situ. Strengths of the study include confirmatory biopsies in cases of clinical clearance. Limitations include a relatively small sample size, a follow-up period of only 12 months, and the lack of a control group.

The active ingredient of *E. peplus* has been identified as ingenol mebutate (Ing Meb). The proposed mechanism by which Ing Meb induces clearance of tumor cells is by stimulating inflammation, causing primary necrosis of tumor cells, and recruitment of neutrophils.[1-3] A phase II trial of topically applied Ing Meb in a gel formulation demonstrated efficacy in clearing superficial basal cell carcinoma.[4] Further studies will more clearly define the role of topical Ing Meb and *E. peplus* sap in the treatment of nonmelanoma skin cancer.

D. Fife, MD

References

1. Ogbourne SM, Hampson P, Lord JM, Parsons P, De Witte PA, Suhrbier A. Proceedings of the first international conference on PEP005. *Anticancer Drugs.* 2007;18:357-362.
2. Li L, Shukla S, Lee A, et al. The skin cancer chemotherapeutic agent ingenol-3-angelate (PEP005) is a substrate for the epidermal multidrug transporter (ABCB1) and targets tumor vasculature. *Cancer Res.* 2010;70:4509-4519.
3. Challacombe JM, Suhrbier A, Parsons PG, et al. Neutrophils are a key component of the antitumor efficacy of topical chemotherapy with ingenol-3-angelate. *J Immunol.* 2006;177:8123-8132.
4. Siller G, Rosen R, Freeman M, Welburn P, Katsamas J, Ogbourne SM. PEP005 (ingenol mebutate) gel for the topical treatment of superficial basal cell carcinoma: results of a randomized phase IIa trial. *Australas J Dermatol.* 2010;51:99-105.

A randomized, multicentre study of directed daylight exposure times of 1½ vs. 2½ h in daylight-mediated photodynamic therapy with methyl aminolaevulinate in patients with multiple thin actinic keratoses of the face and scalp
Wiegell SR, Fabricius S, Stender IM, et al (Univ of Copenhagen, Denmark; Clinic of Dermatology, Charlottenlund, Denmark; Uppsala Univ, Sweden; et al)
Br J Dermatol 164:1083-1090, 2011

Background.—Actinic keratoses (AKs) are common dysplastic skin lesions that may differentiate into invasive squamous cell carcinomas.

Although a superior cosmetic outcome of photodynamic therapy (PDT) is advantageous compared with equally effective treatments such as cryotherapy and curettage, the inconvenience of clinic attendance and discomfort during therapy are significant drawbacks. Daylight-mediated PDT could potentially reduce these and may serve as an alternative to conventional PDT.

Objectives.—To compare the efficacy of methyl aminolaevulinate (MAL)-PDT with 1½ vs. 2½ h of daylight exposure in a randomized multicentre study.

Methods.—One hundred and twenty patients with a total of 1572 thin AKs of the face and scalp were randomized to either 1½- or 2½-h exposure groups. After gentle lesion preparation and application of a sunscreen of sun protection factor 20, MAL was applied to the entire treatment area. Immediately after, patients left the clinic and exposed themselves to daylight according to the randomization. Daylight exposure was monitored with a wristwatch dosimeter and patients scored their pain sensation during treatment.

Results.—The mean lesion response rate at 3 months was 77% in the 1½-h group and 75% in the 2½-h group ($P = 0 \cdot 57$). The mean duration of daylight exposure was 131 and 187 min in the two groups. The mean overall effective light dose was $9 \cdot 4 \, J \, cm^{-2}$ (range $0 \cdot 2 - 28 \cdot 3$). Response rate was not associated with effective daylight dose, exposure duration, treatment centre, time of day or time of year during which the treatment was performed. Treatment was well tolerated, with a mean ± SD maximal pain score of $1 \cdot 3 \pm 1 \cdot 5$.

Conclusions.—Daylight-mediated MAL-PDT is an effective, convenient and nearly pain-free treatment for patients with multiple thin AKs. Daylight-mediated PDT procedures were easily performed and 2 h of daylight exposure resulted in uniformly high response rates when conducted in the period from June to October in Nordic countries.

▶ "Daylight-mediated" methyaminolevulinate (MAL) photodynamic therapy (PDT) provides a reasonable and effective alternative approach to "standard" MAL-PDT for grade 1 actinic keratoses (AKs) because it minimizes some of the drawbacks to in-office PDT, including pain, time patients spend in the office waiting and while being treated, occupied treatment rooms, and the expense of office personnel time required to perform PDT. Not mentioned in the article, although important to a number of patients, is the convenience afforded by a limited downtime necessary to heal postprocedure (generally 7 days). This compares favorably to other AK "field treatments" that require weeks to months of experiencing visible redness and crusting in the area where medication (ie, 5-fluorouracil, imiquimod) was applied.

It will be interesting to see how this technique will be adopted in areas of the world with higher ambient solar insolation. Alternatively, rainy days could create scheduling problems as well. The findings in this article also open the door for the evaluation of lower concentrations of aminolevulinic acid-based photosensitizers that could be used on a daily basis for medical and cosmetic purposes.

G. Martin, MD

Sun-Induced Nonsynonymous p53 Mutations Are Extensively Accumulated and Tolerated in Normal Appearing Human Skin
Ståhl PL, Stranneheim H, Asplund A, et al (Royal Inst of Technology, Stockholm, Sweden; Univ Hosp, Uppsala, Sweden; et al)
J Invest Dermatol 131:504-508, 2011

Here we demonstrate that intermittently sun-exposed human skin contains an extensive number of phenotypically intact cell compartments bearing missense and nonsense mutations in the *p53* tumor suppressor gene. Deep sequencing of sun-exposed and shielded microdissected skin from mid-life individuals revealed that persistent p53 mutations had accumulated in 14% of all epidermal cells, with no apparent signs of a growth advantage of the affected cell compartments. Furthermore, 6% of the mutated epidermal cells encoded a truncated protein. The abundance of these events, not taking into account intron mutations and mutations in other genes that also may have functional implications, suggests an extensive tolerance of human cells to severe genetic alterations caused by UV light, with an estimated annual rate of accumulation of ∼35,000 new persistent protein-altering p53 mutations in sun-exposed skin of a human individual.

▶ Irregular epidermal turnover starts with mutations, leading to consequences of aberrant epidermal hyperplasia, such as actinic keratosis, actinic cheilitis, and even poikilodermatous changes. If the p53 tumor suppressor gene is considered the regulator of that atypical turnover, then the mutation of p53 is the equivalent to the police force going on strike allowing the floodgates of epidermal crimes to commence. The larger problem, as demonstrated in the study population, is that the population of mutations in shielded skin and exposed skin was very similar.

Using the same analogy, the study shows that the location of the mutations on the genome is equally important as the quantity of mutations. A mutation upstream or at a hotspot location will have a significant impact on pathogenesis, similar to the concept that the floodgates of mutations may proceed once these initial events have occurred.

Many patients forget that on a cloudy or colder day sunscreens should be part of their daily routine, but the rationale is that harmful mutagenic ultraviolet light exposure is independent of visible sunlight and temperature. This is even more essential for the patient who has had extensive solar exposure or a previous skin cancer.

N. Bhatia, MD

Heightened Infection-Control Practices are Associated with Significantly Lower Infection Rates in Office-Based Mohs Surgery
Martin JE, Speyer L-A, Schmults CD (Univ of Texas Med Branch, Galveston; Brigham and Women's Hosp, Boston, MA)
Dermatol Surg 36:1529-1536, 2010

Background.—Reported infection rates for Mohs micrographic surgery (MMS) range from less than 1% to 3.5%.

Objective.—To determine whether lower infection rates are possible for MMS with a consistently applied infection-control regimen.

Methods.—A series of 832 consecutive patients with 950 tumors undergoing MMS formed the cohort for a retrospective study of infections before and after a program of heightened infection-control practices at a single-surgeon academic Mohs practice. The sterility upgrade included jewelry restrictions, alcohol hand scrub before stages and reconstruction, sterile gloves and (during reconstruction) sterile gowns for staff, and sterile towels and dressings for patients during Mohs stages.

Results.—Infection rate was 2.5% (9 infections/365 tumors) before the sterility upgrade and 0.9% (5 infections/585 tumors) after, a statistically significant difference ($p = .04$).

Conclusion.—MMS already has low rates of infection, but this study shows that rigorous infection-control practices can significantly affect infection rates.

▶ This article illustrates the low infection rate with Mohs micrographic surgery with the clean surgery approach that has been used extensively for several years even up until today. Proper emphasis on good surgical judgment, proper surgical technique, and assessment of the general health of the patient supports the low surgical infection rate, which is always a laudable goal. Effectiveness of individual methods and their role in surgical management is unclear. Their proposed follow-up study addressing these issues will be welcomed. In addition, the comparison of academic center patients with private office or auxiliary surgery center patients was not addressed. In hospital settings and practices with more patients than expected, such efforts will likely be beneficial. Mohs surgeons should consider at least the use of scrubless alcohol-based hand rubs before being gloved, removal of jewelry, and fresh, clean nonsterile gloves, gowns, and drapes during excision. Other specific perisurgical methods may be useful for higher-risk patients, prolonged and complicated cases, and reconstruction. In the current health care environment, it is more important than ever to utilize the most cost-effective, highest quality practices for office-based surgery.

R. Ceilley, MD
B. Kopitzki, DO

Hedgehog Antagonist GDC-0449 Is Effective in the Treatment of Advanced Basal Cell Carcinoma

Amin SH, Tibes R, Kim J-E, et al (Kaiser Permanente Med Ctr, Oakland, CA; Kaiser Permanente Med Ctr, San Rafael, CA; Translational Genomics Res Inst, Phoenix, AZ)
Laryngoscope 120:2456-2459, 2010

Objectives/Hypothesis.—To demonstrate the efficacy of the hedgehog pathway inhibitor GDC-0449 in the treatment of advanced basal cell carcinoma.

Design Study.—Case series.

Methods.—Three patients treated in a referral center for locally advanced basal cell carcinoma, one with metastases, were referred for treatment in a GDC-0449 phase I clinical trial. The treatment was once per day continuous therapy with oral GDC-0449.

Results.—Two patients showed complete clinical and radiologic resolution of disease, whereas one patient had significant reduction in tumor burden with radiologic evidence of slowly progressive local disease. Side effects were taste changes, mild to moderate hair loss, and muscle cramps in one patient.

Conclusions.—GDC-0449 showed significant inhibitory activity in the treatment of advanced basal cell carcinoma.

▶ This study provides much-welcomed good news regarding efforts being put into systemic therapy for the treatment of extensive and metastatic basal cell carcinomas (BCCs). The molecule GDC-0449 is designed to inhibit the activation of smoothened in the Sonic hedgehog—patched (SHH-PTCH) signaling pathway that leads to cell immortality, a method of skin cancer treatment that more directly targets the error in maturation of the basal cells than other current therapies.

The results of the 3 case studies presented show marked improvement in 1 case and complete resolution in 2 others, 1 of which was metastatic. This is highly encouraging evidence for the efficacy of the drug, but of course the sample size is very small and it would be premature to become overly optimistic based on this report alone. Nonetheless, at the very least, this article highlights the great promise this drug shows for patients with basal cell nevus syndrome and metastatic disease.

There are 2 features of this drug that make this report so meaningful. First, the drug is dosed orally, so some of the very limitations that may have kept patients from seeking treatment in the first place are not compounded by obstacles to getting therapy. Second, the aberrant SHH-PTCH pathway is not limited to BCCs, but is also implicated in gastrointestinal tumors and prostate and pancreatic cancer, providing even more hope that an effective therapy may benefit more than 1 patient population.

Some practitioners may never see such severe cases of locally aggressive or recurrent BCCs, and even fewer cases of metastatic disease, but one can foresee that this drug may not be limited to such cases. If the early reports suggestive of minimal side effects, such and dysgeusia, hair loss, and muscle cramps, are all that become evident in phase III trials, this oral therapy may become a useful tool for all dermatologists who have patients with tumors in areas where resection is problematic or in those patients who live rurally and refuse to come for treatment because of constraints of time, distance, or debilitation.

J. M. Suchniak, MD

Occupational ultraviolet light exposure increases the risk for the development of cutaneous squamous cell carcinoma: a systematic review and meta-analysis

Schmitt J, Seidler A, Diepgen TL, et al (Technische Universität Dresden, Germany; Univ Clinic of Heidelberg, Germany)
Br J Dermatol 164:291-307, 2011

Background.—Despite the fact that ultraviolet (UV) light exposure is the most important risk factor for cutaneous squamous cell carcinoma (SCC) there is an ongoing debate concerning the relationship between cumulative work-related UV exposure and SCC occurrence.

Objectives.—To analyse comprehensively the relationship between work-related UV exposure and SCC risk.

Methods.—We conducted a systematic electronic literature search in PubMed (up to 5 May 2010) supplemented by a hand search, which identified 18 relevant studies that were included in the review. Data abstraction and study quality assessment was done independently by two reviewers. Maximally adjusted odds ratios (ORs) and corresponding 95% confidence intervals (CIs) of all included studies were pooled in a random-effects meta-analysis. Sensitivity analysis included meta-regression on study-specific covariates to explore the robustness of the results and to identify sources of heterogeneity between studies. Eighteen studies (six cohort studies, 12 case–control studies) met the eligibility criteria and were included in the systematic review.

Results.—Sixteen studies (89%) found an increased risk of SCC in individuals with occupational UV light exposure compared with individuals without occupational UV light exposure, reaching statistical significance in 12 studies. Two studies found no association between occupational UV light exposure and SCC occurrence. The pooled OR (95% CI) was $1·77$ ($1·40–2·22$) and did not differ significantly between cohort studies [OR (95% CI): $1·68$ ($1·08–2·63$)] and case–control studies [OR (95% CI): $1·77$ ($1·37–2·30$)]. Meta-regression analyses suggested an increasing strength of the association between occupational UV light exposure and SCC risk with decreasing latitude.

Conclusions.—In summary, there is consistent epidemiological evidence for a positive association between occupational UV light exposure and SCC risk.

▶ This article summarizes an extremely comprehensive literature search to analyze the relationship between work-related exposure to solar ultraviolet (UV) radiation and the development of cutaneous squamous cell carcinoma (cSCC). It is the first meta-analysis that comprehensively summarizes the published epidemiological evidence for this relationship and clearly indicates that outdoor work constitutes an independent and relevant risk factor for the development of cutaneous SCC.

CSCC is a common malignancy worldwide with a steadily increasing incidence over recent decades. Although the etiologic role of UV light in the development of SCC is understood, the role of occupational exposure to UV light had not been well established in the literature as an independent variable related to causing of SCC.

This article is of significant relevance for occupational medicine and public health because large proportions of the working population have regular and chronic exposure to UV light. It supports the need for primary prevention strategies, as well as education for the workers and employers, and provides needed data for occupational health experts, health educators, and physicians. The analysis also supports previous research demonstrating the association between occupational UV exposure and development of SCC with an increased incidence correlated with decreasing latitude.

This article is a nice summary to provide evidence and support to implement sun-protective measures for outdoor workers and encourage the importance of regular skin examinations in this population.

E. M. Billingsley, MD

MAL-PDT for difficult to treat nonmelanoma skin cancer
Stebbins WG, Hanke CW (The Laser and Skin Surgery Ctr of Indiana, Carmel)
Dermatol Ther 24:82-93, 2011

With an incidence of over 3.5 million nonmelanoma skin cancers (NMSCs) per year in the United States, there is an increasing need for effective, cost-effective treatments for NMSC. When surgical excision is impractical or not feasible, methyl aminolevulinate photodynamic therapy (MAL-PDT) has demonstrated consistently high long-term cure rates ranging from 70–90%, with superior cosmetic outcomes compared with other treatment modalities. With the exception of invasive squamous cell carcinoma, MAL-PDT has been successful in treating all types of NMSC, especially in patients with multiple comorbidities, field cancerization, and lesions in cosmetically sensitive locations. Herein, a step-by-step description of the procedure for MAL-PDT is provided, followed by a review of outcomes from large clinical trials performed over the past 15 years for each variant of NMSC. After reading this review, clinicians should have a thorough understanding of the benefits and limits of MAL-PDT, and should be able to add this valuable procedure to their armamentarium of therapies for NMSC.

▶ In this excellent review of the use of methyl aminolevulinate photodynamic therapy (MAL-PDT) for nonmelanoma skin cancer (NMSC), we are provided with a thorough overview of the safety and efficacy data, treatment protocols, and lesion type-response parameters. As a nonsurgical option for difficult-to-treat NMSC, specifically superficial basal cell carcinoma (BCC), superficial squamous cell carcinoma (SCC), and nodular BCC in cosmetically sensitive and difficult-to-treat areas, MAL-PDT outperforms alternatives such as cryosurgery, 5-fluorouracil, and topical imiquimod in terms of efficacy and cosmetic outcomes. Additionally, patient satisfaction studies following PDT for the treatment of NMSC, specifically SCC-in-situ (Bowen disease), rate PDT very highly (> 90%).[1] The European experience with MAL PDT over the last decade has provided a strong database to serve as a guideline for U.S.-based dermatologists. Although aminolevulinic acid (ALA) PDT is achieving increased adoption by U.S.-based dermatologists, the adoption of MAL-PDT over the last few years in the United States has been limited for a variety of reasons, and it has not achieved widespread acceptance. Because both prodrugs (MAL and ALA) result in significant levels of the photosensitizing molecule protoporphyrin IX within skin tumors, acquisition of a commercially available light-emitting diode red light source would allow off-label treatment of selective difficult-to-treat NMSC using ALA or MAL.[2]

G. Martin, MD

References

1. Hu A, Moore C, Yu E, et al. Evaluation of patient-perceived satisfaction with photodynamic therapy for Bowen disease. *J Otolaryngol Head Neck Surg.* 2010;39:688-696.
2. Fritsch C, Homey B, Stahl W, Lehmann P, Ruzicka T, Sies H. Preferential relative porphyrin enrichment in solar keratoses upon topical application of delta-aminolevulinic acid methylester. *Photochem Photobiol.* 1998;68:218-221.

Atypical Squamous Proliferation: What Lies Beneath?
Sebastian S, Yanko R, Goldstein GD (Dermatology and Skin Cancer Ctr of Kansas City, Leawood; MD Anderson Department of Facial Plastic Surgery, Houston, TX)
Dermatol Surg 37:395-398, 2011

Background.—Shave biopsies are often performed because of their speed and efficiency, but they have the drawback of not obtaining a deep enough specimen for dermatopathologists to analyze sufficiently in all cases. The pathology report in these cases often documents an "atypical squamous proliferation of undetermined significance" or similar wording. Among the entities that can be beneath an atypical squamous proliferation are squamous cell carcinoma (SCC), warts, irritated seborrheic keratosis, actinic keratosis (AK), or other less-common neoplasms. To better understand the best course of action to take when one receives a diagnosis of atypical squamous proliferation of undetermined significance, a retrospective chart review was undertaken.

Methods.—The charts of 110 patients were reviewed, constituting 46 women and 64 men (average age 69 years). Most biopsies were done on the head and neck (75 biopsies) or the upper extremities (23 biopsies).

A third of the cases (40 lesions) were not studied further because they were noted clinically to have no recurrence or were treated with Mohs micrographic surgery (MMS) based on a high clinical suspicion of cancer and cleared with a single stage, so the underlying pathology was not determined.

Results.—Fifty-eight lesions were re-biopsied and 12 were treated with MMS and cleared in two or more stages. The underlying diagnosis was AK in 29% of cases, SCC in 20%, and SCC in situ in 7%. Twenty-four percent of cases had normal skin and 16% had benign neoplasms such as verruca, fibrous papules, seborrheic keratosis, and scars. Basal cell carcinoma (BCC) was found in 4% of cases. However, grouping findings into malignant and nonmalignant lesions, 31% of the time a malignancy was under the atypical squamous proliferation. This is probably conservative because of the third of the cases that had already been excluded as highly suspicious for cancer. Some kind of subsequent clinical treatment was required in 59% of the cases.

Conclusions.—Clinicians often disregard or overlook a diagnosis of atypical squamous proliferation of undetermined significance. Nearly two-thirds of the patients studied required further treatment after repeat biopsy, and a malignant lesion was discovered in a third of the cases. Reports with a finding of atypical squamous proliferation should prompt a deeper repeat biopsy, especially if the lesion persists or is clinically suspicious for skin cancer.

▶ Atypical squamous proliferation is an occasional diagnosis on a pathology report. This often confounds the clinician with uncertainty in terms of what management approach to take in addressing this condition, as it is known that it can overlie cancerous and benign conditions. Sebastian et al performed a chart review of 110 patients to determine what exactly was found beneath the reports of atypical squamous proliferations in these charts. The information reported is helpful and important to all practitioners dealing with similar pathology nomenclature. In 31% of cases, an underlying malignancy was found-a squamous cell carcinoma (SCC), a squamous cell carcinoma in situ (SCCIS), or even basal cell carcinoma. In addition, actinic keratosis was found 29% of the time. More telling was that 59% of the cases that were read as atypical squamous cell proliferation were postulated as requiring clinical treatment of some form. Given these data, it is recommended that a deeper rebiopsy of any lesion read as atypical squamous proliferation be considered. While this study only reviewed 110 patient charts and is by no means exhaustive or definitive, it is persuasive enough evidence to consider a deeper rebiopsy as a viable management option for these lesions or at least defined clinical follow-up. Overall, this study helps further elucidate a topic of potential uncertainty and provides a reasonable appropriate course of management based on the presenting data. This is a very practical article.

B. D. Michaels, DO
J. Q. Del Rosso, DO

A Unique Basaloid Proliferation Encountered During Mohs Surgery: Potential Pitfall for Overdiagnosis of Basal Cell Carcinoma

Patel NS, Johnston RB, Messina JL, et al (Univ of South Florida, Tampa, FL)
Dermatol Surg 37:1180-1188, 2011

Background.—Several well-documented neoplasms resemble basal cell carcinoma (BCC) and can complicate surgical management in facial zones. Two cases of follicular-based basaloid proliferation (FBP), which are extremely rare, were reported.

> *Case Reports.*—Case 1: Man, 47, had biopsy-proven BCC of the right nasofacial sulcus and underwent five stages of Mohs surgery. The final diagnosis claimed free deep margins but involvement of all peripheral margins, so the patient was referred for further assessment and possible treatment. Physical examination revealed a 2.5- × 2.0-cm triangular open wound over the right alar rim. Both the nose sidewall and the nasolabial area were involved, and granulation tissue was seen at the wound base. The right alar rim was contracted superiorly about 1 cm, with no nodularity in the surrounding area. Review of the Mohs tissue sections revealed the first two stages had a centrally located BCC with nodular and micronodular histologic patterns but stages 3, 4, and 5 did not. All five stages showed peripheral skin edges with multiple foci of basaloid proliferation. Radiating strands of basaloid epithelium with keratinous cysts were embedded in fibroblastic stroma and attached to several preexisting hair follicles. No further resection was done.

> Case 2: Man, 58, had six stages of Mohs surgical resection for a right medial canthus BCC. Physical examination showed a 2.2-cm open wound with granulation tissue at the base. Histopathologic review revealed a nodular-type BCC on the first and second stages not seen on later stages. Stages 3 to 6 had basaloid proliferation with radiating strands of basaloid epithelium branching out from hair follicles and surrounded by fibromucinous stromal change. The strands were connected to the hair follicles' metrical portion and demonstrated no atypia. No further resection was done.

Analysis.—Characteristics of FBP are a multifocal, multishape basaloid proliferation usually involving the follicular epithelium. It is often found in aggregates with a smooth or uneven ouline and fairly uniform cells that may have peripheral palisading. FBP has a vertical orientation, axial distribution, folliculocentricity, and normal surrounding stroma. The prominent, tightly adherent basement membrane (BM) stains positively with periodic acid-Schiff (PAS) stain. Minor histologic criteria include no epidermal attachments, keratin cysts, single-cell necrosis or dyskeratosis, mitotic figures, or basal cell melanin.

In contrast to FBP, BCC is arranged horizontally, often has a myxoid-appearing stroma, has no axial distribution centered on the follicle, has a disorganized reticular pattern, can extend beyond superficial tissue, and lacks the distinct hyaline BM appearance of FBP. Clefts are common with BCC. Infundibulocystic BCC is often difficult to distinguish from FBP, but is typically less than 5 mm in diameter, limited to the face, and lacks multicentricity. BCC with follicular differentiation can also have mitotic figures, single-cell necrosis, squamous differentiation with keratin cysts, and epidermal attachments. Other entities to be distinguished from FBP are trichoblastoma, trichoepithelioma, basaloid follicular hamartoma, tumor of follicular infundibulum, fibrofolliculoma, trichodiscoma, Birt-Hogg-Dube syndrome, trichofolliculoma, and follicular induction overlying dermatofibromas.

Conclusions.—Mohs surgeons and dermatopathologists rarely see FBP so its differentiation can be challenging. If a conclusive diagnosis cannot be reached based on histologic evaluation, permanent sections, clinical evaluation, and comparison with the original lesion may be needed.

▶ Nonmelanoma skin cancer (NMSC) is the most common malignancy in the United States. Basal cell carcinoma (BCC) is the most common NMSC. BCCs that occur in areas associated with a high recurrence rate may warrant Mohs micrographic surgery (MMS). However, many other entities can mimic BCCs. This report describes 2 cases of an unusual type of folliculocentric basaloid proliferation (FBP), which can look similar to BCC. FBP is a rare entity characterized by multicentric follicular-based growths of basal cell-like epithelium. This entity can be a diagnostic pitfall because it may lead to additional unnecessary stages of MMS. In FBP, the cells are uniform and remain in a vertical direction with a normal surrounding stoma. This is in contrast to BCCs that often project horizontally with surrounding a myxoid stromal appearance. Infundibulocystic BCC has a radiating configuration but is not multicentric, like FBP. Trichoblastoma (TB) is a benign epithelial proliferation of follicular germ cells, unlike FBP. TB produces a nodular mass effect and is not always found in relation to mature follicles. TB is also found much deeper than FBP. Trichoepithelioma is said to be a superficial or mature form of TB. Basaloid follicular hamartoma (BFH) demonstrates basaloid cell proliferation with squamous differentiation, sometimes with keratin horn cysts and abortive hair follicles. Also, patients with BFH may have a systemic illness, such as systemic lupus erythematous, alopecia, and cystic fibrosis. Fibrofolliculomas exhibit elongated trabeculated strands of epithelium from a dilated follicular infundibulum. Trichofolliculoma is a cystic neoplasm of hair follicles with a keratin-filled cavity lined by squamous epithelium with a granular layer. Follicular induction is a reactive proliferation of the epidermis and hair follicles in response to stimuli, demonstrating multifocal basaloid buds from the dermoepidermal junction. FBP can be easily mistaken for BCC, and because it is so rare, it is important to be able to differentiate it from other similar basaloid proliferations.

G. K. Kim, DO

J. Q. Del Rosso, DO

Vascular Complications After Treatment with Low-Dose Isotretinoin in Two Elderly Patients

Sambandan DR, Ratner D (Columbia Univ, NY; Columbia Univ Med Ctr, NY)
Dermatol Surg 37:726-728, 2011

Background.—Oral retinoids can be used to treat nodular acne or psoriasis, or for the chemoprophylaxis of nonmelanoma skin cancer (NMSC). This chemoprophylaxis can be designed to decrease morbidity from multiple primary tumors and actinic keratosis or to decrease mortality from a single high-risk tumor. Lower doses of oral retinoids are used for chemoprevention than for acne (0.25 to 0.5 mg/kg/day rather than 0.5 to 2 mg/kg/day, respectively). However, oral retinoid therapy manifests mucocutaneous, ophthalmic, gastrointestinal, and rheumatologic side effects and may also affect coagulation. Two elderly patients received low-dose oral isotretinoin for NMSC chemoprevention and developed potentially life-threatening conditions.

Case Reports.—Case 1: Man, 79, had a history of multiple NMSCs, hyperlipidemia, hypertension, and left common femoral artery endarterectomy. He had undergone femoral above-knee popliteal artery bypass 1 year previously and was taking 75 mg/day of clopidogrel. To reduce the number and severity of his skin lesions, he was given 10 mg of isotretinoin orally every other day to minimize side effects. He developed nightly leg pain and could not walk within 2 weeks. Ultrasound verified thrombosis of the bypass graft. The isotretinoin effectively cleared the skin lesions, but was discontinued because it may have contributed to the graft thrombosis. He gradually improved over the course of 2 months but still had difficulty walking.

Case 2: Man, 82, had psoriasis, multiple NMSCs, congestive heart failure, rheumatic heart disease, and a prosthetic aortic valve and was taking 4 mg/day of warfarin. A year previously he had undergone photodynamic therapy that temporarily improved his facial lesions but more lesions developed. During 3 weeks of 10-mg/day oral isotretinoin for NMSC chemoprevention, he developed personality changes, epistaxis, dry lips, and a shorter attention span when reading. No laboratory changes were noted and his international normalized ratio (INR) remained therapeutic, so the isotretinoin was continued. After 6 weeks he had increased irritability, pruritus, dry eyes and lips, greater lower extremity edema, and shortness of breath, plus difficulty controlling his INR. Skin lesions were reduced in extent and severity, but isotretinoin was discontinued. Symptoms persisted for several days. He developed bilateral 2+ pretibial pitting edema, right lung base rales, and penile and scrotal edema. The increased congestive heart failure (CHF) symptoms was treated with hydrochlorothiazide and a change from furosemide to torsemide. Two weeks later he had gained about 8 pounds and had jugular venous distention; his condition did not improve with higher torsemide dosing. He was hospitalized to manage the worsening CHF symptoms unresponsive to oral diuretics.

Conclusions.—The benefits of giving oral retinoids must be balanced against the risks of adverse effects. Both patients had preexisting vascular risk factors. Although the isotretinoin achieved good cutaneous improvement, both patients suffered potentially life-threatening adverse reactions, even with low doses of this agent. It is possible that older adults have delayed drug metabolism and difficulty clearing even low doses of oral retinoids, putting them at greater risk for developing thrombosis. Vascular risk factors must be analyzed before prescribing oral retinoids, especially in older patients.

▶ Oral retinoids can be used as a chemoprophylaxis on nonmelanoma skin cancer (NMSC). However, oral retinoids, despite their efficacy, can have many side effects. This is a case report of 2 elderly patents who received low-dose oral isotretinoin for NMSC and developed potentially life-threatening sequelae afterward. The first patient was a 79-year-old man with a history of multiple NMSCs, hyperlipidemia, hypertension, and left common femoral artery endarterectomy with a popliteal artery bypass. He was started on oral isotretinoin 10 mg every other day to minimize the risk of developing more NMSCs. Shortly after being on isotretinoin, the patient developed a graft thrombosis, and oral isotretinoin was discontinued. The second patient was an 82-year-old man with a history of psoriasis, multiple NMSCs, congestive heart failure (CHF), rheumatic heart disease, and a prosthetic aortic valve. Oral isotretinoin was discontinued because the patient was experiencing increased irritability, pruritus, dry eyes, increased lower extremity edema, and shortness of breath. Although isotretinoin was discontinued, the patient developed worsening of his congestive heart failure that became refractory to oral diuretics. There have been cases of cerebrovascular accidents and thromboembolic disorders described during treatment with high-dose isotretinoin therapy. Although oral isotretinoin is not definitively the cause of adverse events in these 2 cases, the possibility cannot be ruled out. However, in both cases, the patients had multiple medical issues and were on various other medications, and to claim that isotretinoin was the cause of these adverse events would not be prudent. The benefits of initiating an oral retinoid must be evaluated carefully according to each patient's medical background. Each clinician must evaluate the benefits versus the risks of starting an oral retinoid, including in patients with underlying disorders, such as hyperlipidemia, hypertension, and prior thromboembolic events. Further vigilance regarding a possible increased risk of adverse events when oral isotretinoin is used in patients with these underlying risk factors is warranted.

G. K. Kim, DO
J. Q. Del Rosso, DO

Use of Reflectance Confocal Microscopy to Differentiate Hidrocystoma from Basal Cell Carcinoma

Willard K, Warschaw KE, Swanson DL (Univ of New Mexico, Albuquerque; Mayo Clinic, Scottsdale, AZ)
Dermatol Surg 37:392-394, 2011

Background.—It is important to distinguish pigmented basal cell carcinoma (BCC) from benign entities such as hidrocystomas. Reflectance confocal microscopy (RCM) is a noninvasive, real-time modality for imaging skin at cellular levels. It is the only noninvasive modality for visualizing details needed for histologic analysis and can be used at bedside. RCM permits the assessment of neoplastic and inflammatory processes and differentiates benign from malignant lesions. A hidrocystoma was distinguished from BCC using RCM.

> *Case Report.*—Woman, 65, had an asymptomatic lesion of 6 months' duration on the right upper lip medial to the nasolabial fold. The 2-mm blue papule had indeterminate characteristics on dermoscopy, necessitating a distinction between various entities, including BCC and hidrocystoma. RCM showed the papule was a homogenous cystic structure bounded by normal-appearing adnexal tissue. A shave biopsy specimen revealed a small, thin, superficial unilocular cyst in the upper dermis with one or two layers of cuboidal cells, an appearance typical of hidrocystoma.

Analysis.—Hidrocystomas are benign cystic tumors of the dermal apocrine or eccrine ducts usually seen in adults. They can be single or multiple and usually have a dome-shaped, translucent, pale blue appearance. Single hidrocystomas are noted in both genders, but multiple lesions are more common in the periorbital and malar regions in women. Microscopically the lesions consist of unilocular cysts with a single cavity of one to two layers of cuboidal cells. Apocrine gland lesions can emit decapitation secretions; eccrine lesions have no epidermal contact. RCM uses near-infrared light from a diode laser to focus on microscopic targets at various depths horizontally to a maximum of about 200 μm in the papillary and upper reticular dermis. Mosaic reconstructions of BCC using RCM allow the differentiation of BCC and hidrocystoma features.

Conclusions.—RCM can clearly distinguish the discrete, homogenous featureless hidrocystoma from the tumor islands, peritumoral dark clefts, tumor silhouettes, bright cells, prominent mucinous edema, and dense stromal collagen of BCC. Its noninvasive nature makes it especially useful for differentiating these conditions.

▶ Reflectance confocal microscopy (RCM) is a noninvasive means of evaluating microscopic characteristics of suspected skin malignancies. Willard et al report a case in which RCM was successfully used to differentiate a hidrocystoma from a basal cell carcinoma (BCC). The characteristic features of the hidrocystoma were a "homogenous, cystic structure abutted by normal-appearing adnexal structures." In contrast, the RCM features of a BCC include "tumor islands surrounded by peritumoral dark clefts, tumor silhouettes, bright cells, and prominent vasculature." The suspected diagnosis of hidrocystoma based on RCM findings was confirmed by histopathologic examination. This article was helpful in demonstrating a noninvasive way to differentiate a benign from a malignant growth. However, a major flaw in the analysis was that the reflectance confocal images compared did not scrutinize a cystic BCC, which may look very different from a traditional BCC. In addition, this is a case report of 1. A study with more lesions and comparing RCM of hidrocystoma to cystic basal cells is needed before we can make any sweeping conclusions.

A. Torres, MD, JD

Trends in the incidence of basal cell carcinoma by histopathological subtype
Arits AHMM, Schlangen MHJ, Nelemans PJ, et al (Maastricht Univ Med Centre, The Netherlands; Maastricht Univ, The Netherlands)
J Eur Acad Dermatol Venereol 25:565-569, 2011

Background.—As a result of the high prevalence, basal cell carcinoma (BCC) causes a significant and expensive health care problem.

Objective.—In this study, we evaluate the proportional increase in BCC by histological subtype over the last two decades.

Methods.—We retrospectively reviewed all primary histological confirmed BCCs diagnosed in the Maastricht University Medical Centre in The Netherlands in the years 1991, 1999 and 2007.

Results.—An annual increase of the number of BCCs of 7% for both genders was shown. The age-standardized incidence rates for BCC increased between 1991 and 2007 from 54.2 to 162.1 per 100 000 men and from 61.7 to 189.8 per 100 000 women. The proportion of superficial BCC increased significantly from 17.6% to 30.7%.

Conclusion.—The incidence of BCC is continuing to increase this century. The observed shift to the superficial histological subtype, which can be treated non-surgically, might reduce the workload in the busy dermatologists practice.

▶ Skin cancers overall are the most prevalent type of cancer, with basal cell carcinoma (BCC) being the most common type among skin cancers. Given its high prevalence and significance as a health care problem, Artis et al provide a retrospectively reviewed study on the increasing incidence of BCC. Although the review was based in the Netherlands, its findings should also be noted by others worldwide. The report reviewed changes in the incidence of BCC between 1991, 1999, and 2007, principally for nodular, infiltrative, and superficial subtype BCCs (although more attention was given to superficial BCC in the article). What Artis et al found in the review was an overall increase in BCC. The most common histological subtype of BCC remained the nodular form, but there was a "significant" increase in the proportion of both superficial BCC and infiltrative BCC during this time. However, the increase from 1999 to 2007 was less than the increase from 1991 to 1997, which was hypothesized to be due to better health awareness and health-seeking behaviors. Other interesting findings included a lower percentage of BCC found on the head and neck region (decreasing from 73.9% in 1991 to 44.3% in 2007) and a higher percentage of BCC found on the trunk (increasing from 17.6% in 1991 to 45.3% in 2007). The reasons postulated for the increased proportion of superficial basal cell carcinoma (sBCC) was 2-fold: sBCC develops from intense intermittent sun exposure rather than chronic sun exposure, and there has been an increase in recreational sun exposure since the 1970s. This might also explain why sBCCs are more commonly seen on the trunk. The other advanced hypothesis is that BCCs may progress from superficial to nodular to infiltrative forms, and this, combined with a heightened awareness of skin malignancies, has resulted in an observed increase in the proportion of sBCCs due to earlier detection. Given the higher relative percentage of sBCC, the authors postulate that this may cause some relief to dermatologists given that it is less costly and time-consuming to treat than other forms. In general, the study provides interesting insight into the continuing prevalence of BCCs and the continued need for educating patients on sun exposure and photoprotection.

B. D. Michaels, DO

J. Q. Del Rosso, DO

Topical methyl aminolevulinate photodynamic therapy for management of basal cell carcinomas in patients with basal cell nevus syndrome improves patient's satisfaction and reduces the need for surgical procedures

Pauwels C, Mazereeuw-Hautier J, Basset-Seguin N, et al (Paul-Sabatier Univ and Toulouse Univ-Hosp, Toulouse, France; Paris-VII Univ and Saint-Louis Hosp AP-HP, Paris, France)
J Eur Acad Dermatol Venereol 25:861-864, 2011

Background.—In basal cell nevus syndrome, basal cell carcinomas occur in early life. The treatment of basal cell carcinomas requires surgical excisions and may lead to unaesthetic scars. Photodynamic therapy (PDT) is a validated treatment of skin cancers, with good cosmetic outcomes.

Objectives.—The aim of the study was to evaluate patient's satisfaction, cosmetic outcome and number of surgical excisions before and after PDT, in patients with basal cell nevus syndrome treated with PDT.

Methods.—A cross-sectional evaluation of all patients with basal cell nevus syndrome, treated with PDT for basal cell carcinomas. A questionnaire evaluated satisfaction, cosmetic outcomes for surgery and PDT. The number of surgeries before and after PDT was noted and efficacy was evaluated.

Results.—Seven patients were evaluated; 85% of patients were satisfied with PDT vs. 55% for surgery. The average visual analogue score for the cosmetic result was 8.42/10 for PDT vs. 6.3/10 for surgery. The mean number of surgical excisions was 4.4 during the 6 months before the first session of PDT and 0.57 after.

Conclusion.—Methylaminolevulinate-photodynamic therapy seems an interesting option for the treatment of basal cell carcinomas in patients with basal cell nevus syndrome.

▶ In patients with multiple basal cell carcinomas (BCCs), particularly those with basal cell nevus syndrome, cosmetic outcomes take on greater importance because of the number and location of the tumor burden. Therapeutic options involving surgery invariably result in scarring that may be unsightly, particularly in patients prone to hypertrophic scarring or keloid formation. Topical 5-fluorouracil (5-FU) and imiquimod therapy for superficial BCC can be lengthy and can involve compliance and cost issues. Although approved by the Federal Drug Agency, the use of topical 5-FU is not supported by a strong body of data for treatment of superficial BCC. Response of nodular BCC to topical imiquimod based on available data is significantly lower than that with established conventional approaches (surgical methods, radiation therapy, temperature-monitored cryosurgery), durations of therapy are more prolonged, and recurrence appears to be higher when nodular BCCs are treated.[1] From a patient satisfaction standpoint, this study confirms that methyl aminolevulinate photodynamic therapy (MAL-PDT) can result in a superior cosmetic outcome and achieve high patient satisfaction with acceptable cure rates compared with surgical procedures. It should be noted that therapeutic outcomes were measured by observation at 12 months and did not involve either biopsy confirmation or an evaluation at 5 years with or without biopsy. Establishment of long-term cure rates with MAL-PDT is an important goal. The authors' conclusion that "PDT seems not to prevent further BCCs" may be misleading because the study was designed to evaluate individual lesion clearance and not field therapy chemoprevention. Future studies looking at the role of MAL-PDT in the chemoprevention of BCCs in patients with multiple BCC should help to determine its value for the prevention of BCC.

G. Martin, MD

Reference

1. Love WE, Bernhard JD, Bordeaux JS. Topical imiquimod or fluorouracil therapy for basal and squamous cell carcinoma: a systematic review. *Arch Dermatol.* 2009;145:1431-1438.

Merkel cell carcinoma: our experience with seven patients in Korea and a literature review
Woo K-J, Choi Y-L, Jung HS, et al (Sungkyunkwan Univ School of Medicine, Seoul, South Korea; Seoul Natl Univ College of Pharmacy, Seoul, South Korea)
J Plast Reconstr Aesthet Surg 63:2064-2070, 2010

Background.—Merkel cell carcinoma (MCC) is a rare but malignant cutaneous neuroendocrine carcinoma. As MCC has primarily been reported in Caucasians, MCC cases in Korea have not yet been reported. The purpose of this study was to retrospectively review our experience with the surgical treatment of MCC in Korea and to study its management and outcome.

Method.—We retrospectively reviewed seven MCC case files between 2000 and 2008 from a single institution. We analysed patient characteristics, tumour location and size, staging, treatment methods and outcomes. We performed polymerase chain reaction (PCR) to detect Merkel cell polyomavirus (MCPyV) from formalin-fixed paraffin-embedded tissue specimens.

Results.—Two patients had stage I tumours, four patients had stage II tumours and one patient had a stage III tumour. Wide local excision with a clear resection margin was the primary modality of treatment in all cases. Adjuvant radiotherapy and chemotherapy were performed for selected patients. Recurrence was observed in two out of the seven cases during the follow-up period. MCPyV was detected by PCR in all seven cases.

Conclusion.—MCC is an aggressive skin cancer, and pathologic lymph node evaluation is important for staging. Wide excision is the primary modality of treatment, but adjuvant radiotherapy could be positively considered if the tumour is large and the lesion is not confined to the dermis. MCPyV was detected by PCR in all cases, which suggests that MCPyV is also a putative aetiological agent in the carcinogenesis of MCC in Korea.

▶ Merkel cell carcinoma (MCC) is a rare neuroendocrine carcinoma of the skin with an apparent higher incidence in the elderly white population. Although there are few reports of MCC in Asians, published cases in the Korean population have been absent overall. This retrospective review of 7 patients from a single Korean medical institution between 2000 and 2008 found Merkel cell polyoma virus detected in all subject samples. Patients were treated with wide local excision, with local recurrence in 2 out of the 7 cases. Those with recurrence were stage II, with tumor size greater than 6 cm. Clinically, lesions may present as erythematous or violaceous papules or nodules usually in the head and neck region or on the extremities. Diagnosis is confirmed by biopsy (histology and immunohistochemical evaluation). Margin-negative wide local excision seems to be the mainstay of treatment. Adjuvant radiotherapy is recommended for tumors larger than 1.5 cm, those with vascular or perineural invasion, those with positive margins, patients with residual disease, or regional lymph node involvement, as stated by the authors. The use of sentinel lymph node biopsy (SLNB) is controversial; however, in a recent study of 346 MCC patients, researchers suggest that it is reasonable to undergo SLNB if the lesion is greater than 1.0 cm.[1]

S. Bellew, DO

J. Q. Del Rosso, DO

Reference

1. Stokes JB, Graw KS, Dengel LT, et al. Patients with merkel cell carcinoma tumors ≤1.0 cm in diameter are unlikely to harbor regional lymph node metastasis. *J Clin Oncol.* 2009;27:3772-3777.

Recurrence of Basosquamous Carcinoma after Mohs Micrographic Surgery

Skaria AM (Univ of Geneva, Vevey, Switzerland)
Dermatology 221:352-355, 2010

Background.—The recurrence rate of basal cell carcinoma (BCC) after Mohs micrographic surgery (MMS) is well documented. Only little is published concerning the recurrence rate in relation to the different histologic subgroups.

Objective.—To analyze the recurrence rate of the different histologic groups and subgroups after MMS.

Subjects and Methods.—We investigated 1,000 cases of epidermal tumors in a private center of MMS including BCC, squamous cell carcinoma and basosquamous carcinoma (BSC) treated by MMS from 1998 to 2007 in a retrospective study. The cases where analyzed regarding the histologic groups and subgroups. The mean follow-up time was 59.55 months.

Results.—The recurrence rate of epidermal tumors in this study was about 2.5% and comparable to that in the literature. Interestingly we observed a relatively high incidence and recurrence rate of BSC compared to other studies.

Conclusion.—BSC seems to be highly aggressive and subject to recurrence even after MMS. The classical approach to stop further excision once the excision is total should be reevaluated (Table 1).

▶ This small study looked at recurrence rates after Mohs surgery for basal cell carcinoma (BCC), squamous cell carcinoma (SCC), and basosquamous cell carcinoma (BSqC). BSqC is a confusing term and entity and has been debated in the literature for years. For this study, BSqC was diagnosed using the World Health Organization definition of 2005 as a BCC with infiltrative growth with areas of keratinization or intercellular bridge formation in the setting of a prototypic proliferative reaction. The clinical behavior and prognosis of BSqC is reported to be worse with higher rates of both recurrence and metastasis when compared with BCC, and the overall biologic behavior has been described as more similar to SCC than BCC.

Table 1 shows the breakdown of the 1000 tumors treated and the recurrence rate based on the specific histology. BSqC had a higher recurrence rate than SCC or BCC with aggressive growth pattern. Although a small study, this seems to support that BSqC, as defined in this article, is a more aggressive

TABLE 1.—Recurrence Rates of the Different Histologic Groups and Subgroups

Histology	Total	Recurrence	Recurrence, % (to Specific Histology Group)
BCC			
Nonaggressive growth pattern	206	1	0.5
Aggressive growth pattern	650	14	2.1
BSC	56	5	8.9
SCC	88	5	5.6

tumor than BCC. Some investigators have postulated this may be due to rupture of the basement membrane in these tumors.

This article suggests that physicians treating patients with a diagnosis of BSqC should be aware of the challenging nature of these tumors. In general, aggressive treatment is indicated initially, and these patients should be watched carefully for recurrence of the tumor.

E. M. Billingsley, MD

Mohs Micrographic Surgery for Hidradenocarcinoma on a Rhinophymatous Nose: A Histologic Conundrum

Rubenzik M, Keller M, Humphreys T (Thomas Jefferson Univ, Philadelphia, PA)
Dermatol Surg 36:2075-2078, 2010

Background.—Nodular hidradenoma (NH) is a rare eccrine sweat gland tumor that can be difficult to distinguish from the malignant form, nodular hidradenocarcinoma (HC). Both are characterized by lobular aggregations of cells in the dermis with various proportions of basaloid polyhedral and round clear cells. Cases also show lumina, cystic spaces, and foci of keratinization, but cellular atypia and an infiltrative pattern are indicative of HC. Standard excision of HC is often followed by local recurrence, but Mohs micrographic surgery (MMS) for malignant eccrine neoplasms improves cure rates substantially. HC can occur along with rhinophyma, making the evaluation of margins from frozen sections of HC difficult.

Case Report.—Man, 83, had a persistent nodule of the left nasal ala that had recently grown. A previous biopsy revealed clear cell pathology that was interpreted as basal cell carcinoma with clear cell change, and the neoplasm was referred for MMS. The clinical appearance was of an ill-defined erythematous nodule surrounded by areas of diffuse textural changes characteristic of rhinophyma. The debulking specimen taken during surgery demonstrated extensive sebaceous gland hyperplasia and deep dermal aggregates of basaloid vacuolated cells. First-stage Mohs layers stained with toluidine blue and hematoxylin and eosin (H&E) showed a diffuse dermal proliferation of clear cells studded with horn cysts and fibroplasia. Minimal cytologic atypia was noted on frozen sections. When the debulking and first-layer sections were evaluated as H&E-stained permanent sections, it was clear that there were mixed collections of pleomorphic keratinizing epithelium and nodular ductal epithelium, leading to a diagnosis of HC. The margins had infiltrating tumor with focal keratinization, sebaceous hyperplasia, and fibrosis. The patient underwent definitive re-excision, with horizontally embedded permanent sections showing negative margins. The patient remains disease free after 18 months.

Conclusions.—NH and HC can both recur after wide local excision in up to 50% of cases. However, MMS is associated with a low rate of recurrence for malignant eccrine neoplasms. Modifying the traditional Mohs technique by performing horizontally embedded permanent H&E-stained sections increases the accuracy of margin evaluations.

▶ This is a well-written case report that reminds us of a rare but important carcinoma that can easily be mistaken for rhinophyma or difficult to diagnoses within the lobular proliferations of phymatous changes.

It also illustrates some of the pitfalls of using frozen sections for certain neoplasms, specifically when evaluating melanocytes, sebocytes, and clear cells. When attempting to evaluate these cell types, sending the specimen for permanent sections can dramatically increase the ease and accuracy of diagnoses. When faced with a rhinophymatous nose, the Mohs micrographic surgeon should be aware of this entity, and if there is any question, the block should be processed for paraffin-embedded sections. This article also reinforces Mohs micrographic surgery as an excellent treatment option for this rare tumor, of which there has not been any recurrences reported in the literature.

R. Ceilley, MD

B. Kopitzki, DO

Need to Improve Skin Cancer Screening of High-Risk Patients
Garg A, Geller A (Boston Univ School of Medicine, MA)
Arch Dermatol 147:44-45, 2011

Background.—Among the barriers that have been identified to primary care physicians (PCPs) performing full skin examinations (FSEs) are time constraints, competing morbidities, and patient embarrassment or reluctance to undress. Added to this may be a knowledge gap concerning who qualifies as a high-risk patient. Methods to improve the situation have been suggested, especially since there is a shortage of PCPs and a coming health care overhaul that will provide care for millions of patients for the first time.

Professional Roles.—Dermatologists can play an important role by training current and future PCPs to identify patients at high risk for advanced melanoma, which is white men over age 50 years. In addition, they can spend more time screening patients with multiple risk factors and less time with low-risk patients. The performance of FSEs should remain among the tasks of PCPs and dermatologists, but other specialists who see high-risk patients may be able to improve early detection rates by integrating an FSE into their routine. These specialists should be able to recognize and triage suspicious lesions.

Reaching Medical Students.—Medical students who have not yet declared a specialty were shown a short film illustrating how to incorporate an FSE into the normal physical examination. Their response was that the integrated examination took less time than had been anticipated and that they strongly intended to incorporate this approach into their routine visit regardless of what specialty they chose. Most graduating medical students do not meet the established American Association of Medical College guidelines for competency in dermatology, but improved competency is possible by integrating experience-based teaching strategies into core curricula and structured practical learning activities.

Patient Approaches.—Patients may request screenings if they are made more aware of the skin cancer problem and if advocacy campaigns can be established to highlight skin cancer risks. Office-based information about the importance of physician-directed skin examinations may help overcome patient embarrassment. Trained staff can knowledgeably approach patients, explain the relevance of skin cancer screening, address expressed concerns, and offer the FSE.

Conclusions.—A coordinated national strategy is needed to screen highrisk individuals for skin cancer, much like what has been established for breast cancer, cervical cancer, and colorectal cancer. The approach must include PCPs, specialists, policy makers, and government supporters.

▶ Ideally, a full body skin examination should be offered and performed on all patients at high risk for developing skin cancer. Drawbacks to a full body skin examination include (1) patient embarrassment and/or reluctance to such an exam and (2) possible time constraints, considering the potential addition of millions of patients entering the new health care overhaul. Dermatologists should take the lead to train primary care physicians and select specialist (eg, cardiologist, nephrologist) in performing a full body skin examination.

It may also be helpful to train other professionals such as nurses regarding skin examination because they may notice lesions of concern that they can point out to the physician.

J. L. Smith, MD

Lip cancer in renal transplant patients

López-Pintor RM, Hernández G, de Arriba L, et al (Complutense Univ, Madrid, Spain; et al)
Oral Oncol 47:68-71, 2011

The aims of this study were to establish the incidence of lip cancer (LC) in a population of renal transplant patients (RTPs), identifying possible risk factors and predictable variables, and to describe the clinical appearance, treatment, and course of LC in this group. The study included 500 patients (307 men, 193 women; mean age 53.63 ± 13.42 years, range 19—95 years; mean period since transplant 59.66 ± 55.81 months, range 4—330 months). Incident cases of LC were ascertained retrospectively from outpatient records. All LC lesions were sampled by biopsy and examined histopathologically. Six of the men (1.2%) suffered lower LC, and LC cases showed significant differences on univariate analysis for tobacco habit, tobacco consumption, and sun exposure. All patients who had LC were taking prednisolone and cyclosporine A (CsA) at the time of LC diagnosis. The median interval for LC incidence after renal transplant was 80.50 ± 31.25 months. Five of six LCs were squamous cell carcinomas. Multiple logistic regression showed that the LCs were not significantly associated with any independent risk factor. The results show that the appearance of LC in RTPs is associated with immunosuppressant treatment, sun exposure, and tobacco and indicate that these patients should avoid unprotected exposure to sunlight and smoking. Because of the high incidence of LC in RTPs, periodic checking of the lips is important to ensure prompt diagnosis and correct management of LC. Our data suggest that the clinical profile of LC in this patient group is similar to that of the general population.

▶ Renal transplant (RTP) patients are at increased risk for development of nonmelanoma skin cancer (NMSC) including on the lip region, posttransplant lymphoproliferative disease, Kaposi sarcoma, carcinomas of the vulva and perineum, and a variety of systemic malignancies. The current retrospective study of 500 RTP patients from Madrid, Spain, found 6 men with cancer involving the lower lip, 5 squamous cell carcinomas (SCC), and 1 basal cell carcinoma (BCC). Carcinoma of the lip usually arises at the vermillion border of the lower lip. Most lip carcinomas in this study displayed an ulcerative pattern. All patients were being treated with prednisolone and cyclosporine A (CsA) as immunosuppressive therapy related to their RTP. As stated by the authors, a study of lip carcinomas in RTP patients on different immunosuppressant drugs is hard to assess. The duration of therapy is significant, and it is difficult to determine whether any one type of immunosuppressive agent increases the risk of lip carcinoma (especially SCC) more than any others because agents are usually used in combination. Given the high risk of lip carcinomas in RTP patients, periodic evaluation of the skin, including careful examination of the lips, and patient education on sun, tanning bed, and smoking avoidance, should be routine and consistently reinforced. Early detection and treatment of NMSC is important to stress to any organ transplant patient and their caretakers.

S. Bellew, DO
J. Q. Del Rosso, DO

Factors associated with large cutaneous squamous cell carcinomas
Renzi C, Mastroeni S, Passarelli F, et al (Istituto Dermopatico dell'Immacolata, Rome, Italy)
J Am Acad Dermatol 63:404-411, 2010

Background.—Large cutaneous squamous cell carcinoma (SCC) is associated with a higher risk of disfigurement, local recurrence, and metastasis; however, little is known about factors associated with tumor size at diagnosis.
Objectives.—We sought to evaluate factors associated with SCC size, including diagnostic/treatment delay and patient and tumor characteristics.

Methods.—We studied a stratified sample of 308 patients with SCC recently treated at a dermatologic referral center in Italy. Medical records were reviewed and telephone interviews conducted. Multiple logistic regression was used to examine factors associated with SCC size.

Results.—With univariate analyses, among both invasive and in situ cases, SCC greater than 2 cm was significantly associated with male gender, tumors arising in chronic lesions, and tumors located on not easily visible sites. Long delay before surgical removal was significantly associated with large SCC size only for invasive SCC ($P < .001$). Among patients with invasive SCC, when controlling for age and gender, multivariate analysis showed a significantly higher likelihood of SCC greater than 2 cm with a total delay longer than 18 months before surgical removal (odds ratio = 4.18; 95% confidence interval 2.45-7.13) and for tumors arising in chronic lesions (odds ratio = 6.42; 95% confidence interval 3.13-13.2).

Limitations.—The study was cross-sectional and based on a single center.

Conclusions.—Long total delay in removal significantly increased the likelihood of invasive SCC greater than 2 cm. Our findings highlight the importance of early detection and treatment to prevent large invasive SCCs, which are associated with a higher risk of disfigurement, recurrence, and metastasis. Particular attention should be paid to chronic skin lesions and not easily visible body sites during physician- and patient-performed examinations.

▶ Squamous cell carcinoma (SCC) is the second most common skin cancer seen in clinics today. When the tumor is at an advanced stage, SCC can often be associated with significant morbidity and higher risk for metastasis, especially when present in certain anatomic locations such as the lip. This cross-sectional study examined the factors associated with SCC tumor characteristics, diagnosis, and treatment in 308 patients at a single dermatologic referral center. The authors concluded that SCCs associated with a long delay before treatment were more likely to be invasive and larger than 2 cm. SCCs arising in chronic skin lesions also pose greater risk. Those in sites not easily visualized by the patient may also be more problematic. Invasive SCCs were more frequently found on the scalp, whereas SCCs in situ were more common on the lips. Perhaps the delay in seeking treatment is a result of SCCs occurring in areas not readily visible to patients, or perhaps SCCs arising in chronic lesions are perceived by patients as being benign because of their long-standing nature. Limitations of the study include that the data came from a single institution and that the data had a cross-sectional design. However, the study highlights the importance of early detection and treatment of SCCs. Particular attention should be paid to difficult-to-see areas and to patient's education regarding the importance of physician evaluations of changes in chronic lesions.

S. Bellew, DO
J. Q. Del Rosso, DO

Ungual and periungual human papillomavirus–associated squamous cell carcinoma: a review

Riddel C, Rashid R, Thomas V (Univ of Texas at Houston)
J Am Acad Dermatol 64:1147-1153, 2011

Background.—Human papillomavirus (HPV)—associated squamous cell carcinoma (SCC) and SCC in situ are often reported in the genital region. The association of HPV with SCC in the ungual and periungual skin is less well recognized, and verrucous lesions may undergo years of therapeutic attempts without a diagnostic biopsy.

Objectives.—To review the epidemiology, associations, and role of HPV in digital SCC and SCC in situ.

Methods.—The English-language literature reporting HPV-associated SCC and SCC in situ of the digits was reviewed.

Results.—HPV-associated SCC and SCC in situ were almost equally represented. The patients' ages ranged from 22 to 89 years, with men affected twice as often as women. HPV16 was the most common subtype. The tumors presented as persistent verrucae, present for an average of 5.3 years. Immune suppression was documented in only 6.8% of patients. Approximately 6% of cases required digital amputation.

Limitations.—Most of the information was obtained from case reports, some of which had limited data regarding the exact location of the tumor and the diagnostic and treatment course. HPV subtyping is not commonly performed in these tumors, which limited the number of reports that could be evaluated.

Conclusions.—The majority of digital HPV-associated SCCs or SCCs in situ involves the nailbed region. The clinical appearance is most commonly that of a periungual verruca. Tumors have a higher rate of recurrence after excision than SCC in other sites. Periungual and subungual warts caused by high-risk HPV subtypes pose a risk for malignant transformation in both immunocompetent and immunocompromised hosts.

▶ Human papillomavirus (HPV)-associated digital squamous cell carcinoma (SCC) and SCC in situ are potentially overlooked diagnoses among patients with persistent periungual/ungual verrucae, especially adults. Although not as well recognized as HPV-associated tumors in the genital region, HPV-associated digital SCC and SCC in situ are very important to recognize. Calling attention to this important tumor, Riddell et al provide a complete literature search and review of the epidemiology and characteristics of digital HPV-associated SCC and SCC in situ. Of note, periungual verrucous mass is the most common presentation of digital SCC and SCC in situ (other presentations included longitudinal melanonychia, subungual tumors, onycholysis, and paronychia). These tumors, when presenting as verrucae, are present on average for approximately 5.3 years. Most were treated unsuccessfully with a variety of modalities used to treat verrucae. In addition, the most common HPV-associated subtype was HPV 16—a known HPV subtype that is associated with development of squamous malignancy. The third digit of the hand was most commonly affected. These tumors tend to be locally aggressive and can be difficult to treat, thus indicating a need for early diagnosis. They can also occur irrespective of the immune status of the patient, as many affected individuals are immunocompetent. There was no predilection for SCC or SCC in situ found in these digital tumors, with both equally represented among patients. Given the potential aggressiveness of these tumors and the frequent delay in diagnosis of SCC lesions, a high degree of suspicion is warranted, especially in cases of refractory or recurrent periungual verrucae in adult patients. If a digital lesion is not resolving with therapy, a saucerization biopsy encompassing adequate width and depth should be considered. Overall, Riddell et al provide a thorough analysis of ungual and periungual HPV-associated SCC lesions and a good source of review on this topic.

B. D. Michaels, DO

J. Q. Del Rosso, DO

Epidermal Growth Factor Receptor Inhibitors in the Treatment of Nonmelanoma Skin Cancers

Khan MH, Alam M, Yoo S (Northwestern Memorial Hosp, Chicago, IL)
Dermatol Surg 37:1199-1209, 2011

Background.—A better understanding of the molecular pathways that characterize cell growth, apoptosis, angiogenesis, and invasion has provided novel targets in cancer therapy. Epidermal growth factor receptor (EGFR)-mediated signal transduction has been one of the most studied pathways in carcinogenesis. The phosphorylation of EGFR activates multiple biological processes, including apoptosis, differentiation, cellular proliferation, motility, invasion, adhesion, DNA repair, and survival. EGFR is a transmembrane tyrosine kinase receptor involved in the proliferation and survival of cancer cells. EGFR is the first molecular target against which monoclonal antibodies have been developed for cancer therapy.

Objective.—To review the mechanisms underlying the effects of EGFR in nonmelanoma skin cancer (NMSC) and their potential role as targeted therapies in the treatment thereof.

Conclusions.—EGFR plays an important role in tumorigenesis of NMSC, especially metastatic squamous cell carcinoma, via mechanisms similar to those of other visceral tumors. Pharmacologic inhibitors of EGFR pathway of tumor production may offer an effective therapeutic strategy to block tumor growth.

▶ The signaling pathway involving the activation of epidermal growth factor receptors (EGFR) has been shown to play an important role in the growth and survival of many tumors. Recent studies have shown that the capability of blocking this receptor provides novel opportunities in the treatment of solid tumors. This is a review of literature evaluating the EGRF pathway and its potential role in nonmelanoma skin cancer (NMSC). This signaling pathway is important in the development of cutaneous epithelial malignancies. Cetuximab is one of the most extensively studied anti-EGFR monoclonal antibodies that is FDA approved for the treatment of squamous cell carcinoma (SCC) of the head and neck (local and metastatic), including in those unresponsive to chemotherapy. It has gained popularity with inoperable NMSC. Panitumumab is a fully human IgG2 monoclonal antibody directed against EGFR. Matuzumab is similar to cetuximab and panitumumab and has been shown to have antitumor activity. Tumor response has been reported in esophageal SCC, head and neck SCC, cervical carcinoma, ovarian carcinoma, and colorectal carcinoma. Gefitinib has been shown to inhibit intracellular activation and phosphorylation of EGFR, leading to cell arrest or apoptosis. Although it has been used for visceral tumors, its role in NMSC remains to be studied. EGFR inhibitors exhibit a variety of adverse side effects such as follicular eruption, painful fissures, and hypertrichosis with trichomegaly. The full extent of EGFR inhibitor use in cancer therapy has yet to be unveiled, because the EGFR signaling pathway appears to be one of the several pathways essential in malignant progression. The use of EGFR inhibitor therapy is likely to increase as more information is gathered and as potential uses expand based on additional research. They may also have a potential benefit in combination with radiotherapy and chemotherapy.

G. K. Kim, DO

J. Q. Del Ross, DO

The Role of Sirolimus in the Prevention of Cutaneous Squamous Cell Carcinoma in Organ Transplant Recipients
LeBlanc KG Jr, Hughes MP, Sheehan DJ (Med College of Georgia, Augusta)
Dermatol Surg 37:744-749, 2011

Skin cancers are common in organ transplant recipients (OTRs). In this review, we discuss the epidemiology of and risk factors for cutaneous neoplasms, particularly squamous cell carcinoma (SCC) in OTRs. The pathogenesis of SCC is reviewed, as well as the potential mechanisms for tumor progression and metastasis associated with two commonly used immunosuppressive medications: tacrolimus and cyclosporine. Finally, we discuss the mechanism of action and potential preventative use of sirolimus, a member of a newer class of immunosuppressants, the mammalian target of rapamycin inhibitors.

▶ Organ transplant recipients (OTRs) are in a chronic immunocompromised state and have higher rates of developing nonmelanoma skin cancer. This is a review of the literature discussing the role of immunosuppressive medications in OTRs. Tacrolimus and cyclosporine exert their immunosuppressive effects through inactivation of calcineurin. This prevents expression of several cytokine genes and enhances the expression of transforming growth factor β. Sirolimus (also known as rapamycin) is a bacterial macrolide antibiotic produced by a strain of *Streptomyces hygroscopicus* used primarily as an immunosuppressant. Clinical data have shown beneficial effects of inhibitors of mammalian targets of rapamycin (mTOR). There are also studies showing the clinical benefits of mTOR inhibition on cancer development in OTRs. The combination of sirolimus and mycophenolate mofetil has been shown to decrease the rate of skin cancer development. The most commonly reported side effects with sirolimus are aphthous ulcers, edema, acneiform eruptions, hyperlipidemia, thrombocytopenia, leukopenia, and delayed wound healing. Although most of the literature involving the use of sirolimus is in renal transplant recipients, similar benefits may be seen in other solid organs as well. Sirolimus immunosuppression is still debated, and larger-scale prospective studies are needed to confirm results.

G. K. Kim, DO

J. Q. Del Rosso, DO

Retinoids for Chemoprophylaxis of Nonmelanoma Skin Cancer

Carr DR, Trevino JJ, Donnelly HB (Wright State Univ, Dayton, OH)
Dermatol Surg 37:129-145, 2011

Background.—Skin cancer cases are increasing, with the most common form being nonmelanoma skin cancers (NMSCs). This is accompanied by an increase in morbidity and mortality associated with basal cell and squamous cell carcinomas (BCCs and SCCs). Chemoprevention is used to help high-risk groups avoid developing disease. For NMSC, retinoids, which are natural or synthetic compounds whose biologic activity is similar to that of vitamin A, is used for chemoprevention. The high-risk populations that may benefit from retinoid chemoprevention, the mechanism of action of retinoids, current retinoid chemoprophylaxis treatments, and relevant side effects were outlined.

Patients at Risk.—A higher risk for NMSC is associated with organ transplant recipients (OTRs), immunosuppressive drug use, human immunodeficiency virus (HIV) infection, psoralen and ultraviolet A (UVA) light therapy, chemical exposure, chronic lymphocytic leukemia and non-Hodgkin's lymphoma, and genetic syndromes. Among the genetic syndromes involved are xeroderma pigmentosum, nevoid basal cell carcinoma syndrome (NBCS), oculocutaneous albinism, dystrophic epidermolysis bullosa, Bazex syndrome, Rombo syndrome, and epidermodysplasia verruciformis.

Mechanism of Action.—There are three generations of retinoids (nonaromatic, monoaromatic, and polyaromatic) and two main families: retinoic acid receptors (RARs) and retinoid X receptors (RXRs). Each family has three isoforms. Receptors must dimerize to achieve transcription. The expression of retinoid receptors depends on anatomic location, presence of inflammation, and disease state. It is believed that retinoids primarily target the promotion and progression stages of carcinogenesis.

Treatments.—Treatment regimens are designed for OTRs and non-OTR high-risk patients. For OTRs, etretinate can significantly lower the numbers of NMSCs that develop. A combination of low-dose etretinate and topical tretinoin cream significantly lowered NMSC numbers in three-quarters of patients compared to topical tretinoin cream only, which improved the outcomes in just two-thirds of patients. Acitretin has also significantly reduced NMSC numbers. However, a rebound phenomenon is common, with higher numbers of NMSCs developing after retinoid therapy was discontinued. Patients with a higher incidence of NMSC before treatment had a greater decrease in NMSC numbers that developed. Both subjective and objective improvements have been reported. Duration of efficacy remains to be determined, as does the usefulness of topical retinoids against actinic keratosis (AK).

Isotretinoin used as chemoprevention for non-OTRs with xeroderma pigmentosum significant reduced NMSCs, but unfortunately their numbers increased substantially once therapy was discontinued. Lower doses are used for long-term administration to avoid severe mucocutaneous and laboratory side effects. Retinol and isotretinoin have produced results comparable to placebo with respect to BCCs or SCCs in several studies of patients with multiple BCCs or SCCs. Retinol 25,000 IU daily for up to 5 years for patients with more than 10 AKs and two or fewer SCCs or BCCs produced a statistically significant decline in SCC numbers but did not affect BCC numbers. Side effects were marginally higher with retinol than with placebo. Psoriatic patients who received prophylactic UVA have higher rates of SCC and, to a lesser extent, BCC. Retinoids have reduced SCC numbers in these patients but had no effect on BCCs. Case reports supply the only data on the effectiveness of isotretinoin and etretinate for patients with NBCS. Two showed no efficacy but three showed active regression of a quarter to three-quarters of the BCCs. Good results are reported for topical retinoids against AKs.

Adverse Effects and Monitoring.—With systemic retinoid use, adverse effects are usually mild, related to the dosage received, and more likely to develop early in the course of therapy. Anticipatory guidance can improve patient adherence to therapy with systemic retinoids. Patients should be prepared to expect mucocutaneous symptoms, laboratory abnormalities, musculoskeletal abnormalities, ocular abnormalities, teratogenicity, and neuropsychiatric effects. Topical retinoids may produce erythema, peeling, burning, stinging, and pruritus, but these effects tend to diminish with time.

Conclusions.—Better prevention and treatment strategies are needed to address the increased incidence of NMSCs, particularly among high-risk populations. Chemoprophylaxis, especially with retinoids, offers promise as an efficacious approach to diminish the numbers of NMSCs that develop in these patients. Further research is needed to better understand these agents' efficacy and optimal dosing.

▶ This is one of the best articles I have read in a long time, and it was great to see a reminder that there are more populations of immunosuppressed patients and other clinical scenarios that warrant consideration for chemoprevention than just organ transplant recipients. Chemoprevention of nonmelanoma skin cancer (NMSC) is high on the list of possible uses for oral retinoid therapy, although many dermatologists either do not do this or do not want to deal with managing side effects, long-term management considerations, or the insurance constraints on the approval of off-label use. My thinking is that we are not going to see an approved indication for this use, nor is anyone going to want to be in the placebo arm of a controlled clinical trial in which NMSC is the endpoint and they may be in the placebo group. After reading this article, it makes sense why using systemic retinoids to modify the progression of NMSC in high-risk patients should be more common. See how many patients fit the criteria for this use in your practice and then evaluate the obstacles measured against the potential outcomes.

N. Bhatia, MD

Margin Detection Using Digital Dermatoscopy Improves the Performance of Traditional Surgical Excision of Basal Cell Carcinomas of the Head and Neck
Carducci M, Bozzetti M, Foscolo AM, et al (Centro Ortopedico di Quadrante Hospital, Omegna, Italy; Castelli Hosp, Verbania, Italy; et al)
Dermatol Surg 37:280-285, 2011

Background.—Dermatoscopy is a simple, inexpensive, noninvasive procedure designed to evaluate pigmented lesions. It may be useful to preoperatively determine the appropriate surgical margins of basal cell carcinoma (BCC), which is a slowly growing, locally invasive malignant skin tumor. Clearing the margins is important to avoid incomplete surgical excision. The preoperative determination of appropriate margins using digital dermatoscopy was compared to results obtained via clinical examination.

Methods.—Eighty-four patients (mean age 70.6 years) with histologically confirmed BCCs were evaluated clinically or dermatoscopically to detect involvement of their surgical margins. Group 1 consisted of 21 women and 19 men who had clinical assessment, whereas group 2 included 21 women and 23 men whose margins were evaluated via digital dermatoscopic evaluation. The percentages of tumor-free margins were compared between the two groups.

Results.—Eight of 40 clinically analyzed specimens and three of 44 patients analyzed using the dermatoscope had histologic margin involvement. The difference between groups was statistically significant. In group 1, six nodular BCCs and two infiltrative or morpheaform BCCs had margins involved, whereas in group 2, two infiltrative and one nodular BCC had such involvement. The difference was significant only for the nodular type. None of the superficial BCCs demonstrated margin involvement.

Conclusions.—Digital dermatoscopic evaluation provided a simple, reproducible, safe, and inexpensive way to analyze surgical margins in BCCs. The presurgical evaluation of tumor margins via digital dermatoscope greatly improved the surgical performance with respect to nodular BCCs of the head and neck.

▶ Standard excision for basal cell carcinoma (BCC) has shown to have recurrence rates ranging from 4% to 14%, and the rate of positive margin involvement is highly dependent on the selection of surgical margins. The larger the surgical margin, the lower the recurrence rate. It is usually possible to obtain low recurrence rates at the expense of wider surgical margins and greater sacrifice of normal tissue. This is usually not a problem when dealing with BCC on the trunk and extremities, especially with well-defined clinical margins or less locally aggressive histologic growth patterns. However, wider surgical margins are often not possible on the facial region without adverse consequences. Therefore, tissue-sparing techniques, such as Mohs micrographic surgery, are usually preferred, with cure rates approaching 99% for primary BCC. This study found a significant reduction in recurrences of nodular BCC after determining the clinical and surgical margins using digital dermatoscopy alone as opposed to clinical margin assessment with only the naked eye. In each case, 3-mm surgical margins were then used to excise the defect. Digital dermatoscopy is cost-effective and relatively easy to learn how to use. While the results of the study are impressive, it would be interesting to know what the average defect sizes were between the 2 groups. The dermatoscope group usually had a margin that extended past the obviously visible clinical margin, and an additional 3 mm of tissue was then excised according to the authors. It is possible that some of the improvement in recurrence rates may have been attributable to this larger amount of tissue excised after use of the dermatoscope. The use of 3-mm surgical margins on the face may not be tissue sparing in all cases. The Mohs technique usually utilizes 1- to 2-mm margins past the clinical margin and with subsequent layers as required based on histologic evaluation of horizontal sections. While the results appear impressive, and this technique may be quite useful on the trunk or extremities, the resulting defects on the face might be larger than they need to be in many cases and could require more extensive repairs and morbidity. It would also be necessary to evaluate long-term recurrence rates with this approach.

R. I. Ceilley, MD

B. A. Kopitzki, DO

Slowly-Developing Facial Nerve Paralysis

Boß C, Wehner-Caroli J, Roecken M, et al (Eberhard Karls Univ, Tübingen, Germany)
Dermatol Surg 37:389-391, 2011

Background.—Basal cell carcinoma (BCC) is the most common type of skin cancer in humans and usually do not metastasize. However, if BCCs are not treated they can extend to connective tissue, cartilage, muscles, and bones. Deep infiltration is particularly likely with BCCs along embryonic fusion planes. These also are more likely to recur because it is so difficult to excise them completely. A patient with a retroauricular BCC was reported.

Case Report.—Man, 65, reported facial nerve paralysis of 7 months' duration. It was initially thought to be inflammatory in nature, but systemic corticosteroids had no effect. The patient remembered having had a retroauricular nodule that had grown slowly for 17 months. He had facial nerve paralysis of the right face. The corner of his mouth drooped and he could not raise his eyebrow, close his eye tightly, purse his lip, or smile on the right side. Physical examination revealed a retroauricular fibrin-coated 15- × 25-mm ulcer behind his right ear. On biopsy, this basaloid epithelial tumor had infiltrated the dermis and subcutis, with extensive fibrosis of the peritumoral stroma and central tumor necrosis. No connection to the epidermis was found, and peripheral palisading and stromal retraction were minimal to absent. Tumor cells expressed BER-EP-4 but not cytokeratin 20. The clinical diagnosis was deeply infiltrating BCC. Imaging revealed the tumor had infiltrated the right pinna, auditory channel, parotid gland, sternocleidomastoid muscle, and stylomastoid foramen. Surgical debulking was performed followed by radiotherapy. Excision included the pinna, part of the external auditory channel, and the facial nerve, which was replaced by the great auricular nerve. Plastic surgery reconstruction was required, including a bilobed flap from the neck, auditory canal restoration, lid weight implantation, and median canthoplasty.

Conclusions.—Most BCCs are readily removed via surgical resection, but if they are left untreated or recur after incomplete treatment, they tend to expand and infiltrate underlying tissues. The resultant damage can be severe, presenting a challenge for reconstruction and cure. The highest incidence of perineural invasion occurs with BCCs of the cheek and periauricular region. Often the presenting symptoms are subtle, requiring the physician to carefully inquire about the possibility of a BCC and do a thorough neurologic examination. Tumors should be suspected when facial paralysis develops slowly or is atypical. Ideal management requires the expertise of a cutaneous surgeon and a radiation oncologist. Three-dimensional histologic surgery with paraffin sections to cover all the margins of resected tissue should reveal any remaining tumor roots and has achieved a cure rate of 99% for most primary cancers, with a slightly lower rate for recurrent lesions.

▶ Basal cell carcinoma (BCC) is the most common skin cancer in the world, affecting anywhere from 20 to 300 per 100 000 people. BCC rarely metastasizes and is amenable to treatment by surgical methods. However, when left untreated, the tumor may extend deeper into connective tissue, cartilage, muscle, or underlying bone. This was illustrated in the current case report of BER-EP-4 + deeply infiltrating BCC with negative cytokeratin-20 marker who developed facial nerve paralysis over 7 months. A biopsy of the retroauricular nodule showed a basaloid epithelial tumor infiltrating the dermis and subcutis with central necrosis and peritumoral fibrosis with no connection to the epidermis. The patient was treated with surgical debulking method followed by radiotherapy. Of note, BCC in the periauricular region and cheek have the highest risk of perineural invasion. Furthermore, all patients with slowly developing or otherwise atypical facial paralysis should be evaluated for possible tumor growths invading the perineural space.

S. Bellew, DO
J. Q. Del Rosso, DO

Eighteen Years of Experience in Mohs Micrographic Surgery and Conventional Excision for Nonmelanoma Skin Cancer Treated by a Single Facial Plastic Surgeon and Pathologist

van der Eerden PA, Prins MEF, Lohuis PJFM, et al (Lange Land Hosp, Zoetermeer, The Netherlands; Tergooi Hosps, Blaricum, The Netherlands; Netherlands Cancer Inst—Antoni van Leeuwenhoek Hosp, Amsterdam)
Laryngoscope 120:2378-2384, 2010

Objectives/Hypothesis.—To determine and compare the efficacy of Mohs micrographic surgery (MMS)- and conventional excision (CE)-confirmed resection of nonmelanoma skin cancers (NMSCs).

Study Design.—Retrospective cohort study.

Methods.—A retrospective cohort study of NMSCs treated in a tertiary referral center by a single facial plastic surgeon and a group of five histopathologists over an 18-year period. The treatment modality was either MMS or CE. The primary outcome measure was recurrence of disease. The secondary outcome measure was the size of resulting surgical excision defect.

Results.—Between 1990 and 2008, 795 patients were treated with MMS and 709 with CE. The median follow-up period for MMS was 24 months and for CE 16 months. Disease recurred in 6/795 and 7/709 patients, respectively ($P = .78$). Analysis of the resection defects with general linear models adjusted for localization and primary or recurrent disease showed significantly smaller defects after MMS ($P = .008$).

Conclusions.—This study demonstrates that: 1) MMS and CE are safe in terms of recurrence rates in NMSCs; 2) MMS can be performed adequately by an experienced facial plastic surgeon in close collaboration with a group of pathologists; and 3) the advantage of MMS is that resection defects can be minimized in important aesthetic and functional areas, such as the nose and eyelid, possibly facilitating the reconstruction.

▶ This article concludes that conventional excision (CE) and Mohs micrographic surgery (MMS) are equivalent in terms of recurrence rates. Indeed, the statistics do suggest nearly the same recurrence rates. Unfortunately, the median follow-up for MMS was 24 months and for CE only 16 months, making a direct comparison less accurate. Furthermore, there were many more patients having follow-up for more than 5 years in the MMS group. Thus, there may be more recurrences in the CE group, but they are more likely to be lost to follow-up.

It is also difficult to draw direct comparisons between the MMS and CE groups. The MMS group consists of the more high-risk sites in the H zone of the central face as well as any more aggressive histopathologic tumor subtypes. The more forgiving areas of the cheek, temple, and forehead were assigned to the CE group. It is entirely plausible to imagine a higher recurrence rate for the CE group had it been used on the nose or on more aggressive tumors.

The slow staged excision technique can be adequately performed by an experienced facial plastic surgeon and an experienced dermatopathologist, but cost may be considerably higher. Major disadvantages to the patient are that the repair usually needs to be done on a subsequent day and the patient may be required to return for multiple paraffin-embedded sections. Processing the tissue with a combination of peripheral and vertical sectioning has an advantage over bread-loafing but still lacks the 100% margin control of a true horizontal MMS section. One of the most significant advantages of MMS is that it is tissue sparing. This study further emphasizes this important point. A follow-up study with 5-year assessment is needed.

R. Ceilley, MD

Skin cancer education and early detection at the beach: a randomized trial of dermatologist examination and biometric feedback

Emmons KM, Geller AC, Puleo E, et al (Dana-Farber Cancer Inst, Boston, MA; Harvard School of Public Health, Boston, MA; Univ of Massachusetts, Amherst; et al)
J Am Acad Dermatol 64:282-289, 2011

Background.—There are limited data on the effectiveness of skin cancer prevention education and early detection programs at beaches.

Objectives.—We evaluate 4 strategies for addressing skin cancer prevention in beach settings.

Methods.—This prospective study at 4 beaches included 4 intervention conditions: (1) education only; (2) education plus biometric feedback; (3) education plus dermatologist skin examination; or (4) education plus biometric feedback and dermatologist skin examination. Outcomes included sun protection behaviors, sunburns, and skin self-examinations.

Results.—There was a significant increase in hat wearing, sunscreen use, and a reduction in sunburns in the education plus biometric feedback group (odds ratio = 1.97, 1.94, and 1.07, respectively), and greater improvements in knowing what to look for in skin-self examinations (odds ratio = 1.13); there were no differences in frequency of self-examinations. Skin examinations plus biometric feedback led to greater reductions in sunburns. The dermatologist examinations identified atypical moles in 28% of participants.

Limitations.—Inclusion of only one beach per condition, use of self-report data, and a limited intervention period are limitations.

Conclusions.—Education and biometric feedback may be more effective than education alone for impacting sun protective attitudes and behaviors in beachgoing, high-risk populations.

▶ As skin cancer worldwide continues to escalate, a key component in attempting to reverse this trend is education. However, as this study illustrates, education alone has its shortcomings.

This prospective study performed at 4 beach locations included 4 interventional methodologies:

1. Education alone.
2. Education plus biometric feedback (use of a Dermascan to highlight sun damage).

3. Education plus dermatologist skin examination.

4. Education plus biometric feedback and dermatologist skin examination.

These results indicate that education plus biometric feedback was more effective than education alone in affecting the behavior of beachgoing, potentially high-risk populations and their attitudes toward sun protection.

The Dermascan is a unique device that demonstrates subsurface pigmentation and irregularities that can augment the traditional educational approach to sun protection in high-risk groups.

An incidental yet important finding in this study was that 28% of participants evaluated by a dermatologist had an atypical mole requiring further evaluation.

J. L. Smith, MD

Sclerosing Squamous Cell Carcinoma of the Skin, an Underemphasized Locally Aggressive Variant: a 20-Year Experience
Salmon PJM, Hussain W, Geisse JK, et al (Skin Cancer Inst, Tauranga, New Zealand; Univ of California at San Francisco)
Dermatol Surg 37:664-670, 2011

Background.—Desmoplastic (sclerosing) responses to a variety of neoplasms have been documented but rarely evaluated in association with primary cutaneous squamous cell carcinoma (SCC). We report a distinctive variant of SCC demonstrating an infiltrative growth pattern and stromal desmoplasia.

Methods.—Cases were identified through a retrospective review of our dermatopathology and dermatologic surgery databases. After initiation of the study, additional cases were identified prospectively. Neoplasms were scored microscopically for specific histopathologic parameters and reactivity with selected histochemical and immunohistochemical stains. Clinical follow-up data were obtained through a review of medical records or contact with the patient's referring physicians.

Results.—Seventy-three carcinomas from 72 patients were identified (46 men, 26 women; median age 76, range 45–91). The original pretreatment biopsies were available in 69 of 73 cases. All lesions developed on sun-damaged skin, with the cheek constituting the most common site. The clinical presentation was typically as a sclerotic plaque. All neoplasms extended into the reticular dermis or subcutaneous fat, and perineural invasion was identified in 53 cases (73%). Patients who underwent standard excisional surgery experienced a recurrence rate of 80%; 9% of those treated with micrographic surgery experienced postoperative recurrences. Metastasis or carcinoma-related death was not observed in any patient during the follow-up period (median 36 months).

Conclusions.—Our results suggest that desmoplasia is uncommonly found in association with cutaneous SCC but helps define a locally aggressive variant of carcinoma. In light of the infiltrative nature of desmoplastic

SCC of the skin and the high incidence of perineural invasion, micrographic surgery is the surgical modality of choice.

▶ The goal of this retrospective and prospective review of 20 years of dermatologic surgery cases was to define and characterize what the authors term, *sclerosing squamous cell carcinoma (SCC)*. It was noted that desmoplasia, the induction of a densely collagenous stroma, has been studied in other tissues and specialty fields, but information is lacking within cutaneous oncology. The authors present a defined criteria list to characterize the lesions of inclusion. Most specifically for their definition was the requirement for stromal changes encompassing 50% or more of the neoplasm. Also of note was the exclusion of other tumors (such as adenosquamous carcinoma) through special stains.

Among the 73 cases determined to be desmoplastic SCC, unsurprisingly, the greatest number were on the head region of heavily sun-damaged older men with a prior history of skin cancer. An unexpectedly high percentage of surgically excised lesions (80%) and micrographically excised lesions (9%) recurred. However, the margins of standard excision were not reported and would be of interest. Radiotherapy improved both surgical and nonsurgical outcomes in only a few patients.

Histologically, almost one-quarter of cases demonstrated subcutaneous involvement on the original biopsy, with 1 additional case involving penetration into skeletal muscle. In addition, almost three-quarters of tumors were perineural on the original biopsy. As their original criteria required, all lesions showed significant marked desmoplasia.

The authors also pose the question of whether the stromal changes enhance the invasiveness of the tumor or are a reactive and host-protective process to an aggressive tumor. Supporting evidence is provided for both arguments. Regardless, as they suggest, any tumors with the invasive histologic properties, which they have characterized as sclerosing SCC, and certainly those with subcutaneous or perineural invasion, would be best managed with Mohs micrographic margin control surgery to minimize recurrence, and incorporation of adjunctive radiation therapy with these tumors would need to be further evaluated.

A physician dealing with skin cancer needs to be aware of this locally, very aggressive form of cutaneous SCC and its proper management.

A. E. Rivera, DO
R. I. Ceilley, MD

Photodynamic therapy of multiple actinic keratoses: reduced pain through use of visible light plus water-filtered infrared A compared with light from light-emitting diodes

von Felbert V, Hoffmann G, Hoff-Lesch S, et al (RWTH Aachen Univ, Germany; Johann Wolfgang Goethe Univ, Germany)
Br J Dermatol 163:607-615, 2010

Background.—Photodynamic therapy (PDT) with methyl aminolaevulinate (MAL) is an effective treatment for multiple actinic keratoses (AKs). Pain, however, is a major side-effect.

Objectives.—To compare pain intensity, efficacy, safety and cosmetic outcome of MAL PDT with two different light sources in an investigator-initiated, randomized, double-blind study.

Methods.—Eighty patients with multiple AKs grade I–II were assigned to two groups: group 1, MAL PDT with visible light and water-filtered infrared A (VIS + wIRA); group 2, MAL PDT with light from light-emitting diodes (LEDs), with a further division into two subgroups: A, no spray cooling; B, spray cooling on demand. MAL was applied 3 h before light treatment. Pain was assessed before, during and after PDT. Efficacy, side-effects, cosmetic outcome and patient satisfaction were documented after 2 weeks and 3, 6 and 12 months. Where necessary, treatment was repeated after 3 months.

Results.—Seventy-six of the 80 patients receiving MAL PDT completed the study. Patient assessment showed high efficacy, very good cosmetic outcome and high patient satisfaction. The efficacy of treatment was better in the group of patients without spray cooling ($P = 0\cdot00022$ at 3 months, $P = 0\cdot0068$ at 6 months) and showed no significant differences between VIS + wIRA and LED. VIS + wIRA was significantly less painful than LED: the median of maximum pain was lower in the VIS + wIRA group than in the LED group for PDT without spray cooling. Pain duration and severity assessed retrospectively were less with VIS + wIRA than with LED, irrespective of cooling.

Conclusions.—All treatments showed high efficacy with good cosmetic outcome and high patient satisfaction. Efficacy of treatment was better without spray cooling. VIS + wIRA PDT was less painful than LED PDT for PDT without spray cooling.

▶ In this investigator-initiated, randomized, double-blind study of 2 light sources, a light-emitting diode (LED) red light with and without cooling and visible light + water-filtered infrared A (VIS + wIRA) were studied during and after methyl aminolevulinate (MAL) photodynamic therapy (PDT) for the treatment of actinic keratoses. The red light chosen for the study has been the standard light source used with MAL PDT. The introduction of VIS + wIRA as a light source was based on a variety of observations during its use other than for PDT. Some of the observations regarding VIS + wIRA include increasing tissue oxygen partial pressure, temperature, and metabolism, all of which theoretically should enhance PDT. The findings that the VIS + wIRA light source and LED without spray cooling were equivalent when efficacy, cosmetic outcome, and patient satisfaction were evaluated does establish VIS + wIRA as a viable alternative to LED light. The observation that VIS + wIRA patients experienced less pain during PDT than patients treated with LED without cooling is a significant observation. Pain management during the PDT procedure is a very important factor in determining a patient's ability to complete the therapy with an adequate dose of light as well as the patient's willingness to be retreated when necessary. Of interest is the observation that patients undergoing cooling during LED MAL PDT experienced less efficacy. This might be attributed to the suppression of protoporphyrin IX re-accumulation during PDT caused by lowering the skin temperature. Future studies using VIS + wIRA as the activating light source for PDT are eagerly anticipated.

G. Martin, MD

Liquid Nitrogen: Temperature Control in the Treatment of Actinic Keratosis
Goldberg LH, Kaplan B, Vergilis-Kalner I, et al (DermSurgery Associates, Houston, TX; Assuta Med Ctr, Tel Aviv, Israel)
Dermatol Surg 36:1956-1961, 2010

Background.—Actinic keratoses (AKs) are in situ epidermal tumors that may progress to invasive squamous cell carcinomas. Liquid nitrogen is used during cryotherapy to freeze the epidermis and upper dermis and is the standard treatment for individual AKs.

Objective.—To evaluate the efficacy of a cryosurgery device incorporating an infrared sensor to measure the temperature at the skin surface while spraying liquid nitrogen on the surface of the skin during the treatment of AKs.

Methods & Materials.—Thirty-six patients with 180 thin AKs were treated with liquid nitrogen spray to a temperature of −5°C using the sensor to control the temperature at the skin surface. Patients were evaluated for cure rate, side effects, and healing time.

Results.—At the 1-week follow-up, 66.7% of the lesions were cleared. By the 6-week follow-up, there was a 100% cure rate. Side effects were limited to redness, blistering, crusting, oozing, and ulceration at the 1-week follow-up and were resolved by the 6-week follow-up. No recurrence of AK, scarring, or hypopigmentation was noted.

Conclusion.—Cryotherapy with an integrated sensor for temperature control is an effective, safe, and precise treatment, allowing for a 100% short-term cure rate of AKs.

▶ Actinic keratosis (AK) is a prevalent in situ epidermal tumor. Although various treatment options exist, liquid nitrogen cryotherapy is the standard for ablative treatment of individual AKs. Goldberg et al, however, sought to determine the effectiveness of cryotherapy using an attached infrared sensor. The infrared sensor was used to measure the skin surface and, ultimately, the length of spray. Their results are both interesting and useful. They evaluated 36 patients with 180 thin AKs. Liquid nitrogen was sprayed on the individual lesions until a skin temperature of −5°C was achieved and then stopped (determined by the infrared sensor). With this temperature there was not only a 66.7% cure rate by week 1, but a 100% cure rate at 6 weeks. Treatment was also noted to be safe and have limited side effects, with no patients experiencing scarring or hypopigmentation. This study is important in that with utilizing this device, it eliminates the need for estimating the appropriate time necessary to treat individual AKs. With this device, skin surface temperature can be used to adequately measure the appropriate amount of cryotherapy needed to effectively treat effectively AKs, decrease variability in treatment time for individual AKs, and still have the noted safety benefit with some mitigation of side effects. This article provides useful data on yet another effective treatment modality for AKs and, thus, is a beneficial study. The practical use of the device in real world practice needs to be evaluated.

B. Michaels, DO
J. Q. Del Rosso, DO

17 Nevi and Melanoma

Absence of *BRAF* and *HRAS* mutations in eruptive Spitz naevi
Gantner S, Wiesner T, Cerroni L, et al (Univ of Regensburg, Franz-Josef-Strauss-Allee, Germany; Med Univ of Graz, Austria; et al)
Br J Dermatol 164:873-877, 2011

Background.—Eruptive Spitz naevi have been reported rarely in the literature. In solitary Spitz naevi, *BRAF* and *HRAS* mutations, as well as increased copy numbers of chromosome 11p have been identified.

Objectives.—To investigate the genetic changes underlying eruptive Spitz naevi.

Methods.—We report on a 16-year-old boy who developed multiple disseminated eruptive Spitz naevi within a few months. We analysed *BRAF, HRAS, KRAS* and *NRAS* genes in 39 naevi from this patient for hotspot mutations. Furthermore, comparative genomic hybridization analysis was performed in three lesions.

Results.—None of the Spitz naevi displayed a mutation in the analysed genes, and no chromosomal imbalances were observed.

Conclusions.—Our results indicate that the typical genetic alterations described in solitary Spitz naevi appear to be absent in eruptive Spitz naevi. Yet unknown alternative genetic alterations must account for this rare syndrome.

▶ Eruptive Spitz nevi are rare, and the associated genetic alterations have not been thoroughly investigated. In solitary Spitz nevi, genetic alterations in the *BRAF* and *HRAS* mutation have been reported. There has also been an increase in amplification in the 11 p chromosome reported in literature. Given the rare incidence of eruptive Spitz nevi, there is a lack of information on the genetic composition of these lesions. This is a case report of a 16-year-old boy with eruptive Sptiz nevi who had 39 nevi removed for cosmetic purposes. Investigators were able to removal these lesions, which were available for genetic analysis. There were 39 melanocytic lesions removed (37 Spitz nevi, 1 dysplastic nevus, 1 lentiginous nevus) and analyzed for *BRAF, HRAS, KRAS*, and *NRAS* mutations by SNaPshot multiplex assays. Genetic analysis of *CDKN2A* gene associated with FAMMM (familiar atypical multiple mole melanoma) syndrome was also performed, but no germline mutation was detected. The analysis of these lesions revealed no significant chromosomal imbalances in the Spitz nevi, and there was no increase of 11 p observed. The eruptive Spitz nevi in this patient showed a complete absence of all genetic alterations that have been reported in solitary Spitz nevi. Since this is 1 case report of eruptive Sptiz nevi, there may be other genetic alterations that are unknown or not yet discovered. It may be difficult to analyze genetic alterations observed in eruptive Spitz nevi since it is so rare and not all patients are willing to go through the process of removing enough of them to be analyzed.

G. K. Kim, DO

J. Q. Del Rosso, DO

A new era: melanoma genetics and therapeutics

Ko JM, Fisher DE (Harvard Med School; Boston, MA)
J Pathol 223:241-250, 2011

   We have recently witnessed an explosion in our understanding of melanoma. Knowledge of the molecular basis of melanoma and the successes of targeted therapies have pushed melanoma care to the precipice of a new era. Identification of significant pathways and oncogenes has translated to the development of targeted therapies, some of which have produced major clinical responses. In this review, we provide an overview of selected key pathways and melanoma oncogenes as well as the targeted agents and therapeutic approaches whose successes suggest the promise of a new era in melanoma and cancer therapy. Despite these advances, the conversion of transient remissions to stable cures remains a vital challenge. Continued progress towards a better understanding about the complexity and redundancy responsible for melanoma progression may provide direction for anti-cancer drug development.

▶ The future of melanoma treatment seems to be related to the identification, understanding, and manipulation of biological and genetic pathways. This article summarizes current treatments and several agents in development that have shown some degree of success. Interferon alfa-2b, interleukin (IL)-2, as well as dacarbazine and related compounds remain the leading compounds topping 20% improvement in survival, despite having no effect in mortality and being limited by their toxicity. Recent agents targeting molecular pathways, including the RAS signaling cascade, which in turn affects other pathways such as MAPK and PI3 kinase/AKT, have been implicated in melanoma survival, proliferation, and progression. RAS farnesyl transferase inhibitors (ie, tipifarnib) target *NRAS* mutations present in only 15% of melanomas. *BRAF* mutations are more common (approximately 50% of all melanomas). Selective *BRAF* inhibitors (ie, sorafenib) have shown great activity in combination with chemotherapeutic agents. PLX4032 has 30-fold selectivity for *BRAF*, and the results have been promising even as a single agent in patients with *BRAFV600E* mutation. Progression-free survival does not appear to be durable (6.2 months on average) because of more than one mechanism resulting in resistance, suggesting the need for combination therapy rather than single *BRAF* inhibitor monotherapy. Downstream *BRAF/MEK* inhibitors have shown some efficacy but at toxic levels. Anthrax toxin, a selective *MEK1* and *MEK2* inhibitor is being tested in melanoma trials. *KIT* mutations such as *c-KIT* are susceptible to imatinib or sorafenib treatment because of inhibition of MAPK, PI3-AKT, and JAK-STAT pathways, although they have limited central nervous system penetration and induction of additional *KIT* mutations as a mechanism of drug resistance. Rapamycin inhibits the PI3K/AKT/mTOR pathway but has failed to demonstrate clinical efficacy. Other approach includes targeting antiapoptotic proteins such as Bcl-2, Bcl-xL, and XIAP, which are overexpressed in melanomas and may confer resistance to chemotherapy. In a phase III study, oblimersen, which targets mitochondrial Bcl-2 failed to improve overall survival. Of the agents targeting angiogenic factors (ie, vascular endothelial growth factor, IL-8, basic fibroblast growth factor, and platelet-derived growth factor) such as bevacizumab, sorafenib, and axitinib, only the latter has demonstrated activity as a single agent. Finally, the anti-CTLA4 antibody ipilimumab has shown some clinical benefit. The article shows the progress made in recent years on identifying genetic, immunologic, and molecular pathways implicated in the development, perpetuation, and resistance to therapy of melanoma cells, some of them with the potential of becoming targets of breakthrough drugs. However, that has not happened yet, and it seems that we still must rely on the combination of therapies and, in the future, personalized melanoma treatments.

B. Berman, MD, PhD

S. Amini, MD

Lentiginous Melanoma In Situ Treatment With Topical Imiquimod: Need for Individualized Regimens

Missall TA, Hurley MY, Fosko SW (Saint Louis Univ School of Medicine, MO)
Arch Dermatol 146:1309-1310, 2010

Background.—Melanoma in situ, lentiginous type (LM) is the most prevalent subtype of in situ melanoma and is increasing in incidence. LM is a precursor lesion for invasive malignant melanoma, lentiginous type (LMM). Patients with LM who have nonsurgical treatment are limited to irradiation and its adverse effects. Recurrence rates after standard treatments range from 8% to 20%. A new treatment that is effective against LM, provides local control, prevents progression to LMM, and lowers mortality and morbidity is sought. Some studies have reported success with imiquimod 5% cream. A case series was reported.

Method.—The 15 LM lesions in 14 patients received topical imiquimod five to seven times a week, with histologic tissue samples obtained before, during, and after treatment. Treatment was adjusted based on clinical responses. Imiquimod therapy was discontinued once there was clinical resolution of the tumor, lack of any inflammatory response, and no residual tumor found on the biopsy specimens.

Results.—Treatment lasted 12 to 20 weeks and included 47 to 106 applications (average 79.5 applications). Follow-up averaged 15.9 months (range 0 to 32 months). LM was clinically cleared from all 14 patients.

Conclusions.—The response to imiquimod varied from patient to patient, probably because of multiple factors. Included would be genetic heterogeneity, immune status, and size and location of the lesion. Thus a predetermined protocol for imiquimod treatment is unlikely to be suitable for all patients. Treatment must be adjusted to achieve an effective immune response. Patients should be closely observed to ensure the inflammatory reaction has resolved and tumor is cleared both clinically and histologically.

▶ Imiquimod's antitumoral properties due to its ability to enhance innate and cell-mediated immune responses have been recognized for many years. It stimulates interferon (IFN)-alpha; tumor necrosis factor (TNF)-alpha; interleukin 1, 2, 6, 8, and 12; toll-like receptors 7 and 8; FasR (CD95) and (Bcl-2)-associated X (Bax) protein, both involved in apoptotic pathways; caspases 9 and 3, involved in mitochondrial death and apoptosis; E-selectin, participant in immunosurveillance; and reduction of T-regulatory cells expressing the transcription factor FOXP3. Both concentrations of imiquimod cream (5% and 3.75%) have been approved by the US Food and Drug Administration for the treatment of actinic keratosis and external genital warts, and imiquimod 5% cream for superficial basal cell carcinoma BCC. Off-label imiquimod 5% cream has been used with some success in the treatment of Bowen disease, invasive squamous cell carcinoma, bowenoid papulosis, vulvar intraepithelial neoplasias, cutaneous T-cell lymphoma, cutaneous extramammary Paget disease, actinic cheilitis, and malignant melanoma, particularly melanoma in situ. The present case series demonstrates what others have shown before in multiple uncontrolled and retrospective studies, case series, and case reports, which is that imiquimod induces clinical and histological clearance of most melanomas in situ, with low recurrence rates in patients who are poor surgical candidates or whose melanoma is not suitable for the standard surgical management. What's lacking in the present case series are data related to local skin reactions and adverse events, and their influence in the management of these patients. Because no statistical conclusion can be drawn from the study, at this point imiquimod should not be used as a first-line treatment or as a monotherapy and must be considered as an adjuvant in the management of lentiginous melanomas.

B. Berman, MD, PhD

S. Amini, MD

Frequencies of *BRAF* and *NRAS* mutations are different in histological types and sites of origin of cutaneous melanoma: a meta-analysis

Lee J-H, Choi J-W, Kim Y-S (Korea Univ Ansan Hosp, Gyeonggi-Do)
Br J Dermatol 164:776-784, 2011

Background.—There have been conflicting data regarding the prevalence and clinicopathological characteristics of *BRAF* and *NRAS* mutations in primary cutaneous melanoma.

Objectives.—To solve this controversy, this study used a meta-analysis to evaluate the frequencies of *BRAF* and *NRAS* mutations, and the relationship between these mutations and clinicopathological parameters of cutaneous melanoma.

Methods.—Data from studies published between 1989 and 2010 were combined. The *BRAF* and *NRAS* mutations were reported in 36 and 31 studies involving 2521 and 1972 patients, respectively. The effect sizes of outcome parameters were calculated by odds ratios (OR).

Results.—*BRAF* and *NRAS* mutations were reported in 41% and 18% of cutaneous melanomas, respectively. The mutations were associated with histological subtype and tumour site, but not with age and sex. The *BRAF* mutation was frequently detected in patients with superficial spreading melanoma (OR $= 2 \cdot 021$; $P < 0 \cdot 001$) and in melanomas arising in non-chronic sun-damaged skin (OR $= 2 \cdot 043$; $P = 0 \cdot 001$). In contrast, the *NRAS* mutation was frequently evident in patients with nodular melanoma (OR $= 1 \cdot 894$; $P < 0 \cdot 001$) and in melanomas arising in chronic sun-damaged skin (OR $= 1 \cdot 887$; $P = 0 \cdot 018$).

Conclusions.—This pooled analysis shows that the incidences of *BRAF* and *NRAS* mutations in cutaneous melanomas differ according to histological type and tumour location based on the degree of sun exposure.

▶ This article provides an important summary of the reported patterns of oncogene mutations in different melanoma variants as well as locations. As these potential targets for therapy become better recognized and correlated to variations of melanoma, treating metastatic disease becomes more plausible. The data suggest that *BRAF* mutations were linked closer to superficial spreading melanomas, with minimal invasive depth, and on central anatomic locations but unrelated to photo damage. In comparison, the presence of *NRAS* mutations was linked closer to nodular melanomas from sun-damaged skin and more often on the extremities.

Therefore, can we conclude that metastatic disease from those original primary tumors will be responsive to chemotherapeutic agents against these targets? Does the article also suggest that screening for these mutations should be part of routine management?

N. Bhatia, MD

The Expanding Melanoma Burden in California Hispanics: Importance of Socioeconomic Distribution, Histologic Subtype, and Anatomic Location
Pollitt RA, Clarke CA, Swetter SM, et al (Stanford Univ Med Ctr and Stanford Cancer Ctr, CA; Northern California Cancer Ctr, Fremont, CA; et al)
Cancer 117:152-161, 2011

Background.—The incidence patterns and socioeconomic distribution of cutaneous melanoma among Hispanics are poorly understood.

Methods.—The authors obtained population-based incidence data for all Hispanic and non-Hispanic white (NHW) patients who were diagnosed with invasive cutaneous melanoma from 1988 to 2007 in California. By using a neighborhood-level measure of socioeconomic status (SES), the variables investigated included incidence, thickness at diagnosis, histologic subtype, anatomic site, and the relative risk (RR) for thicker (>2 mm) versus thinner (≤2 mm) tumors at diagnosis for groups categorized by SES.

Results.—Age-adjusted melanoma incidence rates per million were higher in NHWs ($P < .0001$), and tumor thickness at diagnosis was greater in Hispanics ($P < .0001$). Sixty-one percent of melanomas in NHWs occurred in the High SES group. Among Hispanics, only 35% occurred in the High SES group; and 22% occurred in the Low SES group. Lower SES was associated with thicker tumors ($P < .0001$); this association was stronger in Hispanics. The RR of thicker tumors versus thinner tumors (≤2 mm) in the Low SES group versus the High SES group was 1.48 (95% confidence interval [CI], 1.37-1.61) for NHW men and 2.18 (95% CI, 1.73-2.74) for Hispanic men. Patients with lower SES had less of the superficial spreading melanoma subtype (especially among Hispanic men) and more of the nodular melanoma subtype. Leg/hip melanomas were associated with higher SES in NHW men but with lower SES in Hispanic men.

Conclusions.—The socioeconomic distribution of melanoma incidence and tumor thickness differed substantially between Hispanic and NHW Californians, particularly among men. Melanoma prevention efforts targeted to lower SES Hispanics and increased physician awareness of melanoma patterns among Hispanics are needed.

▶ As I read this article and evaluated the epidemiology and the analysis of melanoma in this ethnic group of skin types III, IV, and V, there was one recurring caveat that we all observe periodically in the dermatology clinic: Patients with darker skin types, independent of ethnicity, do not think about wearing sunscreens. More often than not in these groups, there is a perceived sense of immunity from risks of sunburn and skin cancer. As a result, more work that must be done in addition to the messages from the article that we must incorporate more prevention strategies and melanoma awareness. Dermatologists and public health officials need to address the myth that patients with darker skin types have built-in solar protection and, therefore, do not need sunscreen or to incorporate sun-awareness behaviors. This is something that has to start with parents and adult patients because they need to set examples for their children, but it also has to be part of a strategy in the dermatology clinic so that we are addressing it with all skin types and not just those we perceive are high risk. We often tell patients to think of sunscreen like toothpaste for the skin and prevent problems rather than wait for them, such as with dental caries. In that same example, education about skin cancer prevention has to be in a format that makes enough impact to change behavior patterns. As the article demonstrates, tumors may be less common, but their presentations were more severe. Is that an observation that needs to serve as a teaching point for skin cancer prevention in this group? How does that message get translated to behavior modification? The next question should be clear: how do we get that message through to our patients as dermatologists? Hopefully those answers will be just as clear.

N. Bhatia, MD

"Clark/dysplastic" nevi with florid fibroplasia associated with pseudomelanomatous features

Ko CJ, Bolognia JL, Glusac EJ (Yale Univ School of Medicine, New Haven, CT)
J Am Acad Dermatol 64:346-351, 2011

Background.—Melanocytic nevi may exhibit histologic features in common with cutaneous melanoma, creating diagnostic difficulties.

Objective.—We sought to assess the clinical behavior of melanocytic nevi with pseudomelanomatous features in association with dermal fibrosis.

Methods.—Forty-two melanocytic nevi with pronounced fibrosis and associated pseudomelanomatous changes were collected and studied clinically and histologically.

Results.—The fibrosis was centrally located and laminated in appearance. It imparted a trizonal appearance: a junctional component with prominent single cells and/or irregular nests, underlying fibrosis, and a mature dermal component. No recurrence or metastases were evident over an average follow-up period of 2 years.

Limitations.—The follow-up period was short.

Conclusions.—The central location and laminated appearance of the fibrosis suggest that this may represent the extreme end of a spectrum of fibroplastic changes in "Clark/dysplastic" nevi. Adjacent features of "Clark/dysplastic" nevi and limitation of pseudomelanomatous features to the perifibrotic focus are important in accurately identifying these lesions. Although melanocytic nevi with exaggerated fibroplasia may show foci with melanoma-like features, they do not appear to exhibit aggressive clinical behavior.

▶ This is an interesting article that characterizes a particular variant of dysplastic/ atypical nevus with central florid fibroplasia and features that overlap significantly with melanoma. As the authors duly note, such lesions have been described already within the literature as "sclerosing nevus with pseudomelanomatous features," "nevus with regression-like fibrosis," and "non-surgically traumatized nevus." The authors describe 42 dysplastic nevi with a central area of pronounced fibrosis that yielded a trizonal appearance with: (1) a junctional area with prominent single cells/irregular nests, (2) underlying fibrosis, and (3) a mature dermal component with lateral bookends of a dysplastic nevus. Pseudomelanomatous features included irregular dermal nests (81%), flattened rete ridge pattern (69%), prominent confluence of junctional nests (57%), cytologic atypia (40%), follicular extension (31%), and pagetoid scatter (24%). Importantly, this variant of a dysplastic nevus appears to manifest normal zonation with HMB-45 and a low proliferative index by Ki67.

Still, the challenging nature of the cases is emphasized not only by the features outlined above, but also by the fact that in 1 patient with a history of melanoma, re-examination of the earlier malignant diagnosis prompted some doubt as to the veracity of the diagnosis and speculation that this type of lesion may, in fact, be the patient's signature nevus. In fact, in the timely report of similar nevi with fibrosis and pseudomelanomatous features by Fabrizi et al,[1] 7 of 19 cases were mistaken initially for melanoma.

With 2 years of follow-up, these authors observed no malignant behavior. However, this follow-up period is short, and, in 25 cases, the nevus was re-excised regardless. The number of nevi with actual known-positive surgical margins is not specified.

Understandably, much of the discussion focuses on whether these nevi instead represent an unwittingly traumatized nevus with reactive features characteristic of the pseudomelanomatous features of recurrent nevi. This is a valid criticism, and the issue was addressed, and considered likely, in the series detailed by Fabrizi et al. Nevertheless, the authors of this series feel strongly that a pattern of frank scarring was lacking.

Furthermore, one might argue that if it were simply minor and unnoticed trauma, why would it always occur centrally? Would the trauma not also occur laterally, yielding some cases that were not bookended by more classic-appearing dysplastic nevus? However, this brings up another important limitation not directly addressed, and that is that the files of this particular dermatopathology laboratory were culled specifically for nevi with this exact pattern—in essence, there is some element of a self-fulfilling prophecy.

Therefore, it might be of interest for these authors or other investigators to search large-tissue repositories to locate nevi with similar features in which the changes are not only central in location, but this leads to another "sticky-wicket," for a nevus with such changes laterally might be classified as an asymmetric process diagnosed, either correctly or incorrectly, as melanoma; this most likely would not appear in a search directed at nevi alone. Therefore, perhaps the ultimate illustrative study would compare these nevi to melanoma with similar changes—hopefully cases biologically proven to be malignant.

Finally, there is an interesting comment attributed to Dr Wallace Clark, who reviewed the lesions with one author prior to his death. He reportedly remarked that he had seen similar such lesions, most often on the backs of elderly men. This is also the commonest site of melanoma in this same population, and as the lesions in this report are thin, with pseudomelanomatous changes extending, on average, to just 0.5 mm, and as survival for a melanoma of this depth might be in excess of 85% to 95%, long follow-up time and a large sample size might be necessary before firm conclusions are made.

W. A. High, MD, JD, MEng

Reference

1. Fabrizi G, Pennacchia I, Pagliarello C, Massi G. Sclerosing nevus with pseudome-lanomatous features. *J Cutan Pathol*. 2008;35:995-1002.

Comparison of Classification Systems for Congenital Melanocytic Nevi

Turkmen A, Isik D, Bekerecioglu M (Gaziantep Univ Med Faculty, Turkey; Yüzüncü Yil Univ Med Faculty, Van, Turkey)
Dermatol Surg 36:1554-1562, 2010

Background.—Congenital melanocytic nevi (CMNs) are found in approximately 1% of newborn infants, but these represent only a small proportion of the total population of nevi. They vary widely in size, from a small spot to a large area. Later in childhood, these lesions become thickened, verrucous, and hairy. Giant CMNs predispose to malignant melanoma, with a reported incidence of 2% to 31%.

Objective.—To compare three different classification methods of the CMNs to determine which is most accurate.

Participants and Methods.—Sixty patients were included in the study (34 male, 26 female), with an average age of 17.4 (range 3−32). The nevi were evaluated using three different classification methods: total area of the nevus (in cm^2), greatest nevus dimension, and percentage of nevus surface area to total patient body surface area. An appropriate treatment procedure for each case was applied, and participants were followed from 1997 to 2007.

Results.—Malignant transformation was noted in 15.4% of participants with congenital nevi, which was confirmed histopathologically after excision.

Conclusion.—We recommend the calculation of total nevus area as the most useful method for assessment of the risk of developing melanoma in a CMN.

▶ Giant congenital melanocytic nevi (CMN) are reported to have the greatest inherent potential risk for melanoma development within CMN. This makes proper identification of giant CMN important. Currently, 3 systems exist for classifying CMN. The 3 methods include classification based on total nevus surface area, greatest nevus diameter, and percentage of nevus surface area to total body surface area. Given the necessity for accurately diagnosing CMN, Turkmen et al compared the different classifications systems and determined the most useful method for assessing the risk of developing melanoma in these CMN. Overall, the article meets its objective and provides useful practical considerations into which method would be most beneficial to practitioners. According to the study, total surface area and nevi diameter both detect a similar number of giant CMN, because both methods detected a higher number of giant CMN than the method using total body surface area. Also, using either total surface area or nevi diameter, both had a similar percentage of giant CMN that had risk of malignant transformation. However, when considering operative intervention, using total surface area provides more adequate information regarding preoperative clinical size than total nevi diameter. Thus, on the whole, this study provides rational data to practitioners on the use of total surface area as the most useful parameter for classifying CMN, especially giant lesions.

B. D. Michaels, DO

J. Q. Del Rosso, DO

Impact of Melanoma on Patients' Lives Among 562 Survivors: a Dutch Population-Based Study

Holterhues C, Cornish D, van de Poll-Franse LV, et al (Erasmus MC, Rotterdam, the Netherlands; Comprehensive Cancer Centre South, Eindhoven, the Netherlands; et al)
Arch Dermatol 147:177-185, 2011

Objective.—To assess the impact of melanoma on the health-related quality of life of patients from the general population up to 10 years after diagnosis and its determinants.

Design.—A cross-sectional Dutch population-based postal survey among patients with melanoma for the years 1998 to 2008 using the Eindhoven Cancer Registry.

Main Outcome Measures.—The 36-Item Short-Form Health Survey (SF-36), Impact of Cancer (IOC) questionnaire and specific melanoma-related questions. The SF-36 scores of the cases were compared with normative data. Multiple linear regression models were used to identify associated factors of SF-36 and IOC scores.

Results.—The response rate was 80%. The mean age of the 562 respondents was 57.3 years; 62% were female, and 76% had a melanoma with a Breslow thickness of less than 2 mm. The SF-36 component scores of patients with melanoma were similar to those of the normative population. In a multiple linear regression model, stage at diagnosis, female sex, age, and comorbidity were significantly associated ($P < .05$) with the physical and mental component scores. Women were significantly more likely to report higher levels of both positive and negative IOC. Time since diagnosis, tumor stage, and comorbidity were significant predictors of negative IOC scores. Women seemed to adjust their sun behavior more often (54% vs 67%; $P < .001$) than men and were more worried about the deleterious effects of UV radiation (45% vs 66%; $P < .001$).

Conclusion.—The impact of melanoma seems to be specific and more substantial in women, suggesting that they may need additional care to cope with their melanoma optimally.

▶ This well-designed, cross-sectional, population-based study of Dutch melanoma survivors attempted to assess the impact of melanoma on health-related quality of life (HRQoL) measures. The authors compared the responses of 562 Dutch melanoma survivors with responses of the general Dutch population to a 36-Item Short-Form Health Survey (SF-36), Impact of Cancer (IOC) questionnaire and questions directly related to melanoma. The most compelling results of the study were that female gender was most strongly associated with lower SF-36 scores and more dramatic response to melanoma-specific items. These results suggest that women may have more negative and extreme physical and psychological effects from melanoma compared with men. Men were less likely to change their sun-exposure habits than women. In clinical practice, more attention may need to be given to female melanoma patients to ensure that they are psychologically coping well with their disease, including obtaining psychological evaluation and counseling, if necessary. In addition, men may need more encouragement to adopt better sun exposure and protection habits. The study is limited to a Dutch population, and the results may not be generalizable to individuals from other countries and cultures.

D. Fife, MD

A Phase 2 Trial of Dasatinib in Advanced Melanoma

Kluger HM, Dudek AZ, McCann C, et al (Yale Univ School of Medicine, New Haven, CT; Univ of Minnesota, Minneapolis; et al)
Cancer 117:2202-2208, 2011

Background.—Inhibiting src kinases (non-receptor tyrosine kinase signaling intermediates) reduces melanoma cell proliferation and invasion. Dasatinib inhibits c-kit, PDGFβR, and EPHA2 and src kinases c-src, c-Yes, Lck, and Fyn. A phase 2 trial of dasatinib in melanoma was conducted to assess response rate (RR), progression-free survival (PFS), and toxicity.

Methods.—Adults with stage 3/4 chemotherapy-naïve unresectable melanoma were eligible. Dasatinib was initially administered at 100 mg twice daily continuously to 17 patients. Due to toxicity, the starting dosage was decreased to 70 mg twice daily. Tumor assessments occurred every 8 weeks.

Results.—Thirty-nine patients were enrolled, 36 of whom were evaluable for activity and toxicity. Five, 4, and 3 patients had acral-lentiginous, ocular, or mucosal primaries, respectively. Two patients had confirmed partial responses lasting 64 and 24 weeks (RR 5%). Three patients had minor responses lasting 136, 64, and 28 weeks, and 1 patient who was responding discontinued due to noncompliance. The median PFS was 8 weeks; the 6-month PFS rate was 13%. One patient with an exon-13 c-kit mutation had a partial response, whereas disease in another patient with an exon-11 c-kit mutation progressed. Common toxicities were fatigue, dyspnea, and pleural effusion.

Conclusions.—Daily dasatinib has minimal activity in unselected melanoma patients, excluding those with c-kit mutations. The study did not meet the prespecified endpoints of 30% response rate or 6-month PFS. Dasatinib was poorly tolerated overall, often requiring dose reduction or interruption. Because activity was observed in a small subset without c-kit mutations, identifying predictive biomarkers is important for future development of dasatinib in melanoma alone or in combination trials.

▶ Currently, there are few options for the treatment of advanced nonresectable melanoma. Although there have been some advances in metastatic melanoma with therapies directed at the BRAF mutation, these patients tend to develop resistance over time and not all metastatic melanomas express the BRAF gene. Dasatinib is a inhibitor of several tyrosine kinases that aid in tumor progression. This is a single-arm phase 2 trial of dasatinib used on 39 patients with confirmed stage 3/4 melanomas of cutaneous, mucosal, or ocular origin. Patients with brain metastasis were excluded. Dasatinib was initially started at 100 mg twice daily and decreased to 70 mg twice daily because of toxicity. The endpoints were disease progression or adverse toxicities. Confirmation of tumor regression was observed after 4 cycles in 5 patients. In this study, the overall response rate was greater than 20%. The most common adverse effects were fatigue (n = 35, 97%) and dyspnea (n = 31, 86%). There was also activity seen in a subset of patients (14%) without the c-kit mutation, and therefore a biomarker-based preselection of patients may be beneficial in the future. The authors concluded that dasatinib had minimal activity in unselected melanoma patients, and the doses used in this study were poorly tolerated.

G. K. Kim, DO

J. Q. Del Rosso, DO

An immunohistochemical comparison between MiTF and MART-1 with Azure blue counterstaining in the setting of solar lentigo and melanoma *in situ*

Hillesheim PB, Slone S, Kelley D, et al (Univ of Louisville, KY)
J Cutan Pathol 38:565-569, 2011

Background.—Evaluation of cutaneous pigmented lesions can be diagnostically challenging and represents an activity often supplemented by immunohistochemistry. Immunohistochemical studies typically employ 3,3'-diaminobenzidine (DAB) resulting in brown staining of both melanocytes and melanin. Difficulty may thus arise in distinguishing different cell types in heavily melanized lesions. Azure blue counterstaining has been used in conjunction with melanoma antigen recognized by T-cells (MART-1) to differentiate melanocytes from melanin by highlighting the latter blue-green. Microphthalmia transcription factor (MiTF) represents an alternative immunomarker that shows nuclear reactivity, which facilitates ease of interpretation.

Methods.—Twenty examples of solar lentigo and melanoma *in situ* (MIS) were independently evaluated utilizing MiTF and MART-1/Azure blue for melanocyte quantification. Melanocyte counts were averaged over five high-power fields ($\times$ 400) to obtain a mean melanocytic count.

Results.—There was no significant difference in the mean melanocytic count between MART-1/Azure blue and MiTF as assessed in the solar lentigo group and as assessed independently in the MIS group. MiTF nuclear staining facilitated interpretation and required less laboratory preparation, as an additional counterstain was not necessary.

Conclusions.—MiTF is as effective as MART-1/Azure blue in identifying melanocytes in the context of solar lentigo or MIS. On the basis of our results, we favor expanding the use of MiTF as an immunohistochemical marker, as it provides an efficient alternative to MART-1 with Azure blue counterstaining in the evaluation of cutaneous pigmented lesions.

▶ This investigation examined the use of immunostains with a 3,3'-diaminobenzidine (DAB) brown-chromogen system for melanoma antigen recognized by T-cells (MART-1) versus microphthalmia transcription factor (MiTF) for the study of junctional melanocytic processes (lentigines and melanoma in situ) in which the MART-1 stain was enhanced by use of an Azure blue counterstain.

In brief, in darkly pigmented processes, use of MART-1 with an Azure blue counterstain has the advantage of staining melanin a blue-green color, which lessens the risk of confusion of the brown melanin with the affirmative brown staining of melanocytes when one uses a brown DAB immunohistochemical detection system. This is particularly true, as the MART-1 stain can also lead to cytoplasmic staining of granule in melanophage and pigmented keratinocytes. MiTF has an advantage of being a relatively specific nuclear-based stain that the authors hypothesized would allow for detection of melanocytes without the added expense and complexity of the Azure blue counterstain.

While the number of cases is small (20 solar lentigines, 20 melanoma in situ, and 6 actinically damaged pieces of control tissue from excision tips), there was a similar number of melanocytes recognized at the dermoepidermal junction using either the MART-1/Azure blue staining technique or MiTF staining technique, respectively. The authors concluded that MiTF staining is more economical and technically less demanding than MART-1/Azure blue staining and provides similar diagnostic efficacy.

While the article is well done, and the results compelling, like all studies based on immunohistochemistry, there are some important caveats, including the fact that these results were obtained using a certain brand and batch of immunostains, performed on a certain brand of autostaining machine, by a laboratory that has certain protocols and methods of antigen retrieval and staining.

At our large academic dermatopathology laboratory, where we perform more than 28 000 immunostains per year, we have found, in our own hands, that MiTF is a more fickle and technically demanding stain for our operators and technicians, and I feel quite certain we would not be able to obtain the same data. Furthermore, at our large laboratory, we use nearly exclusively aminoethylcarbazole, which is a red chromagen, for all our pigmented processes, which eliminates the need for the Azure blue stain, thereby placing all immunostains on equal footing. This is probably the emerging trend among larger dermatopathology laboratories with particular expertise in pigmented processes, as it also affords the capability of performing unique double-stains, such as a combined MART-1/Ki67 stain, such that the proliferative index of melanocytes alone can be assessed.

Lastly, while it was previously thought that MiTF would not stain histiocytic or inflammatory conglomerations (inflammatory pseudonesting), recent reports suggest that it may, on occasion, mark such material in a nonspecific way, similar to that of MART-1/Melan A, and hence, it may not be as a specific for nuclear marking only of melanocytes, as once thought.[1]

W. A. High, MD, JD, MEng

Reference

1. Abuzeid M, Dalton SR, Ferringer T, Bernert R, Elston DM. Microphthalmia-associated transcription factor-positive pseudonests in cutaneous lupus erythematosus. *Am J Dermatopathol.* 2011;33:752-754.

AJCC melanoma staging update: impact on dermatopathology practice and patient management

Piris A, Mihm MC Jr, Duncan LM (Massachusetts General Hosp, Boston; Brigham and Women's Hosp, Boston, MA)

J Cutan Pathol 38:394-400, 2011

Changes in the 2010 American Joint Commission on Cancer melanoma staging guidelines include the evaluation of primary tumor mitotic index (mitogenicity) and the recognized prognostic significance of a single melanoma cell in a sentinel lymph node. These revised criteria have important practice implications for dermatopathologists as well as for dermatologists, oncologists and surgeons who treat patients with cutaneous melanoma.

▶ This article summarizes important revisions to the 2009/2010 American Joint Commission on the Cancer (AJCC) staging system for melanoma. Chief among these changes is elevation of mitotic index (measured as mitosis/mm^2) to covariate status for thin melanoma (< 1 mm depth), along with Breslow thickness and ulceration. As the authors duly note, this decision was based on study of more than 10 000 thin melanomas in which 10-year survival rate decreased from 95% to 88% for thin, nonulcerated melanoma when just a single dermal mitosis was detected.

Determination of mitotic index is to occur using the "hot-spot" technique in which a focus of greatest mitotic activity is located, and then one moves outward to assess the number of mitoses per millimeter squared. Specifically, the presence of even a single dermal mitosis, even in a melanoma with an area of more than 1 mm^2, is to be reported as 1 mitosis per millimeter squared, while a melanoma without any detectable mitosis is to be reported as zero mitoses per millimeter squared.

Therefore, considering that currently, staging guidelines treat nonulcerated, thin melanoma without less than 1 mitosis per millimeter squared (zero) as T1a disease, and nonulcerated, thin melanoma with ≥1 mitosis per millimeter squared as T1b disease, the net result, at its most basic level, is establishment of a somewhat binomial variable, with either zero mitoses or ≥1 mitosis per millimeter squared as the 2 possible outcomes.

This places some stress on the dermatopathologist, as merely a single mitotic figure alters the stage for all melanoma less than 1 mm in depth. Furthermore, while sentinel lymph node (SLN) procedures are not without controversy, the authors present an interesting table (Table 4 in the original article) that outlines the general management for the National Comprehensive Cancer Network based on the 3 factors of depth, mitotic index, and ulceration.

Clearly, this table does not consider the patient's age and the likelihood the patient will actually consent to radical node dissection if a sentinel node is positive, and these type of data also have to factor in to any decision on SLN mapping. Nevertheless, ultimately, the dermatologist performing a biopsy, and who is medicolegally responsible for acting on the result (or making the appropriate referral), will want to be certain that these 3 key pieces of data (Breslow depth, mitotic index, and ulceration) are specifically and clearly commented on in every final report of thin melanoma (< 1 mm).

Of somewhat lesser day-to-day importance for a dermatologist is the fact that the new 2009/2010 AJCC guidelines treat even a single parenchymal melanoma cell in a lymph node, even if only detected by immunohistochemical techniques, but so long as it is cytologically atypical, as a "positive" lymph node result (stage III disease).

W. A. High, MD, JD, MEng

Cigarette smoking and malignant melanoma: a case-control study
Kessides MC, Wheless L, Hoffman-Bolton J, et al (Johns Hopkins Univ School of Medicine, Baltimore, MD; Med Univ of South Carolina, Charleston; Johns Hopkins Univ Bloomberg School of Public Health, Baltimore, MD)
J Am Acad Dermatol 64:84-90, 2011

Background.—Several previous studies have reported inverse associations between cigarette smoking and melanoma. Often these studies have not adjusted for ultraviolet (UV) exposure history, skin type, or number of blistering sunburns, which could confound the observed associations between cigarette smoking and melanoma.

Objective.—We sought to assess whether this reported inverse association persists after adjusting for UV exposure, skin type, and number of blistering sunburns.

Methods.—We conducted a population-based case-control study (82 patients with melanoma, 164 control subjects). Two control subjects were matched to each patient by age, sex, race, and skin type. Conditional logistic regression models were fit to assess the association between cigarette smoking history and melanoma, with additional adjustments for UV exposure and sunburns.

Results.—Compared with never smoking, both former (odds ratio 0.43, 95% confidence interval 0.18-1.04) and current (odds ratio 0.65, 95% confidence interval 0.19-2.24) smoking were inversely associated with melanoma, but the associations were not statistically significant.

Limitations.—The number of cutaneous nevi was not assessed in this study. In addition, the relatively small number of patients limits the statistical precision of the observed associations.

Conclusions.—After matching for age, sex, race, and skin type, and further adjusting for UV exposure and number of sunburns, cigarette smoking was not statistically significantly associated with melanoma risk, but the results were consistent with previous observations of an inverse association.

▶ Cigarette smoking has been associated with many cancers such as lung, bladder, pancreatic, and kidney. Some researchers suggest that smoking may be inversely related to melanoma risk. This is a case-control study of cigarette smoking and the risk of melanoma. The authors controlled for age, sex, skin type, sun exposure, and sunburn history. Other studies have been done but have not controlled for sun exposure, skin type, or both. In this study, researchers found that results were not statistically significant, and the observed associations were consistent with previous observations, with an inverse association between past and current cigarette smoking and melanoma shown in this study. Also, results showed that correlations between regular sunscreen use, regular sun protective clothing use, and lifetime sun exposures and melanoma were not statistically significant ($P > .05$ for each). This study found that there may be other more confounding variables that have a stronger and statistical significance. The relatively small number of melanoma cases was 1 limitation. The researchers did not have information on complete body examination among study participants. In conclusion, this study found that there may be an inverse relationship between cigarette smoking and risk of melanoma.

G. K. Kim, DO

J. Q. Del Rosso, DO

Clinical and histologic characteristics of malignant melanoma in families with a germline mutation in CDKN2A

van der Rhee JI, Krijnen P, Gruis NA, et al (Leiden Univ Med Ctr, The Netherlands; et al)
J Am Acad Dermatol 65:281-288, 2011

Background.—About 10% of cutaneous malignant melanomas (CMM) occur in individuals with a family history of melanoma. In 20% to 40% of melanoma families germline mutations in CDKN2A are detected. Knowledge of the clinicohistologic characteristics of melanomas and patients from these families is important for optimization of management strategies, and may shed more light on the complex interplay of genetic and environmental factors in the pathogenesis of melanoma.

Objective.—We sought to investigate the clinical and histologic characteristics of CMM in CDKN2A-mutated families.

Methods.—Clinical and histologic characteristics of 182 patients with 429 CMM from families with a founder mutation in CDKN2A (p16-Leiden mutation) were compared with 7512 patients with 7842 CMM from a population-based cancer registry.

Results.—Patients with p16-Leiden had their first melanoma 15.3 years younger than control patients. The 5-year cumulative incidence of second primary CMM was 23.4% for patients with p16-Leiden compared with 2.3% for control patients. The risk of a second melanoma was twice as high for patients with p16-Leiden who had their first melanoma before age 40 years, compared with older patients with p16-Leiden. Unlike control patients, there was no body site concordance of the first and second melanoma in patients with p16-Leiden and multiple primary melanomas. Patients with p16-Leiden had significantly more superficial spreading, and less nodular and lentiginous melanomas.

Limitations.—Ascertainment of patients with p16-Leiden was family based. The study was performed in families with a founder mutation, the p16-Leiden mutation.

Conclusion.—Our findings are consistent with a pathogenic pathway of melanoma development from nevi, starting early and ongoing throughout life, and not related to chronic sun exposure.

▶ A family germline mutation in CDKN2A (p16-Leiden mutation) has been detected in patients with a family history of melanoma. This is a study comparing the clinical and histologic characteristics of 182 patients with 429 cutaneous melanomas (CM). These patients were from the families with a germline mutation in CDKN2A and were compared with the control group from the Leiden population-based cancer registry (7512 patients with 7842 CM). The authors found that with patients with p16-Leiden, the diagnosis of CM was made before the age of 40 years and was also a significant risk for development of a second CM ($P = 0.011$). In addition, the 5-year cumulative incidence of a second CM was found to be 23.4% in the p16-Leiden population and 2.3% in control population. Also, a diagnosis of a first CM at a young age (< 40 years) was also associated with a double risk of multiple primary melanomas in the p16-Leiden population. In the p16-Leiden population, a high proportion of superficial spreading CM and lack of lentiginous CM was observed. They concluded this may be evidence that those in the p16-Leiden population developed CM from the nevus pathway as opposed to through chronic sun exposure. One drawback was that the CDKN2A mutation in the general CM population can be as low as 0.2% to 2.0% and may not provide a high yield for screening all CM patients. This study suggests that those with multiple primary CMs should be identified and genetically tested for closer surveillance. The authors found that those with a CDKN2A mutation in this large case control study tend to follow the nevus pathway with CM development and suggest that further studies are needed.

G. K. Kim, DO

J. Q. Del Rosso, DO

Melanocytic Nevi with Spitz Differentiation: Diagnosis and Management
Ahmadi N, Davison SP, Kauffman CL (Georgetown Univ Hosp, Washington, DC)
Laryngoscope 120:2385-2390, 2010

Objectives.—Melanocytic proliferations with Spitz differentiation present a difficult clinicopathologic dilemma, as their spectrum ranges from benign to malignant. Distinct entities include Spitz nevus, atypical Spitz nevus, and Spitzoid melanoma. Their histopathologic differentiation can be challenging, and cases of Spitzoid melanoma initially diagnosed as benign Spitz nevi are reported in the literature. The goal of this article is to discuss the diagnostic tools (including comparative genomic hybridization), which may be helpful in differentiating benign Spitz nevi from malignant melanoma with Spitzoid features, and to propose an appropriate management strategy for each entity.
Study Design.—Retrospective case reports.

Methods.—Medical records of patients referred for suspicious nevi were reviewed. Data regarding demographics, site, pathology reports, and treatment were reviewed.

Results.—Four patients with three distinct diagnoses involving Spitz differentiation were identified. The pathologic interpretation of these biopsies was difficult and multiple dermatopathologists were involved. All four patients underwent excision with or without sentinel node biopsy.

Conclusions.—Otolaryngologists, plastic surgeons and dermatopathologists will encounter patients who have melanocytic lesions with Spitz differentiation at some point in their career. The management of these patients is significantly impacted by the histopathologic diagnosis, and should not be undertaken until it is confirmed, possibly with comparative genomic hybridization. In our experience, it is not unusual to have multiple independent pathologic examinations. We believe that a team approach between the surgeon and the dermatopathologist is crucial when diagnosing and managing patients with Spitz lesions.

▶ In this series of case reports, the authors outline the difficulties in differentiating between benign Spitz nevi, atypical Spitz nevi, and Spitzoid melanoma. This article is primarily an overview rather than an in-depth review. The authors briefly discuss the histopathologic and histochemical staining features that can assist in differentiating various Spitz nevi. They mention comparative genomic hybridization as a promising evolving technology that may further assist in differentiating Spitz nevi. Unfortunately, the article concludes that there is currently no technique that unequivocally differentiates atypical Spitz nevi from Spitzoid melanoma.

S. M. Purcell, DO

Melanomas Detected in a Follow-up Program Compared with Melanomas Referred to a Melanoma Unit

Salerni G, Lovatto L, Carrera C, et al (Hosp Clinic Barcelona, Spain)
Arch Dermatol 147:549-555, 2011

Objective.—To compare melanomas diagnosed in patients included in follow-up programs with melanomas diagnosed in patients referred to a melanoma unit.

Design.—Retrospective analysis of 215 consecutive melanomas diagnosed between 2007 and 2008.

Setting.—Melanoma Unit, Hospital Clinic of Barcelona, Barcelona, Spain.

Patients.—The study included 201 patients (105 men and 96 women), 40 of whom were included in a follow-up program in our unit and 161 of whom were referred for evaluation.

Main Outcome Measures.—Clinical (ABCD algorithm), dermoscopic (ABCD rule of dermoscopy), and main histologic characteristics were evaluated in both groups.

Results.—Most melanomas diagnosed in follow-up did not fulfill some of the ABCD criteria, and only 12.0% fulfilled all 4 ABCD criteria, in contrast with 63.6% of the melanomas referred for evaluation ($P < .001$). The total dermoscopy score was lower in melanomas diagnosed in follow-up (5.04 vs. 6.39, $P < .01$), and 36% were misclassified as benign in this group according to the total dermoscopy score. Seventy percent of melanomas diagnosed in follow-up were in situ; among invasive melanomas, the Breslow index was significantly lower in the group of melanomas diagnosed in follow-up, with a mean (range) of 0.55 (0.25-0.90) mm vs 1.72 (0.25-13.00) mm ($P < .001$).

Conclusions.—The inclusion of patients who are at high risk for melanoma in follow-up programs allows the detection of melanomas in early stages, with good prognosis, even in the absence of clinical and dermoscopic features of melanoma. In the general population without specific surveillance, melanoma continues to be diagnosed at more advanced stages.

▶ Digital dermoscopy is being increasingly used to assess how a melanocytic lesion may change over time. As more information is accumulated, identifying groups that are at high risk may also help improve the detection of melanoma at an early stage. This is a retrospective analysis of 215 consecutive melanomas diagnosed between 2007 and 2008. There were 40 patients included in the follow-up unit, and 161 were referred for evaluation. Twenty-four patients (60%) included in the follow-up group were diagnosed as having melanoma before the study began compared with only 8 (5%) who were from the referred unit ($P < .001$). Atypical mole syndrome was found more frequently in the follow-up with a higher nevi count ($P < .01$). Irregular borders, multiple colors, and a diameter larger than 6 mm were found more frequently in referral malignant melanomas (RMMs) than in follow-up malignant melanomas (FUMMs) ($P = .02$, $P < .001$, and $P < .01$). The FUMM lesions demonstrated less asymmetry ($P < .001$) than the RMM lesions overall, with fewer abrupt borders ($P = .001$), a variety of colors ($P < .001$), and fewer dermoscopic structures ($P = .001$). In the FUMM, 19 melanomas (38%) were diagnosed because of changes in follow-up by dermoscopy. A significantly lower proportion of melanomas in the FUMM group were Clark II or III compared with that in the RMM group, and none of the FUMMs were Clark IV or V ($P < .001$). Among the invasive melanomas, the Breslow index was significantly lower in the FUMM group, with a mean of 0.53 mm compared with 1.74 mm in the RMM group ($P < .001$). In this study, only 50% of FUMMs, but almost 90% of RMMs, were classified correctly according to the total dermoscopy score. A limitation of this study was the age of the 2 groups, which was disparate. The inclusion of patients who were at high risk for melanomas in follow-up programs selects for the detection of melanoma at early stages even in the absence of clinical and dermoscopic features of melanoma, as the index of suspicion is higher and the threshold for biopsy is lower. This study also revealed the increasing trend in the diagnosis of thin melanomas in this population. This may be because of early recognition and identification of high-risk individuals with the additional assistance of dermoscopic assessment.

G. K. Kim, DO

J. Q. Del Rosso, DO

Marital Status and Stage at Diagnosis of Cutaneous Melanoma: Results From the Surveillance Epidemiology and End Results (SEER) Program, 1973-2006

McLaughlin JM, Fisher JL, Paskett ED (Ohio State Univ, Columbus)
Cancer 117:1984-1993, 2011

Background.—We evaluated the effect of marital status on risk of late-stage cutaneous melanoma diagnosis.

Methods.—Information about melanoma patients was obtained from Surveillance Epidemiology and End Results (SEER), 1973-2006. A multivariable logistic regression model was used to estimate relative risks of late-stage disease at diagnosis.

Results.—After exclusion criteria, 192,014 adult melanoma patients remained for analyses. After adjustment for age, race, year of diagnosis, tumor histology, anatomic site, socioeconomic status, and SEER site, the relationship between estimated risk of late-stage melanoma diagnosis and marital status was dependent on sex ($P < .0001$ for interaction). Although unmarried patients had a higher risk of being diagnosed at a late stage among men and women, the magnitude of the effect varied by sex. Moreover, among married, single, and divorced or separated patients, men had more than a 50% increase in risk of late-stage diagnosis when compared with women. Widowed men and widowed women, however, were not statistically different in their stage at diagnosis.

Conclusions.—Results from this study are important and may be used by clinicians and public health practitioners interested in increasing the proportion of melanoma patients diagnosed at an early stage through screening, perhaps by specifically targeting unmarried individuals in addition to having broad-based skin cancer prevention programs.

▶ Early diagnosis of melanoma is crucial. Previous studies have identified individual predictors associated with greater likelihood of melanomas being diagnosed at a late stage. Those factors have included male patients, individuals of older age, nonwhites, cigarette smokers, low socioeconomic status, the uninsured, those on public assistance programs (ie, Medicaid), and patients living in areas with fewer dermatologists. McLaughlin et al provide an interesting article that analyzes an additional potential factor for the risk of late-stage malignant melanoma diagnosis: marital status. Based on their research, they found that unmarried individuals were more likely to be diagnosed with late-stage disease. In addition, although not the primary objective of the study, they also revealed that of patients who were either married, single, divorced, or separated (not widowed), men had a greater than 50% increase in the risk of being diagnosed with late-stage melanoma. Given that early detection is essential for all clinicians, the data from this study certainly provide practitioners with important additional insight. Although it remains important to screen all patients for the potential for melanoma, perhaps based on the results of this article, there should be an even more heightened awareness in unmarried individuals, in addition to individuals with the previously identified variables. To this end, the article meets its objective and provides dermatologists with further important information in their goal toward early detection of melanoma.

B. D. Michaels, DO

J. Q. Del Rosso, DO

The "spaghetti technique": an alternative to Mohs surgery or staged surgery for problematic lentiginous melanoma (lentigo maligna and acral lentiginous melanoma)
Gaudy-Marqueste C, Perchenet A-S, Taséi A-M, et al (Hôpital Ste Marguerite, Marseille, France; Hôpital La Conception, Marseille, France; Hôpital La Timone, Marseille, France)
J Am Acad Dermatol 64:113-118, 2011

Background.—Lentigo maligna (LM) and acral lentiginous melanoma (ALM) are often large and clinically ill defined. The surgical challenge is to spare tissue while still achieving clear margins.

Objective.—We sought to provide a retrospective assessment of a two-phase surgical technique for lentiginous melanomas (MM) not suitable for en bloc resection.

Methods.—In the first phase, a narrow band of skin, "the spaghetti", is resected just beyond the clinical outline of the MM, immediately sutured, and sent for pathological examination without removing the MM. The same procedure is repeated beyond the segments which are shown to be not tumor free and so forth until the minimal tumor-free perimeter is outlined. No operative wound is left between operative sessions. In the second phase, the MM resection and reconstruction are performed at the same time.

Results.—In 21 patients with LM (n = 16) or ALM (n = 5), the mean operative defect size was 27.5 cm^2 (range, 1.97-108.4 cm^2). The mean number of steps in the procedure was 1.55 (1-4). Grafts were used for reconstruction in all cases. The relevance of the "spaghetti"-defined outline was confirmed in 19 of 21 patients. After a median follow-up period of 25.36 months (range, 0-72 months), the local control rate was 95.24% with one case (4.76%) of in-transit invasive recurrence after 48 months.

Limitations.—This study was performed at a single center and included a limited number of patients. The follow-up time was relatively brief.

Conclusion.—The "spaghetti technique" is simple and reliable for LM and ALM. Unlike Mohs surgery, it does not require specific training of surgeons or pathologists. Unlike staged surgery, it does not leave patients with an open wound on the face or soles before final reconstruction.

▶ This is a novel technique designed to be tissue sparing with complete margin control using en face paraffin-embedded vertical sections. This technique is evaluated in this article for lentiginous melanomas, including both lentigo maligna (LM) and acral lentiginous melanoma (ALM). The margins used are 3 to 5 mm beyond the clinically visible pigment in a shape similar to the lesion. This is in contrast to the square technique that uses a square, triangle, or hexagon using

5- to 10-mm borders beyond the clinical lesion. Thus, there is likely some tissue sparing that may occur with the "spaghetti technique." With both techniques, the defect is immediately sutured, which theoretically might "seed" the tissue with tumor, although this has never been proven and the lesion is usually in situ at the periphery. While 95% local control is impressive, the mean follow-up was only 25 months, which the authors do point out, so it is difficult to draw firm conclusions at this time. Nevertheless, all new concepts need to start somewhere, and, if pilot studies show high promise and low risk, further studies are warranted. This technique is likely easier on the patient when compared with staged excisions and "slow Mohs," as the patient is not sent home with a large open wound. Mohs micrographic surgery has been shown to provide good cure rates and same-day reconstruction and is tissue sparing, but it does require specialized training for evaluation of melanomas such as LM and ALM histologically. More specifically, not all Mohs micrographic surgeons are comfortable using frozen sections for LM. The spaghetti technique appears to be a useful technique to obtain margin control in the treatment of lentiginous melanomas, with further study warranted.

R. Ceilley, MD

B. Kopitzki, DO

Sun exposure before and after a diagnosis of cutaneous malignant melanoma: estimated by developments in serum vitamin D, skin pigmentation and interviews

Idorn LW, Philipsen PA, Wulf HC (Univ of Copenhagen, Denmark)
Br J Dermatol 165:164-170, 2011

Background.—Previous studies on ultraviolet radiation (UVR) exposure before and after a diagnosis of cutaneous malignant melanoma (CMM) have been based primarily on questionnaires. Objective measures are needed.

Objectives.—To assess changes in UVR exposure in patients with CMM using objective surrogate parameters in a descriptive study.

Methods.—Ten patients recently diagnosed with CMM during the 5 months (autumn and winter) preceding study start in February 2009; 21 patients diagnosed from 12 months to 6 years before study start; and 15 controls, who matched the recently diagnosed patients on age, sex, residential area, constitutive skin type and occupation completed the investigations. UVR exposure before and after diagnosis of CMM was assessed using measures of serum 25-hydro vitamin D [25(OH)D], skin pigmentation and by interviews. Winter 25(OH)D was used as a surrogate parameter of UVR exposure the previous summer — the summer before CMM diagnosis in recently diagnosed patients.

Results.—Winter 25(OH)D was significantly higher among recently diagnosed patients compared with controls ($P = 0·02$, $R^2 = 0·60$) and patients diagnosed up to 6 years earlier ($P = 0·01$). The increase in 25(OH)D during the summer after diagnosis was significantly lower for recently diagnosed patients than for controls ($P = 0·005$, $R^2 = 0·51$) and patients diagnosed up to 6 years earlier ($P = 0 \cdot 008$). No difference was found in summer 25(OH)D between the groups.

Conclusions.—Our findings suggest that patients with CMM had a higher UVR exposure the summer before diagnosis than did controls and patients diagnosed up to 6 years earlier, and that after diagnosis UVR exposure fell to the level of controls in patients with CMM.

▶ The authors offered an interesting way to evaluate sun exposure by measuring 25-hydroxy vitamin D, 25(OH)D, in study subjects. Authors attempted to see if the serum level of 25(OH)D level correlates with recent and past diagnosis of cutaneous melanoma (CM) diagnosis. Collected evidence only showed that more sun exposure relates directly to a diagnosis of CM. The method used offers a possible objective way to measure sun exposure. The study, however, is small, and hence results cannot be generalized to larger population. Besides serum levels of 25(OH)D, the authors also used recall questionnaire answers by study subjects, which pose recall bias of the collected evidence. Because we don't know the necessary length of time between sun exposure and a rise in the level of serum 25-D(OH), how vitamin D-rich foods affect serum 25(OH)D levels, and interference between sunscreen application and the 25(OH)D serum level, the accuracy of this parameter as a measurement of sun exposure is a bit questionable and does not really offer any definitive data for us to discuss with patients.

K. Nguyen, MD

Circulating Benign Nevus Cells Detected by ISET Technique: Warning for Melanoma Molecular Diagnosis
De Giorgi V, Pinzani P, Salvianti F, et al (Univ of Florence, Italy)
Arch Dermatol 146:1120-1124, 2010

Background.—The notion that only malignant melanoma cells circulate and diffuse is shared by oncologists and pathologists. Isolation by size of epithelial tumor cells (ISET) allows the identification of circulating tumor cells by filtration according to size.

Observations.—During a study of identification of circulating melanoma cells using ISET, blood samples from a 69-year-old man with an atypical melanocytic lesion on his back were evaluated. Binucleated and multinucleated cells that fulfilled the criteria for circulating tumor cells were found. The morphological features were similar to those of the excised skin tissue specimen, and the patient was subsequently diagnosed as having a congenital melanocytic nevus. *BRAF* (V600E)-mutated DNA was detected in both plasma and formalin-fixed tissue specimens, and the blood samples demonstrated an increase in tyrosinase messenger RNA levels.

Conclusion.—The finding that benign nevus cells may circulate in blood brings into question the value of tyrosinase or other melanocytic markers as a molecular surrogate for circulating melanoma cells.

▶ There is increasing interest in the use of peripheral blood assays in the diagnosis and monitoring of melanoma. Such technologies include not only isolation by size of epithelial tumor cells (ISET), a technique based on filtering and cytologic examination, but also measurement of messenger RNA (mRNA) for tyrosinase by real-time PCR (rtPCR), used as a surrogate for the presence of actual melanoma cells in the peripheral blood.

Herein, the authors detail a case where nevus cells were identified in peripheral blood by ISET analysis, and rtPCR was positive for elevated tyrosinase mRNA, yet the patient suffered only from a congenital nevus, completely excised, and he was free of disease with 2 years of follow-up.

Certainly, one does not need to practice dermatopathology for long to become keenly aware of the occurrence of benign ectopy of nevus cells in lymph nodes. In fact, this may occur in up to 20% of lymph nodes sampled in melanoma-related procedures; perhaps more rare, but also observed, is the occurrence of nevus cells within lymphatic ducts in the skin. Is it not implausible to think these cells might occasionally find their way into the peripheral circulation as well?

Of particular interest, the nevomelanocytes were present only in peripheral blood drawn after the excisional procedure and diminished with the passage of time. As the authors duly note, this finding suggests that the surgical procedure was a key factor in tumor shedding, and such a phenomenon has occurred in other entities, including breast, colorectal, and prostatic cancer. Furthermore, the mere presence of the cells in the circulation is no guarantee that metastatic disease of any kind will ensue, as without supporting stroma, many cells may undergo apoptosis via a process called anoikis.

Perhaps this case raises issues related to more common skin cancers as well, such as basal cell carcinoma (BCC) and squamous cell carcinoma (SCC). While curettage and electrodesiccation is used in treatment of small and well-differentiated SCC, concern has been voiced on occasion regarding any theoretical potential for hematogenous or lymphatic seeding from such maneuvers.[1] This concern has apparently not risen to the same level with BCC (or is at least unvoiced), and certainly BCC is better recognized as a stromal-dependent neoplasm than SCC. Personally, I might anticipate further intriguing investigation in this arena.

Regardless, the case report suggests that nevus cells from a congenital nevus, but also, potentially, nevus cells of atypical or even borderline lesions, may enter peripheral circulation, particularly after excision. Ultimately, this will complicate investigations by ISET or related technology, particularly if a biochemical marker common to all melanocytic processes (benign or malignant), such as tyrosinase, is used as a surrogate.

W. A. High, MD, JD, MEng

Reference

1. Giesse JK. Comparison of treatment modalities for squamous cell carcinoma. *Clin Dermatol.* 1995;13:621-626.

Management and outcome of metastatic melanoma during pregnancy

Pagès C, Robert C, Thomas L, et al (Université Paris VII, France; Institut Gustave-Roussy, Villejuif, France; Université Claude Bernard Lyon 1, France; et al)
Br J Dermatol 162:274-281, 2010

Background.—Although metastatic melanoma occurrence during pregnancy challenges the physician in several ways, only a few studies have been published.

Objectives.—Our aim was to investigate therapeutic management together with maternal and fetal outcomes in pregnant women with advanced melanoma.

Methods.—A French national retrospective study was conducted in 34 departments of Dermatology or Oncology. All patients with American Joint Committee on Cancer (AJCC) stage III/IV melanoma diagnosed during pregnancy were included. Data regarding melanoma history, pregnancy, treatment, delivery, maternal and infant outcomes were collected.

Results.—Twenty-two women were included: 10 AJCC stage III and 12 stage IV. Abortion was performed in three patients. Therapeutic abstention during pregnancy was observed in three cases, 14 patients underwent surgery, four patients received chemotherapy and one patient was treated with brain radiotherapy alone. The median gestational age was 36 weeks amenorrhoea. Neither neonatal metastases nor deformities were observed. Placenta metastases were found in one case. Among 18 newborns, 17 are currently alive (median follow up, 17 months); one died of sudden infant death. The 2-year maternal survival rates were 56% (stage III) and 17% (stage IV).

Conclusions.—Faced with metastatic melanoma, a majority of women chose to continue with pregnancy, giving birth, based on our samples, to healthy, frequently premature infants. Except during the first trimester of pregnancy, conventional melanoma treatment was applied. No serious side effect was reported, except one case of miscarriage after surgery. Mortality rates do not suggest a worsened prognosis due to pregnancy but larger prospective controlled studies are necessary to assess this specific point.

▶ Knowledge and standard-of-care therapy for patients with melanoma during pregnancy is not well studied. In the past, researchers have thought that melanoma during pregnancy was considered a worse prognosis; however, this may not be the case. This is a study evaluating the management of metastatic melanoma during pregnancy together with maternal and fetal outcome. There were 22 women with stage III and stage IV melanomas; 14 patients underwent surgery, 4 patients received chemotherapy, and 1 patient was treated with radiotherapy alone. The most common was superficial spreading melanoma followed by nodular melanoma. Three patients (14%) chose therapeutic abortion because of information on poor prognosis of metastatic melanoma. Although many of these patients were faced with metastatic melanoma, their infants, although some were premature, were healthy. There were no neonatal metastases or deformities observed. There was only 1 case of placental metastasis found in this study, but this did not affect the health of the infant. Surgery in this study was deemed to be the easiest and safest for treatment of melanoma with few side effects but with 1 individual having a miscarriage after surgery. This study also suggested that CT scans may be acceptable during pregnancy. Radiotherapy during pregnancy may be harmful for the fetus, and its efficacy is poor in melanoma. In this study, 2 pregnant women received radiotherapy for symptomatic brain metastases (second trimester). Pregnancy is not considered to be an absolute contraindication to radiotherapy. Among 18 infants, 17 are currently alive with a median follow-up of 17 months. One died from sudden infant death. This study is of value since there is little information and few studies evaluating melanoma metastases during pregnancy to guide clinicians in decision making and management.

G. K. Kim, DO
J. Q. Del Rosso, DO

Sentinel Lymph Node Biopsy or Nodal Observation in Melanoma: a Prospective Study of Patient Choices

Grange F, Maubec E, Barbe C, et al (Hôpital Robert Debré, Reims, France; Hôpital Bichat, Paris, France; Hôpital Maison Blanche, Reims, France; et al)
Dermatol Surg 37:199-206, 2011

Background.—There is no consensus regarding the therapeutic utility of sentinel lymph node biopsy (SLNB) versus that of nodal observation (NO) in melanoma.

Objective.—To prospectively evaluate a standardized counseling procedure and its effect on patient choices to undergo SLNB or NO.

Methods.—In four centers, patients with melanoma eligible for SLNB or NO received a complete counseling procedure that included verbal information from dermatologists and surgeons, a detailed information sheet, and a written consent form. Data collected included patient and tumor characteristics, counseling conditions, and specialties of informing doctors. Factors influencing patients' choices were studied using multivariate analysis.

Results.—Of 343 consecutive patients, 309 were offered SLNB and NO and received complete verbal and written information from a dermatologist alone (62%) or in association with a surgeon (38%). Approximately half took advice from trusted persons, and half asked for additional time before making a decision; 268 (86.7%) ultimately decided to undergo SLNB. Multivariate analysis showed that older patients, those with a head and neck melanoma, and those informed without a surgeon present were more likely to prefer NO.

Conclusions.—This counseling procedure was easily implemented in clinical practice. Patients favored SLNB but were able to understand uncertainties and express preferences.

▶ Sentinel lymph node biopsy (SLNB) for cutaneous melanoma (CM) is used for pathologically staging regional lymph node basins in patients with clinical stage I/II melanoma.[1] The sentinel lymph node is thought to be the node that is first to receive lymph draining from the site of the primary CM. The current prospective study from France found 86.7% (268 of 309) of patients elected to proceed with SLNB rather than nodal observation when presented with both options. As stated by the authors, these results may have been influenced by the manner in which surgeons offered SLNB favorably, and patients may have been referred strictly for SLNB to the recruiting centers that routinely perform them. Patients were also not asked the reason for their decisions. Nevertheless, even with a positive sentinel lymph node biopsy result, current evidence does not exist that directly correlates elective lymph node dissection with improvement in the overall survival of the patient. It is advisable, however, to discuss with all patients with CM whether SLNB is indicated in their case. If SLNB is chosen, patients should be counseled on the complications, limitations, potential value, and cost of the procedure.

S. Bellew, DO

J. Q. Del Rosso, DO

Reference

1. Stebbins WG, Garibyan L, Sober AJ. Sentinel lymph node biopsy and melanoma: 2010 update part I. *J Am Acad Dermatol*. 2010;62:723-734.

Topical Imiquimod for Periocular Lentigo Maligna

Demirci H, Shields CL, Bianciotto CG, et al (Thomas Jefferson Univ, Philadelphia, PA)
Ophthalmology 117:2424-2429, 2010

Purpose.—To evaluate the efficacy of topical imiquimod 5%, a local immune response modifier, in the treatment of periocular lentigo maligna.

Design.—Retrospective, interventional case series.

Participants.—Five consecutive patients with biopsy-proven periocular lentigo maligna.

Methods.—Periocular lentigo maligna was treated with topical imiquimod 5%. The clinical features, treatment schedule, response to treatment, and complications were analyzed retrospectively.

Main Outcome Measures.—Response to treatment and complications.

Results.—The mean patient age was 73 years. The anatomic location of lentigo maligna was the medial canthal area in 2 patients, the lateral canthal area in 1 patient, and the lower eyelid in 2 patients. Topical imiquimod 5% was used for 5 days per week in 3 patients and for 7 days per week in 2 patients. The medication was placed only on the skin and not the globe. The mean duration of treatment was 9 months (range, 1—14 months). Lentigo maligna partially resolved in 3 patients and completely resolved in 2 patients. The most common side effects included localized erythema and discomfort (n = 4), swelling (n = 3), and cutaneous excoriation (n = 2). There were no patients with toxicity to the conjunctiva, cornea, or globe. Treatment was discontinued in 2 patients (one temporarily and the other permanently) because of intolerable local side effects of discomfort, redness, swelling, and cutaneous excoriation. There was no recurrence of lentigo maligna in those with complete or partial response (mean follow-up, 20 months).

Conclusions.—Periocular lentigo maligna seems to respond to topical imiquimod 5% treatment. Topical imiquimod 5% treatment for periocular lentigo melanoma deserves further study.

▶ Topical imiquimod 5% cream, an immune response modifier used to treat some cutaneous malignancies, actinic keratosis, and viral skin diseases, has been proven to be effective in treating periocular lentigo maligna primarily in case reports. In this case series of 5 patients with periocular lentigo maligna, topical imiquimod achieved either partial (n = 3) or complete response (n = 2).

The average age of the patients was 73 years, frequency of use was 1 application 5 or 7 days per week, and the locations included medial canthus, lateral canthus, or lower eyelid. The mean duration of treatment was 9 months. The practicing physician must use caution when using imiquimod for treating lentigo maligna. Considerations that must be addressed are the following:

1. Surgical intervention is the standard of care and treatment of choice for lentigo maligna. However, particularly in the elderly population, some patients may not be suitable surgical candidates because surgery may create anatomical and functional complications.

2. Pre- and posttreatment biopsy must be adequate (sufficient sample size that correlates with the most suspicious area of the lesion), and multiple biopsies may be needed to make certain an invasive component is not present.

3. Recurrence is possible; hence long-term follow-up is essential. Photographic documentation may also be helpful.

In conclusion, topical imiquimod 5% cream is a safe and reasonable alternative to surgery for periocular lentigo maligna in selected cases. A brisk inflammatory response is to be anticipated, and prolonged treatment over several months is likely to be needed.

J. L. Smith, MD

Prognostic value and clinical significance of halo naevi regarding vitiligo
van Geel N, Vandenhaute S, Speeckaert R, et al (Ghent Univ Hosp, Belgium)
Br J Dermatol 164:743-749, 2011

Background.—Vitiligo and halo naevi can present together or separately. Whether they are different entities remains unclear.

Objectives.—To assess the clinical significance of halo naevi, both with respect to the future development of vitiligo, and to the clinical profile and course of vitiligo.

Methods.—In total, 291 patients were included in this study: patients with only halo naevi (group 1; $n = 40$), patients with generalized vitiligo without halo naevi (group 2; $n = 173$) and patients with generalized vitiligo with halo naevi (group 3; $n = 78$).

Results.—Patients with only halo naevi (group 1) reported significantly less associated autoimmune disease ($P = 0.001$), were less likely to have a family history of vitiligo ($P = 0.013$) and were less likely to have presence of Koebner phenomenon ($P < 0.001$) compared with patients with generalized vitiligo (groups 2 + 3). Multiple halo naevi (≥ 3) were significantly more frequently observed ($P = 0.002$) in patients from group 1 compared with patients from group 3. In group 3, halo naevi were reported prior to the development of vitiligo in 61% (mean ± SD time interval of 33.7 ± 5.17 months). No significant correlation was observed between the presence of halo naevi and the extent, activity or subtype of vitiligo. However, halo naevi in patients with vitiligo significantly reduced the risk for associated autoimmune diseases, and age at onset of vitiligo was significantly lower compared with patients with vitiligo without halo naevi ($P < 0.001$).

Conclusions.—Our results support the hypothesis that halo naevi can represent a distinct condition. In a subset of patients, the occurrence of halo naevi may be an initiating factor in the pathogenesis of vitiligo.

▶ We all have young patients with halo nevi because they are fairly common. However, there is that subset of patients with halo nevi that concomitantly have or go on to develop vitiligo. This study attempts to answer the question of how halo nevi and vitiligo are related. The authors examined 291 patients and divided them into 3 groups: those with only halo nevi, those with only vitiligo, and those with both halo nevi and vitiligo. Participants were also given a standardized questionnaire detailing patient demographics, personal history, and family history. Not surprisingly, patients with halo nevi presented at a younger age than those without. There were no associated differences in possible triggers or extent or type of vitiligo. They did find that those with halo nevi and vitiligo were less likely to have other autoimmune diseases associated than those with vitiligo alone. The authors concluded that halo nevus can be a distinct entity, but in susceptible individuals, it may serve as a cofactor with vitiligo.

In another recent report, the presence of halo nevi and leukotrichia in patients with segmental vitiligo was a strong predictive factor for the progression to a mixed pattern of vitiligo.[1] Other risk factors for progression of disease that were identified include segmental vitiligo located to the trunk, Koebner phenomenon, and presence of circulating antithyroid antibodies.

Both of these reports highlight the close association among halo nevi, vitiligo, and autoimmunity. In susceptible individuals without vitiligo, the presence of halo nevi can foreshadow the appearance of vitiligo. In patients who already have vitiligo, halo nevi can be a marker for progression of disease.

A. Zaenglein, MD

Reference

1. Ezzedine K, Diallo A, Léauté-Labrèze C, et al. Halo nevi and leukotrichia are strong predictors of the passage to mixed vitiligo in a subgroup of segmental vitiligo. *Br J Dermatol.* 2011 Oct 27 [Epub ahead of print].

Melanoma Incidence Rates among Whites in the U.S. Military

Zhou J, Enewold L, Zahm SH, et al (United States Military Cancer Inst, Washington, DC; Natl Cancer Inst, Bethesda, MD)
Cancer Epidemiol Biomarkers Prev 20:318-323, 2011

Background.—The U.S. Military and general populations may differ in the exposure to sunlight and other risk factors for melanoma and therefore the incidence rates of melanoma may be different in these two populations. However, few studies have compared melanoma incidence rates and trends over time between the military and the general population.

Methods.—Melanoma incidence rates from 1990 to 2004 among white active–duty military personnel and the general U.S. population were compared using data from the Department of Defense Automated Central Tumor Registry and the National Cancer Institute Surveillance, Epidemiology, and End Results program.

Results.—Age-adjusted melanoma rates overall were significantly lower in the military than in the general population; the incidence rate ratio was 0.75 for men and 0.56 for women. Age-specific rates, however, were significantly lower among individuals younger than 45 years, but significantly higher among those 45 years or older ($P < 0.05$). Melanoma incidence increased from 1990–1994 to 2000–2004 in both populations, with the most rapid increase (40%) among younger men in the military. Melanoma incidence rates also varied by branch of military service; rates were highest in the air force.

Conclusion.—These results suggest that melanoma incidence rate patterns differ between the military and the general population (Table 1).

▶ This interesting study is related to the aspects of prevention of chronic sun exposure. As a veteran with experience as a general medical officer and who has training in and has practiced dermatology in the military, this study substantiates the principles of preventive medicine and sun exposure consequences with a predictable result. I find it significant to see this documented.

As a new population of younger military recruits comes in from the general population, every military member is required to have an annual physical. During the annual physical examination, the general skin evaluation occurs. During the evaluation, those pigmented lesions that are atypical are appropriately biopsied or sent for further evaluation to the available dermatology service in the military health care system. The atypical or dysplastic nevi are removed prior to the development of melanoma. Diagnosis of atypical nevi is not captured by the Automated Central Tumor Registry. The surveillance may be important in decreasing the overall presence of melanoma, which might be demonstrated with this comparison of the general public to the military in this younger age group.

Military personnel are often stationed in climates of extensive sun exposure during active duty periods and may include long periods of sun exposure, creating a higher risk of developing skin cancer, including melanoma. Sunscreen is often provided by the military, or uniforms with some environmental sun protection may be available. It is of interest that although sun damage and

TABLE 1.—Incidence Rates of Melanoma among Whites Aged 20 to 59 Years in the U.S. Active-Duty Military and U.S. General Populations by Gender and Age at Diagnosis, 1990 to 2004

		Military[a]		General Population[b]	IRR[d] (95% CI)
	Count	Rate[c] (95% CI)	Count	Rate[c] (95% CI)	
Gender					
Men	1342	6.96 (6.59−7.34)	16,791	9.17 (8.95−9.40)	0.75 (0.71−0.80)
Women	203	7.73 (6.70−8.88)	16,821	13.86 (13.56−14.18)	0.56 (0.48−0.64)
Age at diagnosis					
20−24	164	2.17 (1.85−2.53)	1,137	5.68 (5.35−6.02)	0.38 (0.33−0.46)
25−29	224	4.45 (3.89−5.08)	2,090	9.55 (9.14−9.97)	0.47 (0.41−0.54)
30−34	272	7.04 (6.23−7.93)	3,218	13.17 (12.72−13.63)	0.53 (0.47−0.61)
35−39	329	10.38 (9.29−11.57)	4,335	17.25 (16.74−17.77)	0.60 (0.54−0.68)
40−44	293	18.90 (16.80−21.19)	5,508	22.58 (21.99−23.18)	0.84 (0.75−0.95)
45−49	170	33.62 (28.76−39.07)	5,923	27.49 (26.79−28.20)	1.22 (1.06−1.44)
50−54	58	49.76 (37.78−64.33)	5,793	32.18 (31.35−33.02)	1.55 (1.21−2.07)
55−59	35	178.48 (124.32−248.22)	5,608	39.17 (38.15−40.21)	4.56 (3.35−6.70)

[a]ACTUR.
[b]SEER-9.
[c]Age-adjusted (active-duty military 1990−2004) and age-specific rates per 100,000 person-years.
[d]IRR comparing rates in the military to the rates in the general population.

sunburn is extremely discouraged even to the point of a potential court martial offense for repeated offenders with significant sunburn, the recreational patterns of off-duty personnel may be a significant factor for development of melanoma. Additional factors such as possible chemical exposures are also discussed briefly in this article.

Additional interesting information is the segregation of military duty occupations. The report of the Air Force as having a higher incidence of melanoma, indicating the possibility of long flight line activities, as well as information regarding additional segregation as to years of service, skin type, and the type of duty discriminating the operational active duty exposure verses recreational exposure would be helpful. This article supports the principles of surveillance and early detection as well as paying attention to chronic sun exposure as a factor related to an increase in incidence of melanoma.

L. Clever, DO

Acral Melanocytic Nevi: Prevalence and Distribution of Gross Morphologic Features in White and Black Adults

Palicka GA, Rhodes AR (Rush Univ, Chicago, IL)
Arch Dermatol 146:1085-1094, 2010

Objective.—To determine prevalence and morphologic features of acral melanocytic nevi in white and black adults.

Design.—Point prevalence survey.

Setting.—Outpatient dermatology clinic.

Patients.—Convenience sample of subjects 18 years or older.

Main Outcome Measures.—Prevalence and morphologic features based on ethnicity, sex, and age.

Results.—Palmar or plantar nevi were detected in 42.0% of blacks (50 of 119) vs 23.0% of whites (79 of 343) ($P < .001$). Palmar or plantar nevi of 6-mm diameter or larger were detected in 3.4% of blacks (4 of 119) vs 0.6% of whites (2 of 343) ($P = .04$). Diffusely black acral nevi were uncommon in whites (0 of 343) and blacks (1 of 119). The prevalence of palmar or plantar nevi increased directly with degree of skin pigmentation ($P < .001$). In whites, this prevalence was greater in women (27.1%, 51 of 188) than in men (18.1%, 28 of 155) ($P = .047$); in subjects younger than 50 years (30.8%, 57 of 185) than in those 50 years or older (13.9%, 22 of 158) ($P < .001$); in subjects with a history of atypical nevus removal than in those without (odds ratio [OR], 3.6; 95% confidence interval [CI], 1.9-6.9); in those with at least 1 extant atypical nevus than in those without (OR, 3.2; 95% CI, 1.7-6.0); and in those with at least 20 nevi of 2-mm diameter or larger than in those without (OR, 3.0; 95% CI, 1.6-5.6).

Conclusions.—Acral nevi appear to be associated with ethnicity, pigmentation, age, and cutaneous melanoma (CM) risk factors. While relatively large and/or very darkly pigmented acral nevi appear to be more common in blacks than in whites, diffusely black acral nevi are uncommon in both groups. These findings are relevant to the assessment of pigmented lesions in the differential diagnosis of acral CM.

▶ The rate of acral cutaneous melanoma compared with other anatomic sites has been noted to be higher in blacks and Asians than in whites. Acral melanocytic nevi are common, but acral cutaneous melanoma is relatively rare and may be a source of confusion for physicians to identify. This is a study of 187 men and 275 women who were at least 18 years old to determine the prevalence and morphologic features of acral melanocytic nevi in white and black adults. Results revealed that the prevalence of palmar or plantar nevi increased directly with the degree of constitutive skin pigmentation ($P < .001$). For subjects with any palmar nevi, 72.3% of whites (34/47) and 71.4% of blacks (25/35) had only 1 palmar nevus; 17.0% of whites and 17.1% of blacks had only 2 palmar nevi, 80.5% of whites and 83.3% of blacks had only 1 plantar nevus. In whites, the prevalence of palmar or plantar nevi in subjects < 50 years old was 2.2-fold greater than in older subjects ($P < .001$). Presence of at least 1 palmar or plantar nevus in whites was significantly associated with a history of atypical nevus removal. Presence of at least 1 palmar or plantar nevus in whites was not significantly associated with having a first-degree blood relative with cutaneous melanoma. Of 258 white subjects included in this analysis, 14 had a personal history of cutaneous melanoma and 19 had a family history of cutaneous melanoma in a first-degree relative. Of the 14 white subjects who had a personal history of melanoma, 29% had a family history of cutaneous melanoma in a first-degree relative. Size, pigmentation characteristics, and ethnicity-related prevalence of acral melanocytic nevi are relevant to the differential diagnosis of cutaneous melanoma on acral surfaces.

The morphologic features of unselected acral nevi is relevant to the predictive value of gross morphologic features used in the differential diagnosis of cutaneous melanoma. This study also revealed that the prevalence of palmar or plantar nevi increases with degree of constitutive skin pigmentation. Also, the prevalence of palmar or plantar nevi ≥ 4 mm in diameter was 4.5 times greater in blacks (11.8%) than in whites (2.6%; $P < .001$), and the prevalence of palmar or plantar nevi of ≥ 6 mm in greatest diameter was 5.8 times greater in black (3.4%) than in whites (0.6%; $P < .04$). Also, subjects who had any acral nevi with dark brown or darker coloration in the largest nevus per subject were less common among whites (3.8%) than in blacks (58%, $P < .001$). Large or very darkly pigmented acral nevi appear to be more common in blacks than in whites, and diffusely black acral nevi are uncommon in both groups.

Limitations to this study were a lack of histopathologic confirmation of acral pigmented lesions as melanocytic nevi. There may also have been an inconsistency in interobserver ability to accurately assess gross morphologic features of acral pigmented lesions. More prospective studies comparing surface microscopic features of pigmented lesions on acral surfaces with histopathologic characteristics need to be completed. This study demonstrated significant differences in prevalence of acral melanocytic nevi according to ethnicity, age, degree of constitutive pigmentation, and sex and significant differences in size of acral melanocytic nevi according to ethnicity.

G. K. Kim, DO
J. Q. Del Rosso, DO

Internet Use and Anxiety in People with Melanoma and Nonmelanoma Skin Cancer

Ludgate MW, Sabel MS, Fullen DR, et al (Univ of Michigan Health System, Ann Arbor; et al)
Dermatol Surg 37:1252-1259, 2011

Background.—People with cancer are increasingly turning to the Internet for health-related information.

Objective.—To compare the patterns of Internet use of people with skin cancer with previous findings by including people with nonmelanoma skin cancer (NMSC) using a comprehensive survey. To evaluate perceived anxiety levels and overall satisfaction after searching the Internet of people with skin cancer.

Methods & Materials.—We conducted a survey study and prospectively collected data from people newly diagnosed with melanoma or NMSC.

Results.—Four hundred fifteen participants with melanoma and 400 with NMSC completed the questionnaire. Internet use and overall satisfaction with the Internet search increased more than 50% in participants with melanoma from 2005. One-third of participants with melanoma, but many fewer participants with NMSC, reported higher anxiety after Internet use. Participants who were younger, female, more highly educated, and diagnosed with melanoma were most likely to use the Internet to search for information about their diagnosis.

Conclusion.—Internet use is prevalent and increasing sharply in individuals with skin cancer. The majority of individuals describe their use of the Internet as a positive experience. Greater anxiety from searching the Internet is more common in individuals with melanoma than in those with NMSC.

▶ Among patients seeking health care information, Internet use is popular in general, and dermatology patients are no exception. Based on the findings of this article by Ludgate et al, Internet use is increasing among patients with skin cancer. More specifically, Ludgate et al sought to determine both anxiety levels and overall satisfaction of patients with melanoma and nonmelanoma skin cancer (NMSC) after they used the Internet to find more information about their disease. The results of their study provide important considerations for dermatologists. In this study, they found that melanoma patients searching the Internet experienced greater anxiety than patients with NMSC. However, overall, the majority of patients did not describe increased anxiety with Internet use, and importantly, the majority of patients described their experience with the Internet as positive. Fortunately, it was also found that most patients viewed the content they found on Web sites with caution. Given the positive experience with the Internet, it is likely that patients will continue to use it to gather supplemental information regarding skin cancer. As the article notes, although Internet use is essentially inevitable, there is room for dermatologists to take a proactive role in recommending content-appropriate Web sites and addressing concerns and questions for patients who use the Internet to gather additional information. Overall, the article provides important insight and awareness indicating that providers treating patients with skin cancers should ensure that patients receive the most appropriate information regarding their skin cancer, including the best websites to access.

B. D. Michaels, DO
J. Q. Del Rosso, DO

18 Lymphoproliferative Disorders

Cutaneous graft-versus-host disease: rationales and treatment options
Chavan R, El-Azhary R (Mayo Clinic, Rochester, MN)
Dermatol Ther 24:219-228, 2011

The treatment of cutaneous graft-versus-host disease (GVHD) is one of the most challenging clinical scenarios in a dermatological practice. Given the significant risk of morbidity and mortality in this patient group, it is important for a dermatologist to understand the pathophysiology of GVHD, as well as their role within a multidisciplinary practice where many immunosuppressants are prescribed. A significant proportion of the patients with GVHD will require a combination treatment regimen in order to stem the progression of their disease. In this review, the stages, type of GVHD and treatment options are reviewed for the dermatologist.

▶ This is an excellent review article on a graft-versus-host disease (GVHD) for dermatologists who are involved with cancer treatment centers. The article succinctly summarizes the available pertinent studies on treatments of this condition as well as practical guidelines on what the authors actually do in their practice. I recommend this article highly for you to keep handy when you are called on to manage a patient with GVHD.

K. Nguyen, MD

Lymphoepithelioma-like carcinoma of head and neck skin: a systematic analysis of 11 cases and review of literature
Welch PQ, Williams SB, Foss RD, et al (Wiesbaden Dental Clinic Command, Germany; Tripler Army Med Ctr, Honolulu, HI; Armed Forces Inst of Pathology, Washington, DC; et al)
Oral Surg Oral Med Oral Pathol Oral Radiol Endod 111:78-86, 2011

Lymphoepithelioma-like carcinoma of the skin (LELCS) is a rare tumor of unknown etiology, low malignant potential, and microscopic resemblance to undifferentiated nasopharyngeal carcinoma. Clinically, it presents as a flesh-colored firm nodule or plaque on the face, scalp, or shoulder of middle-aged to elderly individuals. Histologically, LELCS is composed of islands of enlarged epithelial cells with large vesicular nuclei surrounded and permeated by a dense lymphoplasmacytic infiltrate. LELCS exhibits immunoreactivity with high-molecular-weight cytokeratins and epithelial membrane antigen, indicating the epithelial origin. The differential diagnosis includes basal cell carcinoma, squamous cell carcinoma, lymphoma, pseudolymphoma, and Merkel cell carcinoma. We report 11 cases of LELCS of the head and neck region with discussion of the clinical, histopathologic, immunohistochemical, and therapeutic aspects of this rare cutaneous neoplasm. In addition, we systematically review and compare the findings with the previously published cases of LELCS. This study is the largest case series of LELCS reported in the English-language literature. It attempts to more clearly define the diagnostic criteria for LELCS. Its histomorphologic and immunophenotypic features help distinguish this tumor from similar-appearing malignancies, including metastatic nasopharyngeal carcinoma.

▶ Lymphoepithelioma-like carcinoma of the skin (LELCS) is extremely rare. The differential diagnoses include Merkel cell carcinoma, basal cell carcinoma (BCC), and squamous cell carcinoma (SCC), among other neoplasms. Clinically, the flesh-colored nodule or plaque could easily be mistaken for BCC or SCC. This should remind us to obtain adequate biopsy specimens in such cases. Also, if the histologic report does not match the clinical presentation, further investigation is indicated. Diagnosis of LELCS should prompt a thorough head and neck evaluation and a metastatic workup because of possible association with underlying regions of involvement. Wide local excision or Mohs micrographic surgery appears to be optimal for primary treatment of LELCS. This is another important example of how hard it is to make a clinical diagnosis of something that we aren't aware of and to avoid being complacent because we encounter so many BCC and SCC lesions.

R. Ceilley, MD

B. Kopitzki, DO

A phase II placebo-controlled study of photodynamic therapy with topical hypericin and visible light irradiation in the treatment of cutaneous T-cell lymphoma and psoriasis

Rook AH, Wood GS, Duvic M, et al (Univ of Pennsylvania Med Ctr, Philadelphia; Univ of Wisconsin and Dept of Veterans Affairs Med Ctr, Madison; Univ of Texas MD Anderson Cancer Ctr, Houston; et al)
J Am Acad Dermatol 63:984-990, 2010

Background.—Hypericin is a known photodynamic agent that has been demonstrated to induce apoptosis in normal and malignant B and T lymphocytes, and has potential to treat benign and malignant disorders of the skin, including psoriasis and cutaneous T-cell lymphoma.

Objective.—We wished to test whether topical hypericin was an effective, safe, and well-tolerated therapy for patch or plaque phase mycosis fungoides and for plaque psoriasis.

Methods.—We conducted a phase II placebo-controlled clinical study in patients who had either patch or plaque phase mycosis fungoides or plaque type psoriasis vulgaris. Representative lesions were treated twice weekly for 6 weeks with topically applied hypericin or placebo followed 24 hours later by exposure to visible light at 8 to 20 J/cm^2.

Results.—After 6 weeks of twice-weekly therapy, several concentrations of hypericin resulted in the significant improvement of treated skin lesions among the majority of patients with cutaneous T-cell lymphoma and psoriasis whereas the placebo vehicle was ineffective.

Limitations.—The clinical trial involved a small number of patients.

Conclusions.—Overall, the data from this study support the conclusion that topical hypericin/visible light photodynamic therapy is an effective and well-tolerated alternative to standard psoralen plus ultraviolet A treatment of these disorders.

▶ The clinical application of photodynamic therapy (PDT) using new photosensitizing molecules to treat a wide spectrum of inflammatory, infectious, and neoplastic skin disorders continues to expand. The use of topical hypericin PDT for the treatment of cutaneous T-cell lymphoma (CTCL) and psoriasis in this phase II study demonstrates encouraging results. It offers a less mutagenic alternative to psoralen plus ultraviolet A (PUVA) light therapy. The use of visible light to perform PDT provides a convenience factor for patients because it permits home therapy. Data on disease-free intervals with this therapy were not addressed in this study but will likely be a critical factor in determining patient compliance and acceptance. Currently, the commercially available photosensitizing agents aminolevulinic acid (ALA) and methyl aminolevulinic acid (MAL), which can also be activated by ambient or fluorescent light, have been studied for the treatment of CTCL and psoriasis. The therapeutic efficacy of both drugs has been found to be quite variable. To date, neither the manufacturer of ALA nor that of MAL has sought agency approval for the treatment of CTCL or psoriasis. It will be interesting to follow the development of hypericin PDT as an alternative to PUVA for the treatment of CTCL and psoriasis.

G. Martin, MD

19 Miscellaneous Topics in Cosmetic and Laser Surgery

Accelerated resolution of laser-induced bruising with topical 20% arnica: a rater-blinded randomized controlled trial

Leu S, Havey J, White LE, et al (Northwestern Univ, Chicago, IL)
Br J Dermatol 163:557-563, 2010

Background.—Dermatological procedures can result in disfiguring bruises that resolve slowly.

Objectives.—To assess the comparative utility of topical formulations in hastening the resolution of skin bruising.

Methods.—Healthy volunteers, age range 21–65 years, were enrolled for this double (patient and rater) blinded randomized controlled trial. For each subject, four standard bruises of 7 mm diameter each were created on the bilateral upper inner arms, 5 cm apart, two per arm, using a 595-nm pulsed-dye laser (Vbeam; Candela Corp., Wayland, MA, U.S.A.). Randomization was used to assign one topical agent (5% vitamin K, 1% vitamin K and 0·3% retinol, 20% arnica, or white petrolatum) to exactly one bruise per subject, which was then treated under occlusion twice a day for 2 weeks. A dermatologist not involved with subject assignment rated bruises [visual analogue scale, 0 (least)–10 (most)] in standardized photographs immediately after bruise creation and at week 2.

Results.—There was significant difference in the change in the rater bruising score associated with the four treatments (ANOVA, $P = 0·016$). Pairwise comparisons indicated that the mean improvement associated with 20% arnica was greater than with white petrolatum ($P = 0·003$), and the improvement with arnica was greater than with the mixture of 1% vitamin K and 0·3% retinol ($P = 0·01$). Improvement with arnica was not greater than with 5% vitamin K cream, however.

Conclusions.—Topical 20% arnica ointment may be able to reduce bruising more effectively than placebo and more effectively than low-concentration vitamin K formulations, such as 1% vitamin K with 0·3% retinol (Fig 6).

▶ As noted by the authors, several studies have been done looking at the utility of arnica in reducing bruising. This study uses a higher concentration of arnica

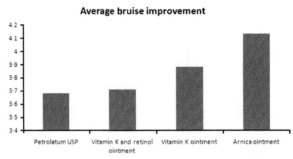

FIGURE 6.—Mean change in bruising level detected by dermatologist rater on visual analogue scale at 2 weeks compared with baseline for each of the four agents. (Reprinted from Leu S, Havey J, White LE, et al. Accelerated resolution of laser-induced bruising with topical 20% arnica: a rater-blinded randomized controlled trial. *Br J Dermatol.* 2010;163:557-563, with permission from John Wiley and Sons www.interscience.wiley.com.)

than what has been used in some previous studies. Although only looking at 16 subjects, the results here add to the evidence that topical arnica may be minimally helpful in reducing post-laser purpura. Fig 6 portrays the reduction in bruising after 2 weeks of twice daily use. Although this bar graph may appear convincing, the study should be critically evaluated to determine whether this effect could translate into clinical practice.

The topical agents evaluated here were applied twice daily for 2 weeks under occlusion. Outside of a study, it is doubtful that a patient would consistently apply an ointment for this long using occlusion. It is even less likely that a patient would do this if the bruise were on the face. Bruising may be somewhat camouflaged by make-up, but an occlusive dressing would be rather obvious. Occlusion is more feasible on nonfacial sites, but on the other hand, most patients aren't as cosmetically concerned about a bruise on a nonfacial site.

It should be noted also that the methods section of the study states that bruising was blindly evaluated immediately after treatment, 1 week after treatment, and 2 weeks after treatment. This is different from what is stated in the abstract. It would have been helpful to also see a diagram similar to Fig 6 but portraying the results at 1 week after treatment.

The medical community needs a better understanding of the pharmacology of arnica in reducing purpura. It is only touched on in this discussion. Additionally, much larger studies are needed. It would also be helpful to quantify the number of days in which bruising can be reduced by using topical arnica.

E. Graber, MD

A Split-Face Comparison of Two Ablative Fractional Carbon Dioxide Lasers for the Treatment of Photodamaged Facial Skin

Ciocon DH, Engelman DE, Hussain M, et al (Skin Laser and Surgery Specialists of New York and New Jersey)
Dermatol Surg 37:784-790, 2011

Objective.—To compare the safety and efficacy of two fractional carbon dioxide (CO_2) laser devices for the treatment of photodamaged facial skin.

Methods.—Eight healthy subjects underwent full-face resurfacing for photodamaged skin with two fractionated CO_2 laser devices using manufacturer-recommended settings for facial rejuvenation. For each subject, one device with a rolling handpiece was used on one side and a second device with a stamping handpiece was used on the other. Patients were evaluated 3 months postoperatively and photographed. A blinded physician investigator assessed the photographs and rated each side for improvement in four categories (wrinkles, pigmentation, skin laxity, and overall appearance). Patient ratings for overall improvement for each side were also recorded.

Results.—All patients had improved on the basis of photographic and clinical assessments at 3 months. No significant differences in patient ratings of overall improvement and physician-measured parameters of clinical improvement were found, although intraoperative times and pain ratings were greater with the laser with the stamping handpiece. No complications were experienced with either device.

Conclusions.—Both fractionated CO_2 resurfacing devices used in the study were safe and effective for the treatment of photodamaged facial skin, but the modality using a stamping handpiece was associated with longer operative times and greater intraoperative pain.

▶ In the field of ablative and nonablative fractional laser treatments, does deep produce better outcomes than superficial? This article would suggest that more superficial treatments have a tendency to give results equal to the deeper fractional carbon dioxide (CO_2) treatment with less pain and less downtime needed. Earlier work has demonstrated that the inflammatory factors generated by the superficial and deep treatments, when the volume of wounded tissue was kept constant, are similar. The outcome of this study supports this contention. In fact, the traditional ablative CO_2 laser therapy is a superficial treatment that wounds 200 to 300 μm of dermal tissue. However, it does so in a nonfractional way, which produces a cutaneous wound that requires more time to heal (downtime) and a greater risk of adverse effects. Recent work by Dr Rox Anderson and colleagues on laser treatment of scars has also supported the concept that deeper is not necessarily better.

E. A. Tanghetti, MD

A study of the efficacy of carbon dioxide and pigment-specific lasers in the treatment of medium-sized congenital melanocytic naevi

August PJ, Ferguson JE, Madan V (Salford Royal Hosp NHS Foundation Trust, Manchester, UK)
Br J Dermatol 164:1037-1042, 2011

Background.—Treatment of medium-sized congenital melanocytic naevi (CMN) can be challenging.

Objectives.—To present the results of treatment of 55 CMN with the carbon dioxide (CO_2) and pigment-specific lasers.

Methods.—CO_2 and Q-switched lasers (frequency-doubled Nd:YAG, Nd:YAG and alexandrite) were used to treat 55 CMN. Patients were treated at 3-month intervals until maximum clearance. Clinical response at 3–6 months after final treatment was graded as poor (< 50%), good (50–75%) or excellent (> 75%). Outcomes were evaluated on case note review and questionnaire.

Results.—Thirty-six of the 55 CMN were macular and 19 were mammillated. Twenty-seven CMN were present on the head and neck. For macular CMN, outcomes were better for truncal CMN. Scarring and pallor were seen in three lower limb macular CMN treated with a CO_2 laser. Mammillated CMN on the head and neck showed most improvement. Pigment-specific lasers were of no additional benefit. Repigmentation occurred in 6% of macular and 21% of mammillated CMN. Partial or complete regimentation of CMN was reported by 46% of patients.

Conclusions.—Compared with macular CMN, mammillated CMN show a marginally better response to laser treatment. CMN on the limbs respond poorly. Pigment-specific lasers do not lighten mammillated CMN. Adverse effects can occur with CO_2 laser treatment of macular CMN on lower limbs.

▶ Treating congenital nevi is fraught with technical and emotional difficulties. This study uses a number of devices to treat a variety of difficult congenital nevi. There was a high rate of recurrence and an unsatisfactory response with nevi on the trunk, especially on the limbs. When surgery is not an option, laser surgery with a combination of devices does make sense, especially on the face where surgical choices are limited. This approach is less than perfect.

E. A. Tanghetti, MD

Early Postoperative Treatment of Thyroidectomy Scars Using a Fractional Carbon Dioxide Laser

Jung JY, Jeong JJ, Roh HJ, et al (Yonsei Univ, Seoul, Korea)
Dermatol Surg 37:217-223, 2011

Background.—Ablative carbon dioxide fractional laser systems (CO_2 FS) have been effectively used to improve the appearance of scarring after surgical procedures, but an optimal treatment time has not been established.

Objective.—To evaluate the efficacy and safety of CO_2 FS in early postoperative thyroidectomy scars.

Methods.—Twenty-three Korean women with thyroidectomy scars were enrolled in this study. All patients underwent a single session of two passes of a CO_2 FS with a pulse energy setting of 50 mJ and a density of 100 spots/cm^2 2 to 3 weeks after surgery.

Results.—Mean Vancouver Scar Scale (VSS) scores were statistically significantly lower after laser treatment. Three months after CO_2 FS treatment of thyroidectomy scarring, 12 of 23 participants showed clinical improvement of more than 51% from 2 to 3 weeks after surgery. The mean grade of clinical improvement based on independent clinical assessment was 2.6 ± 0.9.

Conclusion.—Early postoperative CO_2 FS treatment of thyroidectomy scars is effective and safe.

▶ This article shows that there is use in treating thyroidectomy scars 2 to 3 weeks after surgery with a fractional CO_2 laser. The problem with the study is that there was no control arm, and we have no idea of what the particular scar would be like if it were untreated. The most important point with this study is that this procedure appeared to be safe. In the future, studies such as this should be done with a comparative arm to give us a better perspective on the intervention performed.

E. A. Tanghetti, MD

Complication of Cross-Technique on Boxcar Acne Scars: Atrophy
Weber MB, Machado RB, Hoefel IR, et al (Universidade de Ciências da Saúde de Porto Alegre, RS, Brazil; et al)
Dermatol Surg 37:93-96, 2011

Background.—Up to 80% of young people age 11 to 30 years suffer acne, which is characterized by cornification of the follicular infundibulum, sebaceous hypersecretion and retention, bacterial proliferation, and inflammation. Scarring is the primary complication seen with acne. It causes significant esthetic distress in patients and possibly produces or exacerbates existing psychosocial disorders. Trichloroacetic (TCA) acid has been used to chemically reconstruct skin scars (CROSS method) with good clinical results in the ice pick-n-type scars. These occur with skin damage and are small in diameter but deep. CROSS causes reorganization of the dermis and increases dermal volume by producing collagen, glycoaminoglycans, and elastin when administered in concentrations of 50% to 90% applied directly to the scar. However, complications can occur with this method.

Case Report.—Woman, 28, had suffered acne since age 16 years and was undergoing treatment for severe cystic-nodule acne using ethinyl estradiol-cyproterone acetate oral contraceptives and topical retinoic acid 0.025%. Many ice pick-n-type and boxcar-type scars remained in malar sites, so 80% TCA acid applications were added to the regimen. A sharpened applicator was used to deliver the TCA acid deeply within scars in the left malar region. The result was a whitening of the area. After 30 days the patient expressed satisfaction with the result and had a second application. After 1 month she had areas of atrophy in some of the scars that had been treated and improved appearance in others. The treatment was suspended and the sites observed. Two months later the atrophic areas were less evident and had developed a natural favorable course.

Conclusions.—Compared other treatments, applying high concentrations of TCA acid offers the advantages of shorter recovery time, less disruption of patients' lives, and low cost. However, there are adverse effects of treatment, including erythema, hypopigmentation or hyperpigmentation, scarring, and hypertrophy or atrophy. The atrophy resembles that produced by intralesional corticosteroids and offers a similar course of spontaneous clinical improvement. Physicians should be aware of these drawbacks so they can manage them and guide their patients through the process (Figs 1-3).

▶ This study is of interest because it presents a previously unreported complication of the chemical reconstruction of skin scars (CROSS) technique: atrophy. The photographs illustrate the resultant atrophy and its subsequent resolution

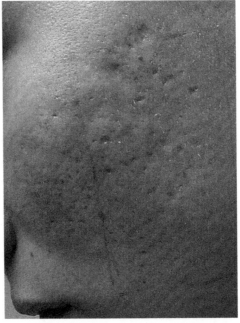

FIGURE 1.—Ice pick— and boxcar-type scars in the malar regions before treatment. (Reprinted from Weber MB, MacHado RB, Hoefel IR, et al. Complication of cross-technique on boxcar acne scars: atrophy. *Dermatol Surg.* 2011;37:93-96, John Wiley and Sons www.interscience.wiley.com.)

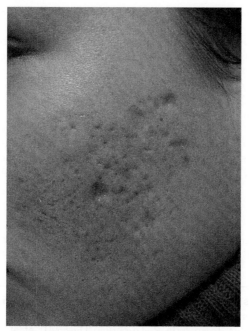

FIGURE 2.—Atrophy in some of the treated scars, after second application. (Reprinted from Weber MB, MacHado RB, Hoefel IR, et al. Complication of cross-technique on boxcar acne scars: atrophy. *Dermatol Surg.* 2011;37:93-96, John Wiley and Sons www.interscience.wiley.com.)

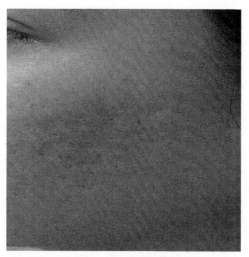

FIGURE 3.—Hypochromic scars 120 days after the first application of TCA acid. (Reprinted from Weber MB, MacHado RB, Hoefel IR, et al. Complication of cross-technique on boxcar acne scars: atrophy. *Dermatol Surg.* 2011;37:93-96, John Wiley and Sons www.interscience.wiley.com.)

(Figs 1-3). The authors state that the trichloroacetic acid (TCA) was applied with a sharpened applicator. However, it is not specified what this applicator was. The CROSS technique can be performed using either a 30-gauge needle or wooden toothpicks of varying sharpness. After the first treatment, the ice pick scar will become both more shallow and more narrow. With subsequent treatments, it may be necessary to use a finer applicator to avoid getting TCA on surrounding normal skin. If TCA does inadvertently touch adjacent normal skin, atrophy may be minimized or prevented by the immediate application of water to that area. The authors state that the atrophy will develop spontaneously, just as corticosteroid-induced atrophy does. It should be noted that atrophy from corticosteroid injections can be corrected by injecting large volumes of saline in the atrophic area.[1] This method may then similarly correct atrophy induced by TCA.

E. Graber, MD

Reference

1. Shumaker PR, Rao J, Goldman MP. Treatment of local, persistent cutaneous atrophy following corticosteroid injection with normal saline infiltration. *Dermatol Surg.* 2005;31:1340-1343.

Keratosis pilaris rubra and keratosis pilaris atrophicans faciei treated with pulsed dye laser: report of 10 cases
Alcántara González J, Boixeda P, Truchuelo Díez MT, et al (Ramon y Cajal Hosp, Madrid, Spain)
J Eur Acad Dermatol Venereol 25:710-714, 2011

Background.—Keratosis pilaris rubra (KPR) and keratosis pilaris atrophicans faciei (KPAF) are both keratinization disorders characterized by erythema and keratotic follicular papules usually located on cheeks, forehead, chin and eyebrows. Topical keratolytics, vitamin D3 analogues, antibiotics, topical and oral retinoids have been used with limited results. As this condition can be socially very limiting, the need for an effective treatment has led to the use of other technologies such as pulsed dye laser (PDL) or intense pulsed light.

Objective.—The aim of this study was to assess the efficacy and safety of PDL in patients with KPR or KPAF.

Methods.—Ten patients with KPR or KPAF were treated with two to seven sessions of PDL at 595-nm wavelength. Laser therapy was performed using a spot size of 7 or 10 mm, a pulse duration of 0.5 or 1.5 ms and a fluence from 5 to 9 J/cm^2. Two dermatologists evaluated treatment effectiveness by means of photographs of the patients before starting and after finishing the therapy.

Results.—Complete resolution of erythema was achieved in three patients; clearance of erythema was >75% in the other seven patients. Transient purpura was present in all patients for about 2 weeks and one patient presented postinflammatory hyperpigmentation for 7 months.

Conclusion.—We consider that PDL is a good option for the treatment of KPR and KPAF. A marked reduction in erythema is achieved in all patients with a low incidence of side effects.

▶ This is an article that has prompted me to reconsider my approach to keratosis pilaris rubra (KPR) and KP atrophicans, both involving the face. My experience with pulsed dye laser at 585 and 595 nm has been disappointing with the typical purpuric doses for 1 to 2 treatments. These authors report a significantly different experience with purpuric settings. The fluences used and the air cooling would suggest that this is a Cynosure device. It is important to identify the brand of laser used, because these instruments do perform differently. Two to 7 treatments were required to achieve the excellent results obtained in this case series, with most patients having 3 to 4 treatments. Of the 10 patients treated, 6 received intermuscular methylprednisolone to avoid significant facial edema. The data given would suggest a cautious approach with multiple treatments to see significant improvement. The patients will have to be aware that purpura lasting up to 2 weeks and significant swelling are to be expected.

E. A. Tanghetti, MD

Contribution of lip proportions to facial aesthetics in different ethnicities: A three-dimensional analysis
Wong WW, Davis DG, Camp MC, et al (Loma Linda Univ Dept of Plastic Surgery, CA)
J Plast Reconstr Aesthet Surg 63:2032-2039, 2010

Background.—Lip augmentations are commonly performed procedures in the United States, with annual numbers surpassing 100 000. While lips contribute to facial beauty, the relative influence of this feature to whole facial appeal has not yet been established. What is also of increasing interest is the consideration of ethnic differences in the evaluation of beauty. However, most current anthropometric measurements refer to Caucasians, and their use in the treatment of Asian American patients would be inappropriate.

Methods.—Three-dimensional models of 197 male and female Caucasian, Chinese and Korean subjects were created using surface-imaging technology. The lips and corresponding faces from these models were ranked according to subjective aesthetic appeal by 20 male and female raters of various ages, occupations and ethnicities. The raters' results were subsequently compared with individually measured lip parameters.

Results.—Rankings between lips and their corresponding whole faces differed greatly. Lips that were rated as the most attractive were smaller than average in midline upper lip surface heights, bilateral paramedian lip surface heights, upper lip angles and volume in the lower lip. Both Asian groups exhibited significantly different lip parameters and lip-projection volumes from that of Caucasians.

Conclusions.—The results from this study suggest that there are indeed measurable differences in the baseline Asian lip morphology as compared with Caucasians. Tailoring lip enhancement treatment to each individual's anatomy, ethnic background and personal goals can optimise outcomes. What is also of interest is that lips did not contribute as much to facial attractiveness as previously thought.

▶ This well-done study is notable in several ways. Primarily, it may change the way physicians approach lip augmentation. In general, this study demonstrated that a thinner upper lip was found to be more aesthetically pleasing. This may cause physicians to favor augmentation of the lower lip rather than the upper lip. Also revealed in this study was a discrepancy between lip and overall face scores in determining overall facial aesthetics. In other words, "lips do not carry as influential a role as previously assumed in the evaluation of an attractive face." An attractive lip does not lead to an overall attractive appearance as other facial features do. This finding may lead physicians to counsel patients to place priority on other facial structures when considering cosmetic improvements. The authors are to be commended for their objective measurements of lips and the varying lip locations from which these measurements were taken. Unfortunately, the lips were measured and viewed from only 1 position. The observers were not asked to evaluate the aesthetic appeal of smiling, frowning, grimacing, or puckering lips. Throughout the manuscript, the authors reiterate the "the current trend of enhancing upper lip volume for increasing youth fullness and beauty." However, the description of this practice as "the current trend" is never cited, thus giving no validity to this claim. I was taught, as I know a number of others have been, that the ideal lip consists of a lower lip that is 1.5 times the volume of the upper lip. Perhaps a study is needed to accurately capture the physician approach to lip augmentation. Regardless, it is not always up to the physician to dictate the patient's treatment. In the arena of cosmetic procedures, the patient needs to be satisfied with the end aesthetic result. Therefore, it is beneficial for the physician and patient to communicate so that the lip augmentation is ultimately pleasing to the patient.

E. Graber, MD

Nonablative 1550-nm fractional laser therapy versus triple topical therapy for the treatment of melasma: a randomized controlled pilot study
Kroon MW, Wind BS, Beek JF, et al (Univ of Amsterdam, The Netherlands)
J Am Acad Dermatol 64:516-523, 2011

Background.—Various treatments are currently available for melasma. However, results are often disappointing.

Objective.—We sought to assess the efficacy and safety of nonablative 1550-nm fractional laser therapy and compare results with those obtained with triple topical therapy (the gold standard).

Methods.—Twenty female patients with moderate to severe melasma and Fitzpatrick skin types II to V were treated either with nonablative fractional laser therapy or triple topical therapy (hydroquinone 5%, tretinoin 0.05%, and triamcinolone acetonide 0.1% cream) once daily for 8 weeks in a randomized controlled observer-blinded study. Laser treatment was performed every 2 weeks for a total of 4 times. Physician Global Assessment was assessed at 3 weeks, 3 months, and 6 months after the last treatment.

Results.—Physician Global Assessment improved (*P* < .001) in both groups at 3 weeks. There was no difference in Physician Global Assessment between the two groups. Mean treatment satisfaction and recommendation were significantly higher in the laser group at 3 weeks (*P* < .05). However, melasma recurred in 5 patients in both groups after 6 months. Side effects in the laser group were erythema, burning sensation, facial edema, and pain; in the triple group side effects were erythema, burning, and scaling.

Limitations.—Limitations were: small number of patients; only one set of laser parameters; and a possible difference in motivation between groups.

Conclusions.—Nonablative fractional laser therapy is safe and comparable in efficacy and recurrence rate with triple topical therapy. It may be a useful alternative treatment option for melasma when topical bleaching is ineffective or not tolerated. Different laser settings and long-term maintenance treatment should be tested in future studies.

▶ This winter-time study showed equal efficacy in using a triple topical therapy consisting of tretinoin, a low-potency topical corticosteroid, and a 5% hydroquinone with a 1550-nm nonablative fractional device. Unfortunately, there was no control group, but the study did show equivalent results with the topical preparation compared with the device alone. From a cost and convenience perspective, topical therapy appears to have distinct advantages.

E. A. Tanghetti, MD

Analysis of Postoperative Complications for Superficial Liposuction: A Review of 2398 Cases

Kim YH, Cha SM, Naidu S, et al (Hanyang Univ, Seoul, Korea; Sein Aesthetic Clinic, Seoul, Korea; Natl Univ Hosp, Singapore; et al)
Plast Reconstr Surg 127:863-871, 2011

Background.—Superficial liposuction has found its application in maximizing and creating a lifting effect to achieve a better aesthetic result. Due to initial high complication rates, these procedures were generally accepted as risky. In a response to the increasing concerns over the safety and efficacy of superficial liposuction, the authors describe their 14-year experience of performing superficial liposuction and analysis of postoperative complications associated with these procedures.

Methods.—From March of 1995 to December of 2008, the authors performed superficial liposuction on 2398 patients. Three subgroups were incorporated according to liposuction methods as follows: power-assisted liposuction alone (subgroup 1), power-assisted liposuction combined with ultrasound energy (subgroup 2), and power-assisted liposuction combined with external ultrasound and postoperative Endermologie (subgroup 3). Statistical analyses for complications were performed among subgroups.

Results.—The mean age was 42.8 years, mean body mass index was 27.9 kg/m^2, and mean volume of total aspiration was 5045 cc. Overall complication rate was 8.6 percent (206 patients). Four cases of skin necroses and two cases of infections were included. The most common complication was postoperative contour irregularity. Power-assisted liposuction combined with external ultrasound with or without postoperative Endermologie was seen to decrease the overall complication rate, contour irregularity, and skin necrosis. There were no statistical differences regarding other complications.

Conclusion.—Superficial liposuction has potential risks for higher complications compared with conventional suction techniques, especially postoperative contour irregularity, which can be minimized with proper selection of candidates for the procedure, avoiding overzealous suctioning of superficial layer, and using a combination of ultrasound energy techniques.

▶ Liposuction is a popular aesthetic procedure, and in recent years, superficial liposuction has been used as an alternative to conventional suction lipectomy. Despite its numerous advantages, superficial liposuction techniques are not without complications and, in fact, have been generally considered as risky. To gain a better understanding of the potential complications and efficacy, an analysis of 2398 patients that had undergone superficial liposuction over a 14-year period was completed. The focus of this review was to provide an informative analysis of the potential postoperative complications that are likely to be seen with the various superficial liposuction techniques, and to that end this analysis of a large number of cases meets its objective. The article also provides some limited guidance on potential correction techniques and treatments for a few of the complications.

Patients were divided into 3 subgroups: those that had power-assisted liposuction alone; those with power-assisted liposuction plus external ultrasonic energy; and those with power-assisted liposuction plus external ultrasonic energy combined with postoperative Endermologie. A range of complications were noted, including contour irregularities, seroma formation, hyperpigmentation, asymmetry, hypertrophic scars, chronic induration, skin necrosis, and infection. The most common complication noted was contour irregularities, which are considered major since they significantly decrease patient satisfaction. Based on the findings, the potential for contour irregularities was decreased significantly by coupling power-assisted liposuction with external ultrasonic techniques. The incidence of contour irregularities was not decreased by a statistically significant rate after the use of Endermologie. In fact, Endermologie did not show any statistically significant differences in any of the aforementioned complications versus use of power-assisted liposuction with external ultrasonic energy. Use of Endermologie was shown, however, to reduce postoperative pain, edema, and ecchymosis.

The most devastating complications associated with superficial liposuction were skin necrosis (4 cases) and infection (2 cases). All of the skin necrosis complications occurred in patients treated with power-assisted liposuction alone and did not occur after the use of external ultrasound. However, the use of ultrasound could not be definitively related to the lack of skin necrosis in subsequent cases. Patients who developed skin necrosis were some of the first patients treated with superficial liposuction, all were smokers, and affected cases involved the lower extremities. Thus, caution should be provided to all patients about smoking, especially for liposuction on the lower extremities.

Overall, the article provides a complete detailed evaluation of the complications associated with superficial liposuction and serves as a good source of review for any practitioner considering the addition of superficial liposuction to their practice, even if it is performed by an associate or partner.

B. D. Michaels, DO

J. Q. Del Rosso, DO

Management of Rhinophyma with Coblation
Roje Z, Racic G (Split Univ Hosp, Croatia)
Dermatol Surg 36:2057-2060, 2010

Background.—Rhinophyma is considered the most severe expression of the final stage of acne rosacea and is progressive and disfiguring to the nasal region. It is most common in Caucasian men age 40 to 60 years but its cause is as yet undetermined. Patients with rhinophyma may seek medical care because of nasal airway compromise or cosmetic deformity. The medical approach may be appropriate early in the progression of rhinophyma, but surgery is the only way to achieve a cure. Cryosurgery, electrosurgery, dermabrasion, scalpel excision, microdebridement, ultrasonic scalpel excision, carbon dioxide laser surgery, argon laser surgery, and yttrium aluminum garnet laser surgery have all been used to manage rhinophyma and achieved similar results in terms of cosmesis and postoperative morbidity. The major complications are hemostasis, uncontrolled tissue destruction, a high scarring rate, and prolonged wound healing times. Coblation surgery is a type of radiofrequency surgery that was originally used for otorhinolaryngologic operations on soft tissues in the head and neck. Coblation produces tissue temperatures between 60° and 70° C without direct contact between the tip of the device and local tissue. The gap between the two is filled with saline solution, which contains the ions that destroy the intercellular bonds in tissues, producing molecular dissociation. Coblation removes the pathologically altered tissue and provides hemostasis through an ablation mode and a coagulation mode. The thermal damage to adjacent tissues is minimal, there is less postoperative morbidity, blood loss intraoperatively is low, and both surgeon and patient tend to be more comfortable.

Case Report.—Man, 70, had rhinophyma for 3 years but had refused treatment previously. There was no nasal obstruction but physical examination revealed diffuse hypertrophy of the sebaceous glands and subcutaneous nasal tissues. Coblation was performed with the patient under general anesthesia. Hypertrophied tissue was debulked to a normal appearance, preserving the pilosebaceous units. A nearly bloodless field permitted excellent visualization, so the procedure lasted just 20 minutes. A thin layer of petroleum jelly and petroleum jelly gauze were applied postoperatively to prevent desiccation. Reepithelialization was accomplished within 2 weeks, with cosmetic results satisfying for both patient and surgeon within 6 months, although the reepithelialized area was hypopigmented.

Conclusions.—Surgery is the definitive treatment for patients with rhinophyma. Coblation surgery accomplishes the removal of excess tissue and achieves acceptable cosmetic results relative to color, texture, and symmetry. The patient has less postoperative pain, less damage to adjacent tissues, less blood loss intraoperatively, and less morbidity postoperatively. The surgeon is afforded a good overall view and control of the surgical site and accomplishes the procedure efficiently and quickly without the need for antibiotics or analgesics postoperatively.

▶ Coblation is another modality that can be used in the management of rhinophyma. We must recognize that physical modalities are important for remodeling fixed phymatous changes.

E. A. Tanghetti, MD

Blinded Evaluation of the Effects of Hyaluronic Acid Filler Injections on First Impressions

Dayan SH, Arkins JP, Gal TJ (Chicago Ctr for Facial Plastic Surgery, IL; DeNova Res, Chicago, IL; Univ of Kentucky, Lexington)
Dermatol Surg 36:1866-1873, 2010

Background.—Facial appearance has profound influence on the first impression that is projected to others.

Objective.—To determine the effects that complete correction of the nasolabial folds (NLFs) with hyaluronic acid (HA) filler has on the first impression one makes.

Methods.—Twenty-two subjects received injections of HA filler into the NLFs. Photographs of the face in a relaxed pose were taken at baseline, optimal correction visit, and 4 weeks after optimal correction. Three hundred four blinded evaluators completed a survey rating first impression on various measures of success for each photo. In total, 5,776 first impressions were recorded, totaling 46,208 individual assessments of first impression.

Results.—Our findings indicate a significant improvement in mean first impression in the categories of dating success, attractiveness, financial success, relationship success, athletic success, and overall first impression at the optimal correction visit. At 4 weeks after the optimal correction visit, significance was observed in all categories measured: social skills, academic performance, dating success, occupational success, attractiveness, financial success, relationship success, athletic success, and overall first impression.

Conclusion.—Full correction of the NLFs with HA filler significantly and positively influences the first impression an individual projects.

▶ With this study, the authors confirm what many of us have already suspected to be true: Hyaluronic acid filler use improves appearance and perception by others. Now we have hard data to substantiate that this is true. It is interesting that first impressions were only significantly better than baseline at 4 weeks after full correction rather than immediately at full correction. This may be due in part to the erythema that is often seen immediately after injection. The temporary discoloration may have undermined the improvement of the fillers. In this study, only those with moderate to severe nasolabial folds were treated. These subjects received a fair amount of filler volume (2.45 mL on average after the initial treatment). It would be interesting to see whether the results of this study would be similar even with more subtle improvements. Additionally, this also causes one to wonder what is the minimal amount of filler needed to cause any improvement on first impression.

E. Graber, MD

Intraepidermal erbium:YAG laser resurfacing: Impact on the dermal matrix
Orringer JS, Rittié L, Hamilton T, et al (Univ of Michigan Med School, Ann Arbor)
J Am Acad Dermatol 64:119-128, 2011

Background.—Various minimally invasive treatments enhance the skin's appearance. Little is known about the molecular mechanisms whereby treatments working at the epidermal level might alter the dermis.

Objective.—We sought to quantify the molecular changes that result from erbium:yttrium-aluminium-garnet (Er:YAG) laser microablative resurfacing.

Methods.—We performed biochemical analyses after intraepidermal Er:YAG laser resurfacing of 10 patients. Immunohistochemical analysis and polymerase chain reaction technology were utilized to measure key biomarkers.

Results.—The basement membrane remained intact after intraepidermal microablation, as demonstrated by laminin γ2 immunostaining. Epidermal injury was demonstrated with acute up-regulation of keratin 16. An inflammatory response ensued as indicated by increases in cytokines interleukin 1 beta (IL-1β) and IL-8 as well as a substantial neutrophil infiltrate. Levels of cJun and JunB proteins, components of the transcription factor AP-1 complex, were also elevated. Up-regulation of extracellular matrix degrading proteinases matrix metalloproteinase 1 (MMP-1), MMP-3, and MMP-9 was noted. A transient increase in keratinocyte proliferation, as indicated by staining for Ki67, was observed. Increased expression of type I and type III procollagen was demonstrated.

Limitations.—The data presented are those that resulted from a single treatment session.

Conclusions.—Although microablation was confined to the uppermost epidermis, marked changes in epidermal and dermal structure and function were demonstrated after Er:YAG laser microablative resurfacing. We demonstrated substantial dermal matrix remodeling, including a degree of collagen production that compares favorably with some more invasive interventions. Dermal remodeling and stimulation of collagen production are associated with wrinkle reduction. Thus these results suggest that the skin's appearance may be enhanced by creating dermal changes through the use of superficially acting treatments.

▶ Dr. Orringer has done a series of articles evaluating the molecular effects of various lasers, light, mechanical, and photodynamic therapy on the skin. He has shown nicely in this study that purely epidermal ablation by an erbium:yttrium-aluminum-garnet laser results in significant dermal changes mediated by a number of factors generated by the epidermal damage. The light lunch-time laser peels do provide benefit. The real question is, how long lived are these changes? This type of wounding may make for an interesting home use device.

This is a thoughtful article that is worth your consideration and study.

E. A. Tanghetti, MD

Adverse reactions caused by consecutive injections of different fillers in the same facial region: risk assessment based on the results from the Injectable Filler Safety study
Bachmann F, Erdmann R, Hartmann V, et al (Charité-Universitätsmedizin Berlin, Germany; et al)
J Eur Acad Dermatol Venereol 25:902-912, 2011

Background.—The combination of different injectable fillers in one area is considered to increase the risk of adverse reactions.

Objectives.—To characterize adverse reactions in patients who received more than one filler in the same facial region.

Methods.—Data (up to July 2009) of the Injectable Filler Safety Study, a German-based registry for adverse filler reactions, was analysed descriptively. All cases were discussed individually.

Results.—In 22 of the 161 patients (13.7%), two or more different fillers were injected consecutively into the same facial region. All patients were female with an average age of 50.6 (SD 13.6) years. In 12 of the 22 patients (54.5%), a specific filler could be attributed to the adverse reactions whereas in the other 10 patients (45.5%), the filler was not clearly attributable to one filler substance causing the adverse reactions.

Conclusions.—With the continuous changes in the filler market, the combination of different fillers in one area becomes more likely. Based on our data, there is not a lot of evidence that the combination of different injectable fillers, specifically biodegradable fillers, in the same region increases the risk of adverse reactions.

▶ In this article the authors make a commendable effort to accurately assess the frequency of adverse events when two fillers are used in the same location. It is difficult to retrospectively interpret these data given interpatient disparities in time between filler injections, types of fillers used, and areas injected. There was also a relatively small data pool to analyze because the adverse events were collected from a limited geographic area. Whereas 22 of the 161 patients with adverse events had 2 fillers, in 7 of these patients a biodegradeable filler had been injected over 2 years before the onset of the reaction. Assuming that the biodegradeable filler would have completely absorbed by 2 years, any adverse event could not be attributed to the combination of fillers. This makes the true incidence of adverse events even lower (15 of 161). In several of the cases, it is plausible that the adverse event was not inherent to the filler or combination of fillers but was instead due to poor filler choice for the anatomic area treated. For example, it is not surprising that nodules would form after treating the lip with a permanent filler. The results here and of other studies do not support the theory that combining fillers may have a deleterious result. Instead, the proportion of adverse events with 2 fillers may mimic the proportion of patients who undergo treatment with 2 fillers. Larger, prospective studies are needed to more accurately evaluate the risk of combining fillers in the same anatomic area.

E. Graber, MD

Enhancing effect of pretreatment with topical niacin in the treatment of rosacea-associated erythema by 585-nm pulsed dye laser in Koreans: a randomized, prospective, split-face trial

Kim TG, Roh HJ, Cho SB, et al (Yonsei Univ College of Medicine, Seoul Korea; et al)

Br J Dermatol 164:573-579, 2011

Background.—Rosacea is a chronic dermatosis that is usually confined to the face. A pulsed dye laser (PDL) system has been proven to be effective in treating rosacea-associated erythema and telangiectasias. Niacin is a cutaneous vasodilator that can increase the chromophore through increased blood flow.

Objectives.—We hypothesized that increased blood flow by pretreatment with topical niacin could enhance the effect of PDL in the treatment of rosacea.

Methods.—Eighteen Korean patients with rosacea were recruited. Three sessions of 585-nm PDL using a subpurpuragenic dose with and without pretreatment with niacin cream were performed on randomly assigned half-faces at 3-week intervals. Erythema was assessed objectively by a polarization colour imaging system, and evaluations were also made by three blinded dermatologists. Patient satisfaction was evaluated using a 10-point visual analogue scale.

Results.—Fifteen patients completed this study. All patients showed an improvement in erythema after three sessions of PDL treatment both with and without niacin pretreatment ($P = 0.023$ and $P = 0.009$, respectively). There was no significant difference in the improvement of objective erythema between the two sides. However, based on physician assessment the overall clinical improvement on the niacin side was significantly higher ($P = 0.005$), and patient satisfaction was also higher on the niacin-pretreated side ($P = 0.007$). There were no remarkable side-effects, with the exception of transient erythema and oedema.

Conclusions.—Pretreatment with topical niacin safely enhanced the effect of 585-nm PDL treatment of rosacea-associated erythema in Koreans. Application of niacin can be helpful in overcoming the relatively lower effect of subpurpuragenic PDL in dark-skinned Asians.

▶ This study is important because it presents a novel, safe technique to enhance the efficacy of pulsed dye laser (PDL) treatment for rosacea. Although the small subject number is not ideal, the investigators used several methods for evaluating efficacy subjectively and objectively. Additionally, the authors eliminated potential confounding variables by using strict exclusion criteria. For example, patients were excluded if they had used any of many topical and oral therapeutic agents. The results may have been more striking if the investigators had used a different (PDL) system. The most commonly used PDL in the United States has a delayed cooling device that delivers a small burst of cryogen spray milliseconds before the laser firing. This spray of cryogen cools and protects the epidermis but also causes vasoconstriction. The particular PDL used in this study delivers concomitant cooling so that rather than a cryogen spray preceding the laser firing, forced cold air is constantly applied to the skin throughout the treatment. This constant cooling may cause further vasoconstriction, thus counteracting the vasodilatory effect of the niacin. If instead a PDL with the burst of cryogen cooling was used in this study, vasoconstriction may have been lessened, thus allowing the pretreatment with niacin to have a more substantial effect. The idea of niacin application before PDL treatment is intriguing and warrants further investigation. The technique introduced by the authors also prompts further thought into other methods whereby target chromophores can be enhanced to maximize laser results.

E. Graber, MD

Acne Scar Treatment with Subcision Using a 20-G Cataract Blade
Ayeni O, Carey W, Muhn C (McMaster Univ, Hamilton, Ontario, Canada)
Dermatol Surg 37:846-847, 2011

Background.—Subcision is a nonoperative technique for managing depressed acne scars. Scar bands within the dermis and subcutaneous tissue are released percutaneously. Release of the fibrous septa in the scar allows the formation of new connective tissue under the scar. Various instruments have been used to perform subcision, beginning with a tri-beveled hypodermic needle and including the commonly used 18-G 1.5-inch Nokor admix needle. The procedure using a 20-G cataract blade was described.

Procedure.—The 20-G microvitreoretinal (MVR) cataract blade incises the skin subdermally and just inferior to the acne scar. The tip of the blade has a dual-bevel arrangement, with blades on both sides. Moving in a back-and-forth sweep, immediate lifting is accomplished. Blood pooling beneath the scar serves as a spacer. The diamond-shaped blade and triangular point allow easy side-to-side motion for cutting, which avoids the tearing or shearing seen with other instruments.

Results.—Most patients have partial response, so one to three treatments may be needed. Patients who have current cystic acne, bleeding disorders, infection, or are using Accutane should not undergo subcision.

Conclusions.—The subcision procedure is enhanced by the use of a 20-G cataract blade. This extremely sharp instrument permits more controlled depth and precision in the incision, is sharp throughout the bevel's length so its cutting distance is greater than with the Nokor needle, and its handle makes it easier to grasp and allows the operator better visualization of the depth and angle of penetration.

▶ Subcision is a technique for elevating atrophic acne scars or surgical scars by inserting a needle under the skin and moving it back and forth in multiple directions to sever any fibrous attachments and create a pocket under the scar. This allows the scar to raise to a more normal level. In clinical trials, it has a reported improvement rate of 25% to 90%.[1-4] Ayeni and colleagues report the use of an instrument that may make subsicion of acne scars more efficient and effective. The authors state that the 20-gauge cataract blade, which is tri-beveled and has very sharp blades on both sides of its tip, cuts the fibrous attachments often found under acne scars more easily than needles currently used for subcision, which are 18-gauge NoKor or standard hypodermic needles. Currently there are no comparative studies evaluating the efficacy of different needles in performing subcision. Anecdotally, I have started using this instrument in my practice for subcision and have found it to be very effective.

D. Fife, MD

References

1. Alam M, Omura N, Kaminer MS. Subcision for acne scarring: technique and outcomes in 40 patients. *Dermatol Surg.* 2005;31:310-317.
2. Balighi K, Robati RM, Moslehi H, Robati AM. Subcision in acne scar with and without subdermal implant: a clinical trial. *J Eur Acad Dermatol Venereol.* 2008; 22:707-711.
3. Aalami Harandi S, Balighi K, Lajevardi V, Akbari E. Subcision-suction method: a new successful combination therapy in treatment of atrophic acne scars and other depressed scars. *J Eur Acad Dermatol Venerol.* 2011;25:92-99.
4. Sage RJ, Lopiccolo MC, Liu A, Mahmoud BH, Tierney EP, Kouba DJ. Subcuticular incision versus naturally sourced porcine collagen filler for acne scars: a randomized split-face comparison. *Dermatol Surg.* 2011;37:426-431.

Treatment of Dermatosis Papulosa Nigra in 10 Patients: a Comparison Trial of Electrodesiccation, Pulsed Dye Laser, and Curettage

Garcia MS, Azari R, Eisen DB (Univ of California at Davis, Sacramento)
Dermatol Surg 36:1968-1972, 2010

Background.—Dermatosis papulosa nigra (DPN) is a common variant of seborrheic keratoses in darkly pigmented individuals. Treatment options include cryosurgery, curettage, electrosurgery, and shave removal.

Objective.—To compare the efficacy and complications of pulsed dye laser (PDL) therapy for the treatment of DPN with those of curettage and electrodesiccation.

Methods and Materials.—Randomized, controlled, single-center, evaluator-blinded trial of 10 patients with at least four clinically diagnosed lesions.

Results.—All 10 patients completed the study. Mean lesion clearance was 96% for curettage, 92.5% for electrodesiccation, and 88% for laser. There was no significant difference between the three treatment modalities. All three techniques had an overall cosmetic outcome of good for most patients. Five of the 10 patients preferred electrodesiccation. Patients rated the laser as the most painful treatment method. The most common adverse outcome was hyperpigmentation. There were no significant differences between the treatment groups for any of the measured outcomes.

Conclusion.—The efficacy of PDL in the treatment of DPN is not significantly different from the already established treatment modalities of electrodesiccation and curettage.

▶ There are various treatment options available for dermatosis papulosa nigra presenting as multiple individual taglike or small papular lesions seen primarily in adult black patients. The lesions are multiple, usually involve the cheeks and periocular region bilaterally, and histologically are seborrheic keratoses. Garcia et al sought to determine if there were better treatment outcomes (both in efficacy and complications) with pulsed dye laser (PDL) versus 2 of the more common means of treatment: electrodessication or focal curettage. Ultimately, there was no difference in efficacy among these 3 modalities, and hyperpigmentation, the most common adverse effect, occurred in all. However, posttreatment hyperpigmentation cleared in all patients in 6 months. It should be noted that curettage had a slightly higher clearance rate, but electrodessication was preferred in 5 of 10 patients. PDL was the painful option. This study was limited by its sample size of only 10 patients. As noted by the article itself, had there been a larger treatment group, there may have been differences among the treatment options. This study thus provides an opportunity for a further, more expansive, investigation on this issue. In general though, this article provides useful and relevant treatment data that are clinically valuable to practitioners on a relatively common dermatologic condition, that is, that PDL offered no advantage over the other 2 conventional methods of treatment in this small group of patients.

B. D. Michaels, DO
J. Q. Del Rosso, DO

Improvement in Nasolabial Folds with a Hyaluronic Acid Filler Using a Cohesive Polydensified Matrix Technology: Results from an 18-Month Open-Label Extension Trial

Narins RS, Coleman WP III, Donofrio LM, et al (Dermatology Surgery and Laser Ctr, White Plains, NY; Tulane Univ, New Orleans, LA; Yale Univ, New Haven, CT; et al)
Dermatol Surg 36:1800-1808, 2010

Background.—Repeat treatments of nonpermanent dermal fillers are used in the long-term treatment of wrinkles and folds and to volumize.

Objective.—To determine the safety and effectiveness of a nonanimal-sourced hyaluronic acid (HA) (which uses a cohesive polydensified matrix

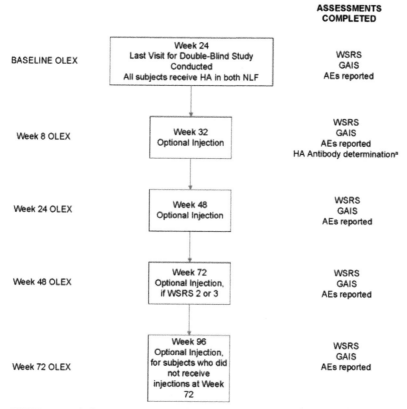

FIGURE 1.—Study flow chart. [a]Serum samples for determination of hyaluronic acid (HA) antibodies were drawn and stored at baseline (of the double-blind study) and again at Week 32. Antibody determinations from the two sets of samples were compared. NLF, nasolabial fold; WSRS, Wrinkle Severity Rating Scale; GAIS, Global Aesthetic Improvement Scale; AEs, adverse events; OLEX, open-label extension study. (Reprinted from Narins RS, Coleman WP III, Donofrio LM, et al. Improvement in nasolabial folds with a hyaluronic acid filler using a cohesive polydensified matrix technology: results from an 18-month open-label extension trial. *Dermatol Surg.* 2010;36:1800-1808, with permission from Blackwell Publishing.)

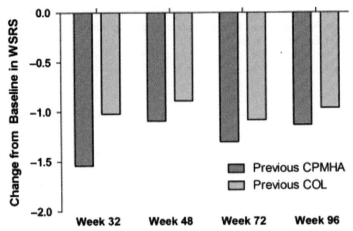

FIGURE 2.—Change from baseline in Wrinkle Severity Rating Scale (WSRS: 0 = absent, 1 = mild, 2 = moderate, 3 = severe, 4 = extreme) during treatment with nonanimal stabilized hyaluronic acid (HA) with cohesive polydensified matrix technology (CPMHA). WSRS score at study entry (double-blind): Previous HA 2.51; Previous bovine collagen (COL) 2.47. (Reprinted from Narins RS, Coleman WP III, Donofrio LM, et al. Improvement in nasolabial folds with a hyaluronic acid filler using a cohesive polydensified matrix technology: results from an 18-month open-label extension trial. *Dermatol Surg.* 2010;36: 1800-1808, with permission from Blackwell Publishing.)

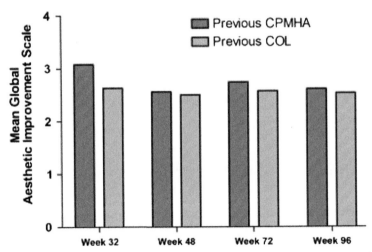

FIGURE 3.—Summary of Global Aesthetic Improvement Scale (GAIS: 0 = worse, 1 = no change, 2 = improved, 3 = much improved, 4 = very much improved) during treatment with nonanimal stabilized hyaluronic acid with cohesive polydensified matrix technology (CPMHA) (treating physician rating). COL, bovine collagen. (Reprinted from Narins RS, Coleman WP III, Donofrio LM, et al. Improvement in nasolabial folds with a hyaluronic acid filler using a cohesive polydensified matrix technology: results from an 18-month open-label extension trial. *Dermatol Surg.* 2010;36:1800-1808, with permission from Blackwell Publishing.)

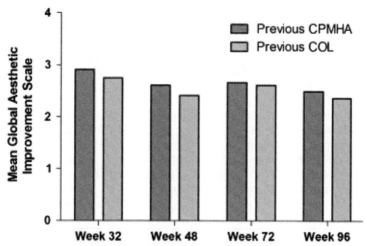

FIGURE 4.—Summary of Global Aesthetic Improvement Scale (GAIS: 0 = worse, 1 = no change, 2 = improved, 3 = much improved, 4 = very much improved) during treatment with nonanimal stabilized hyaluronic acid with cohesive polydensified matrix technology (CPMHA) (subject rating). COL = bovine collagen. (Reprinted from Narins RS, Coleman WP III, Donofrio LM, et al. Improvement in nasolabial folds with a hyaluronic acid filler using a cohesive polydensified matrix technology: results from an 18-month open-label extension trial. *Dermatol Surg.* 2010;36:1800-1808, with permission from Blackwell Publishing.)

TABLE 2.—Summary of Study Injections

| | N, Volume (Mean ± Standard Deviation) | | |
Week	Previous Nonanimal Stabilized Hyaluronic Acid with Cohesive Polydensified Matrix Technology	Previous Collagen	Combined
24	95, 0.71 ± 0.32	95, 1.04 ± 0.50	95, 1.75 ± 0.68
32	7, 0.46 ± 0.16	36, 0.73 ± 0.27	38, 0.78 ± 0.32
48	69, 0.69 ± 0.32	70, 0.75 ± 0.32	70, 1.43 ± 0.55
72	18, 0.67 ± 0.30	18, 0.79 ± 0.40	18, 1.46 ± 0.62
96	58, 0.63 ± 0.24	57, 0.71 ± 0.32	58, 1.32 ± 0.47
24 to 96 (cumulative)	95, 1.75 ± 0.85	95, 2.45 ± 1.23	95, 4.20 ± 1.88

(CPM) technology [CPMHA]) for the treatment of nasolabial folds (NLFs) during an 18-month open-label extension trial.

Methods and Materials.—Ninety-five of 118 subjects continued with this optional open-label extension of a split-face, double-blind trial. All subjects received CPMHA in both NLFs at 24 weeks after treatment in this study and were assessed at weeks 32, 48, 72, and 96. Touch-ups were allowed for optimal correction. Safety was assessed according to reported adverse events (AEs) and serum antibody measurement.

Results.—At all four post-week 24 time points, the severity of the NLFs showed a decrease from baseline on the Wrinkle Severity Rating Scale. The effects persisted in the majority (~80%) of subjects without repeat treatment for at least one interval of 48 weeks. The study filler was well tolerated, with only one related AE (injection site bruising) reported. Little potential for immunogenic reactions was identified.

Conclusion.—This CPMHA is a well-tolerated and effective treatment for at least 48 weeks in the majority of subjects for the correction of moderate to severe NLFs with repeat injections given over an 18-month period (Figs 1-4, Table 2).

▶ This is a very useful article that highlights some important news for those injecting hyaluronic acid (HA) fillers. First, this new HA filler is safe and effective for long-term use in patients. It is a continuation study with repeat injections given to study participants, and its effectiveness with repeat injections was demonstrated. Second, it showed that less volume was needed over time; this is important in maximizing results with fillers.

M. H. Gold, MD

Subcision-suction method: a new successful combination therapy in treatment of atrophic acne scars and other depressed scars

Aalami Harandi S, Balighi K, Lajevardi V, et al (Parsian Laser Clinic, Bandar Abbas, Iran; Tehran Univ of Med Sciences, Iran)
J Eur Acad Dermatol Venereol 25:92-99, 2011

Background.—Among therapeutic modalities of acne scars, subcision is a simple, safe procedure with a different and basic mechanism for correcting atrophic and depressed scars. Subcision releases scar surfaces from underlying attachments and induces connective tissue formation beneath the scar directly, without injury to the skin surface. Therefore, subcision is a valuable method, but due to high recurrence rate, its efficacy is mild to moderate.

Objectives.—To increase the efficacy of subcision, a new complementary treatment of repeated suction sessions was added at the recurrence period of subcised scars.

Methods.—In this before and after trail, 58 patients with mild to severe acne scars of various types (rolling, superficial and deep boxcar, pitted), chicken pox, traumatic and surgical depressed scars were treated by superficial dermal undermining, with mainly 23-guage needles. The protocol for suctioning was: start of suction on third day after subcision for flat and depressing subcised scars and its continuation at least every other day for 2 weeks.

Results.—Forty-six patients followed the protocol completely, had 60—90% improvement in depth and size of scars (significant improvement) with mean: 71.73%. 28.2% of them had '80% improvement or more' (excellent improvement). Twelve patients started suction late and/or had long interval suction-sessions, had 30—60% improvement (moderate improvement) with mean: 43.75%.

Conclusion.—Frequent suctioning at the recurrence period of subcision increases subcision efficacy remarkably and causes significant and persistent improvement in short time, without considerable complication, in depressed scars of the face. Therefore, subcision-suction method is introduced as a new effective treatment.

▶ The authors present a novel method of combining subcision with negative pressure to improve scars. While it appears that the authors achieved excellent results in many of their patients, the methods of evaluating improvement seem somewhat questionable. It is not clearly explained if different criteria were judged or if investigators rated overall improvement. The results were also determined by the investigators and not by blinded observers. However, the similarity between the investigators' and patients' assessments seems to indicate that the ratings were not skewed by having nonblinded evaluators. While the reported results were impressive, the adverse event profile is a bit concerning. The authors state that there was some discoloration for about 2 months in one of the groups. There are no specific numbers given or explanation as to what this discoloration was. Additionally, 22 scars became hypertrophic after treatment. While the authors note that this was only 1.7% of the treated scars, a hypertrophic scar is cosmetically undesirable and conspicuous. Considering that there were only 58 patients in this study, 22 hypertrophic scars are notable. This treatment modality is an interesting concept that needs to be further studied before being widely used on patients.

E. Graber, MD

Split-Face Comparison of Intense Pulsed Light and Nonablative 1,064-nm Q-Switched Laser in Skin Rejuvenation
Huo M-H, Wang Y-Q, Yang X (Plastic Surgery Hosp, Beijing, China)
Dermatol Surg 37:52-57, 2011

Background.—Multiple nonablative skin rejuvenation techniques have been used to improve facial aging.

Objective.—To compare rejuvenation efficiency of intense pulsed light (IPL) with nonablative 1,064-nm Q-switched laser in Asian patients.

Materials & Methods.—Twelve female subjects were enrolled and received five sessions of treatments at 2-week intervals. A split-face study was performed, with IPL applied to the left side of the face and nonablative 1,064-nm Q-switched laser to the right side.

Results.—All assessments showed significant skin rejuvenation. For the improvement of skin texture, pore size, and sebum secretion, similar efficiency from laser and IPL was observed. For lightening of skin tone and macula, the IPL was more efficient than the laser after the first treatment, although no further clinical improvement resulted after three treatments. The laser gradually lightened the skin tone and macula and was ultimately more efficient than the IPL after five treatments.

Conclusion.—A series of IPL and nonablative 1,064-nm Q-switched laser treatments were performed with similar efficiency and safety for the improvement in skin texture, pore size, and sebum secretion. IPL was faster, but nonablative 1,064-nm Q-switched laser was more effective in improving skin tone and macula.

▶ This article is of interest because it is a split-face comparison of 2 commonly used methods of skin rejuvenation. Understanding the different outcomes of these methods would shape our practice of skin rejuvenation. Unfortunately, this study is plagued with weaknesses, making it difficult to reliably interpret the results. The small sample size hinders the study quality as do the few exclusion criteria. Although subjects that used oral retinoids were excluded, no mention was given to whether subjects were prevented from using any topical agents prior to or during treatments. It is difficult to draw conclusions from this study because broad ranges of settings were used rather than a standardized treatment protocol. For example, a range of fluences was used, and the number of treatment passes varied from patient to patient. Because a spectrum of settings was used, there could be misleading results between subjects and within the same subject. For instance, if subject x had the left side of his or her face treated with relatively high intense pulsed light (IPL) settings and the right side of his or her face was treated with relatively low laser settings, one may be falsely led to believe that the IPL treatment is superior. In addition to the lack of standardization of treatment settings, one also has to question the specific settings used for the laser treatment. The authors noted that there was no posttreatment darkening of pigmented lesions after laser treatment as opposed to the darkening that was viewed following IPL treatment. Typically, there is darkening of pigmented lesions for several days following any Q-switched laser treatment. The lack of this finding makes one think that the laser settings were probably too low. In theory, this study is a great idea, but it was poorly executed. Therefore, it is difficult to draw any conclusions from this article.

E. Graber, MD

Granuloma Faciale Treated with 595-nm Pulsed Dye Laser
Fikrle T, Pizinger K (Charles Univ, Pilsen, Czech Republic)
Dermatol Surg 37:102-104, 2011

Background.—The cause of granuloma faciale is unknown, but its manifestations include one or more sharply bordered, infiltrated nodules or plaques that are red-brown in color. This rare, chronic, and benign condition predominantly affects the face of adult Caucasian patients, most notably the cheeks, temples, nose, earlobes, and scalp. Seldom are lesions found in other places and most are asymptomatic. On histopathologic evaluation, the epidermis is normal, but neutrophils and eosinophils accumulate around vessels of the dermis. Early lesions can demonstrate leukocytoclastic vasculitis. Granuloma faciale lesions are persistent and resistant to treatment.

Methods.—Four patients with granuloma faciale were treated with the pulsed dye laser (PDL). All cases had been confirmed histopathologically and all lesions were located on the face. The lesions had been present for 3 to 9 years and were unresponsive to previous treatments with local steroids and cryotherapy. The PDL treatments were delivered using a 7-mm overlapping spot at 9 to 10 J/cm² and a pulse duration of 1.5 ms. The device included an integrated cooling spray. Each patient received treatments 6 to 8 weeks apart, with the number of treatments varying depending on the response. If the lesion did not regress significantly between treatments, once-daily application of a local steroid was added. Follow-up was planned for 6 months.

Results.—Excellent results were achieved, with three of the patients having complete flattening and bleaching of all treated lesions. The PDL was used alone for two patients and combined with steroid cream for two patients. All patients experienced pain with the PDL treatments as well as transient hemorrhage. Two had mild hyperpigmentation, and one had mild central hypopigmentation. These pigmentation distortions resolved in 3 to 4 months. The laser produced no permanent side effects and no recurrence in the three patients evaluated after at least 6 months.

Conclusions.—The PDL produced a marked cosmetic improvement in these patients. Although their granuloma faciale caused minimal subjective health problems, the cosmetic effects were distressing. PDL is accompanied by short-term pain and skin hemorrhage, but none of these effects have been permanent. Lasers other than the 595-nm form have been used, but they were less successful in resolving granuloma faciale lesions.

▶ Granuloma faciale is often poorly responsive to medical therapy. This article reminds us that granuloma faciale usually responds nicely to the pulse dye laser with only a few treatments needed.

E. A. Tanghetti, MD

Percutaneous Collagen Induction Versus Full-Concentration Trichloroacetic Acid in the Treatment of Atrophic Acne Scars

Leheta T, El Tawdy A, Abdel Hay R, et al (Cairo Univ, Egypt)
Dermatol Surg 37:207-216, 2011

Background.—Percutaneous collagen induction (PCI) promotes removal of damaged collagen and induces more collagen immediately under the epidermis. The chemical reconstruction of skin scars (CROSS) method is a focal application of full-concentration trichloroacetic acid (TCA) to atrophic acne scars. The CROSS method has the advantage of reconstructing acne scars by increasing dermal thickening and collagen production.

Objective.—To compare the safety and efficacy of PCI and the 100% TCA CROSS method for the treatment of atrophic acne scars.

Materials and Methods.—Thirty participants were randomly equally divided into two groups; group 1 underwent four sessions (4 weeks apart) of PCI, and group 2 underwent four sessions (4 weeks apart) of 100% TCA CROSS.

Results.—Acne scarring improved in 100% of patients. Scar severity scores improved by a mean of 68.3% ($p < .001$) in group 1 and a mean of 75.3% ($p < .001$) in group 2. The difference in the degree of improvement was not statistically significant between the groups ($p = .47$).

Conclusions.—PCI and 100% TCA CROSS were effective in the treatment of atrophic acne scars.

▶ This study is notable because it confirms the belief that percutaneous collagen induction (PCI) and the trichloroacetic acid (TCA) CROSS technique both work well for treating acne scars. The new information provided in this article is that both treatments work equally well. Not surprisingly, the PCI method worked better for rolling scars and the CROSS method worked better for ice-pick scars. This makes sense because rolling scars have deep fibrous bands pulling down the scars at their apex. To improve these scars, it is necessary to break up the fibrous bands and lay down new collagen, a process that is possible by the PCI technique rather than the CROSS technique. Although it was stated that there was no significant difference in the outcome between the 2 groups, the authors did not specify whether there was a significant difference in the type of scars between the 2 groups. It is very difficult to accurately capture the 3-dimensional nature of atrophic acne scars in 2-dimensional photographs. Therefore, precise means of photography are needed to correctly evaluate the degree of improvement. The camera used in this study was a simple point-and-shoot model, and it was not mentioned whether the photographs were taken in a standardized fashion, if the same photographer took the photographs, and whether similar lighting was used. Although the investigators demonstrated a significant response to both treatments, there could have been an even greater improvement noted if there was a longer follow-up period. Neocollagenesis takes 3 months after completion of the last treatment. The final follow-up for this study was done just 4 weeks after the last treatment. Larger-scale studies with a breakdown of outcomes correlated with acne scar types, standardized photography, and a longer follow-up period would more accurately identify scar improvement from PCI and CROSS.

E. Graber, MD

Evaluation of the Effect of Fractional Laser with Radiofrequency and Fractionated Radiofrequency on the Improvement of Acne Scars

Peterson JD, Palm MD, Kiripolsky MG, et al (Dermatology Cosmetic Laser Associates of La Jolla, San Diego, CA)
Dermatol Surg 37:1260-1267, 2011

Background.—Options for acne scar reduction include peels, subcision, fillers, lasers, dermabrasion, and surgical excision, although not all are applicable in darker skin types. A novel device with a handpiece combining optical and radiofrequency (RF) energies along with a fractionated RF handpiece is available for nonablative resurfacing.

Objectives.—Our primary objective was to evaluate the improvement in acne scars and skin texture. Secondary objectives were determination of patient satisfaction and comfort and evaluation of scar pigmentation improvement. Patients received five treatments at 30-day intervals. Post-treatment follow-up visits were performed 30 and 90 days after the last treatment.

Results.—A 72.3% decrease ($p < .001$) was observed on the acne scar scale from day 1 to 210. From day 30 to 210, investigator-rated changes in scarring, texture, and pigmentation improved 68.2% ($p < .001$), 66.7% ($p < .001$), and 13.3% ($p = .05$), respectively. Patient satisfaction scores showed no significant change over time, although patient-evaluated overall improved scores increased 60% over baseline ($p = .02$).

Conclusion.—This technology may be a useful, nonablative resurfacing treatment for acne scarring. Scarring, texture, and pigmentation improved significantly according to investigator-rated assessment parameters. Although patient satisfaction scores did not improve, overall improvement scores did.

▶ Peterson and colleagues report the findings of a prospective case series of 15 patients who were treated with a unique device that combines a 915-nm diode fractional laser with fractional bipolar radiofrequency. The subjects underwent 5 monthly treatment sessions, each of which consisted of 2 full-face treatments. Initially, the area of scarring was treated with a handpiece combining a diode laser with fractional radiofrequency. Each session then continued with treatment by a novel bipolar radiofrequency handpiece over the same areas. The investigators attempted to obtain objective data by evaluating the total quantitative acne scar scale score during each visit, patient satisfaction scores, and patient overall improvement scores, as well as investigator scores of improvement in scarring, texture, and pigmentation. They demonstrated a 72.3% ($P < .001$) decrease in the acne scar scale as well as an improvement of 68.2% in scarring, a 66.7% improvement in texture, and a 13.3% improvement in pigmentation, all of which were significantly increased from the baseline evaluation. Patients were satisfied with the treatment; however, the level of satisfaction did not increase over the course of treatment from month 2 to month 6.

This is a well-designed pilot study of a new device for acne scars. The results suggest that the device is effective and safe in improving the texture, depth, and overall appearance of the scars. The investigators did not report postinflammatory hyperpigmentation (PIH) in any subjects. They also did not report the exact number of subjects of skin type III or greater (which have the greatest risk for PIH), except for mentioning that all subjects were of skin types II to IV. Limitations of the study include the small sample size of 15, the absence of a control group, and the lack of blinding by the evaluators.

Two additional studies have reported the efficacy of this device for treating acne scars. Ramesh and colleagues[1] evaluated 30 Indian patients of skin types III to V and found similar improvement and no incidence of PIH. A case series of 20 patients whose acne scars were treated with the device was reported by Taub and Garretson,[2] who found a statistically significant improvement in scars. Both of these studies had limitations similar to those of the study by Peterson et al.

In summary, Peterson and colleagues demonstrated a significant improvement in investigator-rated acne scarring, texture, and pigmentation. Patients' satisfaction scores did not improve, although patients' overall improvement scores did. While it would be difficult to perform, a larger split-face controlled study with evaluator blinding would be helpful to evaluate the efficacy of this new technology for treating acne scars.

D. Fife, MD

References

1. Ramesh M, Gopal M, Kumar S, Talwar A. Novel technology in the treatment of acne scars: the Matrix-tunable radiofrequency technology. *J Cutan Aesthet Surg.* 2010;3:97-101.
2. Taub AF, Garretson CB. Treatment of acne scars of skin types II to V by sublative fractional bipolar radiofrequency and bipolar radiofrequency combined with diode laser. *J Clin Aesthet Dermatol.* 2011;4:18-27.

Skin Necrosis of the Nasal Ala after Injection of Dermal Fillers

Kang MS, Park ES, Shin HS, et al (Soonchunhyang Univ Bucheon Hosp, Republic of Korea)
Dermatol Surg 37:375-380, 2011

Background.—The injectable, nonpermanent soft tissue augmentation materials used as dermal filler are usually well tolerated and can be used safely. However, both early and late side effects and complications can occur. Among the early problems are swelling, redness, bruising, and skin necrosis after intradermal or subdermal injections. Later, patients may experience immunologic phenomena such as late-onset allergy, nonallergic foreign body granuloma, and hypertrophic scars. Localized tissue necrosis, although rare, is the worst outcome and results from mechanical interruption of the local vascular supply. Treating physicians must be alert to the development of any compromise to the vascular supply.

Case Report.—Woman, 37, was injected with hyaluronic acid gel to correct wrinkling of the nasolabial fold. She experienced a sharp pain on the right side of the face immediately after injection, and a few hours later she developed a reddish discoloration on the right side of the nose and along the nasolabial fold. Four days after the procedure she demonstrated gangrenous skin necrosis measuring 1.5 × 1.3 cm and eschar in the right nasal alar area. She also had intense erythema in the distribution of the lateral nasal branch and angular artery of the facial artery. She was given intravenous low-molecular-weight heparin 5000 IU and alprostadil for 5 days. Ten days after the dermal augmentation procedure a three-dimensional computed tomogram (3D-CT) showed a suspicious vascular occlusion on the terminal-branch arteriole of the angular artery and compensatory dilation of collateral vessels. Diligent moisturized wound care and daily dressings for 16 days finally produced demarcation of the wound. The necrosis involved the surrounding skin and subcutaneous tissue but had not extended to the lower lateral cartilage. Surgical removal was performed 20 days after the initial procedure. The biopsy specimen revealed severe epidermal necrosis with acute and chronic nonspecific inflammation. Deposits of multi-focal amorphous material were noted in the dermis and vascular lumen. A full-thickness skin graft from the ipsilateral postauricular area was placed. After 3 months, the right nasal ala demonstrated slight contraction.

Conclusions.—Despite the absence of direct filler injection into the nasal alar area, the skin of this area became completely necrotic. The blood supply of the nasal ala appeared to depend strongly on a single arterial branch. 3D-CT angiography showed compensatory dilatation of collateral vessels. It was concluded that the localized skin necrosis resulted from intravascular embolization of the terminal-branch arteriole after an accidental intra-arterial injection of dermal filler.

▶ As the market for cosmetic procedures continues to expand, so does the need for education about outcomes and consequences. The article points out how essential the knowledge of regional anatomy is as an integral component when performing a procedure including injection of dermal fillers. Glabellar necrosis has been recognized as a consequence of therapy for many years but as a result of direct injection. As the case description reveals, embolization and vascular compromise are the main components of the adverse outcome described in this article. The recognition of the initial signs of vascular involvement, as well as proper quality assurance of the techniques described in the discussion section, are very essential in assuring proper placement of the filler substance and understanding where not to place filler.

The authors provide some good teaching points, such as slowing down the injection time, massage at the first sign of blanching, and avoidance of overcorrection, but weekend workshops and preceptorships may not provide these tips to those inadequately trained in details of regional anatomy. Many clinicians are also unfamiliar with the use of hyaluronidase or nitroglycerin paste as well as their roles in rescue during filler injection procedures. Unfortunately, the population of cosmetic surgery providers has expanded from dermatologists and plastic surgeons to general practitioners, physician extenders, nurses, and employees of day spas. The depth of education on facial anatomy varies among these groups and individuals.

After hearing about yet another complication from cosmetic surgery, the reader must now be aware of both the embolic phenomenon and hypersensitivity responses demonstrated in the case discussion. More importantly, the clinician needs to be aware of these potential adverse outcomes regardless of training, simply because the patient who consents to having the procedure needs to know that we know what we are doing.

N. Bhatia, MD

20 Miscellaneous Topics in Dermatologic Surgery and Cutaneous Oncology

Treatment of Striae Distensae Using an Ablative 10,600-nm Carbon Dioxide Fractional Laser: A Retrospective Review of 27 Participants
Lee SE, Kim JH, Lee SJ, et al (Yonsei Univ, Seoul, Korea; Yonsei Star Skin and Laser Clinic, Seoul, Korea)
Dermatol Surg 36:1683-1690, 2010

Background.—Late-stage striae distensae is a type of scar characterized by a loss of collagen and elastic fibers in the dermis. Ablative 10,600-nm carbon dioxide fractional laser systems (CO_2 FS) have been used successfully for the treatment of various types of scars.

Objective.—To investigate the therapeutic efficacy of using CO_2 FS for the treatment of striae distensae.

Methods.—Twenty-seven women with striae distensae were treated in a single session with a CO_2 FS. Deep FX mode with a pulse energy of 10 mJ and a density of 2 (percent coverage of 10%) was used. Clinical improvement was assessed by comparing pre- and post-treatment clinical photographs and participant satisfaction rates.

Results.—The evaluation of clinical results 3 months after treatment showed that two of the 27 participants (7.4%) had grade clinical 4 improvement, 14 (51.9%) had grade 3 improvement, nine (33.3%) had grade 2 improvement, and two (7.4%) had grade 1 improvement. None of the participants showed worsening of their striae distensae. Mean clinical improvement score was 2.6. Surveys evaluating overall participant satisfaction administered after the treatment was completed showed that six of the 27 participants (22.2%) were very satisfied, 14 (51.9%) were satisfied, five (18.1%) were slightly satisfied, and two (7.4%) were unsatisfied.

Conclusion.—Our observations demonstrated that the use of CO_2 FS can have a positive therapeutic effect on late-stage striae distensae.

▶ Striae distensae are exceedingly common and thus far, no perfect treatment has been identified. This study demonstrates the efficacy and safety of fractionated carbon dioxide (CO_2) laser in treating striae distensae. While the authors did show that only 16 of the 27 demonstrated greater than 50% improvement, there are several reasons why these results are more impressive than they might initially seem.

It is not surprising that this laser improves striae distensae, given that it has previously been shown to improve atrophic acne scars.[1] The fractionated laser works by eliminating the damaged collagenous matrix followed by inducing neocollagenesis. The duration of continued neocollagenesis is unknown. Improvement scoring was done just 2 months after treatment, and it is possible that neocollagenesis could continue well past 2 months, thus not capturing the ultimate improvement. Only one treatment was done on each patient. Additional treatments could optimize efficacy. The laser settings were also conservative. Using a pulse energy greater than 10 mJ and a density greater than 10% could induce more neocollagenesis.

It is reassuring to know that none of the striae distensae worsened. This is helpful when counseling patients regarding expected outcomes. As a result of this article, we won't be able to exactly predict the degree of improvement, but we will be able to assure our patients that the striae distensae are not likely to worsen. The paucity of side effects noted may also make others more comfortable to use the fractionated CO_2 laser in nonfacial sites. All the treatments in this study were done off the face, and many physicians are hesitant using any ablative laser on nonfacial skin, given the reduced number of adnexal structures and thus the slower re-epithelialization.

Patients with only Fitzpatrick skin type IV were included in this study. Patients with darker skin are more prone to persistent dyschromias after ablative laser treatment. The authors noted that persistent hyperpigmentation was not observed in any of the patients. However, there was some ambiguity in reporting of the side effects. All the subjects had erythema that lasted from 4 to 8 weeks. The authors note that there were some short-term side effects but don't define the time frame. Included in this side effect profile are transient pruritus, posttreatment crusting or scaling, and oozing. It would have been helpful if the authors quantified the number of subjects who developed posttreatment hyperpigmentation. Instead they say that hyperpigmentation was noted in "several participants but spontaneously resolved within 4 weeks." Overall, this study helped to demonstrate some efficacy in treating striae distensae with fractionated CO_2 laser with only minor side effects, but more insight is needed.

E. Graber, MD

Reference

1. Chapas AM, Brightman L, Sukal S, et al. Successful treatment of acneiform scarring with CO2 ablative fractional resurfacing. *Lasers Surg Med.* 2008;40:381-386.

Achieving Hemostasis After Nail Biopsy Using Absorbable Gelatin Sponge Saturated in Aluminum Chloride

Hwa C, Kovich OI, Stein JA (New York Univ School of Medicine)
Dermatol Surg 37:368-369, 2011

Background.—Nail biopsy can diagnose nail conditions that cannot be identified based on history or clinical appearance alone. Inflammatory or neoplastic conditions are often found using punch nail biopsies. After these procedures, a critical need is postoperative hemostasis, especially in view of the nail bed's rich vascular supply. A way to achieve rapid hemostasis after punch biopsy was described.

Technique.—The method involves the use of an absorbable gelatin sponge saturated in aluminum chloride. Before the digital tourniquet is removed, a 0.5 × 0.5-n-cm section of 12-cm^2, 7-mm deep absorbable gelatin sponge is soaked in aluminum chloride 35% plus isopropyl alcohol. Sterile gauze is held under pressure on the bleeding nail area until bleeding is no longer brisk. The absorbable gelatin sponge is then inserted into the biopsy wound using the wooden part of a sterile cotton swab. More gelatin sponge pieces are packed into the biopsy site until the sponge is flush with the nail plate. The digital tourniquet is removed, leaving the absorbable gelatin sponge in place until the next follow-up visit, which is about 2 weeks after the biopsy. If it is still present, the sponge is removed at that time.

Conclusions.—Hemostasis can be simply and effectively obtained after nail biopsy using absorbable gelatin sponge saturated in aluminum chloride. The combination makes the process dramatically more rapid than using the sponge or the aluminum chloride alone. The process has the advantages of ease of use, accessibility to materials, and rapid effect.

▶ This brief how-to article describes the use of gel foam saturated with aluminum chloride to assist in hemostasis during punch biopsies of the nail unit. Gel foam has been used for hemostasis in punch biopsies of the skin for many years in cases in which the biopsy site is not sutured, and aluminum chloride is commonly used for hemostasis in superficial skin surgery, but the combination of the 2 agents in nail punch biopsies is interesting. More advanced nail surgical procedures would be less amenable to this procedure for achieving hemostasis. Nevertheless, this technique is useful in that it could give novice nail surgeons additional confidence in nail surgery and encourage them to perform more nail biopsies.

P. Rich, MD

A Case of Epithelioid Angiosarcoma of the Scalp Treated With Paclitaxel and Radiotherapy

Kamath S, Bhagwandas K (Princess of Wales Hosp, Bridgend, England; Neath Port Talbot Hosp, England)
Arch Dermatol 147:129-130, 2011

Background.—Angiosarcoma (AS) is a rare malignant tumor of endothelial cells, but cutaneous manifestations are the most common variety. Epithelioid AS (EAS) is a rare histologic variant that can occur in deep tissues and skin. A case was demonstrated.

Case Report.—Man, 67, reported an asymptomatic scalp lesion of 5 months' duration. A 5-cm erythematous plaque was found over the right frontoparietal scalp. Alopecia mucinosa was diagnosed, and a biopsy specimen revealed no follicular mucinosis or epidermotropism. Chronic inflammatory infiltrate was present, and the impression was of actinic keratosis. Oral lymecycline, 408 mg/d, was prescribed for the inflammation. After 6 months the lesion had deteriorated, becoming an erythematous, violaceous nodular plaque. A diagnostic punch biopsy revealed sheets of polygonal cells with marked pleomorphism in both the mid and deep dermis. Immunohistochemical analysis yielded a positive result for focal epithelial membrane antigen, a strongly positive result for vimentin, and negative results for CK, S-1000, HMB-45, and SMA. After the patient developed lymphadenopathy with histologically demonstrated malignant spindle-cell tumor, a further skin biopsy showed sheets of plump pleomorphic spindle-shaped cells and high nuclear pleomorphism with mitotic activity of 17 per 10 high-power fields. CD31 results were positive, and poorly differentiated AS was diagnosed. The patient received weekly paclitaxel for 12 weeks. The left cervical lymphadenopathy resolved in 4 weeks; for the skin lesion, resolution required 3 months. The patient had consolidation radiotherapy as well and achieved clinical remission within 10 months.

Conclusions.—AS is more common in men than women and tends to occur on the legs, trunk, head, and neck. The prognosis is quite poor. The condition is often mistaken for metastatic carcinoma, melanoma, or high-grade lymphoma. A prominent cytoskeleton of intermediate filaments, numerous pinocytic vesicles, small intercellular lumina with microvilli on the surface, and typical vacuoles are found on electron microscopy. Unless there is careful testing with vascular immunohistologic markers, EAS can be mistaken for metastatic carcinoma, amelanotic melanoma, or high-grade lymphoma.

▶ This case report illustrates the difficulty in making the diagnosis of epithelioid angiosarcoma. It provides a good review of the relevant stains that will help to confirm the diagnosis as well as exclude entities in the differential diagnosis, such as metastatic carcinoma, amelanotic melanoma, or high grade lymphoma. Despite the poor prognosis of epithelioid angiosarcomas, it is encouraging that this patient has responded well to paclitaxel and radiotherapy with complete remission at 10 months.

R. Ceilley, MD

B. Kopitzki, DO

The Public's Perception of Dermatologists as Surgeons

Chung V, Alexander H, Pavlis M, et al (Vanguard Dermatology and Skin Cancer Specialists, CO; Hailey, Brody, Casey and Wray, MD, PC Dermatology and Dermatologic Surgery, Atlanta, GA; State Univ of New York at Stony Brook; et al)

Dermatol Surg 37:295-300, 2011

Background.—Dermatologists perform more cutaneous surgical procedures than any other medical specialists, including plastic surgeons, especially for treating skin cancers, but anecdotal evidence suggests that the public may not identify dermatologists as surgeons.

Objective.—Our study was designed to assess the public's perception of expertise in surgery of the skin of three medical specialties: dermatology, plastic surgery, and general surgery. We also investigated whether the physician's specialty biases people when they assess the cosmetic appearance of a surgical scar.

Materials and Methods.—We administered an institutional review board–approved survey to individuals at the Emory Student Center and the Emory Dermatology Clinic. Participants rated the perceived skills and training of the different medical specialties and scored the cosmetic appearance of 16 surgical scars created by a fellowship-trained Mohs surgeon labeled as the work of different specialists.

Results.—Results from 467 participants were overwhelmingly in favor of plastic surgeons ($p<.001$). The physician's specialty did not bias participants in assessing the cosmetic appearance of surgical scars.

Conclusion.—The study population had greater confidence in the surgical skills of plastic surgeons than in those of dermatologists, although participants were objective in rating the cosmesis of surgical scars, regardless of the purported surgeon's specialty. Although dermatologic surgeons must continually refine our surgical expertise, we must also educate the public about the breadth and depth of our work.

▶ The article deftly describes a perception problem within the general public regarding the surgical skills of dermatologists. The authors conclude that dermatologic surgeons need to continuously educate the public about their surgical skills.

I believe that premise is mistaken and is the weakness of the study and its conclusions. The most important aspect of the doctor-patient relationship is the trust that is developed in our in-person encounters. Patients who present to a dermatologic surgeon should have a trusted belief that their physician is the right person for the procedure. The author's results point to this same conclusion. However, the authors try to take this trust factor a step too far. They try to develop the premise that this trust in surgical skills needs to exist prior to a doctor-patient contact, especially as it relates to dermatology. Furthermore, they suggest that an anonymous patient should have the exposure and knowledge base to seek out a dermatologic surgeon. This premise is faulty in that they would not necessarily require a surgeon unless a diagnosis already exists. How would the patient know which course of treatment is necessary? A person having experienced a burn, a car accident, or seeking a facelift should not inherently seek out a dermatologic surgeon for these procedures. By definition, a plastic surgeon will have a perceived elevated skill set when it comes to the public's perceptions about surgical outcome. This is because the term "surgeon" is in their professional title. This is not the case for dermatologists. It would be a difficult task for dermatologic associations to try to break out the difference between a general dermatologist and a dermatologic surgeon and then develop means to publicly educate on those differences. This study does accurately reflect that cosmetic results between dermatologic surgeons and plastic surgeons are almost indistinguishable. It is this fact that dermatologic surgeons need to exploit. By developing a strong and trusted referral physician database in each practitioner's geographic area, those nondermatologist physicians in the area will assist in spreading the word on the skill sets and outcomes expected from dermatologic surgeons.

R. I. Ceilley, MD

The Reconstruction of Male Hair-Bearing Facial Regions

Ridgway EB, Pribaz JJ (Brigham and Women's Hosp, Boston, MA)
Plast Reconstr Surg 127:131-141, 2011

Background.—Loss of hair-bearing regions of the face caused by trauma, tumor resection, or burn presents a difficult reconstructive task for plastic surgeons. The ideal tissue substitute should have the same characteristics as the facial area affected, consisting of thin, pliable tissue with a similar color match and hair-bearing quality.

Methods.—This is a retrospective study of 34 male patients who underwent reconstruction of hair-bearing facial regions performed by the senior author (J.J.P.). Local and pedicled flaps were used primarily to reconstruct defects after tumor extirpation, trauma, infections, and burns. Two patients had irradiation before reconstruction. Two patients had prior facial reconstruction with free flaps.

Results.—The authors found that certain techniques of reconstructing defects in hair-bearing facial regions were more successful than others in particular facial regions and in different sizes of defects.

Conclusion.—The authors were able to develop a simple algorithm for management of facial defects involving the hair-bearing regions of the eyebrow, sideburn, beard, and mustache that may prospectively aid the planning of reconstructive strategy in these cases.

▶ Ridgway and Pribaz discuss the surgical reconstruction of hair-bearing areas of the male scalp. While many of the specific reconstructive procedures described in the article are beyond the expertise of most dermatologic surgeons, the general principles apply to situations encountered by dermatologic surgeons almost daily. Before initiating an excision or a surgical reconstruction, it is important to take into consideration the effect that the procedure will have on important hair-bearing areas, such as the eyebrow, sideburn, mustache, and beard. Importance should be given to planning reconstructions that best maintain the symmetry of these cosmetically important structures and to replace hair-bearing skin with hair of the same length, diameter, density, and orientation. The best reservoir for this type of skin is adjacent hair-bearing skin, if available. The V to Y advancement flap is a well-vascularized flap that can predictably repair small to medium sized defects with hair-bearing skin of similar quality. Single-follicle or hair plug transplants are an option and are most successful if the recipient site is healthy, well-vascularized tissue that has not been damaged by burns or radiation therapy. Valuable location-specific reconstructive algorithms are provided in the article. If the defect is too large for the dermatologic surgeon to reconstruct the area with adequate hair-bearing skin, a referral to a plastic surgeon or ear, nose, and throat/facial plastic surgeon may be indicated. Limitations of this publication are that the sample size is relatively small, all of the reconstructive procedures were performed by one surgeon, and most of the examples given are beyond the expertise of most dermatologic surgeons.

D. Fife, MD

Deroofing: A tissue-saving surgical technique for the treatment of mild to moderate hidradenitis suppurativa lesions
van der Zee HH, Prens EP, Boer J (Univ Med Ctr, Rotterdam, The Netherlands; Deventer Hosp, The Netherlands)
J Am Acad Dermatol 63:475-480, 2010

Background.—Hidradenitis suppurativa (HS) is a chronic inflammatory skin disease, often refractory to treatment. Patients with HS and dermatologists are in need of an effective, fast surgical intervention technique. Deroofing is a tissue-saving technique, whereby the "roof" of an abscess, cyst, or sinus tract is electrosurgically removed. The use of a probe is mandatory to explore the full extent of a lesion.

Objective.—We sought to evaluate the efficacy and patient satisfaction of the deroofing technique for recurrent Hurley I (mild) or II (moderate) graded HS lesions at fixed locations.

Methods.—An open study consisted of 88 deroofed lesions in 44 consecutive patients with HS, treated by a single clinician with a follow-up time of up to 5 years.

Results.—Fifteen of 88 (17%) treated lesions showed a recurrence after a median of 4.6 months. In all, 73 treated lesions (83%) did not show a recurrence after a median follow-up of 34 months. The median patient satisfaction with the procedure rated 8 on a scale from 0 to 10. Of the treated patients, 90% would recommend the deroofing technique to other patients with HS. One side effect occurred in the form of postoperative bleeding.

Limitations.—Some patients were lost to follow-up.

Conclusions.—The deroofing technique is an effective, simple, minimally invasive, tissue-saving surgical intervention for the treatment of mild to moderate HS lesions at fixed locations and it is suitable as an office procedure.

▶ Hidradenitis suppurativa (HS) is a chronic debilitating skin disorder of the apocrine gland-rich body sites including the axillary, inguinal, and anogenital regions. Patients experience recurrent inflammatory nodules and painful abscesses that often lead to fistulas and sinus tract formations. Often refractory to multiple treatment options, the current article investigates the efficacy of the deroofing technique. Surgery is traditionally more efficacious than medical therapy depending on the technique, severity of disease, and extent of fistula or sinus tract involvement. Deroofing is a cost-effective, tissue-saving technique that can be performed in the office with local anesthesia. Best candidates for this treatment are patients with lesions that are at fixed locations and are graded as Hurley stage I or II. In general, the procedure entails injection of local anesthesia, exploration of lesion with a blunt probe, removal of the roof using the probe as guide with an electrosurgical loop, curetting away debris on the floor of the lesion, and then allowing the site to heal by secondary intention. The authors state that overall, 73 of 88 treated patients had no recurrence at 34 months. Deroofing seems to be an underutilized procedure that can provide symptom relief and reduce recurrence at the treated site.

S. Bellew, DO
J. Q. Del Rosso, DO

Cutaneous metastasis of prostatic adenocarcinoma: a cautionary tale
Rattanasirivilai A, Kurban A, Lenzy YM, et al (Boston Univ School of Medicine, MA)
J Cutan Pathol 38:521-524, 2011

With the exception of skin cancer, prostatic adenocarcinoma represents the most common cancer among men in the United States and the second most common cause of cancer mortality. Mortality is often associated with metastatic disease, which in the case of prostatic adenocarcinoma typically involves bones and only rarely affects the skin. Although clinical history and examination, laboratory tests and routine pathology can suggest the prostate as a source of metastatic disease, immunohistochemistry — specifically, for prostate-specific antigen (PSA) — is often used to help establish the diagnosis. We report a case of cutaneous metastatic prostatic adenocarcinoma presenting in the inguinal region of a 78-year-old man 5 years after his initial diagnosis. The case is unusual in that the clinical appearance mimicked a vascular proliferation and in that the metastatic prostatic adenocarcinoma failed to express PSA. Rather, expression of prostatic acid phosphatase was observed.

▶ Metastatic prostatic adenocarcinoma occurs in less than 1% of cases. This is a case report of a 78-year-old man with a previous history of prostate cancer who presented with scrotal swelling and superimposed vesicles. A shave biopsy revealed a dermal infiltration of pleomorphic cells with glandular differentiation. Although the history along with histopathologic findings suggested metastatic prostatic adenocarcinoma, immunohistochemistry for prostate-specific antigen (PSA) was negative. However, false-negative cases of PSA have been reported, typically in poorly differentiated prostate adenocarcinoma. In this case, staining with prostatic acid phosphatase (PAP) can help establish a diagnosis. However, the patient did have a markedly elevated blood PSA at the time of biopsy. Also, the authors in this study ruled out neuroendocrine neoplasm with a negative neural cell adhesion molecule (CD56), chromogranin, and synaptophysin. The authors concluded that this patient's cutaneous metastasis represented a possible malignant clone that had lost its ability to produce PSA on immunostaining but retained the ability to produce PSA in other parts of the body, hence the high blood PSA levels. In conclusion, this is an example of cutaneous prostatic carcinoma with negative immunohistochemistry for PSA and positive PAP. The authors caution using PSA alone in making the diagnosis of prostatic adenocarcinoma metastatic to skin.

G. K. Kim, DO

J. Q. Del Rosso, DO

Digital Block With and Without Epinephrine During Chemical Matricectomy with Phenol

Altinyazar HC, Demirel CB, Koca R, et al (Zonguldak Karaelmas Univ, Turkey; Gazi Univ, Ankara, Turkey)
Dermatol Surg 36:1568-1571, 2010

Background.—Digital block with epinephrine is safe in selected patients. Chemical matricectomy with phenol is a successful, cheap, and easy method for the treatment of ingrown nails.

Objective.—To determine the effect of digital block with epinephrine in chemical matricectomy with phenol.

Material and Methods.—Forty-four patients with ingrown toenail were randomly divided into two groups. The plain lidocaine group ($n = 22$) underwent digital anesthesia using 2% plain lidocaine, and the lidocaine with epinephrine group ($n = 22$) underwent digital anesthesia with 2% lidocaine with 1:100,000 epinephrine. In the postoperative period, the patients were evaluated for pain, drainage, and peripheral tissue destruction and were followed for up to 18 months for recurrence.

Results.—The mean anesthetic volume used in the epinephrine group (2.2 ± 0.4 mL) was significantly lower than the plain lidocaine group (3.1 ± 0.6 mL). There was no statistically significant difference in postoperative pain and recurrence rates, but duration of drainage was significantly shorter in the epinephrine group (11.1 ± 2.5 days) than in the plain lidocaine group (19.0 ± 3.8 days).

Conclusion.—Digital block with epinephrine is safe in selected patients, and epinephrine helps to shorten the postoperative drainage period.

▶ The dogma of avoiding use of epinephrine in digital block anesthesia has been the subject of many articles in the literature in the past several years. This article is another publication documenting safety of epinephrine when performing chemical matrixectomy, and describes some benefits as well, in appropriate patients.

The authors state that the advantages of using epinephrine in these procedures include faster onset of anesthesia, smaller volumes of anesthetic needed, prolonged postoperative pain relief, and less need for tourniquet placement.

Of note, there are no reports of digital necrosis due to use of the standard commercial lidocaine-epinephrine mixture for digital blocks, and there are multiple studies involving thousands of patients supporting the safety of using lidocaine with epinephrine for surgery on the digits.

This is one more piece of evidence to support the idea that for patients without contraindications such as peripheral vascular disease, diabetes, digital infection, or fracture, use of epinephrine in nail surgery is well tolerated and has benefits such as prolonged pain relief, faster onset of anesthesia, and faster recovery. Less bleeding during the procedure is also a significant benefit. Phenol application requires a bloodless field, and hemostasis can also be accomplished much more easily with less trauma to the surgical site. Additionally, there is much less risk of compressive damage due to excessive volumes of anesthetic.

E. M. Billingsley, MD

Mucosal Advancement Flap Versus Primary Closure After Vermilionectomy of the Lower Lip
Sand M, Altmeyer P, Bechara FG (Ruhr-Univ Bochum, Germany)
Dermatol Surg 36:1987-1992, 2010

Background.—Post-vermilionectomy defect closure by a mucosal advancement flap is a wellestablished method, although moderate morbidity may accompany the procedure, especially in elderly patients. The objective of the present study was to compare a simple primary closure (PC) for reconstruction after complete resection of the vermilion (vermilionectomy) with closure using a mucosal advancement flap (MAF).

Methods.—After margin-controlled vermilionectomy, 18 patients with actinic cheilitis ($n = 5$) or squamous cell carcinoma in situ ($n = 13$) of the lower lip were included in the present study. Patients were randomized into one group receiving PC ($n = 8$) and a second group receiving MAF closure ($n = 10$) for reconstruction of the surgical defect on the lower lip. All complications, esthetic outcomes (EOs), and cut–suture times were documented.

Results.—In the MAF group, patients' mean EO score on a 10-point scale was 8.4, and the surgeons' mean EO rate was 7.8. In the PC group the patients' mean EO score was 7.5 and the surgeons' mean EO rate was 6.4 for the reconstruction achieved. The rate of side effects was significantly higher in the MAF group than in the PC group ($p<.05$). The cut–suture times were significantly shorter for PC (29 minutes) than MAF (37.8 minutes; $p<.05$).

Conclusion.—MAF is the method of choice and has good functional and cosmetic outcomes, although elderly patients with different comorbidities that need to be protected from unnecessary strain could potentially benefit from PC.

▶ This article presents a well-designed small study comparing the procedure time, postoperative course, and final outcome of mucosal advancement flaps versus primary closure after lower lip vermillionectomy. The data presented suggest that primary closure (PC) should be considered a reasonable option for some patients. The cosmetic outcome was very acceptable for most patients, and the postoperative course was better tolerated with less bruising and swelling, and fewer complications. The vermillion width was much smaller in the PC group. It is a small study, but the study design is good. The article nicely outlines the techniques used for resection and both reconstructive techniques. Mucosal advancement flap involves significant undermining at the submucosal plane, above the orbicularis muscle. PC involves little to no mobilization of surrounding tissue. Interestingly, no patients received pre- or postoperative analgesics or antibiotics.

PC of the lip following vermillionectomy is a very reasonable reconstructive choice. It can have shorter procedure time, better postoperative course, and reasonable cosmetic outcome. It may be considered especially for patients on anticoagulants and elderly patients with comorbidities. Of course, each case must be evaluated individually.

E. M. Billingsley, MD

Novel method of minimally invasive removal of large lipoma after laser lipolysis with 980 nm diode laser
Stebbins WG, Hanke CW, Petersen J (The Laser and Skin Surgery Ctr of Indiana, Carmel)
Dermatol Ther 24:125-130, 2011

Lipomas are the most common benign tumor of the soft tissue, often presenting as soft, mobile subcutaneous masses. These lesions are often removed for cosmetic reasons, although they may be removed secondary to considerable discomfort or paresthesias. The large majority of lipomas appear as small, solitary lesions that are best removed by surgical excision. However, surgical removal of large (>10 cm) or multiple lesions may result in significant scarring. Tumescent local anesthesia and liposuction of larger lesions has been successful in a number of cases although this technique can be hindered by overly fibrous lesions. Laser lipolysis, performed alone or before liposuction, can further facilitate removal of these lesions. This technique is a minimally invasive and effective method of lipoma removal, resulting in an excellent cosmetic outcome. This report describes step-by-step removal of a large lipoma located on the back, as well as a review of currently employed techniques for minimally invasive treatment of lipomas.

▶ This article is a case report describing a new method to remove a large lipoma, a common benign tumor, that we all encounter in our clinics. The article details the technique of laser liposis, with usage of a 980-nm diode laser to liquify fat cells and to remove a large lipoma with minimal invasiveness to improve ultimate cosmesis. Traditional excision of large lipomas can be cosmetically disfiguring. In this case, the author uses a 980-nm diode laser, but other lasers using different wavelengths are also available on the market. The technology is still new, and many clinicians may not have access to it, but it is useful to know of its existence so we can refer appropriate patients to qualified physicians for treatment if we feel secure that the outcomes are favorable. As the authors pointed out, the technique is operator-dependent, hence seeking a qualified performer of laser lipolysis technique for referral is extremely important to avoid untoward complications for our patients. This new technology can be an additional tool for removal of large lipomas.

K. Nguyen, MD

Preoperative Expectations and Values of Patients Undergoing Mohs Micrographic Surgery
Chuang GS, Leach BC, Wheless L, et al (Med Univ of South Carolina, Charleston)
Dermatol Surg 37:311-319, 2011

Background.—Dermatologists have championed Mohs micrographic surgery (MMS) for its unsurpassed treatment success for skin cancers, safety profile, cost-effectiveness, and tissue-sparing quality. It is unclear whether patients undergoing MMS also value these characteristics.

Objective.—To evaluate patients' preoperative expectations of MMS and identify the factors that may influence such expectations.

Methods.—The study prospectively recruited participants who were newly diagnosed with skin cancer and referred for MMS. A questionnaire listing the characteristics of MMS was given to the participants asking them to score the importance of each characteristic on a 10-point scale. The participants were also asked to provide information regarding their gender, age, subjective health status, education level, family annual income, and their referral source.

Results.—On average, participants placed the highest value, in descending order, on a treatment that yielded the highest cure rate, reconstruction initiation only after complete tumor removal, and the surgeon being a skin cancer specialist. Overall, participants placed high values on characteristics of MMS that dermatologists have long esteemed.

Conclusion.—Our data corroborate that MMS is a valuable procedure that meets the expectations not just of physicians, but also of patients.

▶ Mohs micrographic surgery (MMS) is regarded by dermatologists as an important surgical treatment method for removal of nonmelanoma skin cancer. As noted in the article, it is viewed as such by dermatologists based on many factors, including cost, treatment outcomes, and safety. Chuang et al sought to determine patients' preoperative expectations of MMS and evaluate which, if any, of the characteristics of MMS were also valued by the patient, especially in light of the importance of patient satisfaction in delivering quality health care. Specifically, Chuang et al provided questionnaires to patients and had patients score the importance of certain characteristics of MMS. The results were not only interesting to those who perform MMS but also validated and corroborated the importance of this procedure. Fourteen characteristics of MMS in all were evaluated by patients. The most important characteristics as rated by patients in the questionnaire included that MMS had the highest cure rate (the most important factor), the dermatologist was a skin cancer specialist, and there was confirmation based on histology that the tumor was removed before reconstructive surgery was performed. Other important characteristics included that the pain was well controlled during surgery, pathology results confirmed the successful removal of the skin cancer on the same day, there was a minimal amount of skin removal beyond what is needed to remove the cancer, and MMS may minimize the size of the postsurgical scar. In addition, although it was regarded as important that the surgeons should have completed further training (fellowship) beyond residency, there was no preference whether they were members of the American College of Mohs Surgery or the American Society of Mohs Surgery. The least important characteristics were that patients could be accompanied by friends or family or whether they could eat/drink before and on the day of surgery. Overall, the study simply provides validation that the characteristics that make MMS important to dermatologists are also similarly of importance to patients. Ultimately, this should be reassuring to dermatologists that they are meeting patient expectations and delivering good quality health care with MMS and also ultimately that this modality continues to be a valuable and important procedure in dermatology for the patient.

B. D. Michaels, DO
J. Q. Del Rosso, DO

Risk management in dermatology: an analysis of data available from several British-based reporting systems

Gawkrodger DJ (Royal Hallamshire Hosp, Sheffield, UK)
Br J Dermatol 164:537-543, 2011

Background.—The elimination or reduction of risk is a prime requirement of all healthcare workers. The matter has come to the fore in dermatological practice recently with the widespread use of effective drugs that have significant side-effects (e.g. retinoids, cytotoxic drugs, biologics), the increase in skin surgery, especially for skin cancer, and the extensive use of phototherapies.

Objectives.—To examine the available database from different agencies to which adverse events may be reported over at least a 5-year time frame, categorize the risks, look forward to where as yet unidentified risks might exist, and draw conclusions to improve the safety of dermatological practice. This work came about through a request from the National Patient Safety Agency [to the Joint Specialty Committee of the British Association of Dermatologists (BAD) and Royal College of Physicians] for information on risks to patients receiving treatment or investigation for skin disease.

Methods.—Organizations in the U.K. that receive information about adverse events, whether caused by drugs or procedures in dermatological treatments, were approached for information about reported events over a 5-year (or, in one case, 10-year) time frame up to 2009. Data were received from the National Patient Safety Agency, the Medicines and Healthcare Products Regulatory Agency, the National Health Service Litigation Authority, the Medical Protection Society and the Medical Defence Union. In addition, the results of a survey conducted in 2010 by the BAD of its members concerning potential critical incident reporting were included. The received information was analysed according to category of event and conclusions drawn about how best to manage the risks that were identified.

Results.—Adverse events were divided into the following categories, listed in order of the number of reports received: drug side-effects (biologics and retinoids), phototherapy dosage, drug monitoring (including initial screening), pregnancy prevention programmes, skin cancer follow-up (including acting on reports), dermatopathological reporting and conduct of dermatological surgery (including management of complications, equipment problems, use of lasers, cosmetic procedures and cryotherapy). Critical incidents reported by BAD members often concerned follow-up failures, e.g. of patients receiving systemic drugs or of those with skin cancer.

Conclusions.—Several of the reported adverse events concern systemic failures. Recommendations for risk reduction include the following points: better systems for drug monitoring (including regularity of attendance, provision of sufficient follow-up appointments, acting on results and adequacy of pregnancy prevention programmes); staff training and record keeping for phototherapy; acting on skin cancer multidisciplinary team meeting outcomes (including provision of sufficient follow-up appointments); and adequate training of staff in dermatological surgery including cryotherapy. Regular monitoring of the occurrence of such reports is needed to ensure safe practice and to identify early areas of new risk.

▶ Minimizing the risks associated with dermatologic procedures and treatments is a desired goal for all practitioners. This analysis collected data from 5 different UK agencies, and the claims reported to these agencies over a 5- to 10-year period were reviewed. The highest proportion of claims involved drug-related side effects, but other adverse events included issues with drug monitoring, incorrect phototherapy dosing, lack of follow-up in patients with skin cancers, erroneous dermatopathologic reporting, and complications related to surgical, laser, and cosmetic procedures.

While the types of adverse events reported were not surprising or unusual, it was interesting to see which tended to occur more frequently. However, this was only a review of reported events, and it is generally accepted that adverse events and medical errors tend to be largely underreported. Therefore, the actual number of adverse events may be greater and the types of events that actually occur more frequently may differ.

It may be hypothesized that similar results would be seen in countries such as the United States, but the findings of this report cannot be used to make specific inferences about risk management in the United States because dissimilarities between the health care systems and dermatologic practices could result in different risks and problems in the United States versus the United Kingdom. Thus, a similar analysis would need to be conducted stateside to accurately delineate adverse events and to aid in the development of potential solutions here in the United States. Nevertheless, it is interesting to note that surgery and procedure-related adverse events are on the rise in the United Kingdom concordant with the adoption of these procedures, which should cause those of us in the United States to pause and reflect on our practices.

Finally, suggestions provided in the article to reduce the incidence of adverse effects were essentially just general recommendations. It would have been more helpful if the author gave specific examples of situations in which implemented changes were found to directly correlate with a decrease in the number of adverse events.

A. Torres, MD, JD

Intralesional agents in the management of cutaneous malignancy: A review
Good LM, Miller MD, High WA (Univ of Colorado Health Sciences Ctr, Denver)
J Am Acad Dermatol 64:413-422, 2011

Intralesional agents have a role in the management of cutaneous malignancies. In this article, the efficacy, side effects, strengths, limitations, costs, and practical considerations regarding the use of intralesional agents to treat basal cell carcinoma, squamous cell carcinoma, selected cutaneous lymphomas, and even metastatic melanoma are reviewed. Intralesional administration of 5-fluorouracil, interferon, interleukin-2, bleomycin with electrochemotherapy, and aminolevulinic acid with photodynamic therapy are discussed as treatment modalities in basal cell carcinoma. Interferon (~ 1.5 M IU, 3 times weekly $\times$ 3 weeks) is perhaps the most widely used regimen for basal cell carcinoma. With regard to squamous cell carcinoma, treatment with 5-fluorouracil, methotrexate, interferon, and bleomycin are reviewed. Methotrexate (~ 0.3-2.0 mL of 12.5 or 25 mg/mL, two injections ~ 2 weeks apart) was perhaps the most widely used agent. Interferon (3 M IU $\times$ 3 times weekly for ~ 8.5 weeks) and rituximab (10-30 mg per lesion, 3 times weekly for 1 week, possibly repeated 4 weeks later) are sometimes used in the management of primary cutaneous B-cell lymphomas, whereas in primary cutaneous CD30$^+$ lymphoma intralesional methotrexate (0.4-0.5 mL of 50 mg/mL weekly for 2 weeks) has been used. Finally, the roles of BCG vaccine, cidofovir, rose bengal, and bleomycin with electrochemotherapy for the palliation of metastatic melanoma are reviewed. Intralesional management appears most useful when surgical intervention is not a viable option, for cases in which the cosmetic outcome may be superior, or for situations in which the side effects from systemic chemotherapeutic agents are to be minimized.

▶ Although not always readily considered as a treatment option for cutaneous malignancies by clinicians, there are situations in which intralesional agents are a potential treatment option. These scenarios include when surgery is not a viable option or to avoid the unwanted side effects associated with systemic agents. In this article, Good et al present a thorough review of the different intralesional treatment options for a variety of cutaneous malignancies, including basal cell carcinoma (BCC), squamous cell carcinoma (SCC), various cutaneous lymphomas, and certain situations involving melanoma (extraordinary circumstances). Both the strengths and weakness of different options for individual malignancies are reviewed. Intralesional options reviewed include 5-fluorouracil, interferon, interleukin-2, bleomycin, aminolevulinic acid, methotrexate, rituximab, and mistletoe extract. The indications for each intralesional agent along with published costs and associated side effects are discussed. Overall, the article is informative and provides a complete review on intralesional treatment options, which may provide valid alternatives to add to the clinicians' armamentarium for the treatment of cutaneous malignancies, especially in specific clinical situations.

B. D. Michaels, DO
J. Q. Del Rosso, DO

Significant Differences in Skin Irritation by Common Suture Materials Assessed by a Comparative Computerized Objective Method
Parara SM, Manios A, de Bree E, et al (KAT Hosp, Athens, Greece; Herakleion Univ Hosp, Greece)
Plast Reconstr Surg 127:1191-1198, 2011

Background.—Erythema can be described only through subjective evaluation, except when it is quantified by digital image analysis software.

Using such software, the authors performed comparisons of the erythema produced after skin closure of clean surgical wounds. Five suture materials were compared with respect to the local skin irritation that was caused. Different quantities of erythema are produced by suture material after the skin closure of clean surgical wounds. The authors present an objective method of measuring how unreactive a suture material is in comparison with another when applied to the skin.

Methods.—The suture materials polydioxanone, polypropylene blue, polyamide 6, metallic clips, and polyglactin were compared in the present study. Digital photographs of 100 patients were compared by means of software, evaluating red color superiority (mean value of red color) in the region surrounding the wound.

Results.—The least to most irritation caused to the skin by different suture materials was established for paired data. The Kolmogorov-Smirnov criterion and the Wilcoxon signed rank test were used. Polydioxanone was found to have the best performance, followed in order by polyglactin, polyamide, polypropylene, and metallic clips. Immediately after suture removal, differences between the effects of suture materials were statistically significant on postoperative day 10.

Conclusions.—Absorbable sutures can be used in skin closure of clean surgical wounds and can produce less erythematous reaction than nonabsorbable ones. Digital image analysis is a reliable method of quantitative evaluation of skin erythema resulting after skin closure of surgical wounds.

▶ This well-done study is the first of its kind to use a computer software program to objectively measure postoperative erythema using 5 suture materials. Prior studies had been designed using the subjective evaluation of an examiner. Many surgeons, rightly or wrongly, believe that nonabsorbable suture material is preferable because it is easier to tie, unlikely to break, and elicits minimal host tissue response. The 2 absorbable sutures showed statistically significant less erythema than the nonabsorbable sutures after 10 days. One of these was monofilament and the other braided. This confirms other previously reported studies showing superior outcomes using absorbable sutures for cutaneous closure. It is postulated that the lack of cell-mediated reaction may be the reason for the decreased erythema. Using absorbable sutures, specifically polydioxanone or polyglactin, for subcuticular and cutaneous closure would provide significant cost savings because most closures would only require 1 pack of suture. This would add up to several thousand dollars worth of savings over the course of a year. What is not clear is whether decreased erythema on "postop day 10" translates into a better aesthetic result overall once the scar is complete, but this study nicely lays the groundwork for future research using that as an endpoint.

R. Ceilley, MD

B. Kopitzki, DO

Increased prevalence of left-sided skin cancers

Butler ST, Fosko SW (Saint Louis Univ School of Medicine, MO)
J Am Acad Dermatol 63:1006-1010, 2010

Background.—Previous research has shown an increase in photodamage and precancers on the left side of the face.

Objective.—We sought to determine whether there is a higher frequency of skin cancer development on the left side of the body than the right.

Methods.—The study was a retrospective review of patients with skin cancer referred to our Mohs micrographic surgery and cutaneous oncology unit in 2004.

Results.—When including all types of skin cancers and both sexes, more cancers occurred on the left (52.6%) than the right (47.4%) ($P = .059$), with a stronger trend in men ($P = .042$). There were significantly more malignant melanoma in situ on the left (31/42, 74%) than the right (11/42, 26%) ($P = .002$).

Limitations.—Population was comprised of patients referred to an academic medical center and often for Mohs micrographic surgery.

Conclusions.—There were significantly more skin cancers on the left than the right side in men. This discrepancy was even more profound in malignant melanoma in situ.

▶ The side windows of most automobiles are made of nonlaminated clear glass, which blocks ultraviolet B (UVB) rays but allows for 63% transmission of ultraviolet A (UVA) rays. Correlation between left-sided photodamage and percentage of time spent as the driver of a car has been reported, as has an increased incidence of actinic keratoses on the side of the body correlating with the side of the car on which the subjects sat most of the time. The literature supports the fact that the left side of the head, neck, arm, and hand receives up to 6 times the UV radiation as the right side in those sitting on the left side of the car.

This study looked at 890 patients and demonstrated a significant increase in the percentage of nonmelanoma skin cancers and melanomas in situ that occur on the left sides of men, especially tumors of the head and neck. Trends were also found in women, and they varied with age group. This result is likely associated with changing habits of driving as the subjects aged and were more likely to be the driver than the passenger.

The trend noted in this study—that of increased incidence of nonmelanoma skin cancers and noninvasive melanomas on the left side of the head and neck—supports the need for sun protection while in a car. Tinting the window glass or applying clear film to the glass can block UVA and UVB rays. Doing so could have significant preventive effects on the occurrence of skin cancer, especially in individuals who spend many hours each day in a car. Daily use of sunscreen that blocks UVA and UVB should be encouraged, especially in these patients.

Additionally, this study provides some evidence for the role of UVA in skin cancer. UVB has been well established as an etiologic agent in the development of skin cancer, but these data support the theory that chronic UVA exposure may also be contributory.

E. M. Billingsley, MD

Lesson of the week: When a cyst is not a cyst
Batchelor JM, Handfield-Jones SE (Addenbrooke's Hosp, Cambridge, UK; West Suffolk Hosp NHS Trust, Bury St Edmunds, UK)
BMJ 243:d2844, 2011

Background.—Cystic lesions on the scalp are often but not always benign. Malignant lesions are especially likely in children or elderly patients who have not had any cysts previously. Lesions that are painful, increasing in size, or otherwise atypical should not be simply labeled "benign cysts," as three cases illustrate.

Case Reports.—Case 1: Man, 75, had a lump on his scalp that his general practitioner diagnosed as loculated epidermoid cyst. His medical history included aplastic anemia, but his health was generally good. During excision, the physician found the lesion adhered to the underlying tissues, requiring piecemeal removal. Histologic evaluation was difficult because of the fragmented nature of the sample, but it was clearly malignant. Wide excision was performed by plastic surgeons, and the tumor was found to have features reminiscent of poorly differentiated sebaceous carcinoma. Extensive search was carried out to determine if this was a metastatic lesion, but no primary was found. The patient had no recurrence 12 months after his surgery.

Case 2: Girl, 11, had a lump on the back of her head for 3 months that was painful and increasing in size. It was clinically determined to be an epidermoid cyst and the girl was referred nonurgently to surgery. The procedure was classified as a low priority, so it was 5 months before she had surgery. The lump ruptured when incised, releasing dark red material that was curetted out, and the wound was closed. Histologic evaluation showed a rare giant cell fibroblastoma with myxoid dermatofibrosarcomatous areas. Mohs' micrographic surgery was performed with wide excision, clearing the lesion completely. The final diagnosis was dermatofibrosarcoma protuberans. The patient had no problems after 1 year of follow-up.

Case 3: Woman, 76, was being followed up in the dermatology clinic after removal of a malignant melanoma when she mentioned a scalp lesion present for about 6 years that had recently enlarged. She had already had excision of multiple masses from her scalp at age 28 years, possible bone cancer of her toe at age 40 years, and uterine carcinoma at age 46 years. The scalp lesion was mobile within the skin and did not adhere to underlying tissues. Surgery revealed a solid mass rather than a cyst. Biopsy showed a poorly differentiated carcinoma with a high mitotic rate that was classified as a primary skin adnexal tumor or a secondary deposit from a breast, gynecologic, salivary gland, or bladder primary tumor. Multiple lung metastases were revealed on full-body computed tomography (CT). The tumor shrank considerably with palliative radiotherapy and eight cycles of capecitabine chemotherapy. A year later the lung metastases were completely resolved on CT scans, and the patient remained well after 2½ years.

Conclusions.—The diagnoses in these cases are rare, but the situations point out that malignant lesions should always be considered in the differential diagnosis of scalp lesions. If there is diagnostic uncertainty regarding any skin lesion, the case should be referred to a dermatologist before doing a biopsy unless the uncertainty arises during surgery. At that point a diagnostic biopsy is advisable to guide further treatment. Adherent lesions should not be removed piecemeal, and specimens should always be evaluated histologically.

▶ Batchelor and Handfield-Jones report 3 rare cases in which clinically diagnosed cysts turned out to be, in fact, malignant lesions. The purpose of this brief review was to emphasize the importance for practitioners to always keep in mind the potential for a malignant lesion in the differential for "lumps" on the scalp that may initially appear to be benign cysts. In their discussion, the authors note that a more serious differential for cysts on the scalp should especially be kept in mind in dealing with children, with older patients without a history of prior cystic lesions, and with cystic-appearing lesions that are painful, increasing in size, or have some other atypical feature. Of the 3 cases that were presented and originally thought to be benign cysts, one of the following diagnoses was eventually made: sebaceous carcinoma, dermatofibrosarcoma protuberans, and cutaneous metastases. One of the more important reminders was that any excised cystic lesion on the scalp should be sent for histopathologic interpretation, even if thought originally to be a benign cyst. This advice is very important and relevant, especially as some patients request that specimens not be sent to pathology to reduce possible out-of-pocket costs depending on their insurance coverage type or status. Regardless, all specimens are worthy of histologic evaluation both to confirm the diagnosis for the patient and to avoid medicolegal issues. Overall, this article serves as an important reminder for all practitioners to take the time to carefully assess cysts on the scalp and not just hastily diagnose a cyst as benign without at least considering other possible neoplasms, including a malignant differential. It is our practice to indicate "subcutaneous neoplasm" and then indicate to the patient that a cyst may be suspected clinically; however, surgical removal and histologic evaluation are needed to confirm the diagnosis.

B. D. Michaels, DO
J. Q. Del Rosso, DO

Treatment of minor wounds from dermatologic procedures: a comparison of three topical wound care ointments using a laser wound model

Trookman NS, Rizer RL, Weber T (Colorado Springs Dermatology Clinic PC; Thomas J. Stephens & Associates, Colorado Springs; Beiersdorf Inc, Wilton, CT)
J Am Acad Dermatol 64:S8-S15, 2011

Background.—Topical antibiotic ointments are commonly used for postoperative wound care after dermatologic procedures such as curettage, electrodessication, or shave removals. Antibiotics have the potential to cause allergic contact dermatitis and increase drug resistance and may not be necessary for the treatment of clean surgical wounds.

Objective.—This study compared the wound healing properties of the topical wound care ointments Aquaphor Healing Ointment (AHO) (Beiersdorf Inc, Wilton, CT), Neosporin (Poly/Bac/Neo) (Johnson & Johnson, New Brunswick, NJ), and Polysporin (Poly/Bac) (Johnson & Johnson) using a laser wound model.

Methods.—In this double-blind study, 4 uniform circular erbium/carbon dioxide laser wounds penetrating to the dermis were made in 20 subjects. Each wound was treated 3 times daily for 18 days with AHO, Poly/Bac/ Neo, or Poly/Bac, with one wound left untreated (control). Efficacy and safety were assessed using clinical grading, transepidermal water loss, investigator grading of wound appearance, subjective ranking of wound appearance, and adverse event reporting.

Results.—Significant improvements in erythema (days 7-18), edema (days 4 and 7), epithelial confluence (days 7-18), and general wound appearance (days 7-18) were observed with AHO compared with Poly/Bac/Neo and Poly/Bac ($P \leq .007$). No differences were observed between Poly/Bac/ Neo and Poly/Bac for any clinical parameters. The average transepidermal water loss value on day 4 was significantly less with AHO compared with the other treatments ($P = .0006$). Subjects ranked the treated sites as follows: AHO (best), Poly/Bac, and Poly/Bac/Neo. No adverse events were reported.

Limitations.—This was a small pilot study using a laser wound model to replicate minor wounds.

Conclusions.—AHO demonstrated fast and effective improvements in several wound healing parameters compared with antibiotic-containing treatments.

▶ This is an important article that has a practical implication for every dermatologist. Aquaphor Healing Ointment (AHO) demonstrated rapid improvement in wound healing that was superior to the use of a number of common topical antibiotic preparations. It appears that improvement in epidermal barrier function as manifested by reduction in transepidermal water loss was an important and differentiating characteristic from the effects of other topical preparations. The use of topical antibiotics can in fact lead to resistance, with no benefit over AHO. Because dermatologists deal with wounds on a regular basis, we should pay close attention to these data. We must also be aware that there are rare instances of contact dermatitis to one or more of the ingredients in AHO; however, allergic contact dermatitis is much more common with neomycin and bacitracin.

E. A. Tanghetti, MD

A rare variant of scalp dermatofibrosarcoma protuberans: malignant fibrous histiocytomatous transformation

Görgü M, Sahin B, Ozkan HS, et al (Abant Izzet Baysal Univ, Bolu, Turkey; Ataturk Education and Res Hosp, Izmir, Turkey)
Eur J Plast Surg 34:65-67, 2011

Dermatofibrosarcoma protuberans (DFSP) is a relatively uncommon, local aggressive tumor. Tumor metastasis is rare, and it has equal sex distribution. DFSP usually develops on the trunk and extremities. Scalp DFSP composes less than 5% of all cases. Local recurrence rates are high. Wide local excision and Mohs surgery are options for treatment. Fibrosarcomatous or malignant fibrous histiocytomatous transformation of DFSP are rare conditions. In this article, we described a case of a giant DFSP over the scalp containing malignant fibrous histiocytomatous transformation areas.

▶ Dermatofibrosarcoma protuberans (DFSP) is a rare malignant skin tumor occurring most commonly on the trunk and has been reported in both adults and children. Although DFSP is very locally aggressive and associated with marked subclinical extension, most cases exhibit a low metastatic potential, reported to be < 5%. DFSP with malignant fibrous histiocytomatous transformation are rare variants with a worse prognosis than classic DFSP. The main treatment for DFSP is surgical excision; however, Mohs micrographic surgery has emerged as the preferred surgical method as even wide surgical excision is often fraught with inability to encompass the tumor in its entirety. This is a case report of a 33-year-old woman with a large DFSP with malignant fibrous histiocytomatous transformation located on the scalp. Wide local excision with 5-cm surgical margins was performed, and no hematogenous transformation was found. The histologic grading of the tumor was 2; necrosis, < 50%; and mitosis, 5/10. In most cases, malignant fibrous histiocytomatous transformation zones are usually not CD34 + . Reconstruction was performed with a local scalp flap and a split-thickness skin graft. After 1 year, there was no local recurrence or distant metastasis. This is an interesting case report of a DFSP with malignant fibrous histiocytomatous transformation and successful treatment of an invasive and rare tumor after at least 1 year; however, much longer follow-up is needed to assess cure. Further studies are needed to determine if malignant fibrous histiocytomatous transformations are truly more aggressive than classic DFSP as well as the best treatment options for this DFSP variant.

G. K. Kim, DO
J. Q. Del Rosso, DO

Physicians involved in the care of patients with high risk of skin cancer should be trained regarding sun protection measures: evidence from a cross sectional study

Thomas M, Rioual E, Adamski H, et al (Paul Sabatier — Toulouse 3 Univ and Univ Hosp of Toulouse, France; Univ Hosp of Rennes, France; et al)

J Eur Acad Dermatol Venereol 25:19-23, 2011

Background.—Knowledge, regarding sun protection, is essential to change behaviour and to reduce sun exposure of patients at risk for skin cancer. Patient education regarding appropriate or sun protection measures, is a priority to reduce skin cancer incidence.

Objective.—The aim of this study was to evaluate the knowledge about sun protection and the recommendations given in a population of non-dermatologists physicians involved in the care of patients at high risk of skin cancer.

Materials and Methods.—This study is a cross-sectional study. Physicians were e-mailed an anonymous questionnaire evaluating the knowledge about risk factors for skin cancer, sun protection and about the role of the physician in providing sun protection recommendations.

Results.—Of the responders, 71.4% considered that the risk of skin cancer of their patients was increased when compared with the general population. All the responders knew that UV-radiations can contribute to induce skin cancers and 71.4% of them declared having adequate knowledge about sun protection measures. A proportion of 64.2% of them declared that they were able to give sun protection advices: using sunscreens (97.8%), wearing covering clothes (95.5%), performing regular medical skin examination (91.1%), to avoid direct sunlight exposure (77.8%), avoiding outdoor activities in the hottest midday hours (73.3%) and practising progressive exposure (44.4%).

Conclusion.—Non-dermatologist physicians reported a correct knowledge of UV-induced skin cancer risk factors. The majority of responders displayed adequate knowledge of sun protection measures and declared providing patients with sun protection recommendation on a regular basis. Several errors persisted.

▶ The nondermatologist physicians involved in the questionnaire were deemed by the authors important in the care of high-risk skin cancer patients. This criterion was probably why primary care physicians were excluded from the questionnaire study, which is a major limitation of the survey. The responding physicians ranged in age from 35 to 55 years and surely have heard of various sun protection campaigns against skin cancers that dermatologists have worked so hard to promote to the public. It is, therefore, a bit disheartening to see that only 16% of the responsive doctors recommend to their high-risk patients to practice sun avoidance and to see a dermatologist regularly for skin cancer checks. Thankfully, most of physicians are aware of the detrimental effect of ultraviolet radiation on the skin and its causation in skin cancer, and most of the responsive physicians use sunscreens for photoprotection.

K. Nguyen, MD

A Descriptive Study of Bacterial Load of Full-Thickness Surgical Wounds in Dermatologic Surgery

Saleh K, Sonesson A, Persson B, et al (Lund Univ, Sweden)
Dermatol Surg 37:1014-1022, 2011

Background.—Surgical site infections (SSIs) after dermatologic surgery cause pain, prolong healing, result in unaesthetic complications, and lead to excessive use of antibiotics. The pathogenesis of wound infections is complex and is dependent on bacterial load and diversity, among several factors.

Objective.—To investigate bacterial dynamics at dermatosurgical sites at different time intervals and assess the correlation with postoperative outcomes and to examine different endo- and exogenous factors that may contribute to SSIs.

Methods.—Eighteen patients undergoing skin grafting of the face were studied. The following SSI-related factors were registered: age and sex of the patient, ulceration of the lesion, diabetes, immunosuppressive therapy, smoking, anticoagulative therapy, and use of antibiotic prophylaxis. Wounds from each patient were swabbed preoperatively, intraoperatively, and postoperatively. The bacterial composition of the swabs was then analyzed quantitatively and qualitatively.

Results.—Sixteen of 18 surgical sites contained varying quantities of surface-associated bacteria. Coagulase-negative staphylococci and *Propionibacterium acnes* were the predominant bacteria isolated at all times. Intraoperative analysis was not predictive of SSIs. Use of antibiotic prophylaxis was the only registered SSI-related factor that showed significant variation in bacterial load between pre- and postoperative samples. Postoperative bacterial load was found to be lower than preoperative load in patients who received antibiotics. This was in contrast to patients who did not receive antibiotics, who had significantly higher postoperative levels ($p = .02$). The presence of high postoperative bacterial loads, regardless of the bacterial species isolated, showed a statistically significant positive correlation with a complicated postoperative outcome ($p \le .001$).

Conclusions.—This study provides novel insights into the bacterial dynamics of dermatologic surgery—induced wounds and the variation of this over time. The results highlight the potential relevance of quantifying bacterial loads, as well as determining specific types of bacteria, in dermatologic surgery.

▶ This study examined bacterial loads at 3 time-points in a surgical procedure. Eighteen patients undergoing skin grafting on the face had bacterial loads studied immediately preoperatively, immediately postoperatively, and at 1 week after surgery. Bacterial counts postoperatively correlated with clinical outcome. This is a very small study with several variables not accounted for; however, it serves to raise our attention to several important concepts. The suggestion that a reduction in bacterial load postoperatively would promote wound healing seems intuitive; however, the magnitude of reduction needed that is clinically relevant remains unclear. Use of prophylactic antibiotics is controversial because of concerns of emergence of antibiotic-resistant strains, but perhaps other methods to decrease bacterial load could be implemented. In these patients, wound care consisted of a tie-over dressing that remained in place for a week and an exterior bandage removed 3 days after surgery. Soap and water were used to cleanse the area afterwards. In most patients, the bacterial load 1 week after surgery was much higher than the preoperative bacterial load.

Dermatologic surgeons vary significantly in their wound care and dressings used in skin grafting and perhaps would have very different results in postoperative bacterial counts. Further studies looking at bacterial counts with different wound care regimens and evaluating the effect on outcome would be helpful. The article also brings up the point that even high levels of commensal organisms, such as coagulase-negative staphylococci, can initiate unwanted inflammatory reactions that can affect normal wound healing.

Pathogenesis of wound infections is still not clearly understood, but it does seem, based on this small study, that methods to decrease bacterial loads after surgery can improve healing outcomes.

E. M. Billingsley, MD

Pathologic nodal evaluation improves prognostic accuracy in Merkel cell carcinoma: analysis of 5823 cases as the basis of the first consensus staging system
Lemos BD, Storer BE, Iyer JG, et al (Univ of Washington, Seattle; Fred Hutchinson Cancer Res Ctr, Seattle, WA; et al)
J Am Acad Dermatol 63:751-761, 2010

Background.—The management of Merkel cell carcinoma (MCC) has been complicated by a lack of detailed prognostic data and by the presence of conflicting staging systems.

Objective.—We sought to determine the prognostic significance of tumor size, clinical versus pathologic nodal evaluation, and extent of disease at presentation and thereby derive the first consensus staging/prognostic system for MCC.

Methods.—A total of 5823 prospectively enrolled MCC cases from the National Cancer Data Base had follow-up data (median 64 months) and were used for prognostic analyses.

Results.—At 5 years, overall survival was 40% and relative survival (compared with age- and sex-matched population data) was 54%. Among all MCC cases, 66% presented with local, 27% with nodal, and 7% with distant metastatic disease. For cases presenting with local disease only, smaller tumor size was associated with better survival (stage I, ≤2 cm,

66% relative survival at 5 years; stage II, >2 cm, 51%; $P < .0001$). Patients with clinically local-only disease and pathologically proven negative nodes had better outcome (76% at 5 years) than those who only underwent clinical nodal evaluation (59%, $P < .0001$).

Limitations.—The National Cancer Data Base does not capture disease-specific survival. Overall survival for patients with MCC was therefore used to calculate relative survival based on matched population data.

Conclusion.—Although the majority (68%) of patients with MCC in this nationwide cohort did not undergo pathologic nodal evaluation, this procedure may be indicated in many cases as it improves prognostic accuracy and has important treatment implications for those found to have microscopic nodal involvement.

▶ There have been 5 different staging systems published for Merkel cell carcinoma (MCC) over the last 17 years. In this article, a distinguished panel has published the first consensus staging system that is based on 10-fold more patients than any other prior staging system.

The authors used the National Cancer Database (NCDB) to accumulate 2856 cases, with a median of 64.1 months follow-up, that were used to design the staging system. However, NCDB data do not capture disease-specific survival, and hence relative survival (compared with age- and sex-matched population data of the 2000 US Census) was reported instead. Considering that many patients with MCC are aged (median age 76 years) and many may be immuno-compromised (a recognized risk factor), use of relative survival may overestimate mortality somewhat.

The authors identified and commented on several important factors. Firstly, tumor size (≤2 vs >2 cm) was predictive of survival, although of particular note, patients with the smallest tumors (≤1 cm) had a 5-year survival (69%), which was only modestly better than patients with tumors in the 1.1- to 2.0-cm range (61%). Secondly, about one-third of patients with clinically negative lymph nodes had microscopic involvement, and this suggests that nodal status assessed only by clinical examination must be treated differently than that determined to be negative by histologic inspection.

Lastly, because MCC is rare (~1500 cases/y in the United States), data were captured during a span stretching from 1986 to 2004. Investigative reporting and documentation standards in dermatopathology have changed during this period. For example, cytokeratin-20 immunohistochemical staining, a popular way of diagnosing MCC, was not even introduced in 1994.

Therefore, ultimately, the authors note that additional new histological parameters, such as tumor thickness, lymphovascular invasion, tumor-infiltrating lymphocytes, growth pattern, and extracapsular extension/size of tumor nests, will be studied in the future. In fact, guidelines for the histopathologic evaluation of MCC have been developed by the College of American Pathologists, and in this regard, rapid and widespread adoption by dermatopathologists nationwide would likely facilitate additional future staging/prognostic endeavors pertaining to this malignancy.

W. A. High, MD, JD, MEng

Adjunctive Use of Primary Nasal Tip Closure to Facilitate Local Flap Closure of Challenging Nasal Defects

Gilman L, Fisher G (Virginia Commonwealth Univ, Richmond; Laser and Skin Surgery Ctr of Richmond, VA)
Dermatol Surg 36:2053-2056, 2010

Background.—After Mohs micrographic surgery (MMS), surgeons are often faced with the challenge of closing large nasal tip and dorsum defects. It is important to consider functional preservation and esthetic restoration in these cases. Options for nasal reconstructions include healing by second intention, primary closure, skin grafting, local nasal flap repair, and staged interpolation flap reconstruction.

> *Case Report.*—Woman, 78, had MMS extirpation of a persistent basal cell carcinoma at the nasal tip. It had previously been frozen. After four stages of MMS, all signs of cancer were gone and the defect was ready for repair. All reconstructive options were considered. Given the large size of the lesion, use of an interpolated paramedian forehead flap was considered the best option for achieving functional and esthetic restoration. These flaps are highly vascular and versatile and resemble nasal tissue in contour, texture, and color. The drawback was the morbidity related to the procedure, which is unacceptable to patients who prefer a non-staged procedure or who have no viable donor site. The patient's forehead was determined to be an excellent donor site, but she did not wish to have the interpolation flap. The defect was then modified to convert it to a medium nasal defect that could be closed using a local flap in a single stage. The reconstructive approach combined partial primary closure with a bilobed transposition flap. The patient's appreciable nasal ptosis and wide columella permitted the use of primary nasal tip closure before flap reconstruction. A standard Burow's triangle was excised from the caudal apex of the primary defect, which extended half the distance down the columella. This triangle was closed, then a standard bilobed flap was designed and prepared as usual, with wide undermining in the subnasalis plane. The flap's primary lobe was cut to reflect the defect's shape, but it was 10% to 15% smaller vertically and was left longer horizontally to permit rotational shortening of the flap. Two subcuticular mattress sutures were placed in the dermis and used to mold the shape of the junction to the flap, thus addressing the small Y-shaped deformity at the cephalic margin of the primary closure site.

Conclusions.—This type of closure is especially useful for patients with medium to large nasal defects of the tip and distal nasal dorsum. Primary closure plus local flap closure transforms a large flap into a more manageable size for traditional repair approaches. After partial primary tip closure, either a dorsal nasal or a bilobed flap can be used, but the bilobed flap is more predictable with respect to mobility and final result. Each patient must be assessed individually. Factors contributing to success are precise tissue rearrangement and adjacent tissue laxity and mobility in the tip area. Wider columellar width is also a plus, permitting excision of a wider Burow's triangle.

▶ Repair of large nasal tip and dorsum defects following Mohs micrographic surgery can be challenging. Emphasis must be placed on preserving anatomic function and producing an acceptable cosmetic result, which requires maintenance of symmetry. In this article, the authors illustrate an adjunctive procedure to help facilitate a local flap closure instead of a more extensive surgery such as an interpolation flap. Full thickness grafts are also a valid option; however, cosmetic results are not always optimal. The first step is to excise a Burow's triangle from the caudal apex of the primary defect. Then this defect is closed followed by the execution of a bilobed flap. The primary closure of the distal end of the defect essentially reduces the circumference of the entire wound resulting in a more manageable size to repair using local flaps such as the bilobed or dorsal nasal flap. Appropriate candidates for this procedure should have sufficient columellar width and enough reserve tissue in the caudal nasal tip.

S. Bellew, DO
J. Q. Del Rosso, DO

Article Index

Chapter 1: Urticarial and Eczematous Disorders

Allergic contact stomatitis caused by a polyether dental impression material 75

p-Phenylenediamine sensitization and occupation 75

A prospective multicenter study evaluating skin tolerance to standard hand hygiene techniques 77

A comparative trial comparing the efficacy of tacrolimus 0.1% ointment with aquaphor ointment for the treatment of keratosis pilaris 78

The EU Nickel Directive revisited — future steps towards better protection against nickel allergy 79

Clinically relevant contact allergy to formaldehyde may be missed by testing with formaldehyde 1·0% 80

"Car Seat Dermatitis": A Newly Described Form of Contact Dermatitis 81

Age-related sensitization to p-phenylenediamine 83

A half of schoolchildren with 'ISAAC eczema' are ill with allergic contact dermatitis 84

Allergens responsible for allergic contact dermatitis among children: a systematic review and meta-analysis 85

Advances in allergic skin disease, anaphylaxis, and hypersensitivity reactions to foods, drugs, and insects in 2010 86

Eczema across the World: The Missing Piece of the Jigsaw Revealed 87

Leucoderma after Chinese sofa dermatitis 89

Deodorants are the leading cause of allergic contact dermatitis to fragrance ingredients 90

A Prospective Study of Filaggrin Null Mutations in Keratoconus Patients with or without Atopic Disorders 91

Effectiveness of prevention programmes for hand dermatitis: a systematic review of the literature 92

Genetic variations in toll-like receptor pathway genes influence asthma and atopy 93

Efficacious and safe management of moderate to severe scalp seborrhoeic dermatitis using clobetasol propionate shampoo 0·05% combined with ketoconazole shampoo 2%: a randomized, controlled study 95

Occupational hand eczema caused by nickel and evaluated by quantitative exposure assessment 96

The relevance of chlorhexidine contact allergy 98

Importance of treatment of skin xerosis in diabetes 99

Folic Acid Use in Pregnancy and the Development of Atopy, Asthma, and Lung Function in Childhood 100

The effects of pajama fabrics' water absorption properties on the stratum corneum under mildly cold conditions 101

Preventing eczema flares with topical corticosteroids or tacrolimus: which is best?   103

The role of epigenetics in the developmental origins of allergic disease   104

Utility of routine laboratory testing in management of chronic urticaria/
angioedema   105

Chapter 2: Psoriasis and Other Papulosquamous Disorders

Adalimumab for moderate to severe chronic plaque psoriasis: efficacy and safety of
retreatment and disease recurrence following withdrawal from therapy   107

The Impact of Methodological Approaches for Presenting Long-Term Clinical
Data on Estimates of Efficacy in Psoriasis Illustrated by Three-Year Treatment
Data on Infliximab   108

Efficacy and safety of ABT-874, a monoclonal anti–interleukin 12/23 antibody, for
the treatment of chronic plaque psoriasis: 36-week observation/retreatment and
60-week open-label extension phases of a randomized phase II trial   110

Adalimumab for Treatment of Moderate to Severe Chronic Plaque Psoriasis of the
Hands and Feet: Efficacy and Safety Results From REACH, a Randomized,
Placebo-Controlled, Double-Blind Trial   111

Acute respiratory distress syndrome complicating generalized pustular psoriasis
(psoriasis-associated aseptic pneumonitis)   113

Efficacy of psoralen plus ultraviolet A therapy vs. biologics in moderate to severe
chronic plaque psoriasis: retrospective data analysis of a patient registry   114

Guidelines of care for the management of psoriasis and psoriatic arthritis: Section
6. Guidelines of care for the treatment of psoriasis and psoriatic arthritis: Case-
based presentations and evidence-based conclusions   115

Long-term etanercept in pediatric patients with plaque psoriasis   116

Intermittent etanercept therapy in pediatric patients with psoriasis   118

Psoriasis and melanocytic naevi: does the first confer a protective role against
melanocyte progression to naevi?   119

Chapter 3: Bacterial and Fungal Infections

Treatment of subcutaneous phaeohyphomycosis and prospective follow-up of 17
kidney transplant recipients   121

Severe Refractory Erythema Nodosum Leprosum Successfully Treated with the
Tumor Necrosis Factor Inhibitor Etanercept   122

Methicillin-Resistant Coagulase-Negative Staphylococci in the Community: High
Homology of SCCmec IVa between *Staphylococcus epidermidis* and Major Clones
of Methicillin-Resistant *Staphylococcus aureus*   123

Effect of filaggrin breakdown products on growth of and protein expression by
Staphylococcus aureus   124

Cellulitis: diagnosis and management   126

Comparative Effectiveness of Antibiotic Treatment Strategies for Pediatric Skin
and Soft-Tissue Infections   127

Enterococcus faecalis Complicating Dermal Filler Injection: A Case of Virulent
Facial Abscesses 128

Randomized Controlled Trial of Cephalexin Versus Clindamycin for
Uncomplicated Pediatric Skin Infections 131

Chapter 4: Viral Infections (Excluding HIV Infection)

Intradermal injection of PPD as a novel approach of immunotherapy in anogenital
warts in pregnant women 133

Intralesional Immunotherapy with *Candida* Antigen for the Treatment of
Molluscum Contagiosum in Children 134

Incidence of Postherpetic Neuralgia After Combination Treatment With Gabapentin
and Valacyclovir in Patients With Acute Herpes Zoster: Open-label Study 135

Human Papillomavirus—Induced Lesions on Tattoos May Show Features of
Seborrheic Keratosis 137

A study on the association with hepatitis B and hepatitis C in 1557 patients with
lichen planus 137

Herpes Zoster Vaccine in Older Adults and the Risk of Subsequent Herpes Zoster
Disease 138

Efficacy, safety and tolerability of green tea catechins in the treatment of external
anogenital warts: a systematic review and meta-analysis 140

Herpes Zoster in the Distribution of the Trigeminal Nerve After Nonablative
Fractional Photothermolysis of the Face: Report of 3 Cases 141

Photodynamic therapy of condyloma acuminatum in a child 143

Chapter 5: HIV Infection

Skin disorders in Korean patients infected with human immunodeficiency virus and
their association with a CD4 lymphocyte count: a preliminary study 145

Chapter 6: Disorders of the Pilosebaceous Apparatus

A prospective trial of the effects of isotretinoin on quality of life and depressive
symptoms 147

5 mg/day finasteride treatment for normoandrogenic Asian women with female
pattern hair loss 148

Acne fulminans: explosive systemic form of acne 149

A pilot methodology study for the photographic assessment of post-inflammatory
hyperpigmentation in patients treated with tretinoin 150

Comparison of tretinoin 0.05% cream and 3% alcohol-based salicylic acid
preparation in the treatment of acne vulgaris 152

Antibiotics, Acne, and *Staphylococcus aureus* Colonization 153

A Case of Acne Fulminans in a Patient with Ulcerative Colitis Successfully Treated
with Prednisolone and Diaminodiphenylsulfone: A Literature Review of Acne
Fulminans, Rosacea Fulminans and Neutrophilic Dermatoses Occurring in the
Setting of Inflammatory Bowel Disease 155

Cortexolone 17α-propionate 1% cream, a new potent antiandrogen for topical treatment of acne vulgaris. A pilot randomized, double-blind comparative study vs. placebo and tretinoin 0·05% cream — 155

Alopecia areata: Clinical presentation, diagnosis, and unusual cases — 157

Rosacea − global diversity and optimized outcome: proposed international consensus from the Rosacea International Expert Group — 158

A 6-month maintenance therapy with adapalene-benzoyl peroxide gel prevents relapse and continuously improves efficacy among patients with severe acne vulgaris: results of a randomized controlled trial — 159

A microbial aetiology of acne: what is the evidence? — 160

Does isotretinoin have effect on vitamin D physiology and bone metabolism in acne patients? — 161

Comparison of the epidemiology of acne vulgaris among Caucasian, Asian, Continental Indian and African American women — 162

Cicatricial alopecia — 164

Central hair loss in African American women: Incidence and potential risk factors — 165

Acne-associated syndromes: models for better understanding of acne pathogenesis — 167

Frontal fibrosing alopecia: a clinical review of 36 patients — 168

Combination therapy with adapalene−benzoyl peroxide and oral lymecycline in the treatment of moderate to severe acne vulgaris: a multicentre, randomized, double-blind controlled study — 169

Expert Opinion: Efficacy of superficial chemical peels in active acne management—what can we learn from the literature today? Evidence-based recommendations — 171

Topical and intralesional therapies for alopecia areata — 172

The clinical features of late onset acne compared with early onset acne in women — 173

Low-cumulative dose isotretinoin treatment in mild-to-moderate acne: efficacy in achieving stable remission — 174

Iron deficiency and diffuse nonscarring scalp alopecia in women: More pieces to the puzzle — 176

Staphylococcus epidermidis: A possible role in the pustules of rosacea — 177

Immediate Reduction in Sweat Secretion With Electric Current Application in Primary Palmar Hyperhidrosis — 178

Iron deficiency in female pattern hair loss, chronic telogen effluvium, and control groups — 179

Neurogenic Rosacea: A Distinct Clinical Subtype Requiring a Modified Approach to Treatment — 180

Hair care practices and their association with scalp and hair disorders in African American girls — 182

Effectiveness of conventional, low-dose and intermittent oral isotretinoin in the treatment of acne: a randomized, controlled comparative study — 183

'Follicular Swiss cheese' pattern—another histopathologic clue to alopecia areata — 185

The efficacy of adapalene-benzoyl peroxide combination increases with number of acne lesions | 187

Investigation of optimal aminolaevulinic acid concentration applied in topical aminolaevulinic acid–photodynamic therapy for treatment of moderate to severe acne: a pilot study in Chinese subjects | 188

Alopecia areata as another immune-mediated disease developed in patients treated with tumour necrosis factor-α blocker agents: Report of five cases and review of the literature | 189

A Randomized Trial to Evaluate the Efficacy of Online Follow-up Visits in the Management of Acne | 190

Migrating Hair: A Case Confused with Cutaneous Larva Migrans | 191

Chapter 7: Photobiology

Indoor Tanning — Science, Behavior, and Policy | 193

Clinical evidence of benefits of a dietary supplement containing probiotic and carotenoids on ultraviolet-induced skin damage | 194

Are sunscreens luxury products? | 196

An overview analysis of the time people spend outdoors | 198

Adverse effects of ultraviolet radiation from the use of indoor tanning equipment: Time to ban the tan | 199

Prevalence and Characteristics of Indoor Tanning Use Among Men and Women in the United States | 200

Tomato paste rich in lycopene protects against cutaneous photodamage in humans *in vivo*: a randomized controlled trial | 201

Photo-allergic contact dermatitis caused by isoamyl *p*-methoxycinnamate in an 'organic' sunscreen | 203

A randomized, double-blind, negatively controlled pilot study to determine whether the use of emollients or calcipotriol alters the sensitivity of the skin to ultraviolet radiation during phototherapy with narrowband ultraviolet B | 204

Chapter 8: Collagen Vascular and Related Disorders

A systematic review of drug-induced subacute cutaneous lupus erythematosus | 207

Photoprotective effects of a broad-spectrum sunscreen in ultraviolet-induced cutaneous lupus erythematosus: A randomized, vehicle-controlled, double-blind study | 210

Malignancy in Systemic Lupus Erythematosus: A Nationwide Cohort Study in Taiwan | 211

Aortic aneurysms in systemic lupus erythematosus: a meta-analysis of 35 cases in the literature and two different pathogeneses | 213

Efficacy of tacrolimus 0.1% ointment in cutaneous lupus erythematosus: A multicenter, randomized, double-blind, vehicle-controlled trial | 214

Expression of antimicrobial peptides in different subtypes of cutaneous lupus erythematosus | 215

Current and novel therapeutics in the treatment of systemic lupus erythematosus 217

A New Presentation of Neonatal Lupus: 5 Cases of Isolated Mild Endocardial Fibroelastosis Associated with Maternal Anti-SSA/Ro and Anti-SSB/La Antibodies 218

Retiform Purpura and Digital Gangrene Secondary to Antiphospholipid Syndrome Successfully Treated With Sildenafil 219

Amyopathic Dermatomyositis 221

Mycophenolate mofetil treatment in children and adolescents with lupus 222

Clinical Correlations With Dermatomyositis-Specific Autoantibodies in Adult Japanese Patients With Dermatomyositis: A Multicenter Cross-sectional Study 223

Drug-induced subacute cutaneous lupus erythematosus: evidence for differences from its idiopathic counterpart 224

Antibodies and the Brain: Lessons from Lupus 225

Biologic Therapy for Systemic Sclerosis: A Systematic Review 227

Chapter 9: Blistering Disorders

The role of therapeutic plasma exchange in pemphigus vulgaris 229

Approach to the patient with autoimmune mucocutaneous blistering diseases 230

Pemphigus and Osteoporosis: A Case-Control Study 231

Use of intravenous immunoglobulin therapy during pregnancy in patients with pemphigus vulgaris 232

Therapeutic ladder for pemphigus vulgaris: Emphasis on achieving complete remission 233

Clinical efficacy of different doses of rituximab in the treatment of pemphigus: a retrospective study of 27 patients 234

Chapter 10: Genodermatoses

Cardiac magnetic resonance imaging illustrating Anderson–Fabry disease progression 237

Inherited syndromes 238

Fabry disease in children: correlation between ocular manifestations, genotype and systemic clinical severity 239

Adnexal tumours of the skin as markers of cancer-prone syndromes 240

Chapter 11: Drug Actions, Reactions, and Interactions

A comparative analysis of cetirizine, gabapentin and their combination in the relief of post-burn pruritus 243

Fixed drug eruption caused by etoricoxib – 2 cases confirmed by patch testing 245

A Prospective Self-Controlled Phase II Study of Imiquimod 5% Cream in the Treatment of Infantile Hemangioma 246

Exacerbation of Seborrheic Dermatitis by Topical Fluorouracil   247

Topical calcitriol restores the impairment of epidermal permeability and antimicrobial barriers induced by corticosteroids   249

Allergic contact dermatitis caused by glycyrrhetinic acid and castor oil   250

Allergic contact dermatitis caused by tetrahydroxypropyl ethylenediamine in cosmetic products   252

Chemotherapy-related bilateral dermatitis associated with eccrine squamous syringometaplasia: Reappraisal of epidemiological, clinical, and pathological features   254

Simvastatin-induced myoglobinuric acute kidney injury following ciclosporin treatment for alopecia universalis   256

Stevens—Johnson syndrome and toxic epidermal necrolysis: a review of treatment options   257

Toxic Epidermal Necrolysis with Prominent Facial Pustules: A Case with Reactivation of Human Herpesvirus 7   258

Irritation and allergy patch test analysis of topical treatments commonly used in wound care: Evaluation on normal and compromised skin   259

The risk of infection and malignancy with tumor necrosis factor antagonists in adults with psoriatic disease: A systematic review and meta-analysis of randomized controlled trials   261

The cutaneous and systemic manifestations of azathioprine hypersensitivity syndrome   262

Impact of etanercept treatment on ultraviolet B-induced inflammation, cell cycle regulation and DNA damage   264

Etanercept: An Overview of Dermatologic Adverse Events   265

Occurrence of pustular psoriasis after treatment of Crohn disease with infliximab   266

Ipilimumab: Unleashing the Power of the Immune System Through CTLA-4 Blockade   267

Fas-ligand staining in non-drug- and drug-induced maculopapular rashes   269

Penicillin skin testing in the evaluation and management of penicillin allergy   270

Chapter 12: Drug Development and Promotion

Chemoprevention of Chemically Induced Skin Tumorigenesis by Ligand Activation of Peroxisome Proliferator—Activated Receptor-β/δ and Inhibition of Cyclooxygenase 2   273

Efficacy and Safety Evaluation of a Novel Botulinum Toxin Topical Gel for the Treatment of Moderate to Severe Lateral Canthal Lines   275

Efficacy and Safety of a Novel Botulinum Toxin Topical Gel   276

New Drugs and New Molecular Entities in Dermatology   277

Chapter 13: Miscellaneous Topics in Clinical Dermatology

12-Month Controlled Study in the United States of the Safety and Efficacy of
a Permanent 2.5% Polyacrylamide Hydrogel Soft-Tissue Filler — 279

A Double-Blind, Randomized, Placebo-Controlled Health-Outcomes Survey of the
Effect of Botulinum Toxin Type A Injections on Quality of Life and Self-Esteem — 283

Comparison of Two Botulinum Toxin Type A Preparations for Treating Crow's
Feet: A Split-Face, Double-Blind, Proof-of-Concept Study — 285

Where does the antigen of cutaneous sarcoidosis come from? — 288

The Effect of Combined Steroid and Calcium Channel Blocker Injection on Human
Hypertrophic Scars in Animal Model: A New Strategy for the Treatment of
Hypertrophic Scars — 289

A comparison of wound healing between a skin protectant ointment and a medical
device topical emulsion after laser resurfacing of the perioral area — 291

A comparison of postprocedural wound care treatments: Do antibiotic-based
ointments improve outcomes? — 292

A genome-wide association study to identify genetic determinants of atopy in
subjects from the United Kingdom — 293

Clinical, dermoscopic, and histopathologic features in a case of infantile
hemangioma without proliferation — 294

An Audit of Behcet's Syndrome Research: A 10-year Survey — 296

Targeted treatment of pruritus: a look into the future — 297

A Case of Xanthoma Disseminatum with Spontaneous Resolution over 10 Years:
Review of the Literature on Long-Term Follow-Up — 298

An approach to the patient with retiform purpura — 300

Approach to the hospitalized patient with targetoid lesions — 301

The Modified Patient and Observer Scar Assessment Scale: A Novel Approach to
Defining Pathologic and Nonpathologic Scarring — 301

Bimatoprost Ophthalmic Solution 0.03% for Eyebrow Growth — 302

Early White Discoloration of Infantile Hemangioma: A Sign of Impending
Ulceration — 304

Chronic pruritus — pathogenesis, clinical aspects and treatment — 305

Association of Hearing Loss With PHACE Syndrome — 306

Becker Nevus With an Underlying Desmoid Tumor: A Case Report and Review
Including Mayo Clinic's Experience — 308

Vitamin D-effective solar UV radiation, dietary vitamin D and breast cancer risk — 309

Botulinum Toxin Type A vs Type B for Axillary Hyperhidrosis in a Case Series of
Patients Observed for 6 Months — 309

Effect of Aqueous Cream BP on human stratum corneum *in vivo* — 311

Depth profiling of stratum corneum biophysical and molecular properties — 313

Superantigens in dermatology — 315

Adverse effects of propranolol when used in the treatment of hemangiomas: A case series of 28 infants ... 316

Timolol Maleate 0.5% or 0.1% Gel-Forming Solution for Infantile Hemangiomas: A Retrospective, Multicenter, Cohort Study ... 317

Aesthetic Dermatology for Aging Ethnic Skin ... 318

Development of a Photographic Scale for Consistency and Guidance in Dermatologic Assessment of Forearm Sun Damage ... 319

Gender aspects in skin diseases ... 321

Prevalence of benign cutaneous disease among Oxford renal transplant recipients ... 323

Diagnosis and treatment of the neutrophilic dermatoses (pyoderma gangrenosum, Sweet's syndrome) ... 324

Conceptual Approach to the Management of Infantile Hemangiomas ... 325

Use of complementary and alternative medicine among adults with skin disease: Updated results from a national survey ... 327

Skin Conditions That Bring Patients to Emergency Departments ... 328

Dermatoscopy use by US dermatologists: A cross-sectional survey ... 330

Lichen Planus Occurring after Influenza Vaccination: Report of Three Cases and Review of the Literature ... 331

Nevus simplex: A reconsideration of nomenclature, sites of involvement, and disease associations ... 332

Procedural dermatology training during dermatology residency: A survey of third-year dermatology residents ... 333

Toll-like receptors and skin ... 334

Topical nitroglycerin: A promising treatment option for chondrodermatitis nodularis helicis ... 335

Prospective Study of the Frequency of Hepatic Hemangiomas in Infants with Multiple Cutaneous Infantile Hemangiomas ... 336

Should one offer an unsolicited dermatologic opinion? Ethics for the locker-room dermatologist ... 338

Chapter 14: Pigmentary Disorders

Vitiligo linked to stigmatization in British South Asian women: a qualitative study of the experiences of living with vitiligo ... 341

Vitiligo in children and adolescents: association with thyroid dysfunction ... 342

A prospective, randomized, split-face, controlled trial of salicylic acid peels in the treatment of melasma in Latin American women ... 343

Sequential Treatment with Triple Combination Cream and Intense Pulsed Light is More Efficacious than Sequential Treatment with an Inactive (Control) Cream and Intense Pulsed Light in Patients with Moderate to Severe Melasma ... 344

A Pilot Study of Intense Pulsed Light in the Treatment of Riehl's Melanosis ... 346

Role of apoptosis and melanocytorrhagy: a comparative study of melanocyte adhesion in stable and unstable vitiligo ... 347

Vitiligo 348

A double-blind, randomized, placebo-controlled trial of topical tacrolimus 0·1%
vs. clobetasol propionate 0·05% in childhood vitiligo 350

Future research into the treatment of vitiligo: where should our priorities lie?
Results of the vitiligo priority setting partnership 352

Chapter 15: Practice Management and Managed Care

Mobile teledermatology in the developing world: Implications of a feasibility study
on 30 Egyptian patients with common skin diseases 355

Costs and cost-effectiveness analysis of treatment in children with eczema by nurse
practitioner vs. dermatologist: results of a randomized, controlled trial and
a review of international costs 357

Skin Cancer Prevention Educational Resources: Just a Click Away? 358

Chapter 16: Nonmelanoma Skin Cancer

Alopecia of the Scalp After Ineffective Treatment of Bowen's Disease Using Red
Light 5-Aminolevulinic Acid Photodynamic Therapy: Two Case Reports 363

A cost analysis of photodynamic therapy with methyl aminolevulinate and
imiquimod compared with conventional surgery for the treatment of superficial
basal cell carcinoma and Bowen's disease of the lower extremities 365

Complete Clinical Response to Cetuximab in a Patient with Metastatic Cutaneous
Squamous Cell Carcinoma 366

Expression of the Sonic hedgehog pathway in squamous cell carcinoma of the skin
and the mucosa of the head and neck 368

Evaluation of Patient-Perceived Satisfaction with Photodynamic Therapy for
Bowen Disease 369

Recurrent basal cell carcinoma following ablative laser procedures 370

Bowen's Disease Associated with Human Papillomavirus Infection of the Nail Bed 371

A new American Joint Committee on Cancer staging system for cutaneous
squamous cell carcinoma: Creation and rationale for inclusion of tumor (T)
characteristics 372

A randomized comparative study of tolerance and satisfaction in the treatment of
actinic keratosis of the face and scalp between 5% imiquimod cream and
photodynamic therapy with methyl aminolaevulinate 374

Dermoscopy-guided surgery in basal cell carcinoma 375

Basaloid squamous cell carcinoma of the skin 377

Axillary basal cell carcinoma: additional 25 patients and considerations 378

The sap from *Euphorbia peplus* is effective against human nonmelanoma skin
cancers 379

A randomized, multicentre study of directed daylight exposure times of 1½ vs.
2½ h in daylight-mediated photodynamic therapy with methyl aminolaevulinate in
patients with multiple thin actinic keratoses of the face and scalp 380

Sun-Induced Nonsynonymous p53 Mutations Are Extensively Accumulated and Tolerated in Normal Appearing Human Skin — 382

Heightened Infection-Control Practices are Associated with Significantly Lower Infection Rates in Office-Based Mohs Surgery — 383

Hedgehog Antagonist GDC-0449 Is Effective in the Treatment of Advanced Basal Cell Carcinoma — 384

Occupational ultraviolet light exposure increases the risk for the development of cutaneous squamous cell carcinoma: a systematic review and meta-analysis — 385

MAL-PDT for difficult to treat nonmelanoma skin cancer — 386

Atypical Squamous Proliferation: What Lies Beneath? — 387

A Unique Basaloid Proliferation Encountered During Mohs Surgery: Potential Pitfall for Overdiagnosis of Basal Cell Carcinoma — 389

Vascular Complications After Treatment with Low-Dose Isotretinoin in Two Elderly Patients — 391

Use of Reflectance Confocal Microscopy to Differentiate Hidrocystoma from Basal Cell Carcinoma — 393

Trends in the incidence of basal cell carcinoma by histopathological subtype — 394

Topical methyl aminolevulinate photodynamic therapy for management of basal cell carcinomas in patients with basal cell nevus syndrome improves patient's satisfaction and reduces the need for surgical procedures — 395

Merkel cell carcinoma: our experience with seven patients in Korea and a literature review — 396

Recurrence of Basosquamous Carcinoma after Mohs Micrographic Surgery — 398

Mohs Micrographic Surgery for Hidradenocarcinoma on a Rhinophymatous Nose: A Histologic Conundrum — 399

Need to Improve Skin Cancer Screening of High-Risk Patients — 400

Lip cancer in renal transplant patients — 401

Factors associated with large cutaneous squamous cell carcinomas — 402

Ungual and periungual human papillomavirus–associated squamous cell carcinoma: a review — 404

Epidermal Growth Factor Receptor Inhibitors in the Treatment of Nonmelanoma Skin Cancers — 405

The Role of Sirolimus in the Prevention of Cutaneous Squamous Cell Carcinoma in Organ Transplant Recipients — 406

Retinoids for Chemoprophylaxis of Nonmelanoma Skin Cancer — 407

Margin Detection Using Digital Dermatoscopy Improves the Performance of Traditional Surgical Excision of Basal Cell Carcinomas of the Head and Neck — 409

Slowly-Developing Facial Nerve Paralysis — 410

Eighteen Years of Experience in Mohs Micrographic Surgery and Conventional Excision for Nonmelanoma Skin Cancer Treated by a Single Facial Plastic Surgeon and Pathologist — 412

Skin cancer education and early detection at the beach: a randomized trial of dermatologist examination and biometric feedback — 413

Sclerosing Squamous Cell Carcinoma of the Skin, an Underemphasized Locally Aggressive Variant: a 20-Year Experience   414

Photodynamic therapy of multiple actinic keratoses: reduced pain through use of visible light plus water-filtered infrared A compared with light from light-emitting diodes   415

Liquid Nitrogen: Temperature Control in the Treatment of Actinic Keratosis   417

Chapter 17: Nevi and Melanoma

Absence of *BRAF* and *HRAS* mutations in eruptive Spitz naevi   419

A new era: melanoma genetics and therapeutics   420

Lentiginous Melanoma In Situ Treatment With Topical Imiquimod: Need for Individualized Regimens   421

Frequencies of *BRAF* and *NRAS* mutations are different in histological types and sites of origin of cutaneous melanoma: a meta-analysis   422

The Expanding Melanoma Burden in California Hispanics: Importance of Socioeconomic Distribution, Histologic Subtype, and Anatomic Location   423

"Clark/dysplastic" nevi with florid fibroplasia associated with pseudomelanomatous features   425

Comparison of Classification Systems for Congenital Melanocytic Nevi   427

Impact of Melanoma on Patients' Lives Among 562 Survivors: a Dutch Population-Based Study   428

A Phase 2 Trial of Dasatinib in Advanced Melanoma   429

An immunohistochemical comparison between MiTF and MART-1 with Azure blue counterstaining in the setting of solar lentigo and melanoma *in situ*   430

AJCC melanoma staging update: impact on dermatopathology practice and patient management   432

Cigarette smoking and malignant melanoma: a case-control study   433

Clinical and histologic characteristics of malignant melanoma in families with a germline mutation in CDKN2A   434

Melanocytic Nevi with Spitz Differentiation: Diagnosis and Management   435

Melanomas Detected in a Follow-up Program Compared with Melanomas Referred to a Melanoma Unit   436

Marital Status and Stage at Diagnosis of Cutaneous Melanoma: Results From the Surveillance Epidemiology and End Results (SEER) Program, 1973-2006   438

The "spaghetti technique": an alternative to Mohs surgery or staged surgery for problematic lentiginous melanoma (lentigo maligna and acral lentiginous melanoma)   439

Sun exposure before and after a diagnosis of cutaneous malignant melanoma: estimated by developments in serum vitamin D, skin pigmentation and interviews   440

Circulating Benign Nevus Cells Detected by ISET Technique: Warning for Melanoma Molecular Diagnosis   441

Management and outcome of metastatic melanoma during pregnancy   443

Sentinel Lymph Node Biopsy or Nodal Observation in Melanoma: a Prospective Study of Patient Choices   444

Topical Imiquimod for Periocular Lentigo Maligna   445

Prognostic value and clinical significance of halo naevi regarding vitiligo   446

Melanoma Incidence Rates among Whites in the U.S. Military   448

Acral Melanocytic Nevi: Prevalence and Distribution of Gross Morphologic Features in White and Black Adults   449

Internet Use and Anxiety in People with Melanoma and Nonmelanoma Skin Cancer   451

Chapter 18: Lymphoproliferative Disorders

Cutaneous graft-versus-host disease: rationales and treatment options   453

Lymphoepithelioma-like carcinoma of head and neck skin: a systematic analysis of 11 cases and review of literature   453

A phase II placebo-controlled study of photodynamic therapy with topical hypericin and visible light irradiation in the treatment of cutaneous T-cell lymphoma and psoriasis   454

Chapter 19: Miscellaneous Topics in Cosmetic and Laser Surgery

Accelerated resolution of laser-induced bruising with topical 20% arnica: a rater-blinded randomized controlled trial   457

A Split-Face Comparison of Two Ablative Fractional Carbon Dioxide Lasers for the Treatment of Photodamaged Facial Skin   459

A study of the efficacy of carbon dioxide and pigment-specific lasers in the treatment of medium-sized congenital melanocytic naevi   460

Early Postoperative Treatment of Thyroidectomy Scars Using a Fractional Carbon Dioxide Laser   460

Complication of Cross-Technique on Boxcar Acne Scars: Atrophy   461

Keratosis pilaris rubra and keratosis pilaris atrophicans faciei treated with pulsed dye laser: report of 10 cases   464

Contribution of lip proportions to facial aesthetics in different ethnicities: A three-dimensional analysis   465

Nonablative 1550-nm fractional laser therapy versus triple topical therapy for the treatment of melasma: a randomized controlled pilot study   466

Analysis of Postoperative Complications for Superficial Liposuction: A Review of 2398 Cases   467

Management of Rhinophyma with Coblation   469

Blinded Evaluation of the Effects of Hyaluronic Acid Filler Injections on First Impressions   470

Intraepidermal erbium:YAG laser resurfacing: Impact on the dermal matrix   471

Adverse reactions caused by consecutive injections of different fillers in the same facial region: risk assessment based on the results from the Injectable Filler Safety study   472

Enhancing effect of pretreatment with topical niacin in the treatment of rosacea-associated erythema by 585-nm pulsed dye laser in Koreans: a randomized, prospective, split-face trial 473

Acne Scar Treatment with Subcision Using a 20-G Cataract Blade 474

Treatment of Dermatosis Papulosa Nigra in 10 Patients: a Comparison Trial of Electrodesiccation, Pulsed Dye Laser, and Curettage 476

Improvement in Nasolabial Folds with a Hyaluronic Acid Filler Using a Cohesive Polydensified Matrix Technology: Results from an 18-Month Open-Label Extension Trial 477

Subcision-suction method: a new successful combination therapy in treatment of atrophic acne scars and other depressed scars 480

Split-Face Comparison of Intense Pulsed Light and Nonablative 1,064-nm Q-Switched Laser in Skin Rejuvenation 481

Granuloma Faciale Treated with 595-nm Pulsed Dye Laser 482

Percutaneous Collagen Induction Versus Full-Concentration Trichloroacetic Acid in the Treatment of Atrophic Acne Scars 483

Evaluation of the Effect of Fractional Laser with Radiofrequency and Fractionated Radiofrequency on the Improvement of Acne Scars 484

Skin Necrosis of the Nasal Ala after Injection of Dermal Fillers 486

Chapter 20: Miscellaneous Topics in Dermatologic Surgery and Cutaneous Oncology

Treatment of Striae Distensae Using an Ablative 10,600-nm Carbon Dioxide Fractional Laser: A Retrospective Review of 27 Participants 489

Achieving Hemostasis After Nail Biopsy Using Absorbable Gelatin Sponge Saturated in Aluminum Chloride 491

A Case of Epithelioid Angiosarcoma of the Scalp Treated With Paclitaxel and Radiotherapy 492

The Public's Perception of Dermatologists as Surgeons 493

The Reconstruction of Male Hair-Bearing Facial Regions 494

Deroofing: A tissue-saving surgical technique for the treatment of mild to moderate hidradenitis suppurativa lesions 495

Cutaneous metastasis of prostatic adenocarcinoma: a cautionary tale 496

Digital Block With and Without Epinephrine During Chemical Matricectomy with Phenol 497

Mucosal Advancement Flap Versus Primary Closure After Vermilionectomy of the Lower Lip 498

Novel method of minimally invasive removal of large lipoma after laser lipolysis with 980 nm diode laser 499

Preoperative Expectations and Values of Patients Undergoing Mohs Micrographic Surgery 500

Risk management in dermatology: an analysis of data available from several British-based reporting systems 502

Intralesional agents in the management of cutaneous malignancy: A review   503

Significant Differences in Skin Irritation by Common Suture Materials Assessed by a Comparative Computerized Objective Method   504

Increased prevalence of left-sided skin cancers   506

Lesson of the week: When a cyst is not a cyst   507

Treatment of minor wounds from dermatologic procedures: a comparison of three topical wound care ointments using a laser wound model   509

A rare variant of scalp dermatofibrosarcoma protuberans: malignant fibrous histiocytomatous transformation   510

Physicians involved in the care of patients with high risk of skin cancer should be trained regarding sun protection measures: evidence from a cross sectional study   511

A Descriptive Study of Bacterial Load of Full-Thickness Surgical Wounds in Dermatologic Surgery   512

Pathologic nodal evaluation improves prognostic accuracy in Merkel cell carcinoma: analysis of 5823 cases as the basis of the first consensus staging system   513

Adjunctive Use of Primary Nasal Tip Closure to Facilitate Local Flap Closure of Challenging Nasal Defects   515

Author Index

A

Aalami Harandi S, 480
Abal L, 371
Abdel Hay R, 483
Abou-Bakr AA, 133
Abuabara K, 261
Acler M, 309
Adamski H, 511
Aguayo R, 371
Aguilar M, 365
Ahmadi N, 435
Ahmed AR, 232
Ahuja RB, 243
Akarsu S, 152
Alam M, 405
Alcántara González J, 464
Alexander H, 493
Alio A, 78
Alkhalifah A, 172
Allen LE, 239
Almeida PJ, 83
Almirall M, 189
Almutawa F, 250
Altinyazar HC, 497
Altmeyer P, 498
Amin SH, 384
Ana V, 89
Andersen KE, 90
Andrade P, 245
Arits AHMM, 394
Arkins JP, 283, 470
Asplund A, 382
August PJ, 460
Avitabile G, 237
Ayad M, 355
Ayeni O, 474
Aylward JH, 379
Azari R, 476

B

Babayeva L, 152
Bachmann F, 472
Bai R, 273
Baibergenova A, 328
Bailey E, 126
Balato A, 119
Balato N, 119
Balighi K, 480
Barbe C, 444
Barbier F, 123
Baret I, 252
Basset-Seguin N, 395

Bassioukas K, 85
Bastida J, 137
Batchelor JM, 75, 507
Battafarano DF, 262
Baum S, 229
Bayer ML, 306
Beauchet A, 196
Bechara FG, 498
Beek JF, 466
Bekerecioglu M, 427
Bercovitch L, 338
Bergman H, 190
Berlin JM, 164
Bessis D, 113
Betti R, 378
Bhagwandas K, 492
Bianciotto CG, 445
Bidinger JJ, 262
Birkenfeld S, 137
Boasberg P, 267
Boer J, 495
Boixeda P, 464
Bolognia JL, 425
Bond JE, 301
Bonitsis NG, 85
Boot CRL, 92
Borghi A, 174
Borrego L, 83
Boß C, 410
Botella-Estrada R, 254
Bouilly-Gauthier D, 194
Bovenzi M, 75
Boyd AS, 377
Bozzetti M, 409
Brandt F, 275
Breithaupt AD, 78
Breur JMPJ, 316
Brigo F, 309
Brodell EE, 247
Brodell RT, 247
Brustad M, 309
Bucko A, 159
Butler ST, 506

C

Cacchio PB, 179
Callender V, 165
Callender VD, 318
Calvet J, 189
Camp MC, 465
Carducci M, 409
Caresana G, 375
Carey W, 474
Carr DR, 407

Carrera C, 436
Carrigan CR, 343
Carroll KC, 131
Casabonne D, 323
Cazzaniga A, 275
Cerroni L, 419
Cha SM, 467
Chakkittakandiyil A, 317
Chamorey E, 77
Chang Y-T, 211
Chavan R, 453
Chen AE, 131
Chen JZS, 346
Chen M, 143
Chen W, 167, 321
Chen Y-J, 211
Cheng CE, 162
Chew A-L, 168
Chisholm C, 335
Cho H-H, 370
Cho S, 342
Cho SB, 342, 473
Choi CW, 173
Choi J-W, 422
Choi JW, 148
Choi K, 200
Choi Y-L, 396
Chuang GS, 500
Chung V, 493
Ciocon DH, 459
Clarke CA, 423
Coenraads PJ, 357
Cohen AD, 231
Cohen L, 218
Coleman WP III, 279, 477
Cooper WO, 127
Corcoran G, 277
Cornish D, 428
Cosgrave EM, 239
Cotliar J, 257
Crosti C, 378
Crowley J, 107
Czarnobilska E, 84

D

Dabade TS, 324
Dandine M, 77
Davis DG, 465
Davis EC, 318
Davis MDP, 324
Davison SP, 435
Dayan SH, 283, 470
de Arriba L, 401

533

de Bree E, 504
De Giorgi V, 441
de Graaf M, 316
de Maleissye M-F, 196
de Troya M, 365
Demirci H, 445
Demirel CB, 497
Deng J, 188
Desjardins M, 250
Di Costanzo L, 119
Diamond B, 217, 225
Diener-West M, 131
Diepgen TL, 385
Diffey BL, 198
DiGiorgio C, 135
Dith A, 264
Dommasch ED, 261
Donnelly HB, 407
Donofrio LM, 477
Donovan JC, 176
Dowlatshahi EA, 265
Draelos Z, 158
Draelos ZD, 292
Dreiher J, 137, 231
Dréno B, 158, 169, 171
Droitcourt C, 91
Drolet BA, 332
Duckett LD, 319
Dudek AZ, 429
Duffy KJ, 306
Duncan LM, 432
Dusza SW, 333, 358
Duvic M, 454
Dyga W, 84

E

Eaglstein WH, 277
Eassa BI, 133
Edvardsen K, 309
Eichenfield LF, 116, 118
Eisen DB, 238, 476
El Tawdy A, 483
El-Azhary R, 453
El-Khalawany MA, 133
Eleftheriadou V, 352
Elewski BE, 158
Elias MJ, 302
Ellis AK, 104
Elmets CA, 115
Emmons KM, 413
Enewold L, 448
Engasser HC, 330
Engelman DE, 459
Enns LL, 134
Erdmann D, 301

Erdmann R, 472
Ermertcan AT, 334
Ertugrul DT, 161
Esen F, 296
Evans DM, 293
Evans MS, 134

F

Fabricius S, 380
Fallon PG, 124
Fanelli M, 153
Farasat S, 372
Fay A, 325
Fearmonti RM, 301
Feldman SR, 187
Ferguson JE, 460
Fermont L, 218
Ferran M, 189
Fetil E, 152
Fikrle T, 482
Finner AM, 157
Firoz BF, 141
Fischer TC, 171
Fisher DE, 193, 420
Fisher G, 515
Fisher JL, 438
Flynn V, 335
Forsea A-M, 358
Foscolo AM, 409
Fosko SW, 421, 506
Foss RD, 453
Fox S, 270
Frasson E, 309
Frieden IJ, 317
Friedlander SF, 78
Fuhrmann T, 327
Fujimoto N, 155
Fullen DR, 451

G

Gal TJ, 470
Galante NZ, 121
Gambichler T, 264
Gantner S, 419
Garcia MS, 476
Garg A, 400
Gathers R, 182
Gaudy-Marqueste C, 439
Gawkrodger DJ, 348, 352, 502
Ged C, 91
Geisse JK, 414

Geller A, 400
Geller AC, 413
Gendelman V, 229
Gensch K, 210, 214
Ghali FE, 81
Ghazavi MK, 203
Giardini R, 375
Gillison F, 147
Gilman L, 515
Giunta A, 108
Glick ZR, 332
Glusac EJ, 425
Godoy P, 121
Gohel MDI, 101
Gold MH, 344
Goldberg LH, 141, 417
Goldman MP, 344
Goldstein GD, 387
Gonçalo M, 245
Gonzalez M, 160
Gonzalez ME, 219
Good LM, 503
Goossens A, 252
Gordon KB, 110
Görgü M, 510
Grange F, 444
Grau RH, 207
Grimwood R, 335
Gruis NA, 434
Gruvberger B, 80
Guettrot-Imbert G, 218
Guevara IL, 343
Guillot B, 113
Gunasingam N, 177
Gündüz K, 334
Gupta G, 243
Gupta R, 243
Gürcan HM, 232
Gutta RC, 105
Guy RH, 311

H

Hadgraft J, 313
Haitz K, 135
Hamaguchi Y, 223
Hamid O, 267
Hamilton T, 471
Han J, 143
Handfield-Jones SE, 507
Hanke CW, 386, 499
Hao F, 188
Harbottle A, 201
Harpaz R, 138
Hartmann V, 472

Hauksson I, 80
Haust M, 210, 214
Havey J, 457
Heisterberg MV, 90
Henderson CL, 207
Hernandez D, 123
Hernández G, 401
Hervella M, 89
Heschl B, 114
High WA, 503
Hillebrand GG, 162
Hillesheim PB, 430
Ho N, 350
Hoefel IR, 461
Hoff-Lesch S, 415
Hoffman WY, 304
Hoffman-Bolton J, 433
Hoffmann G, 415
Holterhues C, 428
Hong J-B, 167
Hong SP, 249
Honma M, 258
Horii KA, 336
Hoshino K, 223
Hoteit M, 75
Hu A, 369
Hu XJ, 246
Huang C-Y, 289
Hueso L, 374
Hughes MP, 406
Hughey LC, 301
Humphreys T, 399
Huo M-H, 481
Hurley MY, 421
Hussain M, 459
Hussain W, 414
Hwa C, 491

I

Idorn LW, 440
Iinuma S, 258
Imbriaco M, 237
Imko-Walczuk B, 323
Inzinger M, 114
Irvine AD, 124
Isik D, 427
Iyer JG, 513
Izumi M, 288

J

Jamal S, 227
James WD, 193, 199

Jaouhar M, 215
Jarmuda S, 149
Jeannes C, 194
Jensen P, 96
Jeong JJ, 460
Jiang CH, 246
Joe DH, 298
Johansen JD, 96
Johnson SR, 227
Johnston GA, 203
Johnston RB, 389
Jorizzo JL, 233
Juern AM, 332
Jung D-S, 370
Jung HS, 396
Jung JY, 148, 460
Jung M, 249

K

Kabesch M, 93
Kahn P, 219
Kaltenbach LA, 127
Kamath S, 492
Kang HC, 298
Kang MS, 486
Kanitakis J, 240
Kano Y, 331
Kanwar AJ, 347
Kapke A, 182
Kaplan B, 417
Karadag AS, 161
Katz TM, 141
Kauffman CL, 435
Kaufmann R, 169
Kavanagh GM, 178
Kawakami T, 213
Kawara S, 294
Kazyra I, 222
Keller M, 399
Kelley D, 430
Kennett MJ, 273
Kersey JP, 239
Kessides MC, 433
Keystone JS, 122
Khambatta S, 221
Khan MH, 405
Khemis A, 99
Kim HS, 173
Kim J-E, 384
Kim JH, 234, 342, 489
Kim JY, 191
Kim MR, 234
Kim T-G, 145
Kim TG, 473

Kim Y-S, 422
Kim YH, 234, 467
Kimball AB, 110
Kimura M, 294
Kiripolsky MG, 484
Kloimstein P, 368
Kluger HM, 429
Kluger N, 113
Ko CJ, 425
Ko H-C, 370
Ko JM, 420
Koca R, 497
Kodali S, 343
Kollhorst B, 285
Korman NJ, 115
Kousa P, 98
Kovalyshyn I, 358
Kovich OI, 491
Kreuter A, 215
Krijnen P, 434
Kroon MW, 466
Kroshinsky D, 126
Kuhn A, 210, 214
Kumar R, 347
Kupperman E, 153
Kurata A, 213, 288
Kurban A, 496
Kuwana M, 223

L

Lajevardi V, 480
Lallas A, 140
Lally A, 323
Lammintausta K, 98
Langley RG, 110, 111
Lapolla W, 135
Lautenbach E, 153
Lazovich D, 200
Lazzari R, 224
Leach BC, 500
LeBlanc KG Jr, 406
Lecluse LLA, 265
Lee DH, 173
Lee EH, 333
Lee J-H, 422
Lee JSS, 269
Lee JW, 183
Lee K-H, 145
Lee SE, 489
Lee SJ, 489
Leheta T, 483
Lemos BD, 513
Lenzy YM, 496
Leonardi C, 111
Leow LJ, 177

Letada PR, 363
Leu S, 457
Leung DYM, 86
Leyden JJ, 150
Li Y, 101
Li Y-H, 346
Libutti P, 256
Liippo J, 98
Lim HW, 199
Limiñana JM, 83
Limpens CEJM, 265
Liu J, 346
Lohuis PJFM, 412
Lomonte C, 256
López-Pintor RM, 401
Lovatto L, 436
Lovell CR, 147
Lowe G, 207
Ludgate MW, 451

M

Ma G, 246
Machado RB, 461
Macias ES, 315
Madan V, 460
Magdelijns FJH, 100
Maguiness SM, 304
Mahé E, 196
Malvestio A, 75
Manios A, 504
Mantovani L, 174
Marcy P-Y, 77
Marks SD, 222
Martin JE, 383
Martin L, 365
Martorell-Calatayud A, 254
Marzano AV, 224
Masters R, 363
Mastroeni S, 402
Matts PJ, 313
Maubec E, 444
Maubert Y, 194
Mazereeuw-Hautier J, 395
McCalmont TH, 304
McCann C, 429
McDuffie BC, 164
McFadden J, 79
McGrath EJ, 147
McKenzie NE, 319
McLaughlin JM, 438
McMichael A, 165
Mempel M, 321

Menné T, 90
Menter A, 115
Messalli G, 237
Messina JL, 389
Metz M, 305
Miajlovic H, 124
Mihm MC Jr, 432
Miller K, 366
Miller MD, 503
Minghetti S, 174
Missall TA, 421
Mohammed D, 313
Mommers M, 100
Moneghini L, 378
Monte D, 348
Moore C, 369
Muhn C, 474
Müller CSL, 185

N

Nagore E, 374
Naidu S, 467
Narins RS, 279, 477
Naumescu E, 155
Neel VA, 372
Nehal KS, 333
Nelemans PJ, 394
Nguyen J, 325
Nikkels AF, 95
North ML, 104

O

Obermayer-Pietsch B, 167
Obtulowicz K, 84
O'Connell C, 275
O'Day S, 267
Ogawa MM, 121
Oh S-H, 145
Oh Y, 249
Oiso N, 294
Olsen EA, 165, 179
Orringer JS, 471
Ortonne J-P, 95, 107
Ozkan HS, 510
Öztürk F, 334

P

Pagès C, 443
Palicka GA, 449

Paller AS, 116, 118
Palm MD, 344, 484
Pandey RC, 93
Papoutsaki M, 108
Papp K, 107, 111
Pappert AS, 150
Parara SM, 504
Park ES, 486
Park HY, 298
Park KY, 183
Park MA, 270
Parsad D, 347
Paskett ED, 438
Passarelli F, 402
Patel AB, 283
Patel NS, 389
Pauwels C, 395
Pavlis M, 493
Penders J, 100
Perchenet A-S, 439
Pereira FA, 315
Perkins AC, 162
Perosino E, 171
Persson B, 512
Petersen J, 499
Peterson JD, 484
Philipsen PA, 440
Phillips R, 317
Phumethum V, 227
Pilkington C, 222
Pinzani P, 441
Piris A, 432
Pitman MJ, 128
Pizinger K, 482
Pollitt RA, 423
Polloni I, 224
Pontén A, 80
Pope E, 350
Poulin Y, 159, 187
Pourciau C, 266
Prager W, 285
Prens EP, 495
Pribaz JJ, 494
Price HN, 219
Price V, 168
Prins MEF, 412
Puleo E, 413

R

Racic G, 469
Radojicic C, 105
Ramien ML, 122

Ramsay JR, 379
Raphaël MF, 316
Rashid R, 404
Ratner D, 366, 391
Rattanasirivilai A, 496
Reed KB, 179
Reich K, 95
Renzi C, 402
Reyes MA, 238
Rhodes AR, 449
Riddel C, 404
Ridgway EB, 494
Rietkerk W, 315
Rigel DS, 199
Rioual E, 511
Rittié L, 471
Rivero P, 137
Rizer RL, 259, 292, 509
Rizwan M, 201
Robert C, 443
Rodriguez-Blanco I, 201
Roecken M, 410
Roh HJ, 460, 473
Rohrich R, 279
Roje Z, 469
Rook AH, 454
Rossi AB, 150
Rougier A, 99
Rousso JJ, 128
Rubenzik M, 399
Rucker Wright D, 182
Runge-Samuelson C, 306
Ruppé E, 123

S

Sabel MS, 451
Saboda K, 319
Sagi L, 229
Sahin B, 510
Saleh K, 512
Salerni G, 436
Salmon PJM, 414
Salvianti F, 441
Sambandan DR, 391
Sami N, 230
Samrao A, 168
Sanchez NP, 159
Sand M, 498
Sanmartín O, 254
Sardeli C, 140
Sarnoff DS, 291
Sasseville D, 250
Sato J, 213
Sato NA, 331

Scharschmidt TC, 180
Schimmel EK, 296
Schlangen MHJ, 394
Schmitt J, 385
Schmults CD, 383
Schneider S, 368
Schuttelaar MLA, 357
Schwartz RA, 149
Sciallis AP, 308
Sciallis GF, 308
Sebastian S, 387
Seidler A, 385
Seité S, 99
Serra-Guillen C, 374
Shabrawi-Caelen LE, 185
Shaheen B, 160
Shams K, 178
Shear NH, 328
Sheehan DJ, 406
Sherman W, 366
Shields CL, 445
Shin DB, 261
Shin HS, 486
Shiohara T, 331
Shwayder T, 266
Sicherer SH, 86
Siegfried EC, 116, 118
Silverman RA, 191
Skaria AM, 398
Skellett A, 204
Skrygan M, 215
Sky K, 262
Slone S, 430
Smith E, 247
Smith N, 138, 327
Sonesson A, 512
Soria X, 371
Southwell B, 200
Speeckaert R, 446
Speyer L-A, 383
St Pierre SA, 176
Ståhl PL, 382
Ständer S, 305
Stasko TS, 377
Stebbins WG, 386, 499
Stein JA, 491
Stender IM, 380
Storer BE, 513
Strachan DP, 293
Stranneheim H, 382
Strowd LC, 233
Suhrbier A, 379
Swanson DL, 393
Swetter SM, 423
Swevers A, 252
Swift L, 204

T

Talamonti M, 108
Talarico S, 169
Tan AWH, 269
Tan E, 204
Tan J, 187
Tang Y-W, 377
Tarbox JA, 105
Taséi A-M, 439
Tatsioni A, 85
Tausk F, 327
Taylor SL, 233
Terado Y, 288
Tesse R, 93
Teutonico A, 256
Tey HL, 297
Thomas L, 443
Thomas M, 511
Thomas V, 404
Thompson AR, 341
Thurnher D, 368
Thyssen JP, 79, 96
Tibes R, 384
Tigges C, 264
Tiplica G-S, 155
Tobisawa S, 258
Todd PM, 75
Touboul D, 91
Traidl-Hofmann C, 321
Tran K, 355
Trevino JJ, 407
Trifu V, 155
Trookman NS, 259, 292, 509
Truchuelo Díez MT, 464
Tsang M, 311
Tseng HF, 138
Turkmen A, 427
Tutal E, 161
Tzellos TG, 140

U

Uebelhoer NS, 363
Uenishi T, 155
Uter W, 79

V

Valeròn-Almazán P, 137
van de Poll-Franse LV, 428

van der Eerden PA, 412
van der Rhee JI, 434
van der Zee HH, 495
van Geel N, 446
van Gils PF, 92
van Gils RF, 92
Vandenhaute S, 446
Veierød MB, 309
Venkatesan P, 300
Vercellotti GM, 176
Vergilis-Kalner I, 417
Vermeulen KM, 357
Viles J, 348
Vives R, 89
von Felbert V, 415

W

Wakabayashi M, 155
Wan YI, 293
Waner M, 325
Wang AL, 164
Wang C-B, 211
Wang ECE, 269
Wang Y-Q, 481
Warschaw KE, 393
Warshaw EM, 330
Watson AJ, 190
Weber MB, 461
Weber T, 259, 509

Weger W, 114
Wehner-Caroli J, 410
Weinberg J, 355
Weinstein M, 350
Weiss E, 302
Weiss J, 302
Weitzman D, 137
Welch PQ, 453
West TB, 276
Wheless L, 433, 500
White LE, 457
Whitfeld M, 177
Whitton ME, 352
Wiegell SR, 380
Wiesner T, 419
Willard K, 393
Williams CM, 190
Williams DJ, 127
Williams HC, 87, 103
Williams SB, 453
Wind BS, 466
Wissmüller E, 285
Wittich CM, 221
Wohl Y, 231
Wong A, 122
Wong WW, 465
Woo K-J, 396
Wood GS, 454
Worswick S, 257
Wulf HC, 440
Wysong A, 300

X

Xie J, 143

Y

Yang J-Y, 289
Yang X, 481
Yanko R, 387
Yao L, 101
Yazici H, 296
Yeon JH, 148
Yildirim-Toruner C, 217
Yin R, 188
Yoo KH, 183
Yoo S, 405
Yosipovitch G, 297
Yost JM, 180
Yu E, 369
Yu SS, 372

Z

Zaba R, 149
Zahm SH, 448
Zhou J, 448
Zhu B, 273

Printed and bound by CPI Group (UK) Ltd, Croydon, CR0 4YY

08/05/2025

01864678-0020